Handbook of Experimental Pharmacology

Continuation of Handbuch der experimentellen Pharmakologie

Vol. 68/II

Antimalarial Drugs II

Current Antimalarials and New Drug Developments

Contributors

R. Baurain · P. E. Carson · R. Ferone · C. D. Fitch · W. Hofheinz
A. T. Hudson · R. Leimer · P. Mamalis · M. Masquelier
E. W. McChesney · B. Merkli · W. Peters · R. O. Pick · P. Pirson
R. Richle · K. H. Rieckmann · H. J. Scholer · T. R. Sweeney
A. Trouet · D. Warburton · L. M. Werbel · D. F. Worth

Editors

W. Peters and W. H. G. Richards

Springer-Verlag
Berlin Heidelberg New York Tokyo 1984

WALLACE PETERS, M.D., DSc, FRCP, DTM & H
Professor of Medical Protozoology,
London School of Hygiene and Tropical Medicine,
Keppel Street,
London WC1E 7HT,
Great Britain

WILLIAM H.G. RICHARDS, BSc, Ph. D.
Manager, Scientific Advisory Services,
Wellcome Research Laboratories,
Ravens Lane,
Berkhamsted, Herts. HP4 2DY,
Great Britain

With 150 Figures

ISBN-13:978-3-642-69256-7 e-ISBN-13:978-3-642-69254-3
DOI: 10.1007/978-3-642-69254-3

Library of Congress Cataloging in Publication Data. Main entry under title: Antimalarial drugs. (Handbook of experimental pharmacology; v. 68, 1–2) Includes bibliographies and index. Contents: 1. Biological background, experimental methods, and drug resistance – 2. Current antimalarials and new drug developments. 1. Antimalarials. 2. Malaria–Chemotherapy. I. Peters, W. (Wallace), 1924–. II. Richards, W.H.G. (William H.G.), 1928–. III. Series. [DNLM: 1. Antimalarials–Pharmacodynamics. 2. Antimalarials–Therapeutic use. W1 HA51L v. 68 pt. 1–2/QV 256 A631] QP905.H3 vol. 68, 1–2 615'.1s [616.9'362061] 83-16977 [RC159.A5]
ISBN-13:978-3-642-69256-7

2122/3130-543210

List of Contributors

R. Baurain, Laboratoire de Chimie Physiologique, Faculté de Médecine, Université Catholique de Louvain and International Institute of Cellular and Molecular Pathology, UCL 7539, Avenue Hippocrate, 75, 1200 Bruxelles, Belgium

P. E. Carson, Professor and Chairman, Department of Pharmacology, Rush-Presbyterian – St. Luke's Medical Center, 1753 West Congress Parkway, Chicago, IL 60612, USA

R. Ferone, Group Leader, Department of Microbiology, The Wellcome Research Laboratories, Burroughs Wellcome Co., 3030 Cornwallis Road, Research Triangle Park, NC 27709, USA

C. D. Fitch, Professor, Department of Internal Medicine, Division of Endocrinology, School of Medicine, St. Louis University Medical Center, 1402 S. Grand Blvd., St. Louis, MO 63104, USA

W. Hofheinz, F. Hoffmann-La Roche & Co. Ltd., Pharmaceutical Research Division, 4002 Basel, Switzerland

A. T. Hudson, Department of Therapeutic Chemistry, Wellcome Research Laboratories, Langley Court, Beckenham, Kent BR3 3BS, Great Britain

R. Leimer, F. Hoffmann-La Roche & Co. Ltd., Department of Clinical Research, 4002 Basel, Switzerland

P. Mamalis, Research Associate, Beecham Pharmaceuticals, Research Division, Walton Oaks, Dorking Road, Tadworth, Surrey KT20 7NT, Great Britain

M. Masquelier, Laboratoire de Chimie Physiologique, Faculté de Médecine, Université Catholique de Louvain and International Institute of Cellular and Molecular Pathology, UCL 7539, Avenue Hippocrate, 75, 1200 Bruxelles, Belgium

E. W. McChesney, Research Professor of Toxicology (Ret.), Albany Medical College, private: 14 Alden Court, Delmar, NY 12054, USA

B. Merkli, F. Hoffmann-La Roche & Co. Ltd., Pharmaceutical Research Division, 4002 Basel, Switzerland

W. Peters, Professor of Medical Protozoology, London School of Hygiene and Tropical Medicine, Keppel Street, London, WC1E 7HT, Great Britain

R. O. Pick, Chief, Department of Medicinal Chemistry, Division of Experimental Therapeutics, Walter Reed Army Institute of Research, Walter Reed Army Medical Center, Washington, DC 20012, USA

P. Pirson, Laboratoire de Chimie Physiologique, Faculté de Médecine, Université Catholique de Louvain and International Institute of Cellular and Molecular Pathology, UCL 7539, Avenue Hippocrate, 75, 1200 Bruxelles, Belgium

R. Richle, F. Hoffmann-La Roche & Co. Ltd., Pharmaceutical Research Division, 4002 Basel, Switzerland

K. H. Rieckmann, 70 Pinion Mill Place, Albuquerque, NM 87131, USA

H. J. Scholer, F. Hoffmann-La Roche & Co. Ltd., Pharmaceutical Research Division, 4002 Basel, Switzerland

T. R. Sweeney, 1701 N. Kent Street, Appartment 1106, Arlington, VA 22209, USA

A. Trouet, Professor, Laboratoire de Chimie Physiologique, Faculté de Médecine, Université Catholique de Louvain and International Institute of Cellular and Molecular Pathology, UCL 7539, Avenue Hippocrate, 75, 1200 Bruxelles, Belgium

D. Warburton, May and Baker Limited, Dagenham, Essex RM10 7HS, Great Britain

L. M. Werbel, Pharmaceutical Research Division, Warner-Lambert Company, 2800 Plymouth Road, Ann Arbor, Michigan 48105, USA

D. F. Worth, Pharmaceutical Research Division, Warner-Lambert Company, Plymouth Road, Ann Arbor, Michigan 48105, USA

Preface

The construction of this volume has been guided by two personal convictions.

Experience in the field of experimental chemotherapy, both in the pharmaceutical industry and academia, has convinced us that recent quantum technological advances in biochemistry, molecular biology, and immunology will permit and, indeed, necessitate an increasingly greater use of rational drug development in the future than has been the custom up to now. In Part 1, therefore, we asked our contributors to provide detailed reviews covering the biology of the malaria parasites and their relation with their hosts, the experimental procedures including culture techniques that are necessary to take a drug from primary screening to clinical trial, and an account of antimalarial drug resistance.

Our second conviction is that many research workers are all too loath to learn from the lessons of the past. For this reason we asked the contributors to Part 2 of this volume to review very thoroughly the widely scattered but voluminous literature on those few chemical groups that have provided the antimalarial drugs in clinical use at the present time. Much can be learned from the history of their development and the problems that have arisen with them in man. Some indeed may still have much to offer if they can be deployed in better ways than they are at present. This question has been taken up by several authors.

From about 1963 the threat posed by the increasing failure of chloroquine to cure people infected with *Plasmodium falciparum* led to a rapidly rising crescendo of drug development. Largely under the auspices of the US Army's Walter Reed Army Institute of Research and, latterly, the UNDP/World Bank/WHO Special Programme for Research and Training in Tropical Diseases, this research has led, through well over a quarter of a million compounds in primary screen, to a small handful of more or less new drugs that may help to control the problem for a few years. Paradoxically one of the best new drugs, mefloquine, is a close analogue of that ancient remedy quinine, while a second is another plant derivative known in traditional medicine five times longer than quinine itself, the Chinese compound Qinghaosu or artemisinine. The plant itself, *Artemisia annua* L., was first described as an antipyretic agent 2,000 years ago. Attention is currently being focused, too, on the search for new and better tissue schizontocides for the radical cure of relapsing vivax malaria, a second major problem in many tropical and subtropical areas. Neither mefloquine nor artemisinine possess tissue schizontocidal properties.

The final chapters of this work summarise the intensive research that has been carried out, especially over the past decade, in a number of particularly promising chemical groups from one or more of which, we hope, will emerge the next generation of antimalarials. Once these become available it is vital that we should, for once, try to learn from the lessons of the past and obtain the maximum use possible from them. We have concluded, therefore, with some suggestions concerning the prevention of drug resistance. A major step in this direction, we believe, will be the deployment of rationally selected combinations of antimalarial drugs. While this principle has long been accepted in other antimicrobial fields, e.g., tuberculosis, it has still to prove its value and become accepted (if proven) in the chemoprophylaxis and treatment of malaria.

History has shown that malaria parasites have an uncanny ability to survive in spite of man's best endeavours to eliminate them by drugs or to interrupt their transmission by the use of insecticides to which the vectors become resistant. It is our firm conviction that malaria will be with us for many decades to come, and that we will constantly need to look back to see what has been done before, in order that we can try to do better in the future. That, we believe, fully justifies the considerable effort of all those colleagues who have so generously helped us in the production of this work, including the editorial staff of Springer-Verlag, to all of whom we express our deep gratitude.

WALLACE PETERS
WILLIAM H.G. RICHARDS

Contents

Antimalarial Drugs in Current Use

CHAPTER 1

4-Aminoquinolines. E.W. McChesney and C.D. Fitch
With 4 Figures

CHAPTER 2

Quinine and Quinine Analogues. W. HOFHEINZ and B. MERKLI
With 2 Figures

CHAPTER 3

8-Aminoquinolines. P.E. CARSON. With 3 Figures

Novel Methods of Drug Development

CHAPTER 6

Drug Combinations. W. PETERS. With 3 Figures

CHAPTER 7

Repository Preparations. D.F. WORTH and L.M. WERBEL
With 6 Figures

CHAPTER 8

Cell Targeting of Primaquine

A. TROUET, P. PIRSON, R. BAURAIN, and M. MASQUELIER

Recent Developments in Antimalarials

CHAPTER 9

Drugs with Quinine-like Action. T.R. SWEENEY. With 12 Figures

CHAPTER 10

8-Aminoquinolines. T.R. SWEENEY. With 14 Figures

CHAPTER 11

Lapinone, Menoctone, Hydroxyquinolinequinones and Similar Structures
A.T. Hudson. With 12 Figures

CHAPTER 12

4-Aminoquinolines and Mannich Bases. T.R. Sweeney and R.O. Pick
With 20 Figures

CHAPTER 13

Triazines, Quinazolines and Related Dihydrofolate Reductase Inhibitors
P. Mamalis and L.M. Werbel. With 33 Figures

Prevention of Drug Resistance

CHAPTER 16

Use of Drug Combinations. W. PETERS. With 6 Figures

Contents of Companion Volume 68, Part I

Antimalarial Drugs in Current Use

CHAPTER 1

4-Aminoquinolines

E. W. McCHESNEY and C. D. FITCH

A. Introduction

I. History

Chloroquine (CQ) is generally considered to be one of the most fascinating, useful and versatile drugs developed during the modern era of synthetic organic chemistry (KNOX and OWENS 1966; SAMS 1967). It was first prepared in 1934 by H. Andersag in the Elberfeld-Leverkusen laboratories of the I. G. Farbenindustrie, as part of a programme which included the synthesis of such important compounds as mepacrine, pentaquine, isopentaquine, pamaquine, primaquine, and sontoquine (COATNEY 1963). The objective of this programme was to develop substitutes for quinine which, except for its prompt effect in alleviating the symptoms of an acute attack, is the poorest of antimalarial drugs (WALKER 1949; 1950). The hope in preparing CQ was that it would prove to be less toxic than mepacrine. When this hope appeared not to be realised (COATNEY 1963; see also Table 1), CQ was given only a very limited clinical trial, and it was then abandoned (in favour of sontoquine) as being "too toxic for human use." The magnitude of this error of judgement became apparent when, in the course of the American wartime antimalarial survey (WISELOGLE 1946), CQ proved to be the best of the many compounds which were tested for prophylactic-suppressive activity. Others of this group seemed worthy of further intensive study (see Table 1) including those assigned Survey Nos. (SN) 8137, 9584, 10751, and 13425. Trials in man (BERLINER et al. 1948), involving initially the administration of 200 mg/week, and building up to 600 mg/week by the 5th week, revealed the incidence of side effects to be greatest for SN 9584 and least for SN 8137. Of 32 subjects receiving CQ on the schedule described, 12 had no adverse effects, but 18 reported ocular difficulties. These consisted of blurred vision and seeing haloes around lights. Somewhat similar symptoms were reported in subjects treated by ALVING et al. (1948), on a rather different dosage schedule. The BERLINER and ALVING group reports now appear as indications of problems which were to come, but the former group concluded, nevertheless, that CQ had the most favourable activity/toxicity relationship of the five compounds they tested. Now, more than 30 years later, CQ remains the prophylactic-suppressive antimalarial of choice (Editorial 1976; BRUCE-CHWATT 1977; BARRETT-CONNER 1978), except in those areas of the world where resistance has developed (see Part I, Chap. 16).

Some indication of the remarkable therapeutic versatility of CQ has been documented by REES and MAIBACH (1963), GILES and HENDERSON (1965), KNOX and OWENS (1966) and SAMS (1967). In addition to its activity against several important

Table 1. Structural, antimalarial and toxicity relationships in the 4-aminoquinoline series, as related to quinine and mepacrine[a]

Generic name	Survey No.	Aromatic nucleus	Side chain (R)	Antimalarial activity indices[b]					Oral toxicity[c]		
				A	B	C	D	E	Mouse	Rat	Chick
Mepacrine	390	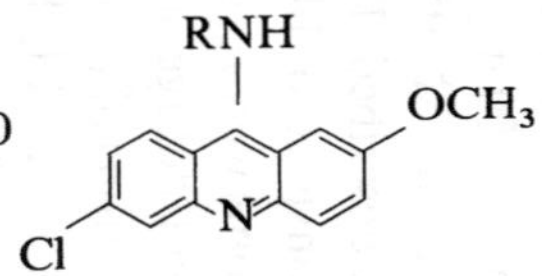	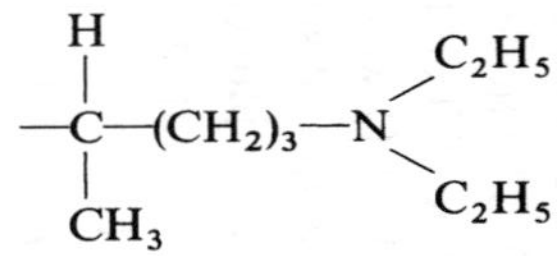	4	15	2–3 (1.7)[d]	1.5	6	4	10	3[d]
Chloroquine	7,618	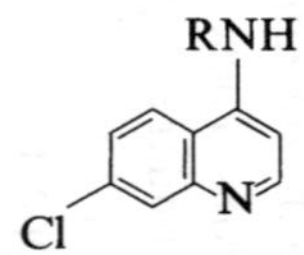	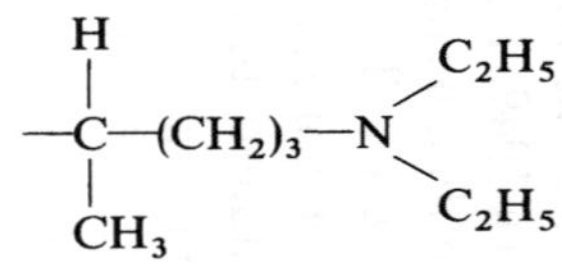	15	60	15 (14.4)[d]	30	10–15	5	5–10	10
				14[e]	32[e]	8[e]	NT	8–15[e]	NT	NT	13[d]
Desethyl-chloroquine	13,616	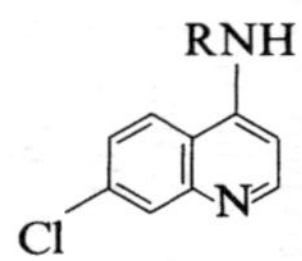	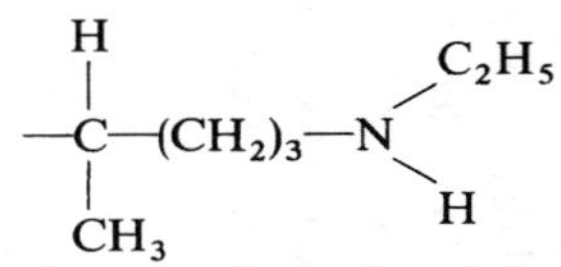	NT	NT	40 (7.2)[d]	NT	4	4	6	18[d]
Bisdesethyl-chloroquine	13,617	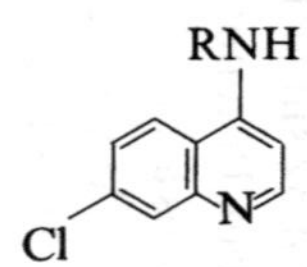	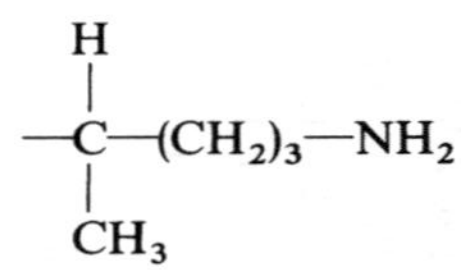	NT	NT	NT	NT	4	NT	NT	NT
Hydroxy-chloroquine		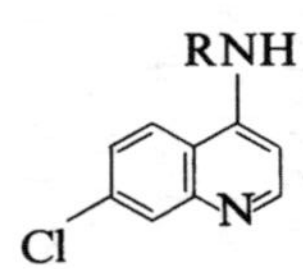	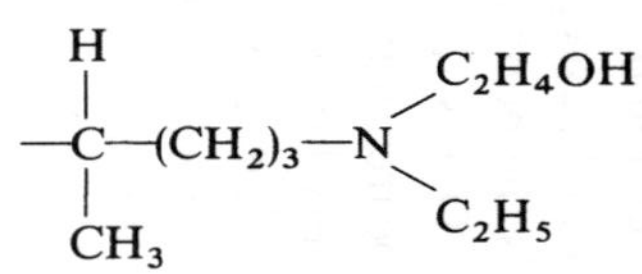	NT	NT	NT	NT	9–21[e]	2[e]	2–4[e]	NT

Oxychloroquine	8,137	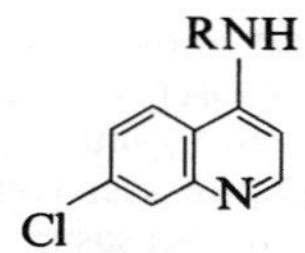	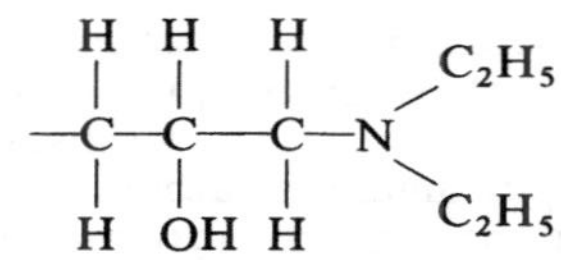	10	6	15–20 (14.4)[d]	30	3	3	4	12 9[d]
Bromoquine	7,373	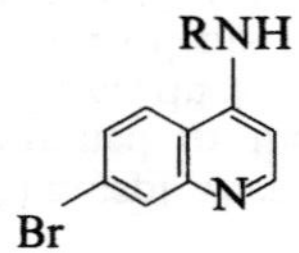	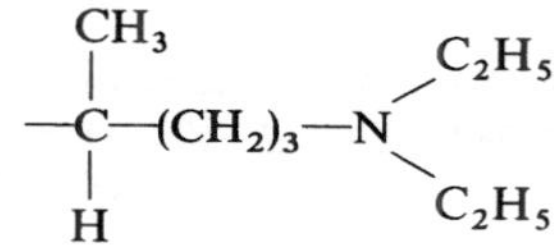	8	30	15 (11.2)[d]	NT	15	4	10	22[d]
	3,294	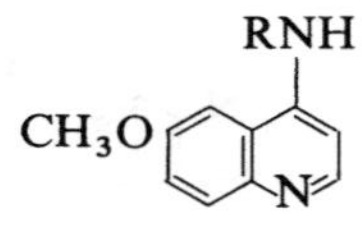	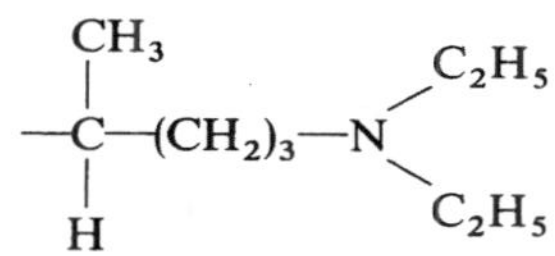	1.5	4	2–3 (12.6)[d]	2	2	3	2.5	15 7[d]
Sontoquine	6,911	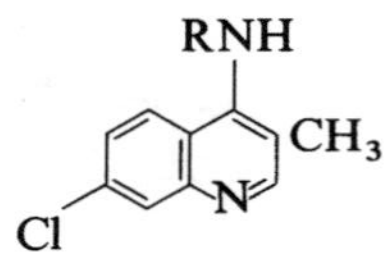	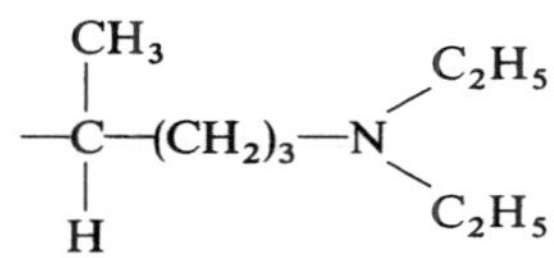	3	15–20	3–4 (3.1)[d]	6	6	5	8–10	8–10 8[d]
Norsontoquine	7,718	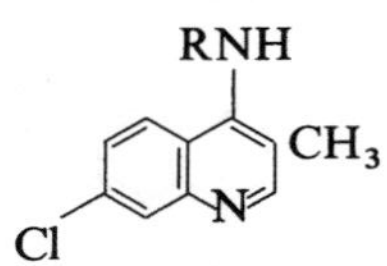	$-(CH_2)_4-N(C_2H_5)_2$	6	15	6	NT	6	3	5[e]	NT
Amodiaquine	10,751	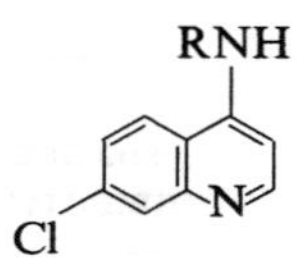	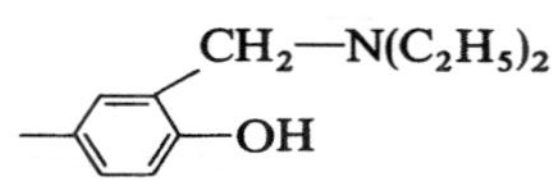	6	30	8–30 (7.2)[d]	30	15	3–4	5	5 4[d]

Table 1 (continued)

Generic name	Survey No.	Aromatic nucleus	Side chain (R)	Antimalarial activity indices[b]					Oral toxicity[c]		
				A	B	C	D	E	Mouse	Rat	Chick
Amopyroquine		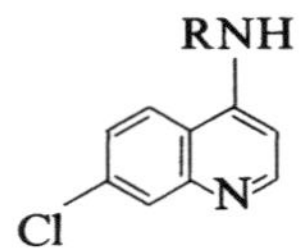	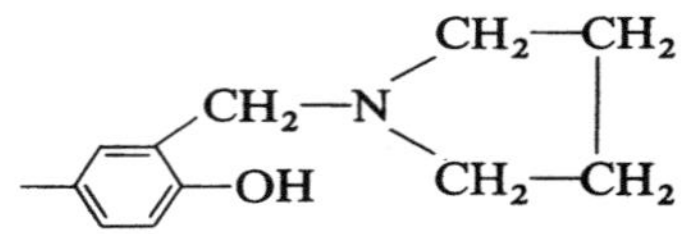	NT	NT	NT	32–37	NT	3–4[f]	9–13[f]	NT
	9,584	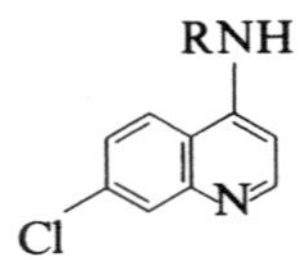	$-(CH_2)_3-N(C_2H_5)_2$	8	30	15–30	30	6	5	8	5 7[d]
	13,425	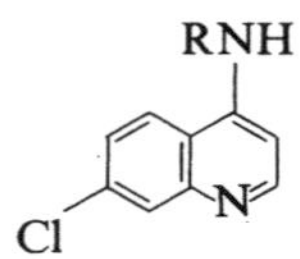	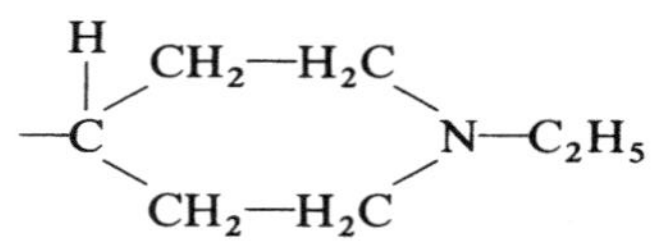	NT	NT	15 (7.2)[d]	NT	8	6	NT	4[d]

[a] Data from WISELOGLE (1946) except where otherwise indicated
[b] These activities were determined in the following assays: A *P. cathemerium*, canary; B *P. cathemerium*, duck; C *P. gallinaceum*, chick; D *P. lophurae*, chick; E *P. lophurae*, duck. In all cases the values given are in terms of quinine equivalents, in the specific test used
[c] Values also given as quinine equivalents
[d] Calculated from the data given in COATNEY et al. (1953). Note that the compounds were usually tested in salt forms (diphosphates, sulphates or hydrochlorides) but in three cases (SN 10,751, 13,425, and 13,616) only the free bases appear to have been available. Toxicity ratios are calculated in terms of the weights of the bases, and of the means of the mean maximum and freely tolerated doses
[e] Data from the files of the Sterling-Winthrop Research Institute
[f] Values estimated from the data of THOMPSON et al. (1958) and of HOEKENGA (1957), in comparison to those given for CQ in Table 2
[g] Compound administered orally two or three times daily; for details of the protocol actually used see WISELOGLE (1946), p. 508

strains of malarial parasites (especially *Plasmodium falciparum*), CQ is of definite value in the treatment of rheumatoid arthritis (RA), discoid and systemic lupus erythematosus, DNA-autosensitivity reaction, polymorphous light eruptions, solar urticaria, recurrent basal cell carcinoma of the skin, and the intestinal forms of amoebiasis. Another established application, not mentioned by the above authors, is in the treatment of porphyria cutanea tarda (GEBEL et al. 1978; CHLUMSKY et al. 1980). REES and MAIBACH (1963) list 26 other conditions, mostly very rare, in which the effectiveness of CQ had at that time neither been proved nor disproved. Its principal adverse effects in man (WENIGER 1979) include ototoxicity, myopathy, and retinopathy.

II. Treatment of Rheumatoid Arthritis

A definite turning point in the fortunes of CQ came in about 1952, when it began to be used on a rather large scale for the treatment of RA (cf. BAGNALL 1957) and the rather closely related lupus erythematosus (GOLDMAN et al. 1953). Complications soon arose, since the dosages used in the treatment of these conditions were in some cases as much as ten times those recommended for malaria prophylaxis. These complications were not immediately evident, but alarming findings began to be reported by 1957. The literature on this subject is much too voluminous to be reviewed in this paper (SCRUGGS 1964); however, some landmark observations may be cited. These were: (a) development of unusual ocular lesions in a patient being treated for lupus erythematosus (CAMBIAGGI 1957), (b) occurrence of corneal deposits in patients being treated for a variety of conditions (HOBBS and CALNAN 1958; ZELLER and DEERING 1958) and (c) description of the syndrome of CQ retinopathy (HOBBS et al. 1959). These, and similar reports, resulted in a marked resurgence of interest in CQ, in an attempt to establish the basic cause(s) of the retinopathy syndrome and, thereby, possibly to develop means of averting it, or of reversing it, once a positive diagnosis had been made. This resurgence of interest has made CQ possibly the most thoroughly investigated drug in the current therapeutic armamentarium, if one excepts aspirin. These investigations have, in themselves, revealed no effective method of dealing with the retinopathy syndrome, other than careful adherence to safe dosage schedules (WOLLHEIM et al. 1978) and frequent monitoring of the patients' ocular functions. However, CQ remains an important anti-RA drug, and the benefits to be derived from its use are considered by many responsible investigators (KERSLEY 1964; HOLLANDER 1965; PERCIVAL and MEANOCK 1968; MACKENZIE 1970; HOLT 1979; MARKS and POWER 1979) definitely to outweigh the risks involved. An alternative drug, hydroxychloroquine (HCQ), is available (see below) for this application and, at 200 mg/day is "the easiest and safest of the antimalarial drugs" (KLINEFELTER 1979).

B. Structure, Antimalarial Activity and Toxicity

I. Compounds Considered

Table 1 lists 13 important members of the 4-aminoquinoline series, along with their structural formulae, their antimalarial activities in one or more of the five standard avian assay procedures, and their relative oral toxicities in mice, rats and chicks. Values for the antimalarial and toxicity parameters have been calculated in relationship to those of quinine (= 1) in the same tests and, except where otherwise indicated, the data are as given in WISELOGLE (1946). Two compounds listed in the table (amopyroquine and hydroxychloroquine) were not available when the wartime survey was in progress, the former having been synthesised later by BURCKHALTER et al. (1948), and the latter by SURREY and HAMMER (1950). Data on mepacrine are included in the table for comparative purposes, although it is not a 4-aminoquinoline. The purpose in synthesizing the 4-aminoquinolines was primarily to effect improvements on mepacrine; therefore, Table 1 indicates the extent to which this objective was achieved.

II. Structure-Activity Relationships

The aromatic nucles in SN 3294 is identical to that in quinine, which represented a logical starting point for the synthetic programme. The amine required for attachment of the side chain of SN 3294 (Novaldiamine) appears to have been readily available from the synthesis of such compounds as mepacrine and pamaquine; hence it was also used in the synthesis of Survey Nos. 6911, 7618 (CQ), and 7373. As regards variations in the nucleus, halogenation in the 7-position (substituting for 6-methoxy) gave favourable activity, but methylation of the 7-chloro derivatives in the 2- or 3-position (as in SN 6911) was detrimental. The side chain of oxy-CQ (SN 8137) also occurs in one active member of the 9-amino-acridine series (7-methoxy, 3-chloro-; SN 186). Although the quinoline nucleus of amodiaquine and amopyroquine is the same as that in CQ, etc., their aromatic side chains resemble those of CQ, etc., only in that there are four carbon atoms between the –4–*N* atom and that in the tertiary amino group. SN 13425 represents something of a structural departure, since in this case the side chain is also cyclic, but aliphatic. The activity/toxicity quotient of this compound was not especially favourable, but it was included in a group of seven for detailed study in man (see below). HCQ differs from CQ only in having a (β-)-hydroxylethyl group in place of ethyl on the –4′–*N* atom. Two compounds listed in Table 1 (desethyl-CQ and bisdesethyl-CQ) were studied in the course of the wartime survey and at least one of them (the former) is a good antimalarial in its own right. These two compounds are of interest now mainly because they are known biotransformation products of CQ (see Sect. E, below).

III. Oral and Parenteral Toxicity

1. Methodology

To conduct a survey of the type described in WISELOGLE (1946) required evaluation of a very large number of compounds, with limited amounts usually available, in a relatively short period of time, and under conditions of testing somewhat similar to the way they were to be used in man (i.e. repeated dosage over a period of days). It was essential, therefore, to design a single, simple protocol which could be expected to yield comparable results in a number of widely separated laboratories. The method which was used in rats to obtain the data in Table 1, column 10, was essentially that described by SMITH (1950). The compounds were given either by stomach tube (for 11 consecutive days, in some cases in divided doses) or in the diet (for 14 days), and the results were evaluated in terms of the daily intakes required to produce 50% suppression of growth. These two methods of administration usually gave essentially equivalent results; for example (SMITH 1950), oxy-CQ was found to be 41% as toxic as CQ by the drug-diet method, while by the stomach tube method it was 45% as toxic.

Oral toxicities of the compounds listed in Table 1, in mice and chicks, were determined in similar short-term assays, as described by BRATTON (1945) and by COATNEY et al. (1953), respectively.

As is pointed out in WISELOGLE (1946), toxicities determined in these ways may indicate relationships among compounds which are considerably different from those based on lethality, since what is being measured may be simply loss of appetite secondary to decreased gastrointestinal motility. In line 1 of Table 1, for example, it is recorded that mepacrine is four times as toxic as quinine in the mouse, and ten times as toxic in the rat. In contrast, BARLOW et al. (1945) found the oral LD_{50} of mepacrine in the mouse to be 558 ± 13 mg/kg, and that of quinine to be 767 ± 14 mg/kg, or a ratio of 1.37 in favour of the latter. Both compounds were administered as hydrochlorides, but the LD_{50} values are given in terms of the bases. These authors found the LD_{50} of mepacrine for rats to be 490 mg/kg; they did not determine this parameter for quinine, but SPECTOR (1956) gives the oral MLD for rats as <500 mg/kg.

2. Therapeutic Indices

These indices, calculated from the data in Table 1 (mean antimalarial activity in assays C and E, divided by the toxicity factor for the mouse), assign the highest value to amodiaquine (SN 10751), and the lowest to mepacrine. A similar calculation, based only on assay method C and the relative toxicities in chicks, would assign the most favourable indices to CQ and oxy-CQ, and the least favourable to SN 9584 and mepacrine.

3. Toxicity Relationships Involving Other Species; Long-Term Tests (21 Days)

In experiments based on a necessarily small number of animals, it is recorded in WISELOGLE (1946) that in the series Survey Nos. 6911, 7373, 7618, 8137, 9584, 10751, and 13425, the tolerated daily oral doses for dogs are all of the order of 30 mg base/kg, and those for monkeys are of the order of 40 mg base/kg, with SN 7618 (CQ) being the most toxic of the series, and SN 6911 and SN 8137 the least. SN 10751 was the only compound in the series which appeared to be less toxic for the dog than for the monkey. In WISELOGLE's (1946) Table 6, data on the relative toxicities of the above seven compounds in four species (mice, rats, dogs, and monkeys) are summarised, with the toxicity of CQ being assigned in each case a value of 1. On this basis, SN 8137 was the least toxic (mean value in the four species, 0.35), and SN 10751 was the second least toxic (mean value, 0.6). However, SN 8137 was the only compound of the series which was not as toxic as CQ in at least one of the four species. It is emphasised in WISELOGLE that CQ has a very steep dose/response curve; therefore, at sublethal doses it has little effect on the well being of the animal. At increased dosages, toxic effects begin to appear rapidly.

Table 2. Animal toxicity of chloroquine and hydroxy chloroquine in acute, subacute and chronic tests

Type of test	Acute LD_{50} (mg base/kg)[a]		Tolerated dose (mg base/kg day)	
	CQ	HCQ	CQ	HCQ
i.v., mouse	25±2[b]	45±2[b]	–	–
i.p., mouse	79[b], 68–78[c]	182[b]	> 40, <155[b,d]	–
Oral, mouse	387±50[b], 1,000[c]	1,880±133[b]	400 = LD_{10}[c]	–
Oral, mouse	390 (343–445)[e]	–	<200[e]	–
	700 (619–792)[e]	–	<270[e]	–
i.m., rat	–	–	> 14[f]	–
i.v., rat	37 (35–40)[g]	–	–	–
i.p., rat	63 (60–66)[g], 87 (61–124)[h]	–	–	–
s.c., rat	118 (108–127)[g]	–	–	–
Oral, rat	608±156[b], <600[c]	–	> 50, <100[b,i]	>250, <400[b,d]
Oral, rat	670 (540–800)[g]	–	50[c,j]	–
Oral, rat	<620[b]	–	> 40, <80[b]	> 80[b,k,l]
Oral, rat	–	–	> 19[m], <80[n]	–
Oral, rat	–	–	>200, <400[o]	–
Oral, rat	–	–	> 7.5, <30[p]	–
Oral, guinea pig	300[b]	–	–	–
i.v., dog	6–8[b], <8[c]	>25[b]	–	–
s.c., dog	< 15[q]	–	–	–
Oral, dog	> 12.5, <50[b]	–	> 12, <20[c,r]	> 20[b,s]
i.v., rabbit	> 12.5, <19.5[b]	12.4[b]	–	–
i.m., rabbit	< 45[t]	–	> 15[t]	–
s.c., rabbit	–	–	> 12[u], >18[v]	–
Oral, rabbit	85[w]	–	> 25[x]	–
i.m., monkey	> 20, <40[y]	–	> 18[z]	–
Oral, monkey	–	–	> 25, <50[c]	> 60[b,aa]
Oral, swine	–	–	> 15, <30[bb]	–

[a] Data given as means ± SE, or 95% confidence limits, where stated
[b] Data from the files of the Sterling-Winthrop Research Institute
[c] Data from WISELOGLE (1946)
[d] Five-day test
[e] Data from HABERKORN et al. (1979); *l* and *d* forms, respectively
[f] Data from FRANÇOIS and MAUDGAL (1964, 1965)
[g] Data from VARGA (1966)
[h] Data form OSIFO and DI STEFANO (1978)
[i] Eleven-day test; complete suppression of growth, but no deaths
[j] Growth depressed 50%
[k] Twenty-one-day test
[l] No suppression of growth
[m] Doses administered 5 days/week for 24 weeks (GRUNDMANN et al. 1972a)
[n] Seven-day test; mortality at 160 mg/kg per day = 10% (VARGA 1968)
[o] Administered as the free base on four consecutive days (SHRIVER et al. 1975)
[p] Two-year test (FITZHUGH et al. 1948)
[q] Data from CHAMBON et al. (1968)
[r] LD_{75} estimated as 20 mg/kg per day
[s] Three-month test
[t] Data from GAMBARDELLA et al. (1955)
[u] Seven-week test (GRUNDMANN et al. 1970)
[v] Two-week test (MURAYAMA et al. 1977)
[w] Data from LARRIBAUD et al. (1961)
[x] Eleven-month test (DALE et al. 1965)
[y] SCHMIDT et al. quoted in CULWELL et al. (1948)
[z] Data from ROSENTHAL et al. (1978)
[aa] Ten-month test
[bb] Data from GLEISER et al. (1969)

4. Toxicity Relationships: CQ vs HCQ

Table 2 lists data on 15 parameters of the acute toxicity of CQ (including data on the D- and L-forms), and 11 parameters of its subacute or chronic toxicity, as determined in various laboratories. For comparative purposes, five parameters of the acute toxicity and four parameters of the long-term toxicity of HCQ are listed. In those cases where the two compounds were directly compared it appears that (overall) HCQ is about half as toxic as CQ, but in the case of some parameters (especially oral-mouse, and i.v.-dog) the margin is much wider. The antimalarial activity of HCQ, in the one type of assay which has been performed (*P. lophurae*, duck), is about equal to that of CQ (see Table 1); therefore, its therapeutic index should be considered conservatively as twice that of CQ. This considerable advantage seems to carry over into man, as reflected in a lower incidence of side effects at comparable dosages (MERWIN and WINKELMANN 1962; HENKIND and ROTHFIELD 1963; MANDEL 1963; KERSLEY 1964; CARR et al. 1968; PERCIVAL and MEANOCK 1968). Single 630-mg doses of HCQ are well tolerated by man, but single 1260-mg doses cause gastrointestinal problems (MCCHESNEY and MCAULIFF 1961; see also LEWIS and FRUMESS 1956; COUNCIL ON DRUGS 1961). The presence of the hydroxyl group on one of the *N*-ethyl groups is obviously responsible for the better tolerance of HCQ. In this connection, it may be noted also that the presence of an hydroxyl group in the side chain has a favourable effect on toxicity (compare the data on SN 8137 and SN 9584 in Table 1).

5. Human Lethal Doses; CQ, HCQ, and Quinine

The lethal dose of CQ for man has been estimated by WENIGER (1979) as about 2 g, or 30 mg/kg, and by TANENBAUM and TUFFANELLI (1980) as perhaps as much as 4 g. These estimates are based on the amounts believed to have been taken in attempted or successful suicides. The relative toxicities of quinine and CQ, as indicated in Table 1 (approximately 1:8), may carry over into man, since it has been reported recently (FRIEDMAN et al. 1980) that a 15.5-g dose of the former, taken in a suicide attempt, proved to be just slightly sublethal. It did, however, result in at least temporary near blindness. HCQ has evidently seldom been taken with suicidal intent, but in one case (GRAHAM 1960) an adult male, with moderate medical assistance, survived a dose of 5.8 g (80 mg/kg) and a plasma level of 6,100 μg/litre.

6. Conclusion

On the basis of its oral LD_{50} value for rats (about 600 mg/kg), CQ would be placed in SPECTOR's (1950) "slightly toxic" group of compounds, but in the case of the human tolerance much more accurately.

C. Methods of Analysis

I. Induced Fluorescence

In connection with the wartime antimalarial survey, the research group of BRODIE developed several very valuable analytical methods, three of which were applicable to compounds of the 4-aminoquinoline series. These were based on: (a) dye-complexing of the bases, (b) UV absorption, and (c) induced fluorescence. The induced fluorescence method (BRODIE et al. 1947 b) involved six distinct steps: (a) extraction of the bases into an organic solvent, using the least polar (for CQ, heptane) or mixture thereof which would extract the free base completely; (b) washing the solvent with water, or an aqueous salt solution, poised at a pH such that the largest possible amount of the biotransformation products, and the least possible amount of the parent compound, would be removed; (c) transfer of the bases into dilute acid; (d) buffering at pH 9.5, with the addition of cysteine (to prevent reaction with dissolved oxygen); (e) UV irradiation in a specially constructed apparatus for 1 h; and (f) reading the fluorescence in a suitable photofluorometer, with specific filters to isolate the activating wave length (e.g. Corning No. 587) and to transmit the fluorescent wave length (e.g. ½ thickness each of Corning Nos. 3389 and 4308). This method, although comparatively unsophisticated by present standards, was by far the best available for about a decade, and it produced a large fund of information on the metabolism of CQ and related compounds. The physical chemistry involved in the fluorescence-induction reaction has been studied recently by LUKASIEWICZ and FITZGERALD (1974), who have demonstrated that CQ is both inherently fluorescent and photochemically unstable. Further, the photoproduct is both photoactive and fluorescent. Maximal sensitivity is achieved by integration of the native fluorescence of the primary photoproduct.

MCCHESNEY et al (1956) revaluated the BRODIE et al. (1947 b) method in some detail, with particular reference to the determination of HCQ. It was found possible to shorten and simplify the procedure somewhat, but basically it remained the same, and no important increase in precision or sensitivity was achieved. In this revised procedure the bases were extracted into ethylene dichloride, after which the solvent was washed with an equal volume of a buffer solution (0.1 *M* each in dipotassium phosphate and boric acid; 1.7 *M* in NaCl), adjusted to pH 7.85 for CQ analysis, and to pH 8.25 for HCQ analysis. In the washing process 8% of CQ, 5% of HCQ, and 71% each of desethyl-CQ and desethyl-HCQ were removed. [Note that in the metabolism of HCQ both of these desethyl compounds are formed (see Sect. V, below); the 71% removal refers to the ethylene dichloride/pH 7.85 combination. Desethyl-CQ is so close to HCQ in extraction properties that it separates only slightly from HCQ, regardless of the pH of the buffer solution (MCCHESNEY et al. 1965 a)].

In the washing step the 5%–8% of parent drugs removed is just about compensated for by that fraction (ca. 30%) of the degradation products which is not removed. If the washing step were repeated four times the amount of degradation products remaining in the solvent phase would be <1%. However, at this point only approximately 72% of the CQ and 78% of the HCQ originally present would remain in the solvent, and correction factors of 1.3–1.4 would have to be applied to the results. To repeat the washing operation four times would be very tedious and time-consuming; furthermore, it is doubtful that the information so obtained would be intrinsically any more valuable, since the inherent experimental error would be increased by 30%–40%.

In a more recent publication (MCCHESNEY et al. 1966), specific solvents and buffer solutions were proposed for the determination of CQ and HCQ, and most of their known degradation products (see Sect. V). Subsequently (MCCHESNEY et al. 1967b), these systems were still further refined so as to give 95%–102% recoveries of CQ and its known metabolites, those recoveries exceeding 100% being accounted for by the relatively high molecular fluorescence of desethyl- and bisdesethyl-CQ. To give some idea of the complexity of the analytical problem involved, it may be noted (McChesney et al. 1965a) that, in the livers of rats receiving CQ for 3 months, the ratio of CQ to desethyl-CQ (as determined by thin layer chromatography) was 88/12. In this case one may calculate readily that application of the single buffer wash method would give a value for CQ about 4% low. However, the situation as regards HCQ metabolism is considerably more complex. In the livers of rats which had received this drug for 3 months the distribution as revealed by TLC analysis was: HCQ, 35%; desethyl-CQ, 22%; desethyl-HCQ plus bisdesethyl-CQ, 34%; unidentified, 8%. In the eyes of the same animals the corresponding percentages were 62, 32, 30, and 0, while in the spleen they were 55, 45, trace, and 0. In these cases it would be impossible, without TLC analysis, to translate the analytical result on any tissue into terms of its actual HCQ content.

II. Spectrophotofluorometry

Introduction of the spectrophotofluorometer (Bowman et al. 1955) made possible the precise and sensitive determination of a wide variety of compounds of biological (Duggan et al. 1957) and pharmacological (Udenfriend et al. 1957) interest, including CQ and HCQ. The single most important component of this instrument was a xenon arc lamp (Hanovia 150 W) which emits radiation of nearly uniform intensity over the range 2,200–8,000 Å. Greatly increased sensitivity and specificity were obtainable by separating (by sets of prisms and slits) the wavelength (if any) at which the compound was activated, and the wavelength(s) (usually 500–700 Å higher) at which it fluoresced. Data given by Udenfriend et al. (1957), for example, show that CQ is activated at 3,350 Å (at pH 11) and fluoresces at 4,000 Å. The "practical sensitivity" of the method was given as 0.05 μg/ml for CQ, and 0.08 μg/ml for oxy-CQ. This method of analysis measures in some degree all degradation products of the 4-aminoquinolines, since none is currently known in which the aromatic nucleus is not intact. However, separate extraction methods are required for the basic and acidic metabolites.

As stated above, the relative molecular fluorescences of CQ, desethyl-CQ and bisdesethyl-CQ are almost, but not quite, identical. The relative molecular fluorescences of the final known degradation product (4-amino-7-chloroquinoline), of the -4′-alcohol and of the -4′-carboxylic acid (see Sect. D.V) are about 50%, 62%, and 15%, respectively, of that of CQ. However, if the acid is converted to its methyl ester its molecular fluorescence increases to 80%–120% of that of CQ (McChesney et al. 1967b), depending on the activating and fluorescing wavelengths used (optimal: 3,150 and 3,950 Å, respectively).

Trenholme et al. (1974) have described a method for the determination of amodiaquine in red cells and plasma, also basing the results on final analysis in the spectrophotofluorometer, with activating and fluorescing wave lengths of 2,500 and 3,900 Å. The important technical difference between this method and that applicable to CQ analysis is that, following extraction of the base into ethylene dichloride at pH 10–11, and transfer therefrom into dilute acid, the solution is buffered at about pH 9.5 and is heated at 100 °C for 30 min. This greatly enhances the fluorescence, which is linear over the range 50–3,000 μg/litre.

The development of the spectrophotofluorometer, then, represented a great step forward, in that it eliminated the troublesome and time-consuming irradiation step, and made the analysis considerably more specific and sensitive by restricting the activating and fluorescing wave lengths to comparatively narrow bands. Coinciding, as it did, with a greatly increased interest in the physiological disposition of CQ and related compounds, the instrument played a very important role in facilitating the production of the large volume of information which was forthcoming in the ensuing 25 years.

III. Gas-Liquid Chromatography

A basic procedure for the determination of CQ by gas-liquid chromatography (GLC) was described by Holtzmann (1965). This method has been modified several times subsequently. In this procedure unmodified CQ base, dissolved in ethyl acetate or toluene, is detected and determined by the electron capture method. Operating temperatures are in the range of 220 °C–250 °C and with SE-30 columns (1%–4%, on DMDCS modifier) on Gaschrom P the method is said to be capable of measuring CQ in the 50- to 100-ng range, while with 1% neopentylglycol succinate as the liquid phase and PVP modifier (2-ft columns), the sensitivity is increased to the 5-ng range. No indication is given by Holtzmann (1965), however, as to whether the various 4-aminoquinoline bases (for example, CQ and desethyl-CQ) would separate satisfactorily in the systems described.

A GLC procedure outlined by Finkle et al. (1971) was intended primarily for forensic purposes. It also uses temperatures in the 220 °C–250 °C range, and an SE-30 column (2.5% on Chromosorb G). Since Finkle et al. (1971) demonstrated that CQ and HCQ separate satisfactorily in their system, it seems likely that CQ and desethyl-CQ would also separate readily, with at worst no more than minor modifications of the operating conditions. However, it remains a matter of speculation as to how effective the method would be when applied to the more complex problem of HCQ metabolism, in which separation of the parent compound from a larger variety of metabolites is required (McChesney, 1983).

In a method described by Viala et al. (1975) CQ base is also determined per se in the vapour phase, on a column of OV-17 on Gaschrom Q, at temperatures of 240 °C–325 °C, using medazepam as an internal standard. The detection limits given for CQ are 0.15 μg/ml in urine, 0.25 μg/ml in blood and 1.5 μg/g in tissue. These limits represent no marked improvement over those obtainable by spectrophotofluorometry, but there may be advantages in terms of extent of separation of parent drugs from degradation products.

The GLC method of Murayama and Nakajima (1977) also determines CQ by electron capture, using a 3% column of OV-17 on Gaschrom Q, and operating temperatures of 260 °C–280 °C. A calibration curve is prepared, using *O*-ethyl-(*p*-nitrophenyl)-phenyl-phosphonothioate as an internal standard. A sensitivity of "a few nanograms" is claimed, but details as to specificity are not available.

IV. Spectrophotometry

JOSEPHSON et al. (1947) described a UV spectrophotometric method for the determination of basic organic compounds in biological materials, but applied it only to quinine analysis. As modified by PROUTY and KURODA (1958) and by MONNET et al. (1964), this method is readily applicable to the determination of CQ and related compounds, based on their absorption at 3,430 Å. However, the sensitivity is low, compared with that of the spectrophotofluorometric or GLC methods (GRUNDMANN et al. 1971, 1972b). Obviously (McCHESNEY et al. 1967b), a biological sample such as urine, which exhibits no absorption at 3,430 Å, cannot contain more than traces of compounds in which the 4-amino-7-chloroquinoline nucleus remains intact.

D. Metabolism

I. General Considerations

Complete information on the metabolism of any xenobiotic includes data on its absorption, tissue distribution, biotransformation, and rate, and routes of excretion. At least 57 publications listed in the bibliography of this review deal with one or more aspects of this problem. As stated above, much of this work was occasioned by a desire on the part of the authors to contribute to an understanding of the retinopathy problem.

II. Absorption

Following oral dosage to man it has been estimated that 8%–10% of CQ may be recovered from the faeces, and in other animals absorption is also nearly complete (LOEB et al. 1946; WISELOGLE 1946; BERLINER et al. 1948; ZVAIFLER et al. 1963). In the case of HCQ, human faecal excretion appears to be considerably higher, i.e. about 25% of a single oral dose. However, in rats receiving three divided oral doses within 24 h, the faecal excretions of CQ and HCQ were essentially equal (McCHESNEY and McAULIFF 1961). In experiments in rats, covering a 216-h period, and based on the excretion of ^{14}C, BARROW (1974) found the faecal output of a single oral dose of [^{14}C]-CQ to be 16.3%. In contrast, the 216-h faecal output of [^{14}C]-amodiaquine, in three different strains of rats, averaged 36% of the doses. Also, in 240 h following a single i.p. injection of [^{14}C]-amodiaquine to rats, BARROW (1974) found faecal excretion of the label to average 30%, while that of rats similarly treated with CQ averaged 19.3%. Also, in a 72-h experiment in guinea pigs, following a single i.p. injection of amodiaquine, faecal excretion averaged 37%, and in dogs receiving 20–40 mg/kg oral doses of the same drug, CHAMBON et al. (1968) found that significant amounts (3% after 17 h; 9% after 24 h; two different animals) appeared in the faeces. A dog which received a 30-mg/kg s.c. dose of CQ died within 20 min, but in that time 0.16% of the dose had already reached the intestine. Subcutaneous doses of 15 mg/kg were tolerated by two dogs, in one of which 2.1% of the dose reached the intestine within 24 h.

Obviously, it is not necessary or correct to assume that all, or even an important fraction, of the faecal excretion of CQ, HCQ or amodiaquine following oral dosage

Table 3. Survey of papers reporting data on the tissue distribution of chloroquine in laboratory animals following various oral or parenteral dosage regimens[a]. Legend see oposite page

Line	Experimental animal (sex)	Route of administration	Dose (mg/kg base)	Doses/days	Order of increasing tissue concentrations[f]	Ref.
1	Albino rat (M, F)	Oral	40	1/1	Mus Eye Hrt Kid Liv = Lng[g] Spl	A
2	Albino rat (M, F)	Oral	40	79/92	Mus Eye Kid = Hrt = Liv Lng Spl	A
3	Pigmented rat (M, F)	Oral	40	79/92	Mus Hrt = Kid Lng = Liv Spl Eye	A
4	Albino rat (M)	Oral	80	1/1	Brn Mus = Tes Hrt Kid Lng = Spl Liv	B
5	Albino rat (M)	Oral	40	7/7	Brn Mus Tes Hrt Kid Lng = Spl = Liv	B
6	Albino rat (M)	Oral	80	7/7	Brn Mus = Tes Hrt Kid Lng = Spl = Liv	B
7	Albino rat (M, F)	Oral	40	27/31	Mus Eye Hrt Liv = Lng Kid Spl	C
8	Pigmented rat (M, F)	Oral	40	27/31	Mus Hrt Kid Lng = Liv Spl Eye	C
9	Albino rat (M, F)	Diet[b]	16.8	224/224	Mus Eye Hrt Liv = Lng Kid Spl	C
10	Albino rat	Oral	25	30/30	Brn Hrt Liv Lng Kid	D
11	Albino rat	Oral	25	10/10	Brn Mus Hrt Liv Lng Kid	E
12	Albino rat	Diet[b]	21[c]	42/42	Mus Brn Hrt Kid Lng Spl Liv	F
13	Albino rat	Oral	2.5	4/1[d]	Hrt Lng = Kid Spl Liv	G
14	Albino rat (F)	Oral	9.5	48/56	Mus Hrt = Ute = Eye Liv = Lng = Kid Spl Adr	H
15	Albino rat (F)	Oral	19	48/56	Eye = Mus Ute Hrt = Lng Spl = Kid = Liv Adr	H
16	Rhesus monkey	i.m.	4	1/1[e]	Fat Brn Mus = Skh = Scl Hrt Spl Kid Bon Lng = Liv Adr ReCh	I
17	Squirrel monkey	i.m.	4[c]	1/1[e]	Brn Fat Mus Skh Bon Lng Liv Hrt	I
18	Rhesus monkey	i.m.	3.7	1/1[e]	Fat Skh Mus Brn Bon Spl Kid Hrt = Lng Adr Pit Liv	J
19	Rhesus monkey	Oral	25	30/30	Brn Spl Hrt Lng Liv	D
20	Mongrel dog	s.c.	15[c]	1/1	Brn Kid Hrt Lng Liv Spl	K
21	Mongrel dog	Oral	10[c] 40	10/10 2/2	Brn Liv Lng Kid Spl	L
22	White rabbit	s.c.	12.2[c]	6/1	Brn Adr Lng Liv Spl Kid	M
23	Chinchilla rabbit (M, F)	s.c.	12.5	42/49	Mus = Ute Tes Hrt = Spl Liv = Lng Adr = Eye Kid	N
24	English guinea pig (M)	s.c.	12.4	12/14	Mus Hrt Liv = Spl Eye Lng Kid	O
25	English guinea pig (M, F)	s.c.	12.4	10/14	Brn Mus Hrt Eye Spl Adr Liv Kid[h]	P

represents unabsorbed material. In addition to the evidence cited above, that these compounds when given parenterally (see also McCHESNEY et al. 1967b) appear in the faeces, VARGA (1966) has demonstrated that in rats receiving 600-mg/kg oral doses of CQ diphosphate (about 0.57 LD_{50}) absorption is complete within 24 h. It has also been shown (VARGA et al. 1975; MINKER and MATEJKA, 1980) that, if steps are taken to reduce the gastric emptying time, or if the drug is given intraduodenally, its accumulation in the gastric mucosa is decreased considerably, and its acute toxicity approaches that when it is administered sc or ip. This finding imply that absorption is more rapid when the drug passes promptly from the stomach into the intestine and that, overall, gastric absorption is of very minor importance.

As regards oral absorption of the free base and various salt forms of CQ, it is generally agreed (FUHRMANN and KOENIG 1955; McCHESNEY et al. 1962; PAULINI and PEREIRA 1963; SCHNEIDER et al. 1963) that soluble salts such as the diphosphate, sulphate, methylene-bis-β-hydroxynaphthoate and a magnesium adsorption complex are about equally well absorbed in man. These conclusions were based on urinary outputs and plasma levels following comparable dosages. It was claimed by FUHRMANN and KOENIG (1955) that the free base and tannate are less well absorbed than the salt forms listed above, but SCHNEIDER et al. (1963) were unable to confirm this conclusion with respect to the free base (either in terms of blood levels at various postmedication intervals, or urinary outputs). Specifically, in 7 days postmedication, five subjects receiving the free base excreted $20 \pm 2.6\%$ of the dose, while five others receiving equivalent amounts of the sulphate excreted 16.8 ± 3.7(SE)% of the dose during that time.

III. Tissue Distribution

1. General Considerations

This problem has been studied under a wide variety of conditions as to species, strain, daily dose, number of doses, route and manner of administration, time elapsed after the final or only dose, etc. The compounds studied include CQ, HCQ, desethyl-CQ, bisdesethyl-CQ, oxy-CQ, sontoquine, norsontoquine, amodiaquine,

References: A, McCHESNEY et al. (1965a); B, VARGA (1968a); C, McCHESNEY et al. (1967a); D, WISELOGLE (1946); E, BERLINER et al. (1948); F, SCHMIDT et al. (1953); G, McCHESNEY and McAULIFF (1961); H, GRUNDMANN et al. (1972b); I, McCHESNEY et al. (1966); J, McCHESNEY et al. (1967c); K, CHAMBON et al. (1968); L, Laboratory data, SN 7618; M, LACAPÈRE et al. (1962); N, GRUNDMANN et al. (1970); O, McCHESNEY et al. (1965b); P, GRUNDMANN et al. (1977)

[a] Animals killed about 24 h after the final or only dose, except where otherwise indicated
[b] Animals killed while still receiving the experimental diets
[c] Results based on one animal
[d] Animals killed 2 h after the final dose
[e] Drug administered in radioactive form; tissue distributions based on ^{14}C content
[f] The symbols (see line 16) refer in order to: fat, brain, muscle, skin-hair, sclera, heart, spleen, kidney, bone marrow, lung, liver, adrenal, and retina-choroid; also pituitary on line 18
[g] Liv = Lng means that although the mean value found for liver was less than that in lung, the difference was not statistically significant
[h] Values for lung not given

Table 4. Tissue-plasma concentration ratios of 4-aminoquinoline antimalarials and degradation products in mammalian species following various dosage regimens[a]. Legend see oposite page

Line	Experimental animal (sex)	Compound	Dose (mg/kg base)	Doses/days	Tissue-plasma concentration ratios in [b]									Ref.
					Brn	Mus	Eye	Hrt	Kid	Liv	Lng	Spl	Adr	
1	Albino rat (M)	CQ	80	7/7	26	47	–	212	314	838	565	633	–	A
2	Albino rat (M, F)	CQ	40	27/31	–	40	69	208	345	490	723	953	–	B
3	Albino rat (M, F)	CQ	40	79/92	–	69	93	515	500	552	763	1,750	–	B
4	Pigmented rat (M, F)	CQ	40	27/31	–	53	3,470	355	411	735	951	1,455	–	B
5	Pigmented rat (M, F)	CQ	40	79/92	–	112	2,720	400	532	733	627	1,215	–	B
6	Albino rat (M, F)	CQ	16.8[c]	224/224	–	11	28	68	158	122	130	403	–	C
7	Albino rat	CQ	25	10/10	31	41	–	150	670	420	640	–	–	D
8	Chinchilla rabbit (M, F)	CQ	12[d]	35/42	–	19	341	135	427	176	178	141	304	E
9	English guinea pig (M)	CQ	12.4	12/14	–	49	462	85	1,780	329	678	339	–	F
10	Rhesus monkey	CQ	4[e]	1/4	13	24	–[f]	50	85	202	193	109	324	G
11	Albino rat (M, F)	HCQ	40	27/31	–	16	33	55	85	132	227	167	–	B
12	Albino rat (M, F)	HCQ	40	79/92	–	18	34	63	125	157	203	358	–	B
13	Pigmented rat (M, F)	HCQ	40	27/31	–	20	1,140	70	95	158	206	203	–	B
14	Pigmented rat (M, F)	HCQ	40	79/92	–	31	2,950	124	194	258	331	565	–	B
15	Albino rat (M, F)	HCQ	48.4	210/210	–	47	79	363	422	707	548	1,140	–	C
16	Albino rat (M, F)	Desethyl-CQ	40	27/31	–	50	108	198	241	568	508	562	–	C
17	Pigmented rat (M, F)	Desethyl-CQ	40	27/31	–	32	1,820	105	181	340	324	558	–	C
18	Rhesus monkey	Bisdes-ethyl-CQ	6.2	1/3[g]	5	5	35	75	183	135	78	85	–	G
19	Albino rat	SN 3,294	25	10/10	6	77	–	93	100	130	150	–	–	D
20	Rhesus monkey	SN 6,911	25[h]	30/30	12	–	–	30	45	97	60	63	–	H
21	Rhesus monkey	CQ	25[h,i]	30/30	[j] 13	–	–	73	58	211	82	54	–	H
					[k] 19	–	–	126	185	1,285	340	383	–	H
22	Rhesus monkey	SN 8,137	25[h]	30/30	19	–	–	24	60	64	41	33	–	H
23	Rhesus monkey	SN 9,584	25[h,i]	30/30	[j] 62	–	–	104	128	185	117	144	–	H
					[k] 265	–	–	315	1,150	2,380	358	585	–	H
24	Rhesus monkey	SN 10,751	25[h]	30/30	76	–	–	144	146	1,340	212	290	–	H
25	Mongrel dog (M)	SN 10,751	40[i]	1/1[m]	tr	6	–	54	338	338	32	125	–	I
26	Albino rat	Amopyro-quine	41.5	1/1[m]	–	5	–	35	155	140	275	300	–	J

amopyroquine, SN 3294, and SN 9584. The species most commonly used for these experiments has been the rat, which is a very suitable animal for the purpose, but mice, dogs, rabbits, guinea pigs and monkeys have also been used. Limited human data, based on autopsy material, are also available. It is obviously impossible, in a review of this scope, to do more than cite the data which seem to be the most representative.

Tissue distribution data may be presented and interrelated in three ways: (a) as a simple order of increasing (or decreasing) affinities, or predilections, as in Table 3; (b) in terms of tissue-plasma concentration ratios, as in Table 4; or (c) in terms of absolute tissue concentrations, as in Table 5. Method (c) has been used herein only in order to include a variety of important observations in which, in some cases, plasma concentrations were not determined.

2. Chloroquine

Far more research effort has been expended on this one compound than on any of the others listed above. The results may be considered as typical of the entire series, except possibly amodiaquine and amopyroquine, which have more complicated metabolic fates (see Sect. D.V2).

a) Rats

α) Tissues/Organs Usually Analysed. These include muscle, heart, kidney, liver, lung, and spleen. In both albino and pigmented rats (Table 3, lines 1–15) this has also most commonly been the order of increasing affinities. Exceptions to this order have involved the liver more than any other tissue (lines 4–6, 10, 12, 13). Strain differences may be a factor in these cases (i.e. Charles River CD versus Wistar), as may sex differences (McChesney et al. 1967a), the size of the daily dose, the length of time on medication and the time elapsed after the final dose (McChesney et al. 1965a; Varga 1968a).

β) Brain. When this tissue has been analysed (see Table 3, lines 4–6, 10, 11; Table 4, lines 1 and 7; Grundmann et al. 1971), it has almost invariably proved

References: A, Varga (1968a); B, McChesney et al. (1965a); C, McChesney et al. (1967a); D, Berliner et al. (1948); E, Grundmann et al. (1970); F, McChesney et al. (1965b); G, McChesney et al. (1966); H, Wiselogle (1946); I, Chambon et al. (1968); J, Thompson et al. (1958)

[a] Animals killed about 24 h after the final or only dose, except where otherwise indicated

[b] The column headings in order are: brain, muscle, eye, heart, kidney, liver, lung, spleen, and adrenal

[c] Drug administered in the diets; concentrations adjusted weekly to food consumption and growth so as to provide the indicated daily intakes

[d] Drug administered s.c. 6 days/week

[e] Drug administered in radioactive form; tissue and blood levels based on ^{14}C analysis; whole blood concentrations assumed to be 3.75 times plasma concentrations

[f] Various parts of the eye were analysed, but concentration in the whole organ was not determined

[g] Animals killed 72 h after dosage

[h] Tissue and plasma concentrations determined by the dye-complexing procedure (Brodie et al. 1947a): for identification of compounds, see Table 1

[i] Values in line k determined by the heptane-fluorescence procedure (Brodie et al. 1947b); it is not known whether the animals in lines [j] and [k] were the same, but it seems doubtful. [l] Values given for free drug only, [m] Results based on one animal only

Table 5. Comparative data on the tissue distribution of some important 4-aminoquinoline antimalarials in rats and dogs following various dosage regimens[a]

Line	Experimental animal (sex)	Compound	Dose (mg/kg base)	Doses/days	Tissue concentrations (mg/kg ± SE) in:[h] Muscle (other)	Eye	Heart	Kidney	Liver	Lung	Spleen	Ref.
1	Albino rat (M)	CQ	20	7/7	7.8 ± 3.0	–	23 ± 7	70 ± 12	112 ± 16	104 ± 18	125 ± 23	A
2	Albino rat (M)	CQ	160	7/7	140 ± 28	–	667 ± 50	720 ± 92	2,345 ± 270	1,160 ± 155	1,320 ± 185	A
3	Albino rat (F)	CQ	19 (s.c.)	10/14	44 ± 11	84 ± 5.8	87 ± 17	196 ± 41	160 ± 25	189 ± 31	312 ± 91	B
4	Albino rat (F)	CQ	19	30/42	17 ± 5.2	–	94 ± 16	243 ± 20	231 ± 29	145 ± 14	268 ± 35	C
5	Albino rat (F)	CQ	19	120/168	55 ± 11	–	290 ± 48	499 ± 86	340 ± 46	312 ± 49	496 ± 58	C
6	Albino rat (M, F)	CQ	40	52/61	13 ± 2.3	38 ± 0.9	95 ± 21	111 ± 4.3	185 ± 5.0	220 ± 22	448 ± 47	D
7	Pigmented rat (M, F)	CQ	40	52/61	34 ± 9.6	863 ± 23	97 ± 12	145 ± 24	186 ± 35	255 ± 43	460 ± 60	D
8	Albino rat (M, F)	HCQ	40	52/61	6.2 ± 0.5	15 ± 0.8	22 ± 4.3	35 ± 4.3	57 ± 5.4	78 ± 5.8	92 ± 8.3	D
9	Pigmented rat (M, F)	HCQ	40	52/61	6.3 ± 0.4	512 ± 37	26 ± 1.1	42 ± 6.0	56 ± 7.4	86 ± 7.4	119 ± 18	D
10	Mongrel dog	CQ	10 40	10/10 2/2	69 (brn)	–	148	254	205	223	376	E
11	Mongrel dog (F)	CQ[b]	15 (s.c.)	1/1	f 1.5 (brn) g 3.2 (brn)	– –	8.7 9.5	27 32	7.3 17	18 20	39 42	F
12	Mongrel dog	Amodiaquine[b]	20	4/4	f 0 (brn) g 0.3 (brn)	– –	1.5 12	0.9 6.7	20 88	4.4 28	6.4 35	F
13	Albino rat	Amodiaquine[c]	164	1/1	–	–	–	26–242	9–130	–	25–48	G
14	Albino rat	Amopyroquine	41.5	8/8	16	–	58	112	200	194	216	H
15	Mongrel dog	Norsontoquin[d]	15.8	78/91	50–78 (brn)	–	–	162–185	288–414	196–238	262–300	I
16	Mongrel dog	HCQ[e]	20.3	78/91	31–49 (brn)	–	–	182–215	328–330	250–267	190–199	I

References: A, VARGA (1968a); B, GRUNDMANN et al. (1971); C, GRUNDMANN et al. (1972a); D, McCHESNEY et al. (1965a); E, Laboratory data, SN 7618; F, CHAMBON et al. (1968); G, BARROW (1974); H, THOMPSON et al. (1958); I, McCHESNEY and McAULIFF (1961)

[a] Animals killed 24 h after final or only dose, except where otherwise indicated; dosage oral except in lines 3 and 11 (s.c.)

[b] Values in line [f] are free drug; those in line [g] are total drug

[c] Animals killed 216 h after single dose; the compound was administered in radioactive form, and the results are expressed as amodiaquine equivalents of the ^{14}C found

[d] Animals killed 2 days after the final dose

[e] Animals killed 5 days after the final dose

[h] Where only one value is given it indicates that the results were based on one animal. brn, brain

to have a lower affinity for CQ than muscle and, therefore, the lowest affinity of any tissue, except possibly fat and bone.

γ) Uterus-Testis. Analyses of these organs (Table 3, lines 4–6, 14, 15) usually place them between muscle and heart in terms of affinities for CQ.

δ) Adrenal Gland. This organ, when analysed (see Table 3, lines 14–15; also GRUNDMANN et al. 1971, 1972a, 1972b), has invariably proved to have an affinity for CQ exceeding all other tissues, including spleen. A possible exception to this generalisation is the eye of pigmented rats; no direct comparison of these two organs seems to have been made.

ε) Skin. This tissue was analysed byMcCHESNEY et al. (1957) in an experiment designed to determine whether CQ might accumulate therein in sufficient concentrations to exert a significant sun-screening effect. The drug was given to male albino rats in three divided doses totalling 10 or 45 mg/kg, over a 24-h period, and the animals were killed at the 26th hour (as in Table 3, line 13). In the lower dose group the ratio of concentrations for skin/liver was 2/12, while in the higher dose group it was 2/11. Assuming that the same ratio would apply to the animals listed in Table 5, line 6, skin would fall just below the eye in the order of increasing tissue affinities. In connection with the results found for the 45 mg/kg group, it is of interest to note that the hepatic concentration found (mean $\pm$SE) was 63 ± 3 mg/kg, while in a much later experiment (McCHESNEY et al. 1965a), in rats receiving single 40-mg/kg oral doses (with killing 24 h later), the level found in this tissue was 61 ± 18 mg/kg. This close correlation emphasises the fact that the metabolism of CQ in the rat is governed by predictable and reproducible pharmacokinetic constants.

φ) Bone. This tissue has customarily been ignored in the various rat experiments. FISCHER and FITCH (1975) have called attention to this omission, and have pointed out the potential importance of bone relative to that fraction of the drug often reported as "not accounted for." These authors analysed representative tissues of adult rats, and of one 8-day old rat, 30 min after the injection of 5 μCi (3-[^{14}C])-CQ. They found in the latter animal tissue concentrations of ^{14}C in the increasing order: bone, muscle, heart, lung, kidney, liver, spleen, adrenal. This is essentially the order which has usually been found (see Table 3, lines 1–15), beginning with muscle. However, as percentage of dose, the principal repositories were: gastrointestinal tract, 18.7; skin, 16.9; muscle, 16.4; liver, 13.3; bone, 11.6; lungs, 8.3; kidney, 3.6; spleen, 2.0; heart, 0.9; other, 4.9. In the adult rats a considerably different percentage distribution was found: liver, 18.2; gastrointestinal tract, 14.7; muscle, 7.6; skin 4.9; bone, 2.0; kidneys, 2.0; lungs, 1.9; spleen, 1.3; heart, trace; other, 1.9. It is evident from these data that bone should not be neglected in the overall accounting, as it has not been in larger species (Table 3, lines 16–18).

η) Eye. The eye was (correctly) regarded as a minor repository of CQ until the retinopathy problem (see Sect. A, above) surfaced. This organ then came to be of the greatest importance, particularly with regard to the localisation of the drug therein. In albino rats (Table 3, lines 1, 2, 4–7, 9–15) eye ranks above muscle, but below heart, in the order of increasing affinities; however, in pigmented rats (lines 3 and 8) eye ranks above all other tissues, except possibly the adrenal gland. Binding of the drug to melanin is clearly the critical factor in determining the wide divergence in response of the two strains (SAMS and EPSTEIN, 1965).

θ) Other Tissues. In a few cases tissues or organs other than any of those mentioned above have been studied. COHÉN et al. (1963), for example, found evidence, in autoradiograms of rats prepared following the injection of [^{14}C]CQ, of considerable accumulations in salivary gland, thymus, hypophysis and frontal sinus. Pituitary gland does not appear to have been studied otherwise as a repository for CQ in the rat, but its strong affinity for the drug has been demonstrated in the rhesus monkey (see Table 3, line 18). *Hair* has been identified as a repository for CQ by BERNSTEIN et al. (1963).

ι) Discussion. At numerous points in Table 3 cognisance has been taken of the fact that, although the mean concentrations given in the literature for two or more tissues in the increasing order may have differed numerically, the differences were not statistically significant. In the following case (GRUNDMANN et al. 1972a) it would be misleading to record the sequence as liver < kidney < spleen when, in fact, the levels reported (as means $\pm$SE) were, respectively, 231$\pm$29, 243$\pm$20, and 268$\pm$35 mg/kg. Reporting the data as in Table 4 (tissue-plasma ratios) or as in Table 5 (actual tissue concentrations) clarifies these relationships, since it not only shows the increasing order, but also gives a definite idea of the magnitude of the differences involved.

The ubiquitous nature of the distribution of CQ in rat tissues is evident from the data cited above. Figure 1 illustrates what appear to be typical results for its distribution in albino rats receiving 40-mg/kg oral doses 6 days/week for up to 3 months, followed by a withdrawal period of 15 days. The sequence of increasing concentrations, i.e. muscle, eye, heart, kidney, liver, lung, spleen, was maintained throughout the treatment period, except at the 3-month interval. At this point heart had overtaken kidney, and there was no significant difference between the levels in kidney and liver (specifically, these values were 215$\pm$40 and 237$\pm$17 mg/kg, respectively). Tissue concentrations after 1 day of treatment were about one-fifth of those observed after 79 doses; this indicates that rapid degradation and/or excretion were occurring, as do the regression rates after discontinuation of treatment. These rates were not uniform: although the tissue levels declined overall by 97% in 15 days (corresponding to a body half-life of 2.8 days), the rates varied from a decrease of 98.5% in spleen to 89.5% in the eye. Data on levels in the eyes of pigmented rats, treated identically, are shown in Fig. 1 for comparative purposes. In these organs the CQ concentration after the 79th dose averaged 911$\pm$61 mg/kg, compared with 39.9$\pm$4.1 mg/kg in the albinos. In the former the 15-day regression rate corresponded to a $t^{1/2}$ of 38 days, compared with 4.8 days in the latter.

Similar graphs could be prepared from the data of GRUNDMANN et al. (1972a, 1972b). In the former experiment female albino rats received 30 mg/kg CQ diphosphate orally, 5 days/week for 24 weeks, with groups killed at 2-week intervals. Total drug retention in the eight organs analysed at these intervals decreased from 6.4% of the administered doses at the 2nd week, to 1.35% at the 24th week, again emphasising rapid turnover. Position in the increasing order occupied by the various tissues shifted somewhat from one interval to another, but averaged as follows:

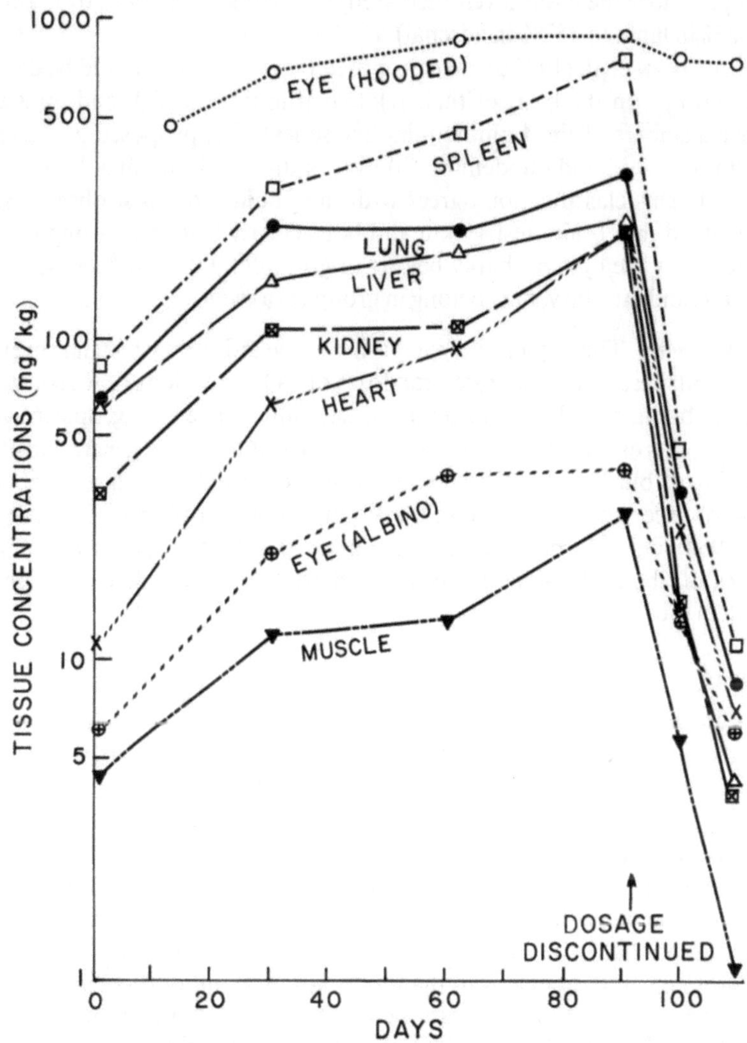

Fig. 1. Tissue concentrations of chloroquine in albino rats of both sexes during and following the oral administration of 40-mg/kg oral doses 6 days/week for 3 months. Data on the eyes of hooded rats receiving the same dosage regimen are included in the figure for comparative purposes (McChesney et al. 1965 a)

brain, 1.0; muscle, 2.0; heart, 3.2; lung, 3.9; liver, 5.4; kidney, 6.2; spleen, 6.4; adrenal, 8.0. (It is to be understood that those tissues assigned whole numbers remained in the same relative positions for the entire 24 weeks; the others shifted positions on one or more occasions.) In Grundmann et al.'s (1972 b) second experiment similar animals received 15- or 30-mg/kg oral doses of CQ diphosphate, 6 days/week for 8 weeks, with groups killed at weekly intervals. At the lower dose level the CQ concentrations in nine representative tissues remained essentially constant, or even declined somewhat, between the 1st and 8th weeks but, in contrast, at the higher dose the tissue levels increased over that same period, by about 200% (from 43% in lung, to 357% in adrenal).

GRUNDMANN et al. (1972b) have proposed that rat tissues should be divided into three groups on the basis of their relative affinities for CQ (and, presumably, for other members of the 4-aminoquinoline series). The proposed groups are: (a) uterus, muscle, eye, and duodenum; (b) liver, kidney, spleen, lung, and heart; and (c) adrenal. This classification agrees with the findings of most observers, but it may be added that brain, testis, skin and bone clearly belong in group (a), and in pigmented rats the eyes probably belong in group (c). Other tissues, such as salivary glands and pituitary, may belong in group (c) as well.

κ) Summary. The sequence of increasing tissue affinities which has been established for rats receiving moderate oral doses of CQ for periods of weeks to several months is: brain, muscle, eye (albino), heart, kidney, liver, lung, spleen, adrenal. Skin, bone, uterus, and testis belong in this series in the same general positions as eye and heart, but they have been studied only occasionally. This distribution is, with minor exceptions, the same as that found for amotriphene (McCHESNEY and BANKS 1960) and chlorpromazine (BERTI and CIMA 1955). These two compounds are bases of about the same molecular weight as CQ, but they are monobasic, rather than dibasic.

b) Monkeys

Results are given in Table 3, lines 16–19, for the relative tissue affinities of CQ in rhesus monkeys, and in one squirrel monkey. The order indicated in lines 16 and 18 differs from that in rats mainly in the lower position of spleen, and the comparatively high positions of bone and liver. It is of particular interest, in connection with the retinopathy problem, to note the very high affinity of CQ for retina choroid, and the comparatively low affinity for sclera (line 16). Results on the one squirrel monkey (line 17) are notable for the fact that the concentration in heart exceeded that in all of the other tissues analysed; otherwise, the relative affinities were much the same as in the rhesus strain. In all of these animals, except the one listed in line 19, the analyses were based on ^{14}C content, but it may be assumed that at least 80% of the ^{14}C was present in the form of unchanged CQ. Analysis by the methods available in 1946 (line 19) gave essentially the same distribution (see also, Table 4, line 21). It is of interest to note, in comparing the results in Table 4, lines 10 and 21a, that in spite of the completely different dosage schedules and methods of analysis, the tissue-plasma ratios were remarkably similar.

c) Dogs

Data reported on the tissue distribution of CQ in dogs (Table 3, lines 20–21, and Table 5, lines 10–11) are rather fragmentary, being based on a few animals and a small number of tissues. It can only be generalised from this limited amount of information that, as in the rat, brain has the lowest affinity for CQ, and spleen the highest. A complicating factor in correlating the data in Table 5, lines 10–11, is the claim of CHAMBON et al. (1968) that in this species, at least, CQ forms an *N*-glucuronide. They report their data, therefore, in terms of "free" and "total" drug.

[Note that WILLIAMS (1959) states that glucuronic acid conjugation of CQ had already been observed, but the structure of the conjugate was unknown at that time.] Since the results described in line 10 of Table 5 did not take the possibility of conjugation into account, what was presumably being measured should be comparable to CHAMBON et al.'s (1968) "free" drug. Even so, it is clear that the values listed in lines 10 and 11 are of completely different orders of magnitude. It is true that the dosage schedules involved, especially in terms of the number of doses given, were quite different. However, if the kinetics of CQ metabolism in rat and dog are at all comparable, it would appear that the differences in tissue concentrations listed in lines 10 and 11 a should be of the order of two fold, not eight- to ten fold. This discrepancy is only partly resolved if line 10 is compared with line 11 b.

CHAMBON et al. (1968) point out that the existence of glucuronic acid conjugation of CQ had escaped other observers; the reason for this may be in part the comparatively small amount of attention accorded to the dog as an experimental animal for the study of the 4-aminoquinolines. If they are correct, it would follow that CQ and related compounds should have relatively short half-lives in the dog. This does indeed appear to be the case: calculating from the plasma levels observed in the dog following i.v. administration (MCCHESNEY and MCAULIFF 1961) it develops that CQ has a half-life of about 2 h, and HCQ of about 3 h. In contrast (see Sect. E, below) these parameters in man are of the order of at least 35–55 h.

d) Rabbits

Data on two strains of rabbits are given in Table 3, lines 22–23, and in Table 4, line 8. (The last two entries are from the same experiment, but with different lengths of time on medication.) The results on the one white rabbit (line 22) seem anomalous in the very low affinity reported for the adrenals, but there is agreement for both strains that the highest affinity is for the kidneys. As was to be expected, from the observations on albino and pigmented rats (for example, Table 5, lines 6, 7), the affinity of CQ for the eyes of the pigmented strain (Chinchilla) was very high. This organ was not analysed in the one white rabbit, but it may be assumed that in this case the affinity was lower.

e) Guinea Pigs

Two experiments have been reported in this species, with the results listed in Table 3, lines 24–25 and Table 4, line 9, the latter two entries being from the same experiment. The strains used in lines 24–25 may have been identical (English), but this is not clear from the information available. However, the different positions assigned to eye and liver in the increasing order suggest that the strains were not the same. The two studies do agree that in the guinea pig the highest affinity of CQ is for the kidneys, and that its affinity for the spleen is definitely lower than it is in such species as the rat.

The hope in conducting the experiment described in Table 3, line 24, was that a high ascorbic acid intake would decrease the extent of deposition of CQ in the eye. This hope, under the experimental conditions at least, was not realised. On the contrary, increasing the ascorbic acid intake to ten times the normal requirement reduced all tissue levels significantly *except* those in the eye (MCCHESNEY et al. 1965 b).

f) Man

Data on the human tissue distribution of CQ are available, mostly from cases in which considerable overdoses were taken, as in accidental poisoning in children or in instances in which the drug was taken by adults with deliberate suicidal intent. In this connection, VIALA et al. (1972) have concluded that CQ intoxication is irreversible if the blood concentration exceeds 4,000–6,000 μg/litre and, as noted above, WENIGER (1979) has estimated that the fatal dose of CQ for man is only of the order of 30 mg/kg. This is a dose which is readily tolerated by rats daily, 6 days/week, for as long as 3 months (McCHESNEY et al. 1965a); therefore, tissue concentrations and distribution in human overdosage cases are not necessarily abnormal. PROUTY and KURODA (1958) did have an opportunity to determine tissue levels in military personnel who were on prophylactic-suppressive CQ medication, but who had died from unrelated causes. These cases ($n=8$) gave the order of increasing concentrations as: brain (mean level, 2.9 μg/g); kidney, heart, spleen, liver (mean level, 24.6 μg/g). In one case of CQ suicide KIEL (1964) found a somewhat different sequence, and much higher levels (given as micrograms per gram in parentheses): heart (40), brain (50), muscle (180), spleen (260), liver (280), lung (580), and kidney (640). Also, in one case of CQ suicide ROBINSON et al. (1970) analysed four tissues, with the following results, in the same terms: brain (16), heart (57), kidney (70), and liver (175). These two sets of results have little in common. VIALA et al. (1972) have presented an extensive review of the literature on this problem, and have given some detailed results on two of their own cases. These cases are consistent with one another in giving the order of increasing tissue affinities (with the concentrations as micrograms per gram in parentheses) as: brain (17), pancreas (75), heart (154–175), lung (193–210), kidney (358–388), liver (441–531), and spleen (532). This order differs from that usually observed in the rat in no important respect, and the absolute concentrations are about the same as have been found in rats after 2–3 months of medication at 40 mg/kg per day (McCHESNEY et al. 1965a).

3. Other 4-Aminoquinolines

a) Hydroxychloroquine

Typical results on this structural analogue of CQ, in rats, are given in Table 4, lines 11–15, and in Table 5, lines 8–9. In Table 5 it is seen that in comparison to CQ (lines 6–7) tissue concentrations of HCQ, when administered in equivalent dosages for equal times, are lower by about 60%. However, in terms of relative affinities (compare, for example, Table 4, lines 3, 12), the increasing order is the same for both drugs (see also McCHESNEY, 1983). This statement applies to the pigmented strain (Table 5, lines 7, 9), as well as to the albinos. LEGROS and ROSNER (1971) determined ocular concentrations of HCQ in albino (Wistar) rats following 2 and 3 months' treatment at about 120 mg base/kg per day, 6 days/week. The concentrations found in the whole eyes for these time intervals were, respectively, 36.7 ± 17.3 and 66 ± 11 μg/g, and the regression rate from the former (found, 0.8 ± 0.1 μg/g after 3 months' withdrawal) indicated a $t^{1/2}$ of about 18 days. These values correlate satisfactorily with those found by McCHESNEY et al. (1965a; see Table 5, line 8), which were, for a daily dose of 40 mg/kg, 15.2 ± 0.8 μg/g after 2 months of medication and 14.8 ± 1.6 µg/g after 3 months. The t½ indicated by the McCHESNEY et al. (1965a) data was 6.6 days, but this calculation is based on observations at shorter intervals (6.3 ± 0.5 µg/g after 8 days and 3.4 ± 0.1 µg/g after 15 days). Another positive correlation with the LEGROS and ROSNER (1971) data is the observation (McCHESNEY et al. 1967a) that after the administration of HCQ in the diet to albino rats at 48.4 mg/kg per day for 30 weeks the mean ocular concentration was 20.2 ± 2.0 µg/g.

In the dog (Table 5, lines 10, 16), the orders of increasing tissue affinities were identical only in terms of the low position of brain; they differed considerably in the relative positions of kidney and spleen. A lower dose of HCQ (10.2 mg/kg per day) in this experiment (McCHESNEY and McAULIFF 1961) gave for HCQ the order: brain, spleen, kidney, adrenal, lung, and liver.

b) Sontoquine

Data for this compound are available only for the monkey (Table 4, line 20). When administered on the same dosage schedule as CQ (line 21), it gave very similar results, the only difference being in the relative positions of spleen and heart.

c) Norsontoquine

This compound has been studied only in the dog, with results given in Table 5, line 15. The experiment was run in parallel with that on HCQ (line 16) but, due to poor tolerance, lower dose levels of norsontoquine had to be used, and even then forced feeding was required to keep the animals alive. The results on the 15.5 mg/kg per day dose level and those at a lower level (7.8 mg/kg per day) together indicate that the order of increasing canine affinities for norsontoquine is: brain, spleen, kidney, adrenal, lung, and liver.

d) Desethyl-CQ

This compound, which is the first and most quantitively important degradation product of CQ, has been studied in both albino and pigmented rats (Table 4, lines 16–17) in a 1-month experiment. The results are readily comparable to those given for CQ (lines 2, 4) and for HCQ (lines 11, 13), since the experiments were run in parallel on animals from the same source. In the albinos the observed order of affinities for desethyl-CQ differed from those for CQ and HCQ only in the relative positions of spleen, lung, and liver, with liver having the highest affinity for desethyl-CQ. However, (see line 16, columns 8, 10), the difference in tissue-plasma ratios, between 562 and 568, is clearly not significant; specifically, as mg/kg ± SE, the results for spleen and liver were 145 ± 27.7 and 147 ± 14.7, respectively. Similar results were obtained for the pigmented strain (line 17), except that the eye had by far the highest affinity for all three compounds. Since in both rodent strains the affinity of liver for desethyl-CQ exceeded that of the lungs, this may be a real difference. An examination of the original data (McCHESNEY et al. 1967a), which also present information on the tissue levels of desethyl-CQ at 1, 5, and 8 days after the final dose, indicates a body half-life of 54 h in both strains of rats, as against about 36 h for CQ.

e) Bisdesethyl-CQ

Data on this compound (Table 4, line 18) were obtained in rhesus monkeys, 72 h after a single oral dose equivalent to 6.2 mg base/kg. The results are qualitatively similar to those obtained in the same strain/species for CQ (Table 3, lines 16, 18) in according low affinities to brain, muscle, and heart, but they differ in the relative positions of lung, spleen, liver, and kidney. However, it must be recognised that the results on CQ in monkeys have not been entirely consistent. Orders of predilection based on one or two animals are much less likely to be truly representative, since with a larger number of animals meaningful standard errors can be calculated and a better indication of the magnitude of individual variations may be obtained.

f) Desethyl-HCQ

As regards tissue distribution, this compound appears to have been studied only by LEGROS and ROSNER (1971), and by these authors only in terms of ocular concentrations in albino rats. After 2 months' treatment at about 240 mg base/kg per day, six days/week, the concentration found was 35.3 ± 2.3 µg/g, while after 3 months at 120 mg base/kg per day it was 32.6 ± 2.8 µg/g. The regression rate indicated following the former (3.8 ± 0.2 µg/g after 3 months' withdrawal) corresponds to a $t^{1/2}$ of about 27 days. The levels, as well as those for HCQ (see above), which were determined without washing the organic phase, would thus include all basic degradation products of HCQ and desethyl-HCQ.

g) Amodiaquine

α) Rats. Results on this compound are rather fragmentary and, therefore, somewhat inconclusive. There appear to be, in fact (Table 5, line 13) only data on three tissues, and these values were obtained by ^{14}C analysis, 216 h after a single dose of the compound. Since presumably little, if any, of the unchanged drug would remain in the organism at this time, the results would not be at all comparable to those obtained for CQ in the same species.

β) Dogs. Results are given for one animal in Table 4, line 25, and for another in Table 5, line 12. Again, rapid metabolism (see Sect. E.II, below) complicates interpretation of the data, in comparison to those obtained for other members of the 4-aminoquinoline series, but it probably does account for the low observed tissue concentrations. The extent of metabolism is evident from a comparison of the values shown in lines 12a and 12b of Table 5. In terms of relative affinities, however, it is clear that those for brain and muscle are very low, while those for liver and kidney are relatively high.

γ) Rhesus Monkeys. In this species (Table 4, line 24) dosage was daily for 1 month, and the method of analysis was such that presumably only the unchanged drug plus the unconjugated primary and secondary amines would be measured. Of the five compounds studied in this way (Table 4, lines 20–24), amodiaquine gave the highest tissue-plasma ratios, by the dye-complexing procedure, especially so in liver. Otherwise, the sequence of increasing tissue concentrations was much the same as that which has usually been observed in the rat, and it agrees with that reported for CQ (line 21) in assigning a high affinity to liver.

δ) Mice. This species has not been used extensively as a subject for tissue distribution studies, probably because it yields insufficient samples of most tissues for satisfactory analysis. BARROW (1974), however, has recorded that in albino mice (Tuck's strain No. 1), killed 5 h after the i.v. injection of (methylene-[^{14}C])-amodiaquine dihydrochloride (dosage not stated), ^{14}C activity was detected chiefly in the intestine, gall bladder and brown fat of the neck. Other repositories were liver, kidneys, lungs, spleen, heart, and possibly salivary gland and thymus. This could well have been the order of increasing affinities, but it is not so stated. After 24 h ^{14}C was found principally in the intestine, brown fat, liver, kidneys, and lungs, while at 48 h radioactivity was localised mainly in the intestine, liver, and kidneys. A high level of biliary excretion is indicated by these observations.

h) Amopyroquine

The data available on this compound have been obtained in albino rats (Table 4, line 26; Table 5, line 14). The method of analysis used was such that it would (presumably) measure only the unchanged drug and the primary (bisdesethyl) amine. The sequence of tissue affinities observed following the administration of eight daily doses (Table 5, line 14), i.e. muscle, heart, kidney, lung, liver, and spleen, is, nevertheless, almost identical to that which has commonly been found for those members of the 4-aminoquinoline series which have aliphatic side chains. (For a further discussion of these findings, see Sect. E.II, below.) THOMPSON et al. (1958) did not analyse the eyes of their animal, but KURTZ et al. (1967) did determine concentrations in that organ of beagle dogs and rhesus monkeys receiving high (8–64 mg base/kg per day and 4.2–42 mg base/kg per day, respectively) doses of amopyroquine for up to 1 year. Specific figures are not given, nor is it clear what mixture of unchanged drug and degradation products was being measured, but it is stated that there were "large accumulations" and that the t½ was in excess of 68 days.

i) SN 3294

This non-chlorinated compound has also been studied in detail only in the albino rat, on one dosage schedule, as indicated in Table 4, line 19. The abbreviated list of tissues for which data are reported indicates a sequence of increasing affinities identical to that usually observed for CQ and HCQ, in that species and strain.

j) SN 8137

This compound, as noted in Sect. B, is the least toxic, in four commonly used laboratory species, of the drugs listed in Table 4, lines 20–24. It (line 22) is characterised, following the administration of equivalent dosages, by relatively low tissue concentrations and by low tissue-plasma ratios. Its pattern of tissue affinities is the same as that of CQ as regards brain and liver, but there are some shifts in the positions of heart, spleen, kidney, and lung in the series.

k) SN 9584

Also, in the rhesus monkey (Table 4, line 23) SN 9584 gave lower tissue-plasma ratios than amodiaquine (line 24), although the tissue levels reported were, with one exception (liver), considerably higher. The pattern of relative tissue affinities is the same as that of the other compounds listed in lines 20–24 only as regards brain (lowest) and liver (highest).

IV. Localisation of 4-Aminoquinolines Within Organs

1. Liver and Kidney

VARGA (1968 b) gave CQ diphosphate to rats in oral doses ranging from 13 to 360 mg/kg, and killed the animals 24 h later. Subcellular localisation was then studied in liver and kidney. In the former organ increasing dosage had little effect on the relative concentrations in the nuclear (about 10% of the total) or microsomal (10% –15%) fractions, but those in the mitochondrial fraction decreased from 69% of the total present to 5%, while those in the soluble fraction increased from 10% to 76%. Similarly, in the kidneys, nuclear and microsomal fractions were almost unaffected by increasing dosage, while the percentage of total renal CQ in the mitochondrial fraction decreased and that in the soluble fraction increased. VARGA concluded that there is no basis for the assumption that the localisation of CQ in these organs is determined by binding to nucleic acids.

2. Eye

The extent to which CQ localises in the eye, and to which specific structures it binds preferentially, are obviously of the greatest importance in connection with the retinopathy problem. This question has been studied largely in experimental animals, but limited human data are available. As early as 1959 PAU and BAÜMER reported the existence of corneal deposits in RA patients being treated with CQ, and they concluded that these deposits were definitely related in composition to the drug or its degradation products.

In early studies in experimental animals (albino and pigmented rabbits) BERNSTEIN et al. (1963) administered 5-mg/kg doses of CQ dihydrochloride, i.v. or i.m., and killed the animals at various intervals thereafter. At the 48-h interval, tissue levels were generally higher in the pigmented strain, and CQ was found in the iris and choroid of that strain only. Similarly, 63 days after the single i.m. doses, CQ was found in the iris and choroid of the pigmented animals, but not in any other tissue of either strain. Following the administration of CQ to pigmented rats for 6 months and to albinos for 14 months (both in the drinking water, at an estimated intake of 70 mg/kg per day), the same authors found large drug concentrations in the iris and choroid of the pigmented strain, with smaller amounts in cornea, retina, and sclera. The level in iris, for example, was 62 times that in retina and sclera, and 87 times that in the liver. In the albino rats, in spite of an intake of more than twice that of the pigmented animals, CQ was found only in retina and sclera, the concentration in the former being about the same as that in liver and hair. The strong affinity of CQ for the iris and choroid, of the pigmented animals only, was very evident. General confirmation of these findings has been reported by other investigators (McCHESNEY et al. 1965 a, 1967 a; GRUNDMANN et al. 1970) in the sense that the eyes of pigmented rats and rabbits accumulate large amounts of CQ relative to those of albinos and release these deposits very slowly on cessation of medication.

FRANÇOIS and MAUDGAL (1964, 1965) were the first investigators to produce CQ retinopathy or keratopathy in experimental animals (rabbits). They accomplished this by i.m. injection of the sulphate three times weekly for 3–7 months, in amounts equivalent to about 7–14 mg Base/kg per day. Of the 18 survivors after 3 months of this treatment, 14 showed definite, but reversible, corneal changes. Although no figures were given for the CQ content of the various ocular structures, at the 3-month or subsequent intervals, CQ "deposits" were demonstrated as being present, on the basis of their fluorescence after UV irradiation. Later FRANÇOIS and MAUDGAL (1967) produced experimental retinopathy in young adult male rabbits which had received i.m. injections equivalent to 2.5 mg base/kg per day for 6–16 months. Fluorescent ocular deposits were detected by the 14th month and lesions were observed in the choroid by the 8th month. Deposition of CQ in the pigment epithelium, specifically, was demonstrated by the development of characteristic fluorescence in this layer.

DALE et al. (1965) attempted to produce a condition comparable to human retinopathy by giving considerably higher daily oral doses of CQ (25 mg/kg; ten times the usual human anti-RA dose) to albino and pigmented rabbits. They also reported no data for CQ concentrations in various parts of the eye, but they did find characteristic pigmentary deposits in the choroid, pigmented epithelium, iris and ciliary body of the pigmented animals only. No changes were seen in the cornea or lens of either strain. These authors did not consider their findings, although very striking, really comparable to those observed in human retinopathy, in that changes other than those in the pigment epithelium were not conspicuous.

Specific localisation of CQ in various parts of the eye was studied by MCCHESNEY et al. (1966), 96 h after the i.m. administration of 4-mg/kg doses of the (-4-[^{14}C])-labelled compound to rhesus monkeys. Very high concentrations were found in retina-choroid (16–37 mg/kg), followed by sclera (1.3–1.5 mg/kg) and optic nerve (0.5–1.8 mg/kg). These levels were accompanied by hepatic concentrations ranging from 6 to 13.6 mg/kg. Traces of CQ were found in the cornea-iris and lens of one of three animals, but none in the vitreous humour. These analyses were based on ^{14}C content, but it is a reasonable assumption that at least 80% of the ^{14}C was present in the form of CQ per se.

The extent of ocular damage induced in swine by the oral administration of CQ, and its localisation in the eye, have been studied by GLEISER et al. (1969). Four animals receiving 31 mg/kg per day of the diphosphate survived for 32–92 days (mean, 65.5), while all animals receiving half this dosage survived for 106 days. The latter pigs were then killed at intervals ranging from 1 to 62 days. In the animals on the higher dose level ($n=3$) concentrations of CQ averaged 550 mg/kg in neuroretina, 2,840 mg/kg in choroid-pigment epithelium and 97 mg/kg in sclera. At the lower dose level ($n=3$) the corresponding values were 452, 2,433, and 53 mg/kg. Withdrawal periods of 1, 6, and 34 days were involved in this case, but no significant downward trend in concentrations was noted with time, except possibly in the sclera. In the one animal killed after the 62-day withdrawal period there was a large decrease in the CQ content of the choroid-pigment epithelium (compared with that in the animal killed after a 1-day withdrawal period) but it is difficult to say whether this was really a significant change. The very striking persistence in these three parts of the eye correlates positively with the slow regression rate noted in the eyes of pigmented rats (see Fig. 1).

ROSENTHAL et al. (1978) were not able to produce the clinical picture of human retinopathy in monkeys, even with i.m. dosages of 16.5 mg/kg per day, 5 days/

week, for 4½ years. On a weight basis this is approximately five times the usual human oral dosage level (MEYER and WEYERBROCK 1979). The ocular lesions which ROSENTHAL et al. did observe (in retina and choroid) were thought, however, to represent an early stage of simian retinopathy. In animals killed after 3–6 months of treatment, large concentrations of CQ plus desethyl-CQ were found in the iris (1,680–3,216 mg/kg), ciliary body (2,070–7,440 mg/kg), and choroid (5,520–14,224 mg/kg). Much smaller amounts were found in the retina (0–24 mg/kg) and sclera (144–342 mg/kg), but none in cornea, lens or optic nerve. Thus, the lesions found did not correlate convincingly with high drug concentrations.

Other attempts at producing retinopathy or keratopathy in experimental animals by the administration of the 4-aminoquinolines (McCONNELL et al. 1964; MEIER-RUGE 1965; KURTZ et al. 1967; LEGROS and ROSNER 1971) have met with varying degrees of success. Thus, McCONNELL et al. (1964) found, after administration of CQ diphosphate in the drinking water, to both hooded and albino rats for 3 months, significant alterations in the a and b waves of electroretinograms. However, neither light nor electron microscopy of retinal sections revealed significant morphological changes, and the ATPase activity of visual pigment extracts was not affected. MEIER-RUGE (1965) did find definite evidence of retinopathy in cats receiving 1.5–6 mg/kg per day CQ diphosphate for 50–250 days. Evidence of retinal changes (light pigmentation of the whole fundus) was seen in 4–7 weeks and retinopathy was completely developed in 7–8 weeks. KURTZ et al. (1967) were able to produce retinal changes in albino rats (females only) and in beagle dogs, but not in monkeys, receiving high doses of amopyroquine for up to 52 weeks. (The drug was not tolerated by female rats at 50 mg base/kg per day, or by the dogs at 65 mg base/kg per day.) It is significant that in the rats the retinae were normal after a medication period of 26 weeks, but lesions did develop in the course either of a withdrawal period of 16 weeks or of continued medication for another 26 weeks. These authors concluded that retinal sensitivity to amopyroquine was related to species differences and not to the melanin content of the eyes. Similarly, LEGROS and ROSNER (1971) confirmed McCONNELL et al. (1964) in finding electroretinographic changes in the eyes of albino rats receiving long-term high doses of HCQ and desethyl-HCQ. The fact that ocular changes in experimental animals are caused by amopyroquine, HCQ, and desethyl HCQ, as well as CQ, means, in effect, that the commonly used term "CQ retinopathy" is really a misnomer.

LAWWILL et al. (1968) determined CQ in several human ocular structures on samples obtained from five subjects who had taken various dosages, followed by a variety of withdrawal periods. In two subjects who had taken 200 mg/week for 6–9 months, and then discontinued medication for 0–30 days, CQ was found in minor amounts (5–100 mg/kg) in the sclera, neuroretina, and choroid-pigment epithelium. However, in two other subjects who had received an additional 550 mg 24 h before surgery, the concentration in choroid-pigment epithelium was much higher (840–880 mg/kg vs 40–100 mg/kg). Perhaps an even more significant finding was a level of 10 mg/kg of CQ in the choroid-pigment epithelium in a subject not known to have taken the drug for the preceding 16 years.

McCHESNEY et al. (unpublished) analysed the eye (supplied by Dr. E. L. DUBOIS) of a human subject who had taken CQ daily for "a considerable period of time", but had then been off medication for about 6 months. These concentrations were found, as milligrams per kilogram: lens and optic nerve, 2; vitreous humour and iris, 6; sclera, 10; cornea, 16; retina, 197; total drug in the eye, 91 μg.

The LAWWILL group (APPLETON et al. 1973) has found no evidence of serious ocular damage in subjects who took 200 mg CQ/week for an average of 7.4 years and it has been concluded (LIFE SCIENCES DIVISION 1969) that retinopathy rarely (if ever) develops unless the total amount of CQ taken exceeds 100 g. TANENBAUM and TUFFANELLI (1980) have set the upper limit of safe dosage somewhat higher (200 g).

Various explanations have been advanced for the adverse effects of CQ and closely related compounds on ocular structures. These include: (a) binding to melanin (SAMS and EPSTEIN 1965; LINDQUIST and ULLBERG 1972; LARSSON and TJÄLVE 1979); (b) irreversible lysosomal damage (ABRAHAM and HENDY 1970); (c) reaction with acidic mucopolysaccharides (MARX et al. 1960); (d) inhibition of aryl sulphatases (HARA 1979); and (e) differential affinities for individual polar lipids, especially those in retinal neurones and Müller cells (DRENCKHAHN and LÜLLMAN-RAUCH 1978). In connection with item (a), LEGROS and ROSNER (1971) emphasise that any physiopathological effect of the quinolines must be attributed to a direct action of the drug on the neuroretina and not to their affinity for melanin, which could, in fact, exert a protective action.

Once it was established that CQ accumulates in the eye in potentially dangerous amounts, and in some patients the condition of retinopathy was diagnosed, it was obviously desirable that methods should be devised for removing the drug from the eye as rapidly as possible. This can only be accomplished by removal of drug from the whole organism, followed by establishment of equilibrium at lower tissue levels. Unfortunately (MCCHESNEY et al. 1965a; see also Fig. 1) spontaneous removal from the eye, especially in pigmented animals, proceeds more slowly than it does from the other tissues. Various methods of accelerating removal of CQ from the tissues have been suggested. One of these (PEREZ et al. 1964) is the administration of large doses of ascorbic acid to release the drug from the melanin-containing tissues. When this method was applied in an ascorbic acid-dependent species (MCCHESNEY et al. 1965b) it was found that, although large ascorbic acid intakes did decrease tissue accumulation of CQ by amounts averaging 50% (14-day experiment), the ocular concentrations were not significantly affected.

Other agents suggested as possible accelerators of CQ excretion in retinopathy cases are ammonium chloride and dimercaprol (BAL). The stimulating effect of the former (LABORATORY DATA SN 7618; JAILER et al. 1947) on CQ excretion is well known. RUBIN et al. (1963) did find some positive effects of both agents on CQ excretion, but PEREZ et al. (1964) were not able to demonstrate any removal of CQ from the iris or choroid of rabbits following treatment with either compound. One reason not to expect dramatic results from the use of ammonium chloride may be implicit in the observations of MURAYAMA et al. (1977). These authors found in rabbits that ammonium chloride did stimulate the excretion of CQ, but only as long as the latter was still being administered.

As matters now stand, therefore, and as is stated in Sect. A, it appears that the only established way of dealing with the human CQ retinopathy syndrome is careful adherence to safe dosage schedules. If this is done, the risk of retinopathy is relatively low (DUBOIS 1978). It has been recommended (TANENBAUM and TUFFANELLI

1980) that the patients' ocular functions (EOG), in any case, should be monitored at about 4-monthly intervals. This is certainly a reasonable precaution; however, GRANIEWSKI-WIJNANDS et al. (1979) doubt that such a precaution is really necessary, providing that the dosage of CQ or its equivalent does not exceed 75 g/year.

3. Ear

DENCKER and LINDQUIST (1975) have studied the accumulation of CQ in the melanin-bearing tissues of albino and pigmented rats, following injection of the ^{14}C-labelled compound. Large accumulations were found in the *stria vascularis* and *planum semilunatum* of the inner ear, but in the pigmented animals only. This accumulation persisted even after an interval of 13 days post-injection.

4. Brain

It has been pointed out frequently above (see Tables 3–5) that brain is a minor repository for CQ in all species. Localisation within the brain has been studied in detail by OSIFO (1979a, 1979b). The animals used were rats, which were killed 1 h after the i.p. injection of 0.1 LD_{50} (8.7 mg base/kg) of CQ. The highest concentrations were found in the hypothalamus (1.28 ± 0.11 mg/kg) and the lowest in medulla, pons, and cortex (0.15±).006), with the other regions (hippocampus, cerebellum, midbrain, and striatum) intermediate at about 0.6 mg/kg. Overall, OSIFO and DI STEFANO (1978) found the concentrations in brain to be about four times those existing concomitantly in plasma, 0.11 times those in heart and 0.014 times those in liver. The ratios reported by GRUNDMANN et al. (1971) for these same quotients were, respectively, 1.9, 0.26, and 0.14, but there is some doubt about the magnitude of the plasma levels in this case.

V. Biotransformation

1. Chloroquine and Close Structural Analogues

Mention is made in WISELOGLE (1946) of biotransformation of the 4-aminoquinoline antimalarials and of the manner in which it proceeds, but the first published detailed studies on this problem (based, in fact, on the same information) were those of TITUS et al. (1948). These authors collected urine samples from subjects who had taken 400-mg doses of CQ, oxy-CQ or SN 9584, and after these samples were made strongly alkaline they were thoroughly extracted with chloroform. On evaporation of the solvent an oil remained. This oil was then subjected to countercurrent distribution between chloroform and 0.2 *M* phosphate buffers of pH 6–7. Further purification of the several fractions so obtained gave large amounts of the unchanged drugs and lesser amounts of the corresponding secondary amines in all three cases. In the case of SN 9584 a further step in metabolism was demonstrated, namely replacement of the terminal diethylamino group with carboxyl. This transformation evidently involved loss of the second *N*-ethyl group, followed by the well-known oxidative deamination reaction. It has been repeatedly demonstrated since 1948 that in the case of CQ the *N*-desethyl compound (desethyl-CQ; SN 13616) is the second most important excretory product following the administration of CQ. However, the development of more sophisticated methods of analysis has revealed that there are, in fact, many other metabolites. These findings serve to explain the observations that, although a considerable fraction of CQ administered to man and animals (McCHESNEY et al. 1966, 1967a) is not recoverable from the tissues and excreta as CQ plus desethyl-CQ, ^{14}C administered as [^{14}C]CQ is recoverable almost quantitatively (McCHESNEY et al. 1966, 1967c).

The complexity of the problem is well illustrated by the fact that an autoradiograph of a pH 9.5 ether extract of a 24- to 48-h urine sample obtained from a monkey following a 4-mg/kg i.m. dose of (3-[^{14}C]-CQ revealed the presence of at least 12 labelled compounds. Those definitely identified, with percentages, were: CQ, 63; desethyl-CQ, 13.6; bisdesethyl-CQ, 0.6; the -4′-alcohol, 1.5; and 4-amino-7-chloroquinoline, 4. Seven (then) unidentified compounds accounted for the remaining 17.5%, of which two made up 14% (McCHESNEY et al. 1966). Some of these unidentified compounds could have been the *N*-oxides postulated by WILLIAMS (1959) and subsequently isolated by ESSIEN (1978) but, under the conditions used for extraction of the bases, neither the -4′-carboxylic acid nor the hypothetical -2′-carboxylic acid (see below) could have been present in the sample chromatographed. However, extraction of the 0- to 4-day urine of another monkey in this group, at pH 5–6 with isopropanol after saturation with sodium sulphate, gave three main fractions which accounted for 29%, 34%, and 37%, respectively, of the total label in the extract. One of these (the 37%) was identified as the -4′-carboxylic acid. Nearly complete conversion of the -4′-alcohol to this acid was demonstrated in the monkey, as was partial conjugation of the alcohol with glucuronic acid. A further observation, not yet explained in structural terms, was that in the urine samples obtained in an experiment involving the administration of (4-^{14}C)-CQ to monkeys, about 8% of the labelled materials travelled with the solvent front in the system used for resolution of the bases (ethyl acetate-isopropanol-20% ammonium hydroxide, 79:15:6), yet eluates of this zone exhibited no absorption at 3,300–3,450 Å.

KURODA (1962) studied the biotransformation of CQ in detail, as revealed by the analysis of liver samples from subjects who had taken excessive doses of the drug and of urine samples from subjects who had taken 0.3- to 0.6-g doses. Paper chromatograms of the liver extracts demonstrated, as expected, the presence of very large amounts of unchanged CQ. Four metabolites were detected, one of which (desethyl-CQ) was more polar than CQ, and another (on the basis of its R_f, colour reaction with iodoplatinate and UV spectrum) was identified as 4-amino-7-chloroquinoline. The other two compounds were tentatively identified as the -4′-alcohol and bisdesethyl-CQ. The relative amounts of these metabolites, especially that of desethyl-CQ, varied with the amount of CQ ingested. Thus, KURODA's (1962) studies demonstrated that degradation of CQ as far as the quinoline nucleus occurred, but did not establish whether there was any transformation beyond that point.

In studies of urine samples from eight systemic lupus erythematosus patients being treated currently with CQ or HCQ, McCHESNEY et al. (1966) found these mean distributions of quinoline bases: (a) for CQ ($n=5$); unchanged drug, 59%; desethyl-CQ, 38%; bisdesethyl-CQ, 3%; 4-amino-7-chloroquinoline, 0; (b) for HCQ ($n=3$); unchanged drug, 69%; desethyl-CQ, 16%; desethyl-HCQ, 12%; bisdesethyl-CQ, 3%; 4-amino-7-chloroquinoline, 0.

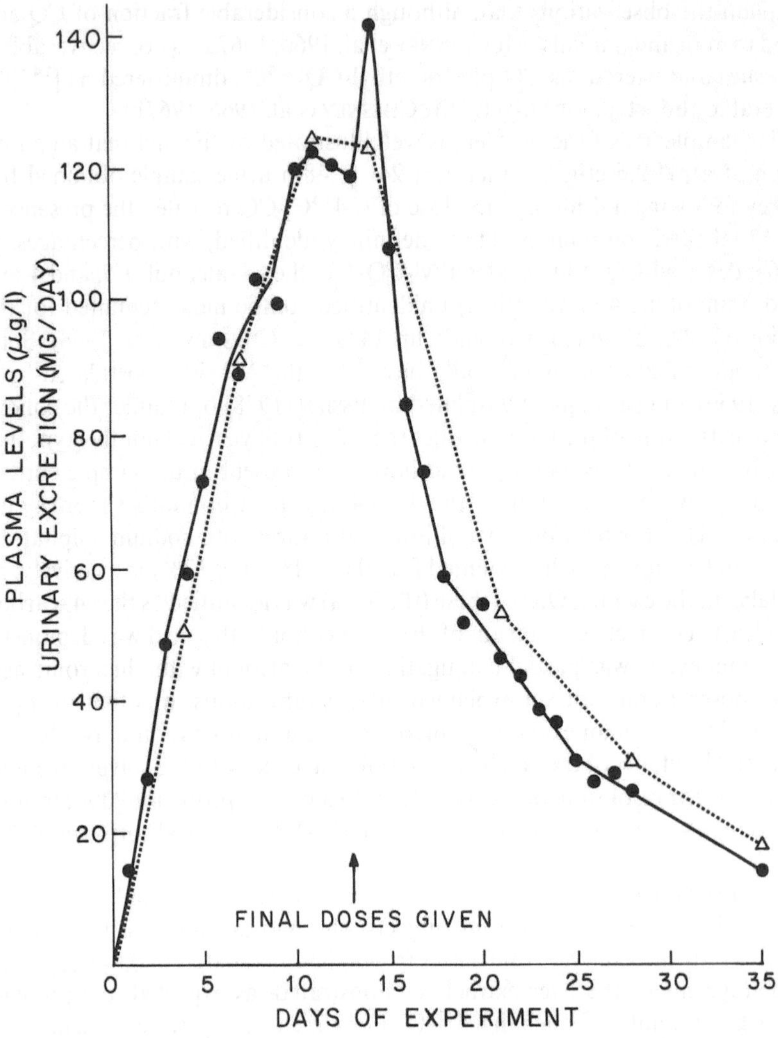

Fig. 2. Mean plasma levels (as µg/l) and urinary excretion (as mg/day of chloroquine plus all determinable degradation products) in eight human subjects (four black, four white) taking two tablets of the diphosphate (500 mg, 316 mg base) daily for 14 consecutive days. *Triangles*, plasma levels; *circles*, urinary excretion. The mean plasma levels were subject to a SE of 11.4±4.5(SD)%, and the urinary outputs to a SE of 10.7±3.7(SD)% of the observed values

Subsequently (McCHESNEY et al. 1967b), methods were developed whereby CQ, desethyl-CQ, bisdesethyl-CQ, the -4′-alcohol, the -4′-carboxylic acid, and 4-amino-7-chloroquinoline could be determined quantitatively in urine with reasonable accuracy.

These methods were applied to the analysis of urine samples from subjects who had taken 310-mg oral doses of CQ as the diphosphate daily for 14 consecutive days. In these subjects plasma levels and urinary outputs appeared to have reached at least temporary plateaux by the 11th day, at 120–125 µg/litre and mg/day, respectively (see Fig. 2). When dosage was discontinued these parameters declined in parallel fashion, at rates which corresponded initially to half-lives of about 160 h. Later the excretion rate decreased somewhat to indicate a half-life of about 17 days. No significant difference in these parameters was noted between white and black subjects (of which there were four each), such as might have been expected if extensive binding to melanin had occurred in the latter group. In this connection, it has been estimated by YOSHIMURA (1964) that the average melanin content of an adult black is about 1 g. No specific figures for white adults have been found, but from the data of WASSERMAN (1965) their total melanin content may be estimated as about 250 mg. If this is a true difference, 750 mg melanin, if completely saturated with CQ, might bind 1.5 g. Since the total amount of CQ ingested per person in these experiments was 4.4 g, it is obvious that no such amount as one-third of the doses was being sequestered in a separate compartment by the black subjects.

Urine was collected from the eight subjects, under close supervision, daily for the first 28 days and then for days 35, 42, and 91. Analysis of the samples obtained for days 5, 10, 15, 20, 25, 35, and 91 gave ratios of unchanged CQ to total determinable quinolines varying only from 0.676 to 0.703. [These ratios are almost identical to those reported by OSIFO (1979a) in rats]. As was expected, desethyl-CQ represented the bulk of the remaining 30%, varying only from 21.4% to 24.1% of the total determinable quinolines. Traces of other degradation products were found, i.e. 0.4%–2.4% as bisdesethyl-CQ, 0%–2.6% as the -4′-carboxylic acid (but in the 5- to 20-day samples only), while the -4′-alcohol and 4-amino-7-chloroquinoline were found at 0.3%–2%, but in the 25- and 35-day samples only. Four unidentified products were detected (bases); they usually accounted for about 5% of the total quinolines, with two of them (designated as A and C) present in every sample analysed but one (D) present in only one of four samples. In the 91-day sample, which was obtained from only one of the subjects, unidentified products made up 16.8% of the total quinolines, in a sample which contained the equivalent of only 1 mg CQ. In this case one product (C) accounted for over half of the 16.8%; it was formed at the expense of desethyl-CQ.

After allowance for the 8%–10% of ingested CQ usually found in the faeces, about 63% of the total dosages were accounted for in this human experiment. Since the urine residues, after extraction of both basic and acidic metabolites, did not absorb in the 3,300–3,450 Å region, it seemed clear that derivatives of CQ, other than those determined, could not be present therein. The important question remaining to be elucidated in connection with CQ metabolism thus appears to be the ultimate fate of the 4-amino-7-chloroquinoline nucleus. WILLIAMS (1959) has suggested that, by analogy to 4-aminoquinoline, this nucleus may be hydroxylated at the 3-position, and then form an ethereal sulphate. It may be noted in this connection (MCCHESNEY et al. 1966) that in one human volunteer who took a 200-mg dose of 4-amino-7-chloroquinoline in 50% propylene glycol, only 7 mg was recovered from the urine within 72 h and, of this, 6.3 mg was present in a conjugated form. The UV absorption spectrum and colour reaction with iodoplatinate of the conjugated material were such as to indicate that no chemical reaction, other than conjugation, had occurred. Since it seems highly unlikely that 97% of the dose was ex-

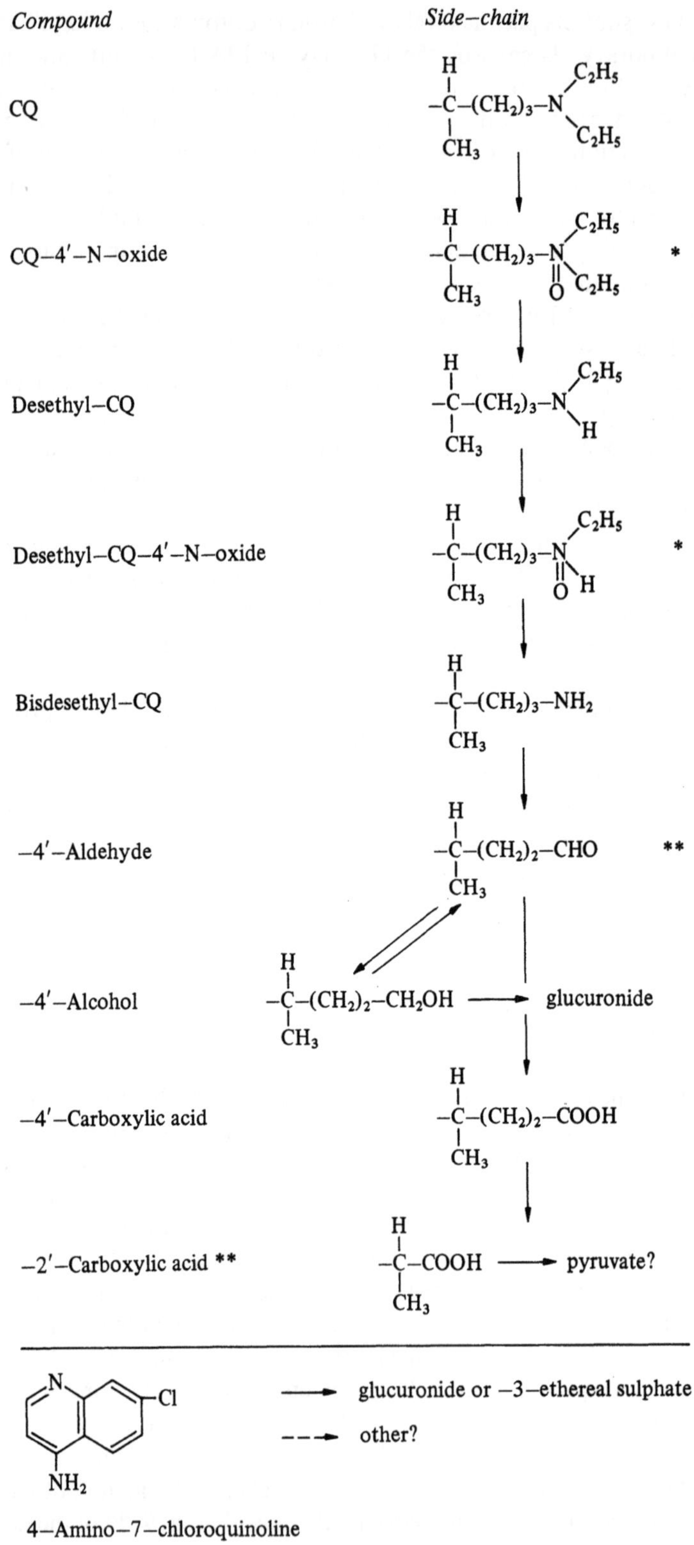
Compound
Side–chain
CQ
CQ–4′–N–oxide
*
Desethyl–CQ
Desethyl–CQ–4′–N–oxide
*
Bisdesethyl–CQ
–4′–Aldehyde
**
–4′–Alcohol
glucuronide
–4′–Carboxylic acid
–2′–Carboxylic acid **
pyruvate?
glucuronide or –3–ethereal sulphate
other?
4–Amino–7–chloroquinoline

creted in the faeces, it appears to follow that the compound was being transformed to derivatives not determinable by the methods used. Administration of (3-[^{14}C])-4-amino-7-chloroquinoline to experimental animals should give a definitive answer to this problem.

Laboratory volunteers also took 300-mg doses of desethyl-CQ base and collected urine for various intervals thereafter. The 0- to 72-h excretion accounted for 6%–8% of the amounts ingested, and analyses of samples collected until the 29th day (by interpolation) indicated that the total determinable urinary excretion in that time was only of the order of 16%. Of the excretory products in the 0- to 8-h samples, 85% was identified as the unchanged compound. At least six other compounds were detected in thin-layer chromatograms; of these, two were identified as the –4′-alcohol and 4-amino-7-chloroquinoline. Bisdesethyl-CQ could have been present in the 6% of bases which did not move from the origin in the system used. Similarly, desethyl-HCQ was given to three subjects in 317-mg doses, as the oxalate, and urine was collected for four intervals up to 72 h. Analysis of these samples revealed the presence only of the unchanged compound, but the mean 72-h excretion accounted for only 3% of the amounts ingested. Acid hydrolysis of the samples released no further amounts of determinable quinolines. It is possible, of course, that the oxalate salt of this compound is poorly absorbed.

In monkeys taking 10-mg/kg oral doses of bisdesethyl-CQ sulphate, 0- to 72-h urinary and faecal excretion and the soft tissues obtained on necropsy at 72 h accounted for only about 7% of the doses. Only the unchanged compound could be detected in urine samples extracted with ethylene dichloride: isoamyl alcohol (9:1, v:v) at pH 10–11, but the –4′-carboxylic acid (which was not determined) could well have accounted for some of the remainder (FLETCHER et al. 1975).

The sequence of steps involved in the metabolism of CQ, which now seems to be well established, is presented in schematic form in Fig. 3. In this scheme the various side chains are to be considered as being substituted for one H atom on the 4-amino group of 4-amino-7-chloroquinoline. Somewhat similar sequences have been proposed by KURODA (1962), by WHITEHOUSE and BOSTRÖM (1965) and by VIALA et al. (1972). Analogous series of steps may be assumed to apply to others of the 4-aminoquinoline compounds which have aliphatic side chains. It is of interest to note here, in connection with CQ (and possibly sontoquine), that the urinary excretion product has a positive optical rotation (WILLIAMS 1959). This suggests that the laevo-rotatory form may be preferentially degraded.

In contrast to other drugs, the metabolism of CQ and closely related compounds results only in gradual and incomplete loss of activity. Thus, desethyl-CQ is a good antimalarial in its own right, and bisdesethyl-CQ, on the basis of the one type of assay which has been performed (see Table 1) retains about half the antimalarial activity of the parent drug. The –4′-alcohol (SN 15063) and 4-amino-7-chloroquinoline (SN 11283) both possess slight activity and therapeutic indices (avian) about 2% of that CQ (COATNEY et al. 1953).

Fig. 3. Sequence of steps involved in the biotransformation of chloroquine in mammalian species. * The di-*N*-oxide may also be formed at this point (ESSIEN 1978). ** Presumably formed, but not yet specifically demonstrated

HCQ differs from CQ in metabolism only in that two different secondary amines are formed in the first step. On the basis of observations in man, as noted above, HCQ is slightly less rapidly degraded than CQ, and it loses the –4′–*N*-hydroxyethyl group slightly more rapidly than the *N*-ethyl. In the rat, however, it appears that HCQ is more rapidly degraded than CQ and that the –4′–*N*-hydroxyethyl group is much more rapidly removed than the –4′–*N*-ethyl (McCHESNEY et al. 1965 a; McCHESNEY, 1983).

2. Amodiaquine and Amopyroquine

The metabolic fate of these compounds has not been studied as thoroughly as that of the 4-aminoquinolines which have aliphatic side chains. Amodiaquine (ADQ) and amopyroquine (APQ) are so similar in structure that they would be expected to follow nearly identical pathways, but this interpretation is complicated by the fact that the secondary amine derived from APQ would presumably have the structure

$$R\ldots\overset{\displaystyle H}{\overset{|}{N}}\text{–}(CH_2)_3\text{–}COOH,\ \text{rather than } R\ldots\overset{\displaystyle H}{\overset{|}{N}}\text{–}C_2H_5,$$

and that the former would not be extractable at high pH values. That the rates and routes of excretion of ADQ and APQ are quite different from those of CQ and closely related compounds is evident from the studies of both BARROW (1974) and of CHAMBON et al. (1968). These authors have shown that, when administered parenterally, ADQ is excreted primarily in the bile, while CQ is excreted principally in the urine. Further, CHAMBON et al. (1968) reported that ADQ is rapidly converted by dogs to a conjugated form (an ether glucuronide involving the phenolic group), while CQ is conjugated to a much lesser degree (supposedly as an *N*-glucuronide). The difference between ADQ and CQ was particularly evident in the latters tissue analyses: in brain, ADQ was 100% conjugated, while in lung, heart, liver, and adrenal the order of conjugation was 80%–90%. In contrast, the conjugation of CQ exceeded 50% only in kidney. The finding of 15%–30% conjugation of CQ in urine, however, seems rather contradictory when compared with the 50% reported for kidney.

In BARROW's (1974) experiments in rats it was found that of the ^{14}C in urine following the administration of [^{14}C]ADQ, 40%–66% was extractable with ether at pH 9–10 and $<5\%$ at pH 2. In the former extract there were at least six labelled compounds, of which unchanged ADQ was only one of four or five minor components. These minor components accounted for $<5\%$ of the ^{14}C in the extracts, while two major components accounted for about 20% and 40%, respectively. Both major components had UV spectra identical to that of unchanged ADQ and it is logical, therefore, to assume that they were the corresponding primary and secondary amines. Thus, in contrast to CQ, where the unchanged drug may account for 65%–70% of the total determinable quinolines in the urine (McCHESNEY et al. 1967 b), in the case of ADQ the unchanged drug evidently represents only 1%–2% of the total. BARROW (1974) also found that, in early samples of bile obtained from a rat which had received [^{14}C]ADQ orally, the unchanged drug accounted for 20% –40% of the total ^{14}C, but by the 12th hour postadministration this fraction had decreased to < 10%, and in the bulked 24 h sample it was only 5%–8%. In agreement with CHAMBON et al. (1968), BARROW (1974) found that the major biliary components gave negative phenolic reactions. Also, although < 5% of the bulked biliary ^{14}C was extractable with ether at pH 9–10, acid hydrolysis increased this fraction to 16%–20% and the largest single component so released was unchanged ADQ. Thus, the most important initial metabolic reaction of ADQ is evidently the formation of the ether glucuronide.

In their studies of APQ, THOMPSON et al. (1958) did not consider metabolic fate in detail, but it is evident from their method of analysis that they were measuring essentially the sum of APQ plus the derived secondary amine. In this sense their results do not indicate an especially rapid degradation and/or conjugation of the former. If, for example, one compares the results for the tissue distribution of APQ and CQ in Table 5, it is seen that the levels given for the former (line 14) are intermediate between those found for CQ (lines 1, 2). The number of doses given in the three cases was almost identical, and the dose level used by THOMPSON et al. (1958) was intermediate between the two used by VARGA (1968 a). Also, if one compares the THOMPSON et al. (1958) results with those of VARGA (1968 a) for his 40 mg/kg per day dosage level, it develops that the former average (mean ± SD) 0.85 ± 0.07 of the latter, with the biggest individual difference being in the liver. These comparisons would not indicate that the metabolism of APQ in the rat is much more rapid than that of CQ. Once past the primary amine stage, APQ would clearly follow the same pathways as ADQ, with conversion of the methylene carbon to carboxyl.

E. Pharmacokinetics

I. Plasma Half-lives

The plasma half-life of CQ is either stated as such in numerous publications, or it may be calculated from data contained therein. These publications, with the estimated $t^{1/2}$ values in hours, include the following: LABORATORY DATA (SN 7618), 65; LOEB et al. (1946), 72; MOST et al. (1946), 120; ALVING et al. (1948), 57; BERLINER et al. (1948), 130; CULWELL et al. (1948), 20; MCCHESNEY et al. (1962), 72; MCCHESNEY et al. (1967 b), 160. Some of the apparent discrepancies in the above are due in part to the different postmedication intervals upon which the estimates were made, and in part to the difficulties involved in measuring very low plasma levels accurately. FRISK-HOLMBERG et al. (1979) have presented data from which conclusions may be drawn regarding peak plasma levels of CQ and its metabolites in man following single oral, repeated oral or parenteral dosage regimens, and the regression rates from these peak levels. They have concluded that the plasma half-life of CQ depends on the dose level, i.e. for a single 250-mg dose they give this value as 3.1 ± 2.6 h; for 500 mg, 43 ± 7.3 h; and for 1,000 mg, 312 ± 94 h. This functional relationship seems doubtful, since it implies that the lower the body burden of CQ the more rapidly physiological disposition proceeds. If anything, exactly the opposite is the case (MCCHESNEY et al. 1967 b, and many others). In a re-examination of the plasma level data of MCCHESNEY et al. (1962), and basing the regression rates only on the 24- to 96-h post-medication periods, the following relationships emerge for CQ; dose 316 mg, $t^{1/2} = 52$ h; dose 465 mg, $t^{1/2} = 50$ h; dose 632 mg, $t^{1/2} = 51$ h;

dose 698 mg, $t_{½}$ = 45 h. Similar calculations for HCQ give these relationships: dose 232 mg, $t_{½}$ = 32 h; dose 313 mg, $t_{½}$ = 51 h; dose 626 mg, $t_{½}$ = 50 h; dose 1,256 mg, $t_{½}$ = 32 h. In these examples no relationship whatever between dose levels and regression rates is evident (cf. also McCHESNEY, 1983).

II. Pharmacokinetic Constants

RITSCHEL et al. (1978) have calculated the important pharmacokinetic constants which apply to CQ and ADQ, and from these constants they have derived optimal dosage regimens for both suppressive and therapeutic antimalarial treatments. They assume a half-life of 53.7 h for CQ, which they calculated from the data of McCHESNEY et al. (1962). For multiple-dosing suppressive treatment they suggest dosages of 85 mg at 48-h intervals rather than the current standard 300 mg/week. This regimen would eventually provide serum levels fluctuating only between 15 and 20 µg/litre (values well within the therapeutic range), as opposed to levels fluctuating between 6 and 35 µg/litre, as provided by the 300-mg/week regimen. In place of the usual multiple-dosing schedule for therapeutic treatment (600 mg at zero hour, followed by 300 mg at 6, 24, and 48 h), RITSCHEL et al. (1978) suggest 1,020 mg at zero hour, followed by 300 mg/day thereafter. The latter schedule would provide a higher peak level (150 as opposed to 80 µg/litre) during the first 6 h, for prompt effect, but beginning with the 9th hour there would be no difference between the blood levels provided by the two dosage regimens.

It may be noted that McCHESNEY et al. (1962) determined the plasma levels provided by CQ and HCQ during and following the administration of a standard multiple-dosing suppressive treatment regimen. For weeks 2–6, 96 h after the weekly doses, the plasma levels found (as means ± SD) were 31 ± 9 mg/litre for HCQ and 15 ± 9 mg/litre for CQ, while at 168 h the corresponding values were 14 ± 8 and 10 ± 5 mg/litre, respectively.

Based on data obtained by the method of TRENHOLME et al. (1974), RITSCHEL et al. (1978) calculated the half-life af ADQ as 49.5 h, and they suggested for suppressive treatment a dosage of 115 mg at 48-h intervals, rather than 400 mg/week. This regimen would provide plasma levels in the range of 80–120 µg/litre, rather than the wider fluctuations of 33–165 µg/litre provided by the 400-mg/week regimen. Similarly, for multiple-dosing therapeutic treatment they suggest 820 mg at zero hour, followed by 180 mg at 6 h and 300 mg at 24 and 48 h, instead of the currently used schedule of 600, 300, 300, and 300 mg at these same intervals. The recommended schedule would provide a higher peak plasma level (200 µg/litre vs 145), but thereafter (by the 9th hour) the plasma-level curves provided by the two dosage regimens would be virtually identical.

F. Modes of Action

I. Introduction

Quinine, mepacrine, 4-aminoquinoline derivatives, and related drugs have a variety of biological effects because they work through a hierarchy of at least three different modes of action. Whether the components of the hierarchy operate independently of each other or in tandem depends on the concentration of drug and the target cell. Using CQ as an example, concentrations of 10^{-7} *M* are sufficient to bind ferriprotoporphyrin IX (FP) and form a toxic complex; concentrations of 10^{-6} *M* or greater inhibit lysosomal function; and concentrations of 10^{-4} *M* or greater permit the drug to bind to major cellular constituents and, presumably, compromise their function. Thus low concentrations of these drugs selectively affect only those cells that produce significant amounts of FP, such as malaria parasites, and other cell types are spared; intermediate concentrations affect cells that produce FP plus all cells that are dependent on lysosomal function; and high concentrations can even kill certain bacteria.

II. The Ferriprotoporphyrin IX Drug Complex

A connection between the presence of haemozoin (malarial pigment) in malaria parasites and the effectiveness of certain antimalarial drugs has been recognised for a long time. Nearly a century ago, MARCHIAFAVA and BIGNAMI (1894) realised that quinine exerts its effect only when malaria parasites actively digest haemoglobin to produce haemozoin, and it has been known for nearly half a century that the gametocytes of *Plasmodium falciparum* which survive quinine or mepacrine treatment exhibit little or no pigment after drug exposure (SINTON 1938; MACKERRAS and ERCOLE 1949). It was no surprise, therefore, to find that CQ and amodiaquine are effective only as blood schizontocidal agents (PETERS 1970).

The relationship of haemoglobin digestion to drug susceptibility is further exemplified by studies of CQ resistance in rodent malarias. CQ resistance occurs spontaneously in *P. yoelii* (WARHURST and KILLICK-KENDRICK 1967) and, as is also true for *P. falciparum* (NGUYEN-DINH and TRAGER 1978), it can be induced in *P. berghei* (JACOBS 1965; PETERS 1965; THOMPSON et al. 1967) and *P. vinckei* (POWERS et al. 1969) by drug exposure. Some CQ-resistant lines of rodent malaria digest haemoglobin and make abundant amounts of haemozoin when they are not exposed to CQ (LADDA and SPRINZ 1969; POWERS et al. 1969). During exposure to CQ, however, their haemozoin production ceases. Certain other CQ-resistant lines of *P. berghei* produce no haemozoin whether exposed to CQ or not. These parasites invariably revert to haemozoin production if they revert to CQ susceptibility (JACOBS 1965; THOMPSON et al. 1967; PETERS 1968). Finally, in this context, it should be noted that the NYU-2 strain of *P. berghei*, which is susceptible to CQ when it infects mice, immediately becomes resistant to CQ when it infects rats (LADDA and SPRINZ 1969). In rats this strain of *P. berghei* infects only reticulocytes, and little or no haemozoin is produced (LADDA and SPRINZ 1969). Haemoglobin digestion apparently is an absolute requirement for CQ susceptibility of malaria parasites. PETERS (1970) and WARHURST (1973) have reviewed this subject comprehensively.

The correct reason for the dependence of CQ susceptibility on haemoglobin digestion was first suggested by studies of the effect of CQ on the morphology of malaria parasites. When susceptible parasites are exposed to CQ or related drugs an early morphological effect is clumping of haemozoin (BOCK 1939). This phenomenon is so impressive and reproducible that WARHURST (1973) has developed it as a tool to study the interactions of antimalarial drugs with CQ-susceptible malaria parasites. Although the biochemical basis for the phenomenon remains to be elucidated, WARHURST and HOCKLEY (1967) and MACOMBER et al. (1967) simultaneously reported that clumping of haemozoin is associated with the formation of autophagic vacuoles within the parasites. In recognition of the importance of their finding, WARHURST and HOCKLEY (1967) entitled their report "Mode of action of chloroquine on *Plasmodium berghei* and *P. cynomolgi*." MACOMBER et al. (1967) concluded their report with the following paragraph:

Our study...suggests that formation of hematin [FP] by the parasite may serve to concentrate the drug within the parasite, particularly in the digestive vesicles. Such an effect would account for the selective toxicity of chloroquine for erythrocytic malaria parasites. The apparently unique concentration mechanism of parasitized erythrocytes for chloroquine as well as the early selective morphological alterations of the digestive vesicles are readily explained by such a process. We have found that chloroquine does not bind to malaria pigment *in vitro*, which suggests that chloroquine would be concentrated only by parasites actively forming malaria pigment. This would account for the inactivity of chloroquine, mepacrine, and quinine on mature gametocytes [of *P. falciparum*]. Our hypothesis also clarifies the consistent correlation which has been observed between the degree of chloroquine resistance (and the accompanying resistance to mepacrine and quinine) of various, independently selected, chloroquine-resistant strains of *P. berghei* and the reduced formation of malaria pigment by such strains, as well as the reduced ability of such parasites to concentrate chloroquine...[1].

Unequivocal experimental evidence confirming the hypothesis that FP is involved in the mode of action of CQ was not forthcoming, however, for another 13 years.

It was known that FP binds nitrogenous bases such as CQ and quinine (COHEN et al. 1964; JEARNPIPATKUL et al. 1980; PHIFER et al. 1966; SCHUELER and CANTRELL 1964) and also that haemoglobin digestion by malaria parasites produces FP (FULTON and RIMINGTON 1953), but it was not until 1980 that FP was finally identified as the receptor responsible for high-affinity accumulation of CQ (CHOU et al. 1980). The identification was made by comparing the process of accumulation to the binding of CQ to FP. The process of accumulation is saturable with an apparent intrinsic association constant (K_A) for CQ of 10^8 M^{-1} in *P. berghei* (FITCH 1969) and of 1.5×10^7 M^{-1} in *P. falciparum* (FITCH 1970). The binding of CQ to pure FP in aqueous solution has a K_A of 2.9×10^8 M^{-1}; in the presence of biological materials the K_A may decrease to values as low as 4.4×10^6 M^{-1} (CHOU et al. 1980). The specificity of accumulation (FITCH 1972; FITCH et al. 1974) indicates that the receptor has the following topography:

(a) A flat surface large enough to accommodate planar ring systems of 30–40 Å^2. The existence of this surface would explain the ability of the receptor to interact with a heterogeneous group of compounds, including derivatives of 4-aminoquinoline, of quinoline-4-methanol, of pyridine, of pyrimidine and of phenanthrene. (b) A chemical grouping in the flat surface that favors interaction with compounds having a nitrogen in their ring system, such as the quinoline derivatives. This would account for increased accumulation of chloroquine with increasing pH... Also, interactions with this grouping would help explain the differing affinities of the receptor for the various compounds with which is interacts. Furthermore, the proximity of the side chain to the nitrogen atom in the ring of 8-aminoquinoline derivatives might hinder interaction with this grouping and account for the failure of primaquine and pamaquine to inhibit chloroquine accumulation competitively. And (c) an anionic site located in the proper geometric relationship to the flat surface to attract the protonated terminal nitrogen atom in the side chain. The existence of this site would explain the higher

1 Reprinted with permission from Nature 214:937–939. Copyright 1967 Macmillan Journals Limited

affinity of the receptor for compounds with a terminal nitrogen in the side chain, and it might explain the apparent restriction on length of the side chain.[2]

FP possesses these topographical features, and it has precisely the specificity predicted from studies of *P. berghei* (FITCH 1972; FITCH et al. 1974; CHOU et al. 1980). These facts identify FP as the receptor responsible for CQ accumulation. For a more detailed discussion of this identification, the papers by CHOU et al. (1980) and FITCH and CHEVLI (1981) may be consulted.

FP is not only the receptor responsible for CQ accumulation, but it is also a toxic compound which lyses erythrocytes (CHOU and FITCH 1980) and other cells, including the protozoan parasite, *Trypanosoma brucei* (MESHNICK et al. 1977). The lysis is due to osmotic effects. In a concentration of 5 μM or less, FP causes nearly total loss of potassium from normal erythrocytes. As the potassium is lost the erythrocytes swell, and they develop an extreme susceptibility to hypotonic lysis (CHOU and FITCH, unpublished), lysing in media having an osmolality as high as 275 mos$M$ (CHOU and FITCH 1980). Increasing the osmolality, with sucrose for example, protects from lysis but does not prevent the potassium loss induced by FP (CHOU and FITCH unpublished). This effect on cation gradients is not reduced when FP is complexed with CQ; instead it appears to be enhanced (CHOU and FITCH 1980).

Abnormal potassium loss from erythrocytes and increased osmotic fragility occur with malarial infection (FOGEL et al. 1966; DUNN 1969) and would be consistent with FP toxicity. Additional evidence consistent with FP toxicity has been obtained recently in studies of *P. falciparum* in culture (FRIEDMAN 1978, 1979; FRIEDMAN et al. 1979). When this parasite is cultured in erythrocytes harbouring abnormal haemoglobins, conditions which accelerate the release of FP (RACHMILEWITZ 1974) cause accelerated potassium loss and kill the parasite. For example, menadione accelerates the release of FP from haemoglobin (CHOU 1980), and the addition of menadione to the culture medium kills *P. falciparum* growing in erythrocytes obtained from subjects with β-thalassaemia (FRIEDMAN 1979). Further documentation of the toxicity of FP for malaria parasites is desirable. Nevertheless, it is reasonable now to conclude that the accumulation of free FP in the infected erythrocyte would be lethal for malaria parasites. From this conclusion, it follows that the ability to sequester FP in haemozoin is required for the survival of those malaria parasites which are obliged to produce FP as they digest haemoglobin to obtain essential amino acids.

As FP is produced by haemoglobin digestion, it apparently exists only transiently before it is sequestered in haemozoin in a complex that makes it innocuous for the parasite and inaccessible to bind CQ (FITCH and CHEVLI 1981). This process of sequestration serves to keep the steady-state concentration of FP low. In the absence of active metabolism, the process of sequestration continues until the concentration of FP drops to very low values. Thus the concentration of the transient accessible form of FP ordinarily is low or undetectable when parasitised erythrocytes are incubated in the cold or in the absence of metabolisable substrate (FITCH et al. 1974), as well as in cell-free preparations of *P. berghei* (FITCH and CHEVLI 1981). It is of interest, therefore, that preincubation of parasitised erythrocytes with CQ

---

2 Reprinted with permission from Journal of Clinical investigation 54:24–33, 1974

increases the concentration of FP sufficiently to permit its detection during a subsequent period of incubation in the cold (Fitch et al. 1978) or in cell-free preparations. The presence of CQ during the preincubation period obviously either accelerates FP production or inhibits FP sequestration.

From our present understanding of the interaction of CQ with FP and of the toxicity of FP and of the FP-CQ complex, the following hypothesis for the mode of action of CQ as an antimalarial drug may be offered. CQ acts by forming a complex with FP that impairs the ability to maintain cation gradients in the parasite, in the host erythrocyte, or in both. The parasites then die either because of the ionic changes or because of outright lysis. This hypothesis synthesises all of the available information about CQ susceptibility of malaria parasites, including the absolute requirement for haemoglobin digestion, and explains the selectivity of CQ as an antimalarial drug. In addition, the haemolytic effect of the FP-drug complex could contribute to intravascular haemolysis and blackwater fever, which have been observed after the administration of antimalarial drugs, especially quinine (Edington and Gilles 1969; Peters 1970).

The possibility that porphyrin-CQ complexes may be important in cells other than those infected with malaria parasites merits further attention. The formation of such a complex probably explains the beneficial effect which occurs after CQ is administered to patients with porphyria cutanea tarda (Scholnick et al. 1973) as liver cells affected by this disease overproduce porphyrins (Chlumsky et al. 1980; Tschudy 1974). As a second example, consideration should be given to the possibility that the formation of an FP-CQ complex would inhibit prostaglandin biosynthesis in vivo. In vitro FP stimulates prostaglandin synthesis (Ogino et al. 1978). CQ inhibits the stimulatory effect of FP (Zenser, personal communication) and this inhibition could explain some of the apparent antagonism of CQ for prostaglandins (Manku and Horrobin 1976). These two examples suffice to emphasise the need for study of the effects of the formation of porphyrin-CQ complexes in various cell types.

III. Inhibition of Lysosomal Function

When the amount of unbound CQ exceeds the low concentration that saturates FP, its selectivity as an antimalarial drug is lost and it begins to function as a lysosomotropic amine. This second mode of action represents an intermediate level in the hierarchy of modes of action. CQ and related drugs are described as lysosomotropic (de Duve et al. 1974) because they accumulate extensively in lysosomes when their concentrations external to the cell and, presumably, in the cytoplasm reach the range of 10^{-6}–10^{-4} M (Allison and Young 1964; Dingle and Barrett 1969; Wibo and Poole 1974). Important changes in morphology and function accompany the accumulation of CQ.

Although much remains to be learned about the process of CQ accumulation in lysosomes (Polet 1976), two mechanisms may play a role. The first mechanism involves a substance associated with lysosomal membranes. This substance has been partially characterised by Dingle and Barrett (1969), who demonstrated that it binds nitrogenous bases. The binding substance may not be present in high enough concentration to account for the large capacity of lysosomes to accumulate

CQ but, if not, it could serve to recognise and facilitate the movement of CQ across the membrane. The second mechanism involves the hypothesis of a proton pump and the accumulation of large quantities of unbound, diprotonated CQ. The arguments in favour of this hypothesis have been presented by DE DUVE et al. (1974) and by OHKUMA and POOLE (1978). These investigators point out that CQ would be trapped inside if lysosomes were able to maintain a high concentration of protons relative to cytoplasm. OHKUMA and POOLE (1978) present evidence of a decrease in proton concentration in lysosomes in response to CQ accumulation, which would be consistent with trapping of the diprotonated species.

As lysosomes accumulate CQ they swell, develop granular inclusion bodies and fuse to form phagolysosomes (FEDORKO et al. 1968). Later they develop lamellar inclusion bodies which are rich in phospholipids (FISCHER and NELSON 1974; KLINGHARDT 1974; FISCHER 1976; LÜLLMANN et al. 1978; RIDOUT et al. 1978; MATSUZAWA and HOSTETLER 1980; STAUBER et al. 1981). The swelling and formation of granular inclusion bodies are easily demonstrable in diverse cell types in tissue culture as well as in vivo. The lamellar lysosomopathy develops with chronic exposure to chloroquine in neurones (FISCHER and NELSON 1974; KLINGHARDT 1974), myocardium (FISCHER 1976; RIDOUT et al. 1978) and skeletal muscle (STAUBER et al. 1981) among other tissues, and it may cause disease in these tissues. For example, some patients receiving long-term treatment with CQ develop a disabling myopathy (WHISNANT et al. 1963). In many other tissues including skin (SAMS and EPSTEIN 1965), adrenal gland (DENCKER et al. 1976; GRUNDMANN et al. 1971; 1972a, 1972b, 1973) and eye (ABRAHAM and HENDY 1970; DRENCKHAHN and LÜLLMAN-RAUCH 1978), which accumulate CQ extensively, certain pathological changes may be due to lysosomotropism.

The swelling and perhaps some of the other morphological abnormalities induced by CQ may reflect pressure changes resulting from accumulation of the osmotically active, diprotonated species of the drug (DE DUVE et al. 1974). In addition, some of the morphological abnormalities may be due to the recently discovered effect of CQ on the assimilation of acid hydrolases by lysosomes (WIESMANN et al. 1975; SANDO et al. 1979; GONZALEZ-NORIEGA et al. 1980; TIETZE et al. 1980). CQ reduces the uptake of these enzymes into fibroblasts in tissue culture by impairing binding at the cell surface, thereby inhibiting enzyme pinocytosis. Furthermore, CQ causes a dramatic loss of endogenous lysosomal enzymes into the medium. It is now known that impairment of binding at the cell surface is not due to direct inhibition by CQ (SANDO et al. 1979) but, instead, is due to depletion of enzyme-binding sites (GONZALEZ-NORIEGA et al. 1980). This discovery led to the hypothesis that CQ impairs recycling of receptors which are believed to be necessary for lysosomal uptake both of exogenous and of endogenous lysosomal enzymes. GONZALEZ-NORIEGA et al. (1980) speculate that CQ accumulation in the lysosome raises the pH sufficiently to inhibit receptor-enzyme dissociation. As a result cell surface and cytoplasmic receptors for the enzymes would be sequestered in the lysosomes. At present there is no information on the possible relationship between impaired assimilation of acid hydrolases and the results of earlier studies, such as the well-known "stabilising" effect of CQ on the lysosome (WEISSMANN 1964) and other evidence of inhibition of lysosomal function (LIE and SCHOFIELD 1973; CRABB et al. 1980; KOBAYASHI et al. 1980).

In the past, much attention has been focused on the hypothesis that CQ functions as a lysosomotropic amine to kill malaria parasites (POLET and BARR 1969; POLET 1970, 1976; HOMEWOOD et al. 1972; DE DUVE et al. 1974). This hypothesis is no longer tenable for unbound CQ, but the FP-CQ complex could be lysosomotropic. In CQ susceptible malaria parasites, the swelling of food vacuoles (lysosomes) and the formation of phagolysosomes, which occur in response to CQ treatment (MACOMBER et al. 1967; WARHURST and HOCKLEY 1967), cannot be attributed to the accumulation of unbound, diprotonated CQ, since it is known that CQ binds preferentially to FP in the concentration range at which it functions selectively as an antimalarial drug (CHOU et al. 1980; FITCH and CHEVLI 1981). It is possible, however, that the FP-CQ complex would selectively damage and cause fusion of the digestive vesicles responsible for haemoglobin digestion (RUDZINSKA et al. 1965). AIKAWA (1972) did find tritium in food vacuoles of malaria parasites isolated from mice treated with tritiated CQ, but he provided no evidence that the tritium remained in the CQ molecule. WARHURST and THOMAS (1975), on the other hand, found no fluorescence in food vacuoles of malaria parasites exposed to 0.3 to 1×10^{-7} *M* mepacrine, but they could not exclude the possibility of quenching of fluorescence under their conditions. More work is needed to determine whether the FP-CQ complex is localised to or selectively damages the food vacuoles of malaria parasites.

IV. Binding to Major Cellular Constituents

The third level in the hierarchy of modes of action of 4-aminoquinoline derivatives and related drugs probably results from binding of these drugs to cellular constituents, including melanin (RUBIN et al. 1965; SAMS and EPSTEIN 1965), phospholipids (HARDER et al. 1980; LÜLLMANN et al. 1980), enzymes (MA and SOURKES 1980) and nucleic acids (PARKER and IRVIN 1952). With the exception of melanin, these constituents have low affinity for CQ (K_A on the order of 10^4 M^{-1}). Consequently, high concentrations of unbound drug would be required in vivo before this mode of action could operate in tandem with the other two. Although melanin has higher affinity for CQ (LARSSON and TJÄLVE 1979), the melanin-CQ complex causes little toxicity unless large doses of CQ are administered for relatively long periods of time, when retinopathy and skin toxicity may become apparent (RUBIN and SLONICKI 1966). Aside from causing undesirable toxic effects, the binding of CQ to cellular constituents could be responsible for a wide variety of other biological responses. Binding of drugs in this group to phospholipids could produce electrophysiological effects, which are known to occur and have been most thoroughly studied for quinidine (BIGGER and HOFFMAN 1980), and could delay the degradation of phospholipids and permit their accumulation in lysosomes (LÜLLMANN et al. 1978). In addition, binding directly to the enzymes undoubtedly explains the inhibition of diamine oxidase (MA and SOURKES 1980) and cathepsin B (WIBO and POOLE 1974) by CQ. Unfortunately, information about the effects of CQ binding to cellular constituents is scanty in most instances.

The most extensive evidence in support of a mode of action resulting from binding to a major cellular constituent is provided by studies of the interaction between CQ and nucleic acids. PARKER and IRVIN (1952) reported that CQ binds to nucleic acids with a K_A of approximately $10^4\ M^{-1}$, and they suggested that this interaction might be involved in the mode of action of CQ. Their observation was confirmed by KURNICK and RADCLIFFE (1962), STOLLAR and LEVINE (1963), COHEN and YIELDING (1965a) and ALLISON et al. (1965). O'BRIEN et al. (1966a) provided hydrodynamic evidence that CQ is intercalated between base pairs of double helical DNA. A structure of the DNA-CQ complex "...in which the 7-chloroquinoline ring is intercalated between base pairs and the cationic side chain protrudes beyond the contour of the double helix and bridges the minor groove by electrostatic attraction of phosphate to both strands..." was proposed (HAHN 1974). For a detailed presentation of the evidence that CQ is an intercalating drug the review by HAHN (1974) may be consulted.

As expected for intercalating drugs, CQ inhibits the DNA-dependent DNA and RNA polymerase reactions in vitro (COHEN and YIELDING 1965b). Using calf-thymus DNA, O'BRIEN and associates (1966b) found an ED_{50} of 2×10^{-4} for DNA polymerase I. Inhibition of RNA polymerase in this in vitro system required a CQ concentration of approximately $10^{-3}\ M$. Similar results were obtained using DNA extracted from *P. berghei* (HAHN 1974). As predicted from these results, inhibition of nucleic acid synthesis and cell death have been observed in model systems using *B. megaterium* (CIAK and HAHN 1966) and *P. berghei* (VAN DYKE et al. 1969; LANTZ and VAN DYKE 1971; FITCH 1977) suspended in media containing 10^{-4} to $3 \times 10^{-3}\ M$ CQ. In fact with $3 \times 10^{-3}\ M$ CQ in the medium, CQ-resistant and CQ-susceptible *P. berghei* are both killed (FITCH 1977). There is no doubt that inhibition of DNA transcription is one of the modes of action of CQ but only at extraordinarily high concentrations of the drug.

Because of the foregoing observations, there was a time when inhibition of DNA transcription was an attractive hypothesis to account for the antimalarial action of CQ (HAHN 1974). No convincing experimental evidence from studies of malaria parasites was produced to support the hypothesis (POLET and BARR 1968), however, and recently it has been shown to be based on a false assumption. For the hypothesis to be tenable, it was necessary to assume that large concentrations of unbound CQ would be maintained in CQ-susceptible malaria parasites. Large amounts of CQ are accumulated in these parasites but not in an unbound form. The drug is bound to FP (CHOU et al. 1980; FITCH and CHEVLI 1981). With this new knowledge, inhibition of DNA transcription as a mode of action of CQ against malaria parasites in vivo is primarily of historical interest.

C. Drug Resistance

On historical account of chloroquine resistance in experimental malaria and in man is given by PETERS (1970) and of experimental techniques used in the study of chloroquine resistance by PETERS (1980), and Part I, Chapt. 18.

The first clues to the reason for CQ resistance were the observations that CQ-resistant *P. berghei* (MACOMBER et al. 1966; FITCH 1969) and *P. falciparum* (FITCH 1970) accumulate less CQ with high affinity than do comparable CQ-susceptible strains. Since high-affinity accumulation is due to binding of CQ to FP (CHOU et al. 1980), it follows that less accumulation represents inaccessibility or absence of

FP. That is to say, CQ-resistant parasites form little or none of the FP-CQ complex. Failure to form the FP-CQ complex eliminates the first level in the hierarchy of modes of action of CQ and, as a result, malaria parasites which do not form the complex are as resistant to the drug as the cells of the host. CQ resistance in malaria, therefore, is due to inaccessibility or absence of FP in the parasitised erythrocyte. In the case of the CQ-resistant line derived from the NYU-2 strain of *P. berghei*, FP is absent because haemoglobin apparently is not degraded (ECKMAN et al. 1977; LADDA and SPRINZ 1969). In the case of CQ-resistant *P. falciparum*, FP obviously is not accessible to bind CQ, although it may be produced (SCHMIDT, personal communication). The reason for the inaccessibility of FP in CQ-resistant *P. falciparum* merits further study.

Acknowledgements. The authors are indebted to Mrs. ELLEN V. MILLER of the Sterling-Winthrop Research Institute for the preparation of Figs. 1 and 2. This review was prepared during the tenure of a grant from the UNDP/WHO Special Programme for Research Training in Tropical Diseases and a contract from the US Army Medical Research and Development Command (DADA 17-72-C-2008) to CDF.

Addendum

Since the chapter on 4-aminoquinolines was completed, the toxicity of FP and a chloroquine-FP complex for *P. berghei* and *P. falciparum* has been verified experimentally (ORJIH et al. 1981; FITCH et al. 1982). In addition, it has been found that a water-soluble substance in malaria parasites detoxifies free FP more effectively than it detoxifies the chloroquine-FP complex (BANYAL and FITCH, 1982). These observations may be incorporated into the new hypothesis to explain the mode of action of chloroquine, as is shown diagramatically in Fig. 4. The diagram indicates that FP released from haemoglobin is rendered non-toxic by binding reversibly to a soluble haem binder. FP also is sequestered irreversibly in a non-toxic form in malaria pigment. At present, it is not known whether the immediate precursor of malaria pigment is free FP, the haem binder-FP complex, or both. Nevertheless, the existence of a soluble haem binder and the process of FP sequestration would protect the parasite from committing suicide by digesting haemoglobin and releasing large quantities of FP. If chloroquine were present, however, it would compete with the soluble haem binder for the formation of a complex with FP

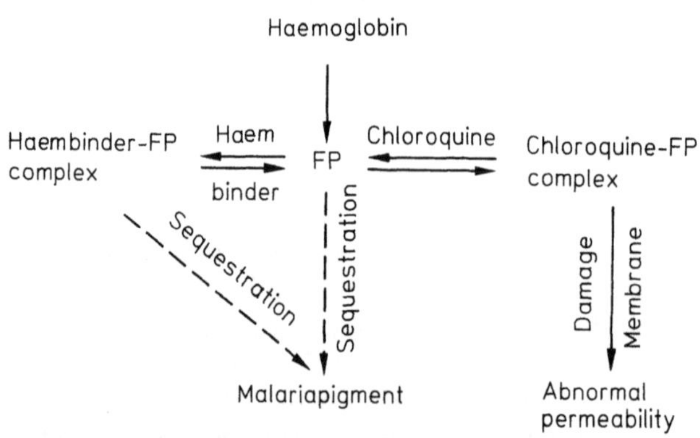

Fig. 4. Diagrammatic representation of a hypothesis to explain the mode of action of chloroquine as an antimalarial drug

(BANYAL and FITCH, 1982. Thus, a toxic chloroquine-FP complex could accumulate, cause abnormal membrane permeability (CHOU and FITCH 1981) and kill the parasite.

References

Abraham R, Hendy RJ (1970) Irreversible lyosomal damage induced by chloroquine in the retinae of pigmented and albino rats. Exp Mol Pathol 12:185–200

Aikawa M (1972) High-resolution autoradiography of malaria parasites treated with ^{3}H-chloroquine. Am J Pathol 67:277–280

Allison AC, Young MR (1964) Uptake of dyes and drugs by living cells in culture. Life Sci 3:1407–1414

Allison JL, O'Brien RL, Hahn FE (1965) DNA: Reaction with chloroquine. Science 149:1111–1113

Alving AS, Eichelberger L, Craige B Jr, Jones R Jr, Whorton CM, Pullman TN (1948) Studies in the chronic toxicity of chloroquine (SN-7618) J Clin Invest 27(Suppl):60–65

Appleton B, Wolfe MS, Mishtout GI (1973) Chloroquine as a malarial suppressive; absence of visual effects, Milit Med 138:225–226

Bagnall AW (1957) The value of chloroquine in rheumatic disease; a 4-year study of continuous therapy. Can Med Assoc J 77:182–194

Banyal HS, Fitch CD (1982) Ferriprotoporphyrin IX binding substances and the mode of action of chloroquine against malaria. Life Sci 31:1141–1144

Barlow OW, Auerbach ME, Rivenburg H (1945) Studies on the pharmacology of atabrine in mice, rats, ducks and dogs. J Lab Clin Med 30:20–31

Barrett-Conner E (1978) Chemoprophylaxis of malaria. Ann Intern Med 89:417–419

Barrow A (1974) The disposition and metabolism of amodiaquine in small mammals. Xenobiotica 11:669–680

Berliner RW, Earle DP Jr, Taggart JV, Zubrod CG, Welch WJ, Conan NJ, Bauman E, Scudder ST, Shannon JA (1948) Studies on the chemotherapy of the human malarias. VI. The physiological disposition, antimalarial acitivity and toxicity of several derivatives of 4-aminoquinolines. J Clin Invest 27(Suppl):98–107

Bernstein H, Zvaifler N, Rubin M, Mansour AM (1963) The ocular deposition of chloroquine. Invest Ophthalmol Vis Sci 2:384–392

Berti T, Cima L (1955) Distribuzione degli aminoderivati fenotiazinici nell' organismo animali; ricerche in diversi specie animali con la cloropromazina. Arch Int Pharmacodyn Ther 100:373–379

Bigger JT, Hoffman BF (1980) Antiarrhythmic drugs. In: Gilman AG, Goodman LS, Gilman A (eds) The pharmacological basis of therapeutics, 6th edn. Macmillan, New York, pp 761–792

Bock E (1939) Über morphologische Veränderungen menschlicher Malariaparasiten durch Atebrineinwirkung. Arch für Schiffs- und Tropen-Hygiene 43:209–214

Bowman RL, Caulfield PA, Udenfriend S (1955) Spectrophotofluorometric assay in the visible and ultraviolet. Science 122:32–33

Bratton AC Jr (1945) A short-term chronic toxicity test employing mice. J Pharmacol Exp Ther 85:111–118

Brodie BB, Udenfriend S, Dill W (1947a) The estimation of basic organic compounds in biological material. V. Estimation by salt formation with methyl orange. J Biol Chem 168:335–339

Brodie BB, Udenfriend S, Dill W, Chenkin T (1947b) The estimation of basic organic compounds in biological material. III. Estimation by conversion to fluorescent compounds. J Biol Chem 168:319–325

Bruce-Chwatt LJ (1977) Prolonged antimalarial prophylaxis. Br Med J 2:1287

Burckhalter JH, Tendick FH, Jones EM, Jones PA, Holcombe WF, Rawlins AL (1948) Aminoalkyl phenols as antimalarials. II. (Heterocyclic-amino)-2-amino-*o*-cresols. J Am Chem Soc 70:1363–1373

Cambiaggi A (1957) Unusual ocular lesions in a case of systemic lupus erythematosus. Arch Ophthalmol 57:451–453
Carr RE, Henkind P, Rothfield N, Siegel IM (1968) Ocular toxicity of antimalarial drugs: long-term follow-up. Am J Ophthalmol 66:738–744
Chambon P, Vo Phi H, Remenant J-M (1968) Enquète expérimentale sur le métabolisme de quelques médicaments antimalariques: chloroquine et amodiaquine. Bordeaux Médical 8:1471–1477
Chlumsky A, Chlumsky J, Malina L (1980) Liver changes in porphyria cutanea tarda patients treated with chloroquine. Br J Dermatol 102:261–266
Chou AC (1980) Oxidant drugs release ferriprotoporphyrin IX (FP) from hemoglobin. Fed Proc 39:2092
Chou AC, Fitch CD (1980) Hemolysis of mouse erythrocytes by ferriprotoporphyrin IX and chloroquine: Chemotherapeutic implications. J Clin Invest 66:856–858
Chou AC, Fitch CD (1981) Mechanism of hemolysis induced by ferriprotoporphyrin IX. J Clin Invest 68:672–677
Chou AC, Chevli R, Fitch CD (1980) Ferriprotoporphyrin IX fulfills the criteria for identification as the chloroquine receptor of malaria parasites. Biochemistry 19:1543–1549
Ciak J, Hahn FE (1966) Chloroquine: Mode of action. Science 151:347–349
Coatney GR (1963) Pitfalls in a discovery: the chronicle of chloroquine. Am J Trop Med Hyg 12:121–128
Coatney GR, Cooper WC, Eddy NB, Greenberg J (1953) Survey of antimalarial agents. US Government Printing Office, Washington, DC
Cohen SN, Yielding KL (1965a) Spectrophotometric studies of the interaction of chloroquine with deoxyribonucleic acid. J Biol Chem 240:3123–3131
Cohen SN, Yielding KL (1965b) Inhibition of DNA and RNA polymerase reactions by chloroquine. Proc Natl Acad Sci USA 54:521–527
Cohen SN, Phifer KO, Yielding KL (1964) Complex formation between chloroquine and ferrihemic acid *in vitro* and its effect on the antimalarial action of chloroquine. Nature 202:805–806
Cohén Y, Lacapère J, Vial M-C (1963) Distribution de la (^{14}C)-chloroquine chez le rat normal et arthritique. Biochem Pharmacol 12(Suppl):174–175
Council on Drugs (1961) New drugs and developments in therapeutics: hydroxychloroquine sulfate. JAMA 178:576
Crabb DW, Jersild RA Jr, McCune SA, Swartzentruber MS, Harris RA (1980) Inhibition of hepatocyte proteolysis and lactate gluconeogenesis by chloroquine. Arch Biochem Biophys 203:49–57
Culwell WB, Cooper WC, White WC, Lints HA, Coatney GR (1948) Studies in human malaria. XX. The intramuscular administration of chloroquine. J Natl Malaria Soc 7:311–315
Dale AJD, Parkhill EM, Layton DD (1965) Studies on chloroquine retinopathy in rabbits. JAMA 193:241–243
deDuve C, deBarsy T, Poole B, Trouet A, Tulkens P, Van Hoof J (1974) Lysosomotropic agents. Biochem Pharmacol 23:2495–2531
Dencker L, Lindquist NG (1975) Distribution of chloroquine in the inner ear. Arch Otolaryngol 101:185–188
Dencker L, Lindquist NG, Tjälve H (1976) Uptake of ^{14}C-labeled chloroquine and an ^{125}I-labeled chloroquine analogue in some polypeptide hormone producing cell systems. Med Biol 54:62–68
Dingle JT, Barrett AJ (1969) Uptake of biologically active substances by lysosomes. Proc R Soc Lond [Biol] 173:85–93
Drenckhahn D, Lüllman-Rauch R (1978) Drug-induced retinal lipoidosis: differential susceptibilities of pigment epithelium and neuroretina toward several amphiphilic cationic drugs. Exp Mol Pathol 28:360–371
Dubois EL (1978) Antimalarials in the management of discoid and systemic lupus erythematosus. Semin Arthritis Rheum 8:33–51
Duggan DE, Bowman RL, Brodie BB, Udenfriend S (1957) A spectrophotometric study of compounds of biological interest. Arch Biochem Biophys 68:1–14

Dunn MJ (1969) Alterations of red blood cell sodium transport during malarial infection. J Clin Invest 48:674–684

Eckman JR, Modler S, Eaton JW, Berger E, Engel RR (1977) Host heme catabolism in drug-sensitive and drug-resistant malaria. J Lab Clin Med 90:767–770

Edington GM, Gilles HM (1969) Pathology in the tropics. Williams and Wilkins, Baltimore

Editorial (1976) Chemoprophylaxis of malaria. Br Med J 2:1215–1216

Essien EE (1978) Metabolism of chloroquine: *N*-oxidation, an important metabolic route in man and its significance in chloroquine metabolism. Nigerian J Pharm 9:63–69

Fedorko ME, Hirsch JG, Cohn ZA (1968) Autophagic vacuoles produced *in vitro*. II. Studies on the mechanism of formation of autophagic vacuoles produced by chloroquine. J Cell Biol 38:392–402

Fink E, Minet G, Nickel P (1979) Chloroquin-enantiomere Wirkung gegen Nagetieremalaria (*P. vinckei*) und Bindung an DNS. Arzneimittelforsch 29:163–164

Finkle BS, Cherry EJ, Taylor DM (1971) Gas-liquid chromatographic system for the detection of poisons, drugs, and human metabolites encountered in forensic toxicology. J Chromatogr Sci 9:393–419

Fischer VW (1976) Evolution of a chloroquine induced cardiomyopathy in the chicken. Exp Mol Pathol 25:242–252

Fischer VW, Fitch CD (1975) Affinity of chloroquine for bone. J Pharm Pharmacol 27:527–529

Fischer VW, Nelson JS (1974) Chloroquine-enhanced cerebellovascular changes in nutritionally imbalanced chicks. Acta Neuropathol (Berl) 29:65–77

Fitch CD (1969) Chloroquine resistance in malaria: a deficiency of chloroquine binding. Proc Natl Acad Sci USA 64:1181–1187

Fitch CD (1970) *Plasmodium falciparum* in owl monkeys: drug resistance and chloroquine binding capacity. Science 169:289–290

Fitch CD (1972) Chloroquine resistance in malaria: drug binding and cross resistance patterns. Proc Helminthol Soc Wash 39 (Suppl):265-271

Fitch CD (1977) Chloroquine susceptibility in malaria: dependence on exposure of parasites to the drug. Life Sci 21:1511–1514

Fitch CD, Chevli R (1981) Sequestration of the chloroquine receptor in cell-free preparations of erythrocytes infected with *Plasmodium berghei*. Antimicrob Agents Chemother 19:589–592

Fitch CD, Chevli R, Banyal HS, Phillips G, Pfaller MA, Krogstad DJ (1982) Lysis of *Plasmodium falciparum* by ferriprotoporphyrin IX and a chloroquine-ferriprotoporphyrin IX complex. Antimicrob Agents Chemother 21:819–822

Fitch CD, Ng RCK, Chevli R (1978) Erythrocyte surface: novel determinant of drug susceptibility in rodent malaria. Antimicrob Agents Chemother 14:185–193

Fitch CD, Yunis NG, Chevli R, Gonzalez Y (1974) High-affinity accumulation of chloroquine by mouse erythrocytes infected with *Plasmodium berghei*. J Clin Invest 54:24–33

Fitzhugh OG, Nelson AA, Holland OL (1948) The chronic oral toxicity of chloroquine. J Pharmacol Exp Ther 93:147–152

Fletcher KA, Baty JD, Price-Evans DA, Gilles HM (1975) Studies on the metabolism of chloroquine in rhesus monkeys and human subjects. Trans R Soc Trop Med Hyg 69:6

Fogel BJ, Shields CE, Von Doenhoff AE Jr (1966) The osmotic fragility of erythrocytes in experimental malaria. Am J Trop Med Hyg 15:269–275

François T, Maudgal MC (1964) Experimental chloroquine retinopathy. Opthalmologica (Basel) 148:442–452

François J, Maudgal MC (1965) Experimental chloroquine keratotherapy. Am J Ophthalmol 60:459–464

François J, Maudgal MC (1967) Experimentally-induced chloroquine retinopathy in rabbits. Am J Ophthalmol 64:886–902

Friedman L, Rothkoff L, Zaks U (1980) Clinical observations on quinine toxicity. Ann Ophthalmol 12:640–642

Friedman MJ (1978) Erythrocytic mechanism of sickle cell resistance to malaria. Proc Natl Acad Sci USA 75:1994–1997

Friedman MJ (1979) Oxidant damage mediates variant red cell resistance to malaria. Nature 280:245–247
Friedman MJ, Roth EF, Nagel RL, Trager W (1979) *Plasmodium falciparum:* physiological interactions with the human sickle cell. Exp Parasitol 47:73–80
Frisk-Holmberg M, Bergkvist Y, Domeij-Nyberg B, Hellstrom L, Jansson F (1979) Chloroquine serum concentrations and side-effects: evidence for dose-dependent kinetics. Clin Pharmacol Ther 25:345–350
Fuhrmann G, Koenig K (1955) Untersuchungen über die Resorption und Ausscheidung der oral anwendbaren Resochin (Chloroquin)-Salze. Zeits Tropenmed Parasitol 6:431–437
Fulton JD, Rimington C (1953) The pigment of the malaria parasite *Plasmodium berghei.* J Gen Microbiol 8:157–159
Gambardella A, Diglio V, Tedeschi G (1955) Intossicazione acuta e cronica da chlorochina. Acta Med Ital Inf Parass 10:12–20
Gebel M, Doss M, Schmidt FW (1978) Chloroquine treatment of porphyria cutanea tarda. Diagn ther porphyrias lead intox intern symp. In: Doss M (ed) Clin Biochem. Springer Berlin Heidelberg New York, pp 133–135
Giles CL, Henderson JW (1965) The ocular toxicity of chloroquine therapy. Am J Med Sci 249:132–137
Gleiser CA, Dukes TW, Lawwill T, Read WK, Bay WW, Brown RS (1969) Ocular changes in swine associated with chloroquine toxicity. Am J Ophthalmol 67:399–405
Goldman L, Cole DP, Preston RH (1953) Chloroquine disphosphate in the treatment of discoid lupus erythematosus. JAMA 152:1428–1429
Gonzalez-Noriega A, Grubb JH, Talkad V, Sly WS (1980) Chloroquine inhibits lysosomal enzyme pinocytosis and enhances lysosomal enzyme secretion. J Cell Biol 85:839–852
Graham JDP (1960) An overdose of Plaquenil. Br Med J I:1256
Graniewski-Wijnands HS, van Lith GHM, Vijfvinkel-Bruin-Enga S (1979) Ophthalmological examination of patients taking chloroquine. Doc Ophthalmol 48:231–234
Grundmann M, Bayer A, Vrublovský P, Mikulíková I (1973) Effect of chloroquine on adrenocortical function. I. Concentration of chloroquine and morphological changes in the suprarenal gland of rats on long-term administration of chloroquine. Z Rheumaforsch 32:306–312
Grundmann M, Mikulíková I, Vrublovský P (1971) Tissue distribution of subcutaneously administered chloroquine in the rat. Arzneimittelforsch 21:573–574
Grundmann M, Mikulíková I, Vrublovský P (1972a) Tissue distribution of chloroquine in rats in the course of long-term application. Arch Int Pharmacodyn Ther 197:45–52
Grundmann M, Vrublovský P, Mikulíková I (1970) Tissue distribution of chloroquine in the rabbit. Arch Int Pharmacodyn Ther 184:366–373
Grundmann M, Vrublovský P, Demková V, Mikulíková I, Pěgřimova E (1972b) Tissue distribution and urinary excretion of chloroquine in rats. Arzneimittelforsch 22:82–88
Grundmann M, Vrublovský P (1977) Tissue distribution of chloroquine in guinea pigs. Acta Univ Palacki Olomouc Fac Med 81:273–279
Haberkorn A, Kraft HP, Blaschke G (1979) Antimalarial activity of the optical isomers of chloroquine. Zeits Tropenmed Parasitol 30:308–312
Hahn FE (1974) Chloroquine (resochin). In: Corcoran JW, Hahn FE (eds) Antibiotics III. Mechanism of action of antimicrobial and antitumor agents. Springer, Berlin Heidelberg New York, pp 58–78
Hara S (1979) Lysosomal arysulfatases in the bovine eye. Nippon Ganka Gakkai Zasshi 83:619–628
Harder A, Kovatchev S, Debuch H (1980) Interactions of chloroquine with different glycerophospholipids. Hoppe-Seylers Z Physiol Chem 361:1847–1850
Henkind P, Rothfield N (1963) Ocular abnormalities in patients treated with synthetic antimalarial drugs. N Engl J Med 269:433–439
Hobbs HE, Calnan CD (1958) The ocular complications of chloroquine therapy. Lancet 1:1207–1209
Hobbs HE, Sorsby A, Freedman A (1959) Retinopathy following chloroquine therapy. Lancet 2:478

Hoekenga MT (1957) Propoquin in the treatment of malaria. Am J Trop Med Hyg 6:987–989
Hollander JL (1965) The calculated risk of arthritis treatment. Ann Intern Med 62:1062–1064
Holt PJL (1979) Chloroquine in rheumatic disease. Lancet 1:502
Holtzmann JL (1965) Detection of nanogram quantities of chloroquine by gas-liquid chromatography. Anal Biochem 13:66–70
Homewood CA, Warhurst DC, Peters W, Baggaley VC (1972) Lysosomes, pH and the antimalarial actions of chloroquine. Nature 235:50–52
Jacobs RL (1965) Selection of strains of *Plasmodium berghei* resistant to quinine, chloroquine, and pyrimethamine. J Parasitol 51:481–482
Jailer JW, Rosenfeld M, Shannon JA (1947) The influence of orally administered alkali and acid on the renal excretion of quinacrine, chloroquine, and sontoquine. J Clin Invest 26:1168–1172
Jearnpipatkul A, Govitrapong P, Yuthavong Y, Wilairat P, Panijpan B (1980) Binding of antimalarial drugs to hemozoin from *Plasmodium berghei*. Experientia 36:1063–1064
Josephson ES, Udenfriend S, Brodie BB (1947) The estimation of basic organic compounds in biological material. VI. Estimation by ultraviolet spectrophotometry. J Biol Chem 168:341–344
Kersley GD (1964) The value and dangers of antimalarial therapy in arthritis, with special relation to ophthalmic complications. Proc R Soc Med 57:669–671
Kiel FW (1964) Chloroquine suicide. JAMA 190:398–400
Klinefelter HF (1979) Antimalarials in rheumatoid arthritis. Hosp Pract 14(Aug):24
Klinghardt GW (1974) Experimentelle Schädigungen von Nervensystem und Muskulatur durch Chlorochin: Modelle verschiedenartiger Speicherdystrophien. Acta Neuropathol (Berl) 28:117–141
Knox JM, Owens DW (1966) The chloroquine mystery, including antimalarial agents in general. Arch Dermatol 94:205–214
Kobayashi M, Iwasaki M, Shigeta Y (1980) Receptor mediated insulin degradation decreased by chloroquine in isolated rat adipocytes. J Biochem (Tokyo) 88:39–44
Kurnick NB, Radcliffe IE (1962) Reaction between DNA and quinacrine and other antimalarials. J Lab Clin Med 60:669–688
Kuroda K (1962) Detection and distribution of chloroquine metabolites in human tissues. J Pharmacol Exp Ther 137:156–161
Kurtz SM, Kaump DH, Schardein JL, Roll DE, Reutner TF, Fisken RA (1967) The effect of long-term administration of amopyroquin, a 4-aminoquinoline compound, on the retina of pigmented and nonpigmented animals. Invest Ophthalmol Vis Sci 6:420–425
Laboratory Data (1946) SN-7618, Department of Medical Research, Winthrop Chemical, New York
Lacapère J, Delaville G, Bonhomme F (1962) Use and mode of action of antimalarials: distribution of aminoquinolines in various tissues. Rev Rhumat 29:252–257
Ladda R, Sprinz H (1969) Chloroquine sensitivity and pigment formation in rodent malaria. Proc Soc Exp Biol Med 130:524–527
Lantz CH, Van Dyke K (1971) Studies concerning the mechanism of action of antimalarial drugs. II. Inhibition of the incorporation of adenosine-5′-monophosphate-^{3}H into nucleic acids of erythrocyte-free malarial parasites. Biochem Pharmacol 20:1157–1166
Larribaud J, Colonna P, Chevrel M, Romani B, Roux J, Pidoux A, Renouf P, Lefebure RY (1961) Intoxication aiguë par la chloroquine absorbée par voie orale; à propos de deux observations. Press Méd 69:2193–2196
Larsson B, Tjälve H (1979) Studies on the mechanism of drug binding to melanin. Biochem Pharmacol 28:1181–1187
Lawwill T, Appleton B, Alstatt L (1968) Chloroquine accumulation in human eyes. Am J Ophthalmol 65:530–532
Legros J, Rosner I (1971) Modifications électrorétinographiques après administration chronique de fortes doses d'hydroxychloroquine et de déséthylhydroxychloroquine chez le rat albinos. Arch Ophthalmol (Paris) 31:165–180

Lewis HM, Frumess GM (1956) Plaquenil in the treatment of discoid lupus erythematosus: preliminary report. Arch Dermatol 73:576–581
Lie SO, Schofield B (1973) Inactivation of lysosomal function in normal cultured fibroblasts by chloroquine. Biochem Pharmacol 22:3109–3114
Life Sciences Division (1969) A study of the pharmacology and toxicology of vision in the soldier. I. Chloroquine and hydroxychloroquine. Life Sciences Research Office, Bethesda Maryland, Contract No DA-HC, 19-68-C0001
Lindquist N, Ullberg S (1972) Melanin affinity of chloroquine and chlorpromazine studied by whole body autoradiography. Acta Pharmacol Toxicol (Copenh) [Suppl] 31:1–32
Loeb RF, Clark WM, Coatney GR et al. (1946) Activity of a new antimalarial agent, chloroquine, SN-7618. JAMA 130:1069–1070
Lukasiewicz RJ, Fitzgerald JM (1974) Comparison of three photochemicalfluorometric methods for the determination of chloroquine. Appl Spectroscopy 28:151–155
Lüllmann H, Lüllmann-Rauch R, Wassermann O (1978) Lipidosis produced by amphiphilic drugs. Biochem Pharmacol 27:1103–1108
Lüllmann H, Plösch H, Ziegler A (1980) Ca replacement by cationic amphiphilic drugs from lipid monolayers. Biochem Pharmacol 29:2969–2974
Ma K, Sourkes TL (1980) Inhibition of diamine oxidase by antimalarial drugs. Agents Actions 10:395–397
MacKenzie AH (1970) An appraisal of chloroquine. Arthritis Rheum 13:280–291
Mackerras MJ, Ercole QN (1949) Observations on the action of quinine, atebrin, and plasmoquine on the gametocytes of *P. falciparum*. Trans R Soc Trop Med Hyg 42:455–463
Macomber PB, O'Brien RL, Hahn FE (1966) Chloroquine: physiological basis of drug resistance in *Plasmodium berghei*. Science 152:1374–1375
Macomber PB, Sprinz H, Tousimis AJ (1967) Morphological effects of chloroquine on *Plasmodium berghei* in mice. Nature 214:937–939
Mandel EH (1963) The side-effects of chloroquine and hydroxychloroquine: results of a comparative study *in vivo*. NY State J Med 63:3111–3113
Manku MS, Horrobin DF (1976) Chloroquine, quinine, procaine, quinidine, and clomipramine are prostaglandin agonists and antagonists. Prostaglandins 12:789–801
Marchiafava E, Bignami A (1894) On summer-autumn malarial fevers. The New Sydenham Society, London (translated by Thompson JH)
Marks JS, Power BJ (1979) Is chloroquine obsolete in the treatment of rheumatic disease? Lancet 1:371–373
Marx P, Brech P, Meisner T (1960) Visual disturbances and eye changes accompanying quinoline therapy in rheumatoid arthritis. Klin Wochenschr 38:443–447
Matsuzawa Y, Hostetler KY (1980) Effects of chloroquine and 4,4′bis-(diethylaminoethoxy)-α,β-diethyldiphenylethane on the incorporation of [^{3}H]glycerol into the phospholipids of rat liver lysosomes and other subcellular fractions, *in vivo*. Biochim Biophys Acta 620:592–602
McChesney EW, Wyzan HS, McAuliff JP (1956) The determination of 4-aminoquinoline antimalarials: revaluation of the induced fluorescence method, with specific application to hydroxychloroquine analysis. J Pharm Sci 45:640–645
McChesney EW, Nachod FC, Tainter ML (1957) Rationale for the treatment of lupus erythematosus with antimalarials. J Invest Dermatol 29:97–104
McChesney EW, Banks WF Jr (1960) The metabolic fate of a new cardiac regulator compound (amotriphene) in rats, dogs, and monkeys. Toxicol Appl Pharmacol 2:206–219
McChesney EW, McAuliff JP (1961) Laboratory studies of the 4-aminoquinoline antimalarials. I. Some biochemical characteristics of chloroquine, hydroxychloroquine, and SN-7718. Antibiot Chemother 11:800–810
McChesney EW, Banks WF Jr, McAuliff JP (1962) Laboratory studies of the 4-aminoquinoline antimalarials. II. Plasma levels of chloroquinoline and hydroxychloroquine in man after various oral dosage regimens. Antibiot Chemother 12:583–594
McChesney EW, Banks WF Jr, Sullivan DJ (1965a) Metabolism of chloroquine and hydroxychloroquine in albino and pigmented rats. Toxicol Appl Pharmacol 7:627–636
McChesney EW, Banks WF Jr, Wiland J (1965b) Effect of ascorbic acid on tissue deposition of chloroquine in the guinea pig. Proc Soc Exp Biol Med 119:740–742

McChesney EW, Conway WD, Banks WF Jr, Rogers JE, Shekosky JM (1966) Studies of the metabolism of some compounds of the 4-amino-7-chloroquinoline series. J Pharmacol Exp Ther 151:482–493
McChesney EW, Banks WF Jr, Fabian RJ (1967a) Tissue distribution of chloroquine, hydroxychloroquine, and desethylchloroquine in the rat. Toxicol Appl Pharmacol 10:501–513
McChesney EW, Fasco MJ, Banks WF Jr (1967b) The metabolism of chloroquine in man during and after repeated oral dosage. J Pharmacol Exp Ther 158:323–331
McChesney EW, Shekosky JM, Hernandez PH (1967c) Metabolism of chloroquine-^{14}C in the rhesus monkey. Biochem Pharmacol 16:2444–2447
McChesney EW (1983) Animal toxicity and pharmacokinetics of hydroxychloroquine sulfate. Am J Med 75 (Suppl): 11–18
McConnell DG, Wachtel J, Havener WH (1964) Observations on experimental chloroquine retinopathy. Arch Ophthalmol 71:552–553
Meier-Ruge W (1965) Experimental investigation of the morphogenesis of chloroquine retinopathy. Arch Ophthalmol 73:540–544
Merwin CF, Winkelmann RK (1962) Antimalarial drugs in the therapy of lupus erythematosus. Mayo Clin Proc 37:253–268
Meshnick SR, Chang K-P, Cerami A (1977) Heme lysis of the bloodstream forms of *Trypanosoma brucei*. Biochem Pharmacol 26:1923–1928
Meyer W, Weyerbrock W (1979) Probleme der Basis-Therapie rheumatischer Erkrankungen mit Chloroquin, Gold und *d*-Penicillamin. Internist (Berlin) 20:426–432
Minker E, Matejka Z (1981) Pharmacological basis of dosage form of two antimalarials: chloroquine and mepacrine. Acta Physiol Acad Sci Hung 57:197–200
Monnet R, Boiteau H, Moussion C (1964) Identification et dosage de la chloroquine dans les milieux biologiques par spectrophotometrie dans l'ultraviolet. Ann Biol Clin (Paris) 22:429–434
Most H, London IM, Kane CA, Lavietes PH, Schroeder EF, Hayman JM Jr (1946) Chloroquine for treatment of acute attacks of vivax malaria. JAMA 131:963–967
Murayama K, Nakajima A (1977) Determination of chloroquine in urine by gas chromatography. Yakagaku Zasshi 97:445–449
Murayama K, Kobayashi K, Futemma M, Nakajima A (1977) Effect of ammonium chloride on the excretion of chloroquine in rabbit urine. Yakugaku Zasshi 97:949–954
Nguyen-Dinh P, Trager W (1978) Chloroquine resistance produced *in vitro* in an African strain of human malaria. Science 200:1397–1398
O'Brien RL, Allison JL, Hahn FE (1966a) Evidence for intercalation of chloroquine into DNA. Biochim Biophys Acta 129:622–624
O'Brien RL, Olenick JG, Hahn FE (1966b) Reactions of quinine, chloroquine and quinacrine with DNA and their effects on the DNA and RNA polymerase reactions. Proc Natl Acad Sci USA 55:1511–1517
Ogino N, Ohki S, Yamamoto S, Hayaishi O (1978) Prostaglandin endoperoxide synthetase from bovine vesicular gland microsomes. J Biol Chem 253:5061–5068
Okuma O, Poole B (1978) Fluorescence probe measurement of the intralysosomal pH in living cells and the perturbation of pH by various agents. Proc Natl Acad Sci USA 75:3327–3331
Olatunde IA (1971) Chloroquine concentrations in the skin of rabbits and man. Br J Pharmacol 43:335–340
Orjih AU, Banyal HS, Chevli R, Fitch CD (1981) Hemin lyses malaria parasites. Science 214:667–669
Osifo NG (1979a) The regional uptake of chloroquine in the brain. Toxicol Appl Pharmacol 50:109–114
Osifo NG (1979b) Drug-related transient dyskinesia. Clin Pharmacol Ther 25:767–771
Osifo NG (1979c) The effect of pyrogen on the *in vivo* metabolism and initial kinetics of chloroquine in rats. J Pharm Pharmacol 31:747–751
Osifo NG, di Stefano V (1978) Enhanced lethality and tissue levels of chloroquine in rats pretreated with pyrogens. Res Commun Chem Pharm Pharmacol 22:513–521

Parker FS, Irvin JL (1952) The interaction of chloroquine with nucleic acid and nucleoproteins. J Biol Chem 199:897–909
Pau H, Baümer A (1959) Resochineinlagerungen in der Kornea. Klin Monatsbl Augenheilkd 135:362–377
Paulini E, Pereira JP (1963) Estudos de sal antimalárico. II. Observações sôbre excreçâo de três derivados de cloroquina. Rev Bras Malariol Doenças Trop 15:47–54
Percival SPB, Meanock I (1968) Chloroquine: ophthalmological safety and clinical assessment in rheumatoid arthritis. Br Med J III:579–584
Perez R, Mansour AM, Rubin M, Zvaifler NJ (1964) Chloroquine binding to melanin: characteristics and significance. Arthritis Rheum 7:337
Peters W (1965) Drug resistance in *Plasmodium berghei,* Vincke and Lips, 1948. I. Chloroquine resistance. Exp Parasitol 17:80–89
Peters W (1968) The chemotherapy of rodent malaria. V. Dynamics of drug resistance, part I: methods of studying the acquisition and loss of resistance to chloroquine by *Plasmodium berghei.* Ann Trop Med Parasitol 62:277–287
Peters W (1970) Chemotherapy and drug resistance in malaria. Academic Press, London
Peters W (1980) Chemotherapy of malaria. In: Kreier JP (ed) Malaria vol I. Academic Press, New York, pp 145–283
Phifer KO, Yielding KL, Cohen SN (1966) Investigations of the possible relation of ferrihemic acid to drug resistance in *Plasmodium berghei.* Exp Parasitol 19:102–109
Polet H (1970) Influence of sucrose on chloroquine-3-H^3 content of mammalian cells *in vitro*: the possible role of lysosomes in chloroquine resistance. J Pharmacol Exp Ther 173:71–77
Polet H (1976) Chloroquine-^3H: mechanism of uptake by Chang liver cells *in vitro.* J Pharmacol Exp Ther 199:687–694
Polet H, Barr CF (1968) Chloroquine and dihydroquinine. *In vitro* studies of their antimalarial effect upon *Plasmodium knowlesi.* J Pharmacol Exp Ther 164:380–386
Polet H, Barr CF (1969) Uptake of chloroquine-3-H^3 by *Plasmodium knowlesi in vitro.* J Pharmacol Exp Ther 168:187–192
Powers KG, Jacobs RL, Good WC, Koontz LC (1969) *Plasmodium vinckei:* production of chloroquine-resistant strain. Exp Parasitol 26:193–202
Prouty RW, Kuroda K (1958) Spectrophotometric determination and distribution of chloroquine in human tissue. J Lab Clin Med 52:477–480
Rachmilewitz EA (1974) Denaturation of the normal and abnormal hemoglobin molecule. Semin Hematol 11:441–462
Rees RB, Maibach HI (1963) Chloroquine: a review of reactions and dermatologic indications. Arch Dermatol 88:280–289
Ridout RM, Decker RS, Wildenthal K (1978) Chloroquine-induced lysosomal abnormalities in cultured foetal mouse hearts. J Mol Cell Cardiol 10:175–183
Ritschel WA, Hammer GV, Thomson GA (1978) Pharmacokinetics of antimalarials and proposals for dosage regimens. Int J Clin Pharmacol Ther Toxicol 16:395–401
Robinson AE, Coffer AI, Camps FE (1970) The distribution of chloroquine in man after fatal poisoning. J Pharm Pharmacol 22:700–703
Rosenthal AR, Kolb H, Bergsma D, Huxsoll D, Hopkins JL (1978) Chloroquine retinopathy in the rhesus monkey. Invest Ophthalmol Vis Sci 17:1158–1175
Rubin M, Bernstein HP, Zvaifler NJ (1963) Studies on the pharmacology of chloroquine: recommendations for the treatment of chloroquine retinopathy. Arch Ophthalmol 70:474–481
Rubin M, Slonicki A (1966) A proposed mechanism for the skin-eye syndrome. Proceedings of the 5th international congress of the collegium internationale neuropsychopharmacologicum Washington, March 1966, pp 661–679 (Excerpta Medica international congress series No 129)
Rubin M, Zvaifler N, Bernstein H, Mansour A (1965) Chloroquine toxicity. In: Drugs and Enzymes (Proceedings of the 2nd International Pharmacological Meeting, Prague, 20–23 August 1963) Pergamon Press, Oxford
Rudzinska MA, Trager W, Bray RS (1965) Pinocytotic uptake and digestion of hemoglobin in malaria parasites. J Protozool 12:563–576

Sams WM Jr (1967) Chloroquine: mechanism of action. Mayo Clin Proc 42:300–309
Sams WM Jr, Epstein JH (1965) The affinity of melanin for chloroquine. J Invest Dermatol 45:482–487
Sando GN, Titus-Dillon P, Hall CW, Neufeld EF (1979) Inhibition of receptor mediated uptake of a lysosomal enzyme into fibroblasts by chloroquine, procaine, and ammonia. Exp Cell Res 119:359–364
Schmidt LH, Hughes HB, Schmidt IH (1953) The pharmacological properties of 2,4-diamino-5-*p*-chlorophenyl-6-ethyl-pyrimidine (daraprim). J Pharmacol Exp Ther 107:92–130
Schneider J, Nenna A, Couture J (1963) Étude comparative de la circulation dans le sang et de l'élimination urinaire de la chloroquine base et du sulfate de chloroquine. Bull WHO 29:417–421
Scholnick PL, Epstein J, Marver HS (1973) The molecular basis of the action of chloroquine in porphyria cutanea tarda. J Invest Dermatol 61:226–232
Schueler FW, Cantrell WF (1964) Antagonism of the antimalarial action of chloroquine by ferrihemate and a hypothesis for the mechanism of chloroquine resistance. J Pharmacol Exp Ther 143:278–281
Scruggs JH (1964) Ocular complications from chloroquine therapy. Tex Med 60:362–365
Shriver DA, White CB, Sandor A, Rosenthale ME (1975) A profile of the rat gastrointestinal toxicity of drugs used to treat inflammatory diseases. Toxicol Appl Pharmacol 32:73–83
Sinton JA (1938) The action of atebrin upon the gametocytes of *Plasmodium falciparum*. Rivista di Malariologia 17:305–330
Smith CC (1950) A short term chronic toxicity test. J Pharmacol Exp Ther 100:408–420
Spector WS (ed) (1956) Handbook of toxicology, vol I. Saunders, Philadelphia
Stauber WT, Hedge AM, Trout JJ, Schottelius BA (1981) Inhibition of lysosomal function in red and white skeletal muscle by chloroquine. Exp Neurol 71:295–306
Stollar D, Levine L (1963) Antibodies to denatured deoxyribonucleic acid in lupus erythematose serum. V. Mechanism of DNA-anti DNA inhibition by chloroquine. Arch Biochem Biophys 101:335–341
Surrey AR, Hammer HF (1950) Preparation of 7-chloro-4-[4-(*N*-ethyl, *n*-2-hydroxyethylamino)-1-methylbutylaminol]-quinoline and related compounds. J Am Chem Soc 72:1814–1815
Tanenbaum L, Tuffanelli DL (1980) Antimalarial agents: chloroquine, hydroxychloroquine and quinacrine. Arch Dermatol 116:587–591
Thompson PE, Olszewski B, Bayles A, Waitz JA (1967) Relations among antimalarial drugs: results of studies with cycloguanil-, sulfone-, or chloroquine-resistant *Plasmodium berghei* in mice. Am J Trop Med Hyg 16:133–145
Thompson PE, Weston K, Glazko AJ, Fisken RA, Reutner TF, Bayles A, Weston JK (1958) Laboratory studies on amopyroquin (propoquin). Antibiot Chemother 8:450–460
Tietze C, Schlesinger P, Stahl P (1980) Chloroquine and ammonium ion inhibit receptor-mediated endocytosis of mannose-glycoconjugates by macrophages: apparent inhibition of receptor recycling. Biochem Biophys Res Commun 93:1–8
Titus EO, Craig LC, Golumbic C, Mighton HR, Wempen IM, Elderfield RC (1948) Identification by distribution. IX. Application to metabolic studies of 4-aminoquinoline antimalarials. J Org Chem 13:39–62
Trenholme GM, Williams RL, Patterson EC, Frischer H, Carson PE, Rieckmann KH (1974) A method for the determination of amodiaquin. Bull WHO 51:431–434
Tschudy D (1974) Porphyrin metabolism and the porphyrias. In: Bondy PK, Rosenberg LE (eds) Disease of metabolism: genetics and metabolism, 7th ed. Saunders, Philadelphia, pp 775–824
Udenfriend S, Duggan DE, Vasta BM, Brodie BB (1957) A spectrophotofluorometric study of compounds of pharmacological interest. J Pharmacol Exp Ther 120:26–32
Van Dyke K, Szustkiewicz C, Lantz CH, Saxe LH (1969) Studies concerning the mechanism of action of antimalarial drugs: inhibition of the incorporation of adenosine-8-^{3}H into nucleic acids of *Plasmodium berghei*. Biochem Pharmacol 18:1417–1425

Varga F (1966) Intestinal absorption of chloroquine in rats. Arch Int Pharmacodyn Ther 163:38–46
Varga F (1968a) Tissue distribution of chloroquine in the rat. Acta Physiol Acad Sci Hung 34:319–325
Varga F (1968b) Intracellular localization of chloroquine in the liver and kidney of the rat. Acta Physiol Acad Sci Hung 34:327–332
Varga F, Fischer E, Szily TS (1975) Effect of gastric emptying time on the intestinal absorption of chloroquine in rats. Pharmacology 13:401–408
Viala A, Durand A, Cano J-P, Jouglard J (1972) La chloroquine: sort dans l'organisme et toxicologie analytique. Eur J Toxicol 5:189–202
Viala A, Cano J-P, Durand A (1975) Determination of chloroquine in biological material by gas chromatography. J Chromatogr 111:299–303
Walker AJ (1949/1950) Malaria therapy, 1950. Bull Tulane Med Fac 9:48–51
Warhurst DC (1973) Chemotherapeutic agents and malaria research. Symp Br Soc Parasitol 11:1–28
Warhurst DC, Hockley DJ (1967) Mode of action of chloroquine on *Plasmodium berghei* and *P. cynomolgi*. Nature 214:935–936
Warhurst DC, Killick-Kendrick R (1967) Spontaneous resistance to chloroquine in a strain of rodent malaria (*Plasmodium berghei yoelii*). Nature 213:1048–1049
Warhurst DC, Thomas SC (1975) Localization of mepacrine in *Plasmodium berghei* and *Plasmodium falciparum* by fluorescence microscopy. Ann Trop Med Parasitol 69:417–420
Wassermann HP (1965) The circulation of melanin – its chemical and physiological significance. S Afr Med J 39:711–716
Weissmann G (1964) Labilization and stabilization of lysosomes. Fed Proc 23:1038–1044
Weniger H (1979) Review of side-effects and toxicity of chloroquine. WHO, Geneva, WHO/MAL 79:906
Whisnant JP, Espinosa RE, Kierland RR, Lambert EH (1963) Chloroquine neuromyopathy. Mayo Clin Proc 38:501–513
Whitehouse MW, Boström H (1965) Biochemical properties of anti-inflammatory drugs. VI. The effects of chloroquine (resochin), mepacrine (quinacrine), and some of their potential metabolites on cartilage metabolism and oxidative phosphorylation. Biochem Pharmacol 14:1173–1184
Wibo M, Poole B (1974) Protein degradation in cultured cells. II. Uptake of chloroquine by rat fibroblasts and the inhibition of cellular protein degradation and cathepsin B_1. J Cell Biol 63:430–440
Wiesmann UN, Didonato S, Herschkowitz NN (1975) Effect of chloroquine on cultured fibroblasts: Release of lysosomal hydrolases and inhibition of their uptake. Biochem Biophys Res Commun 66:1338–1343
Williams RT (1959) Detoxication mechanisms, 2nd edn. Wiley, New York, pp 651–652
Wiselogle FY (1946) A survey of antimalarial drugs, 1941–1945, vol. I. JW Edwards, Ann Arbor, Michigan
Wollheim FA, Hanson A, Laurell C-B (1978) Chloroquine treatment of rheumatoid arthritis: correlation of clinical response to plasma protein changes and chloroquine levels. Scand J Rheumatol 7:171–176
Yoshimura H (1964) Organ systems in adaptation; the skin. In: Handbook of Physiology, Sec. 4. American Physiological Society, Washington, DC, p 113
Zeller RW, Deering D (1958) Corneal complications of chloroquine (Aralen) therapy. JAMA 168:2263–2264
Zvaifler NJ, Rubin M, Bernstein H (1963) Chloroquine metabolism: drug excretion and tissue distribution. Arthritis Rheum 6:799–800

CHAPTER 2

Quinine and Quinine Analogues

W. HOFHEINZ and B. MERKLI

A. Introduction

I. Scope of the Chapter; Literature Review

Quinine, the oldest universally known antimalarial agent, has been the subject of numerous reviews in the past. We do not intend in this chapter to repeat once more all the known facts about quinine, but rather to select and critically discuss those properties which are essential for an assessment of its merits and its defaults in comparison with its modern successors. Since only those properties will be mentioned which contribute to an appraisal and understanding of the antimalarial activity, the therapy of cardiac arrhythmias for which quinidine is one of today's standard drugs will not be dealt with (for a review on antiarrhythmic drugs see BIGGER and HOFMAN 1980).

The most comprehensive account of the fundamental chemotherapeutic and pharmacological properties of quinine and related alkaloids was written by FINDLAY (1951). Other information can be found in reviews by SCHMIDT (1955) and HILL (1963) and in the short but informative summary by ROLLO (1980). As medicinal chemistry texts the monograph by THOMPSON and WERBEL (1972) and the chapter on antimalarials in *Burger's Medicinal Chemistry* by SWEENEY (1979) are recommended. For a comprehensive review of the chemistry of the cinchona alkaloids the reader is directed to SAINSBURY (1978). A detailed account of the structure elucidation, chemical transformation and the first total synthesis, a truly classical chapter of natural products chemistry, was provided by TURNER and WOODWARD (1953) and continued by USKOKOVIĆ and GRETHE (1973) reviewing the more recent achievements in total synthesis. The technical production of quinine was dealt with by STOLL and JUCKER (1953).

For the historically interested reader it might be useful to mention also a comprehensive review (including text references not listed at the end of this chapter) covering all aspects of quinine written at a time when quinine was still the sole antimalarial drug, e.g. FISCHL and SCHLOSSBERGER (1934).

II. Historical Review

Two and a half centuries before the causative agent of malaria was known the curative property of the bark of the cinchona tree had already been exploited. Today, 350 years later, modern medicine must still rely on quinine, the major alkaloid constituent of the bark, as a life-saving medicament in severe cases of falciparum malaria. As no other drug quinine helped to shape today's world, enabling explorers and colonists from Europe to live in tropical countries, and build their colonial empires in spite of lethal tropical malaria.

It is traditionally claimed that the first European to be successfully cured of malaria by the powdered bark of cinchona trees was Juan Lopez, a Jesuit, in the year 1630, and that its rapid acceptance as an antimalarial drug was due to the miraculous cure in 1638 of the countess Anna del Chinchon, wife of the viceroy to Peru. The first of these two events is not conclusively documented and the second must now be dismissed as romantic fiction. Nevertheless it is well established that around 1630 the value of cinchona bark was well known in Peru. The first record of its use is found in Calancha's chronicle, written in 1633 in Lima and published in 1638 in Barcelona. In 1641 the drug was imported into Spain by Juan de Vega, then physician to the Count of Chinchon. The bark first came to be used in Seville around 1642. In 1645 the Jesuit Bartolome Tafur, delegate from Peru, convinced Roman Jesuits of the efficiency of Peruvian bark for treating intermittent fever. From the Jesuit pharmacy in Rome cinchona bark started to be spread quickly all over Europe. By 1669 the bark is described in early German pharmacopoeias and, in 1677, it appears in the London pharmacopoeia as Cortex peruvianus. (For a critical account of the early history of quinine, including historical references, see GUERRA 1977a, b.)

Little was known in Europe about the botanical origin of the bark for almost a century until, in 1738, the French explorer De la Condamine identified the tree from which the bark was taken. He supplied the first botanical description of the plant, drew it and named it quinquina. Based on this description, Carl von Linné in his *Genera plantarum* of 1742 classified it as a representative of a new genus and renamed it *cinchona* – misspelled to honour the Countess of Chinchon.

With the ever increasing domination of the world by European countries the supply of cinchona bark took on increasing importance. This led to a dangerous over-exploitation of the natural sources of the bark in South America and also to attempts by the colonial powers to transfer cinchona trees to other parts of the tropical world. In 1852 an expedition supported by the Dutch government and led by Karl Hasskarl finally succeeded in carrying off large quantities of cinchona seeds and live plants in a Dutch warship and in transporting them to Java in the Dutch East Indies, where the first plantations were established. However, the original plants contained only low amounts of alkaloids, and it was only after the Dutch obtained seeds of a species much richer in alkaloids from the Peruvian cinchona merchant Ledger that the plantations in Java began to flourish. By the end of the nineteenth century Java supplied 90% of the world market of the drug. The occupation of Java during World War II by Japan cut off the rest of the world from these supplies. This event triggered an intensive search to find synthetic drugs with which to replace quinine. These research efforts finally led to a number of new synthetic antimalarials. However, the emergence in the 1960s of *P. falciparum* strains resistant to chloroquine which responded only to quinine renewed the need for quinine which, until today, has remained an essential drug for the treatment of malaria.

The chemical investigation of the cinchona bark began in the early nineteenth century and, up until recent times, its alkaloids have formed a constant focus of interest for generations of organic chemists. In 1820, Pelletier and Caventou isolated the first pure alkaloids from the bark, quinine and cinchonine. With the isolation of cinchonidine in 1847 by Winckler and of quinidine in 1849 by van Hejningen the four major alkaloids became known. The first correct elemental composition of quinine was obtained in 1854 by Strecker. Two years later, Perkin attempted to obtain quinine by synthesis. His attempt failed but yielded the first aniline dye and led to the development of the dye industry. The elucidation of the structure of quinine, one of the major achievements of early organic chemistry, took from around 1870 to 1908. Rabe, who finally elucidated the correct structure of quinine, was also the first to succeed in synthesising dihydroquinine in 1931. Quinine itself was synthesised for the first time in 1944 by Woodward and von Doering (TURNER and WOODWARD 1953). It has continued to attract the attention of organic chemists ever since and, between 1968 and 1973, a number of elegant syntheses were developed, most notably by USKOKOVIĆ and his collaborators at Hoffmann-La Roche Inc. (USKOKOVIĆ and GRETHE 1973).

The synthetic preparation of quinine analogues with simpler structures began in the 1920s, initially at the Bayer AG. It developed into a major research effort in the United States during World War II and later again in the 1960s. Products of these efforts are the well-established drugs chloroquine and primaquine and, recently, probably the most successful quinine substitute, mefloquine (see also Chaps. 1, 3, 9).

B. Chemistry

I. Occurrence

Cinchona alkaloids occur most notably in plants of the genus *Cinchona* and the related genera *Remijia* and *Ladenbergia* of the family Rubiaceae, where they are almost completely located in the bark. Small amounts of cinchona alkaloids have also been found in species of the families Annonaceae, Loganiaceae, and Oleaceae (e.g. in *Olea europea* and *Ligustrum vulgare*). Cinchona species grow wild as trees in the cloud forest of the tropical Andes in South America. Commercial bark is, however, entirely produced in plantations of varieties and hybrids of the species *C. ledgeriana, C. calisaya,* and *C. succirubra.*

About 35 cinchona alkaloids are known. With the exception of a few indole derivatives, they are quinoline compounds with rather similar structures. With respect to their biosynthesis they are all closely related (for a review on the biosynthesis see LEETE 1969).

There are four principal alkaloids (Fig. 1), cinchonidine (Ia), quinine (Ic), cinchonine (IIIa), and quinidine (IIIc), which are usually accompanied by smaller amounts of their dihydro derivatives and traces of the stereoisomeric epi-alkaloids. A common minor alkaloid is cupreine (Ib). The alkaloid content of the bark and the relative proportions of the individual alkaloids vary considerably with the species. The bark of cultivated *C. ledgeriana* contains up to 13.5% of quinine and less than 1.5% of other alkaloids, whereas the alkaloid content of the bark of wild-growing species rarely exceeds 1.5%. The highest quinidine concentrations are found in the bark of *Remijia pedunculata*.

The pure alkaloids are obtained by industrial processes such as those described by STOLL and JUCKER (1953) and VETTER (1936).

II. Structure

The general structure (Fig. 1) consists of two moieties, a quinoline and a quinuclidine ring, linked by a hydroxymethylene bridge. The quinoline ring can be unsubstituted as in cinchonidine and cinchonine or bear a methoxy or hydroxy substituent in position 6′ as in quinine, quinidine or cupreine. The quinuclidine ring always carries a vinyl or an ethyl group attached to position 3.

Each alkaloid has four non-interrelated chiral centres at C-3, C-4, C-8, and C-9. The absolute configuration at C-3 and C-4 is the same for all natural alkaloids and, therefore, four stereoisomers are possible for each substitution type. The stereochemical relationship of these four isomeric series is shown in Fig. 1. Cinchonidine/quinine and cinchonine/quinidine are configurationally identical pairs. The first

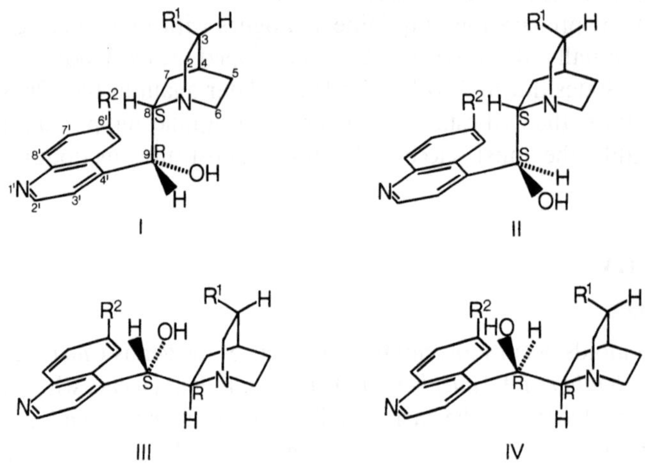

Fig. 1. Structure and absolute configuration of quinine-type cinchona alkaloids

I	a	$R^1 = -CH{=}CH_2$	$R^2 = -H$	cinchonidine
	b		$= -OH$	cupreine
	c		$= -OCH_3$	quinine
	d	$R^1 = -CH_2-CH_3$	$R^2 = -H$	dihydrocinchonidine
	e		$= -OH$	dihydrocupreine
	f		$= -OCH_3$	dihydroquinine
II	a	$R^1 = -CH{=}CH_2$	$R^2 = -H$	epicinchonidine
	b		$= -OCH_3$	epiquinine
	c	$R^1 = -CH_2-CH_3$	$R^2 = -H$	epidihydrocinchonidine
	d		$= -OCH_3$	epidihydroquinine
III	a	$R^1 = -CH{=}CH_2$	$R^2 = -H$	cinchonine
	b		$= -OH$	cupreidine
	c		$= -OCH_3$	quinidine
	d	$R^1 = -CH_2-CH_3$	$R^2 = -H$	dihydrocinchonine
	e		$= -OH$	dihydrocupreidine
	f		$= -OCH_3$	dihydroquinidine
IV	a	$R^1 = -CH{=}CH_2$	$R^2 = -H$	epicinchonine
	b		$= -OCH_3$	epiquinidine
	c	$R^1 = -CH_2-CH_3$	$R^2 = -H$	epidihydrocinchonine
	d		$= -OCH_3$	epidihydroquinidine

two are laevorotatory; the other two are dextrorotatory. All four alkaloids have erythro configuration at C-8 and C-9 as opposed to the *threo* configuration of the epialkaloids.

All quinine-type alkaloids have two basic nitrogen groups. Consequently two series of salts can be obtained with either one or both nitrogens protonated. The latter are usually somewhat more readily soluble in water. Large numbers of different salts of quinine and quinidine are commercially available, the most common being the mono- and dihydrochlorides and the neutral sulphates.

III. Analytical Methods

Numerous methods have been developed for the identification and quantitative determination of cinchona alkaloids in raw materials, crude and pure drugs and in galenic formulations. Representative methods have been described by STOLL and JUCKER (1953) and by VETTER (1936). Today much improved techniques are available including chromatographic separation (TLC and HPLC) and various spectroscopic and colorimetric methods. Publications by VERPOORTE et al. (1980), HAZNAGY (1976), KARAWYA and DIAB (1977), and POUND and SEARS (1975) may serve as leading references.

For the quantitative measurement of quinine and quinidine and their metabolites in body fluids assay methods are needed which are both specific and sensitive. Such methods did not exist until very recently. Older procedures still commonly practised in clinical laboratories use fluorescence spectrometry of acidic sample solutions. These are prepared either by precipitation of proteins with metaphosphoric acid (BRODIE and UDENFRIEND 1943) or by benzene extraction of the biological sample, followed by re-extraction of the basic alkaloids into sulphuric acid (CRAMER and ISAKSSON 1963). Neither of these methods differentiates sufficiently between parent alkaloids and metabolites (GUENTERT et al. 1979 b).

Far better results are obtained if, prior to fluorescence measurement, the samples are separated by TLC (UEDA et al. 1977). The most advanced methods use HPLC separation, which combines specificity, sensitivity and speed. Suitable procedures have been described by BARROW et al. (1980), OCHS et al. (1980), GUENTERT et al. (1979 a), and CONRAD et al. (1977).

C. Mode of Action

I. Activity

1. Activity Against Plasmodium

The therapeutic effect of the cinchona alkaloids is derived entirely from their capacity to check the multiplication of the asexual erythrocytic stages of the parasite. They do not exert any lethal effect on sporozoites and pre-, or secondary exoerythrocytic tissue forms; they are gametocytocidal for *P. vivax* and *P. malariae* but only for early developing stages of *P. falciparum*.

The four major alkaloids all possess significant blood schizontocidal activity but their relative potencies vary with the species of *Plasmodium*. FINDLAY (1951)

Table 1. Activity of quinine in comparison to mefloquine against different *Plasmodium* species

Species	Host	Compound	ED_{90} (mg/kg p.o.)	References
P. berghei (K 173)	Mouse	Quinine · HCl Mefloquine · HCl	153 [a] 5 [a]	MERKLI and RICHLE (1980)
P. falciparum (various strains)	*Aotus* monkey	Quinine Mefloquine	266–>560 [b] 14–28 [b]	SCHMIDT et al. (1978a, b)
P. vivax (two strains)	*Aotus* monkey	Quinine Mefloquine	518–>560 [b] 8–14 [b]	SCHMIDT et al. (1978a, b)

[a] Daily oral dose (given for 4 days)
[b] Total dose (given within seven consecutive days)

and HILL (1963) give the following rating:
P. falciparum (man): quinidine > quinine ≧ cinchonidine > cinchonine
P. vivax (man): quinidine ≧ quinine > cinchonidine = cinchonine
P. gallinaceum (chicken): cinchonine > quinidine > cinchonidine > quinine
P. lophurae (duck): quinine = quinidine > cinchonidine > cinchonine
P. relictum (canary): quinine = quinidine > cinchonidine > cinchonine
P. berghei (mouse): quinidine = quinine = cinchonine
(see Table 2)

Quinine is evidently not the most effective cinchona alkaloid, but has reached a unique position because it just happened to be the first to be isolated and used in pure form, and also because the cultivation of cinchona has fortuitously favoured its production. The level of its activity is, in fact, by no means exceptional. Table 1 summarises a few quantitative data on quinine and compares it with the new and chemically related antimalarial mefloquine.

2. Other Chemotherapeutic Activities

Cinchona alkaloids are slightly active in vitro against bacteria and dermatophytes, but have no effect in systemic infections (GRUNBERG 1968, unpublished data). An interesting synergism with tetracyclines has been reported (TOAMA 1980) which may have some significance when quinine is used in combination with tetracyclines (see Sect. F.II).

Other protozoa such as trypanosomes and trichomonads are not significantly affected (GRUNBERG 1968, unpublished data; BROTHERTON 1978). A slight, though therapeutically not useful, activity has been observed against *Schistosoma mansoni* (PELLEGRINO and KATZ 1974) but not, however, against other helminth parasites.

II. Structure-Activity Relationships

Chemical transformations and degradations of the natural alkaloids have led to numerous structural analogues in the past. More recently total syntheses (USKOKOVIĆ and GRETHE 1973) have resulted in a number of stereoisomers and derivatives which cannot be prepared from the natural alkaloids. Antimalarial effectiveness of a selection of such analogues is shown in Table 2. The comparison of

Table 2. Response of *P. berghei* to natural cinchona alkaloids and some racemic and enantiomeric analogues obtained by synthesis

Compound	Structure	ED_{50} [a, b]	MED [c, d]
		(mg/kg p.o.)	
Cinchonine	IIIa	15	
Quinidine · $^1/_2\,H_2SO_4$	IIIc	22	100
Dihydroquinidine · $^1/_2\,H_2SO_4$ natural enantiomer	IIIf	13>	50
Dihydroquinidine · $^1/_2\,H_2SO_4$ unnatural enantiomer			50
Dihydroquinidine · $^1/_2\,H_2SO_4$ racemate			50
Quinine · HCl	Ic	10	
		39 [e, f]	200
Dihydroquinine · $^1/_2\,H_2SO_4$ natural enantiomer	If	8 [e]	200
Dihydroquinine · $^1/_2\,H_2SO_4$ unnatural enantiomer			200
Dihydroquinine · $^1/_2\,H_2SO_4$ racemate			200
Epiquinine · 2 HCl	IIb	> 100 [e]	
Ro 21-3472 2′,7′-$(CF_3)_2$-dihydrocinchonidine (racemate)	(Id) [g]	3	
Ro 13-5359 2′,7′-$(CF_3)_2$-epidihydrocinchonidine (racemate)	(IIc) [g]	15	
Ro 21-3473 2′,7′-$(CF_3)_2$-dihydrocinchonine (racemate)	(IIId) [g]	1.4	
Ro 13-5360 2′,7′-$(CF_3)_2$-epidihydrocinchonine (racemate)	(IVc) [g]	9	
Ro 21-0960 (racemate)	V	1.6	
Ro 13-4443 (racemate)	VI	2	
Mefloquine (WR 142490; Ro 21-5998) · HCl (racemate)	VII	1.8	
		5.2 [e]	
WR 177602 (Ro 12-9120) · HCl (racemate)	VIII	2.5	

[a] Dose required for 50% reduction of parasitaemia on day 5, given on four consecutive days
[b] Data from HOFHEINZ and RICHLE (1978, unpublished data) unless stated otherwise
[c] Lowest dose given daily on four consecutive days that keeps blood of infected animals free of parasites on day 5
[d] Data from BROSSI et al. (1971)
[e] Data from PETERS et al. (1975)
[f] Subcutaneous application
[g] Structures as shown, with trifluoromethyl groups in the 2′ and 7′ positions of the quinoline ring

these data and of others reported in the literature (see THOMPSON and WERBEL 1972) leads to the following conclusions on the correlation between structure and activity:

1. A hydroxy group on C-9 is essential for activity. If it is replaced by hydrogen or halogen, or acylated, activity is lost (esters which can be cleaved enzymatically are, however, active: PETTIT and GUPTA 1968). Sulphur-containing groups are potentially useful substitutes (KLAYMAN et al. 1973).

2. The quinoline ring tolerates a number of different substituents in the 6′ position as shown by the natural cinchona alkaloids. The introduction of substituents in other positions has been achieved by total synthesis and has resulted in a particularly useful substitution pattern having one CF_3 group in the 2′ and a second one in either the 7′ or 8′ position (i.e. compound V, Fig. 2).

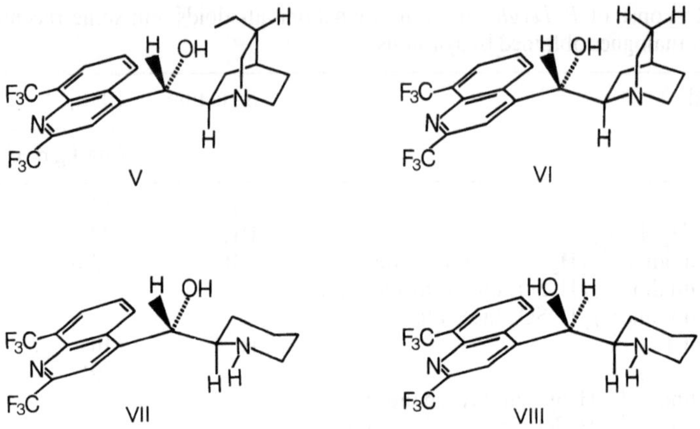

Fig. 2. Structures of quinine analogues (see Table 2). V, Ro 21-0960; VI, Ro 13-4443; VII, mefloquine (WR 142490; Ro 21-5998); VIII, WR 177602 (Ro 12-9120)

3. The quinuclidine ring can be modified drastically. Provided the bond between N-1 and C-8 is not broken and no oxygen functions are introduced, activity is retained. The vinyl group can be saturated, epimerised (BROSSI et al. 1973) or taken off (i.e. compound VI); the double bond can be shifted; or the quinuclidine ring can be opened between N-1 and C-2 to form piperidines (i.e. compounds VII and VIII). All these operations do not fundamentally influence the antimalarial activity.

4. Stereochemistry has variable effects. *Erythro* configuration at C-8 and C-9 seems to be best, although contrary to common belief *threo* isomers (i.e. the epi-alkaloids) are not inactive as illustrated by the 2,7-bis-trifluoromethyl-substituted analogues of the dihydro alkaloids shown in Table 2. The difference in activity of *erythro* and *threo* isomers disappears in the piperidine analogues VII and VIII. The most remarkable observation, however, is that the absolute configuration has no bearing whatsoever on the activity. Both enantiomers, the natural and its unnatural antipode, of dihydroquinine as well as those of dihydroquinidine have the same degree of activity (BROSSI et al. 1971). This rather uncommon fact among biologically active compounds must be taken into account whenever molecular mechanisms of action are discussed, because enantiomers behave as distinctly different molecular species when they associate with chiral material such as happens in substrate-enzyme interaction.

III. Molecular Pharmacology

1. Morphological Changes

DAVIES et al. (1975) have given a detailed description of the effects of quinine on the fine structure of intraerythrocytic *P. berghei*. They observed swelling and vesiculation of outer parasite membranes, swelling of the digestive vacuoles and a decrease of their pigment density. These changes were followed by cytoplasmic degeneration and vacuolisation. It was tentatively concluded that the primary harmful effect was on the mitochondrial functions of the membranes.

Similar ultrastructural changes were observed with various analogues of quinine (DAVIES et al. 1975; PETERS et al. 1977).

2. Parasite Drug Receptors

The modification of the malaria pigment caused by quinine differs characteristically from that observed after exposure to chloroquine. The latter causes a rapid coarsening of the malaria pigment, the chloroquine-induced pigment clumping (CIPC), which can be competitively inhibited by quinine and other cinchona alkaloids (WARHURST et al. 1972). An already established CIPC can be reversed by such compounds (EINHEBER et al. 1976). These observations led to the conclusion that the intraerythrocytic parasites had a specific receptor for quinine- and chloroquine-type drugs, the clumping site, which appeared to be associated with the digestive vacuole.

Infected erythrocytes have the unique capacity to accumulate quinine, chloroquine and similar drugs. The first quantitative studies by POLET and BARR (1968) showed that erythrocytes infected with *P. knowlesi* took up 200 times more dihydroquinine than did normal erythrocytes. FITCH (1972) was able to prove that this accumulation is due to a high affinity site receptor within the parasite. He found that chloroquine uptake was competitively inhibited by quinine and other cinchona alkaloids. The high affinity site and the clumping site are overall very similar. Despite some distinct differences stressed by WARHURST and THOMAS (1975) it is likely that the same receptor serves the pigment-clumping process and the high affinity uptake (CHOU et al. 1980). (See also Part I, Chap. 10, Sect. C and this part, Chap. 1.)

The receptor is localised within the digestive vacuoles of the parasite. It is formed when host haemoglobin is digested to the complex malaria pigment haemozoin, which is accumulated within the vacuoles. In addition to FITCH's group, JEARNPIPATKUL et al. (1980) and JEARNPIPATKUL and PANIJPAN (1980) have proposed that the iron-porphyrin moiety of digested haemoglobin could be the binding site for all fast-acting schizontocides. More recently CHOU et al. (1980) presented convincing evidence that the true receptor is ferriprotoporphyrin IX. This compound is formed transiently by proteolytic degradation of haemoglobin and is finally incorporated into the haemozoin, whereby its binding capacity is lost. According to these authors, ferriprotoporphyrin IX fulfills all criteria for identification as the high-affinity uptake receptor.

The relationship between the binding of quinine to this receptor and the chemotherapeutic effects remains, so far, unclear. The complex may only serve to accumulate the drug within the parasite, but it is also possible that the complex would itself be toxic to the parasite.

3. DNA Binding

For a long time DNA was regarded as the target for the antimalarial action of cinchona alkaloids. Quinine intercalates with DNA and it was therefore considered that it would act as a template poison, inhibiting DNA replication and RNA transcription. Inhibition of DNA synthesis by dihydroquinine has indeed been observed by POLET and BARR (1968). (For a review on quinine-DNA interaction, see HAHN 1979.)

Quinine binds, however, much more weakly than other antimalarials such as mepacrine and drugs like ethidium bromide whose biological action is thought to involve DNA binding. Furthermore, it has been shown that mefloquine (VII) does not intercalate with DNA, although in all respects its pattern of action is the same as that of quinine (DAVIDSON et al. 1977; PETERS et al. 1977). These facts strongly suggest that interaction with DNA is not primarily involved in the antimalarial action of quinine. This conclusion is supported by the rather weak inhibition by quinine of DNA synthesis in erythrocyte-free drug-sensitive *P. berghei* (CARTER and VAN DYKE 1972) and also by the weak effect quinine has on protein synthesis in cell-free ribosome systems of *P. knowlesi* (SHERMAN 1976) when compared with the strong effects of mepacrine and other typical DNA intercalators.

4. Other Interaction with Parasite and Host Structures

LASER et al. (1975) postulated that quinine exerts its antimalarial action by inducing a premature lysis of the parasitised erythrocytes. This lysis could be caused by the formation of a haemolytic complex between quinine and unsaturated fatty acids which are normally bound to proteins.

A recent study by HOMMEL et al. (1979) points out yet another potential mechanism of action. By pretreating erythrocytes with quinine or chloroquine it was possible to suppress their invasion by merozoites. This mechanism could involve binding of the drug to a receptor on the erythrocyte surface, such as the "low affinity site" described by FITCH (1972).

D. Pharmacokinetics and Metabolism

I. Pharmacokinetics

Most of the available information on absorption, distribution and excretion of the cinchona alkaloids was accumulated in the 1940s and has been extensively reviewed by FINDLAY (1951). When given orally the alkaloids are rapidly and almost completely absorbed through the upper intestinal tract. Plasma concentrations reach a maximum after 1–3 h. Peak concentrations of the different alkaloids vary considerably. With the same oral dose quinine gives approximately twice the concentration reached by quinidine and by cinchonidine, and around ten times the concentration reached by cinchonine. A high proportion, at least 70%, of the alkaloids are bound to plasma proteins. Excretion is rapid and almost complete within 24 h, with a half-life of between 5 and 10 h. Most of the excretion products are metabolites and only a small fraction of the administered dose appears unaltered in the urine.

Only a few additional observations on quinine can be found in the more recent literature. SAGGERS et al. (1969) showed that an oral dose of 300 mg results in plasma levels of around 1.5 μg/ml 4 h after application. The elimination half-life was determined at 5.3–5.9 h. Intravenous instead of oral administration leads to considerably higher plasma levels and to significantly increased urinary excretion of the unchanged drug (HALL et al. 1973). This observation suggests that the oral bioavailability of quinine is somewhat lower than is commonly assumed. Increased plasma levels and decreased metabolism are observed during malaria as well as during artificially induced fever, suggesting impaired hepatic metabolism (TRENHOLME et al. 1976).

Because quinidine, used as an antiarrhythmic drug, has a narrow therapeutic index, knowledge of its pharmacokinetic properties was imperative for its rational use. Therefore it is not surprising that the pharmacokinetics of quinidine have been far better studied than those of other related compounds. By and large quinine and quinidine do not differ markedly as far as absorption, metabolism and excretion are concerned, and much of the information on quinidine may also be valid for quinine [for a review on quinidine pharmacokinetics, see OCHS et al. (1980)].

II. Metabolism

As early as 1869 the first metabolite of quinine was isolated from human urine, quinetine, a derivative in which the vinyl group is oxidised to a carboxylic group. Fifty years later, a second acidic product was obtained from urine, haemoquinic acid, the 6-methoxyquinidine-4-ketocarboxylic acid. Whether these acids are true metabolites or rather artefacts is not yet known with certainty (WATABE and KIYONAGA 1972). In a classic investigation BRODIE et al. (1951) found that all four principal cinchona alkaloids are oxidatively metabolised to the 2′-hydroxy compounds and to a varying number of additional, not fully characterised products. A second hydroxylated quinine metabolite was identified by BRODIE as 2-hydroxyquinine but it may, in fact, be 3-hydroxyquinine in analogy with the metabolism of quinidine. The *N*-oxide of quinine has been found as a urinary excretion product after consumption of tonic water (JOVANOVIC et al. 1976). In rabbit urine 2′-hydroxy- and 2′,3-dihydroxyquinine were identified as metabolites (WATABE and KIYONAGA 1972). Recently the urinary metabolites were also studied in rats. Eight metabolites were detected, seven of which could be partially identified, 2′-hydroxy-, 3-hydroxyquinine and cupreine (Ib) as major products and two stereoisomeric pairs of 10,11-dihydrodiols, one pair derived from quinine and the second from cupreine (Ic and Ib with R^1=–CHOH–CH_2OH), as minor products (BARROW et al. 1980). All metabolites are present both free and conjugated.

The metabolic oxidations take place in liver microsomes (SAGGERS et al. 1969; WATABE and KIYONAGA 1972). It can safely be assumed that all metabolites are chemotherapeutically inactive.

The metabolic transformation of quinidine has received far more attention. Next to 2′-hydroxyquinidine identified by BRODIE et al. (1951), (3*S*)-3-hydroxyquinidine has been identified as a major metabolite in human urine (PALMER et al. 1969; CAROLL et al. 1974, 1976; BEERMANN et al. 1976). Cupreidine (IIIb) formed by oxidative demethylation (DRAYER et al. 1976) and an additional, not fully characterised hydroxyquinidine, have also been found in human urine (GUENTERT et al. 1979a). In rat urine altogether nine metabolites were isolated but only partly identified (BARROW et al. 1980).

When steady-state serum levels of the three major quinidine metabolites in cardiac patients were measured, it was found that antiarrhythmic activity is not lost by metabolic oxidation (DRAYER et al. 1978).

E. Toxicity

I. Introduction

A remarkable discrepancy exists between the extremely vast century-old experience with adverse reactions of quinine, collectively called cinchonism, and the scarcity of pertinent studies using the methods of modern science. Comprehensive descriptions of cinchonism are contained in the reviews by FINDLAY (1951) and ROLLO (1980). The first systematic studies on the experimental pharmacology of the various cinchona alkaloids were initiated in the United States during World War II and were summarised by SCHMIDT (1955). The present treatise is largely based on these papers and attempts to add relevant recent findings. Essentially, the focus is put on quinine used as an antimalarial drug, whereas quinidine which is mainly used for indications other than malaria, particularly for cardiac arrhythmias, is more or less neglected.

II. Animal Tolerance

1. Acute and Subchronic Toxicity

a) Single Dose

The available data are scarce and sometimes incomplete. Figures for three animal species are summarised in Table 3.

b) Repeated Doses

When quinine (hydrochloride) was given orally once a day on five consecutive days, the "LD_{50}", which was determined 10 days after the last dose, was 550 ± 80 mg/kg in mice and 490 ± 80 mg/kg in rats (BAECHTOLD 1979).

c) Daily Doses for 2–5 Weeks

The report by SCHMIDT (1955) contains the following data on rats, dogs, and rhesus monkeys: Quinine given to rats orally for 2 weeks was tolerated without any adverse effects in daily doses up to 600 mg/kg. Significant weight loss was noted with daily doses of 900 mg/kg, whereas 1,200 mg/kg was lethal for most of the animals. Death appeared to result from anorexia and starvation.

In dogs treated orally for 5 weeks the highest daily dose not producing any adverse effects was 80 mg/kg, and 160 mg/kg per day produced blindness as a result of degenerative changes in the optic nerve, all the animals succumbing to convulsions after 16–19 days of treatment. The quinine plasma level measured before death was 6–10 mg/litre.

Mentioning experiments with monkeys only briefly, SCHMIDT states that daily doses of 480 mg/kg of quinine have to be administered to produce blindness in this species (plasma levels >25 mg/litre). Despite the similarity of the toxic symptoms observed by SCHMIDT (1955) in all three species, the doses provoking them are quite different. These findings are explained by the interspecies differences of concentrations that quinine reaches in different organs of the animals. In species such as the chicken or dog (KELSEY et al. 1943; HIATT and QUINN 1945), the levels of the alkaloid in the liver, spleen, kidney, intestinal mucosa and lung are often 10–40

Table 3. Acute toxicities of quinine and related alkaloids (single dose)

Species	Compound	Route of administration	Observation time	LD_{50} (mg/kg)	References
Mouse	Quinine · HCl	p.o.	24 h	910 ± 140	BÄCHTHOLD (1979, unpublished data)
	Quinine · $^1/_2$ H_2SO_4	p.o.	NS	1100	HILL (1950)
	Quinine · HCl	i.p.	72 h	210 ± 8	BROSSI et al. (1971)
	Quinine · HCl	i.v.	72 h	125	GRUNBERG (1968, unpublished data)
	Dihydroquinine · $^1/_2$ H_2SO_4	i.p.	72 h	210 ± 12	BROSSI et al. (1971)
	Quinidine · HCl	p.o.	24 h	500	JÄGER (1957, unpublished data)
	Quinidine · HCl	s.c.	24 h	290	JÄGER (1959, unpublished data)
	Quinidine · HCl	i.v.	24 h	72	JÄGER (1957, unpublished data)
	Dihydroquinidine · $^1/_2$ H_2SO_4	i.p.	72 h	192 ± 2	BROSSI et al. (1971)
Rat	Quinine · HCl	p.o.	24 h	1100 ± 170	BÄCHTOLD (1979, unpublished data)
	Quinine · HCl	s.c.	5 days	790 [a]	SCHROEDER (1913)
Rabbit	Quinine · HCl	p.o.	5 days	790 [a]	SCHROEDER (1913)

NS, not specified

[a] Minimum lethal dose

times the concentration in the plasma. However, in the monkey the quinine concentrations in these tissues were rarely more than five times the level of the drug in the plasma. Since tissue levels in man are similar to those found in monkeys, it is understandable that man tolerates quinine at plasma levels which cause blindness in the dog.

2. Chronic Toxicity

FLAKS (1978) treated male albino rats (150 g starting weight) over a period of 15 months with quinine sulphate at 0.1% in the drinking water (estimated daily dose: ~110 mg/kg). He reported the following observations. Out of 48 rats, 28 were still alive after 15 months and 15 were killed for histology. Histological examination showed that bile canaliculi were often enlarged and dilated. These changes probably indicate that chronic administration of quinine affects both the parenchyma and the Kupffer cells of the liver. No evidence of liver necrosis was found. The only other sign of toxicity due to treatment was the presence of minimum tubular cell necrosis in the renal cortex of some rats during the early part of the experiment. In the author's opinion, death of the animals was not explained by this low-grade hepatotoxicity of quinine.

3. Carcinogenicity

In the above-mentioned study, which was continued for a total of 20 months (FLAKS 1978), no tumor was found in any tissues of the quinine-treated rats.

4. Teratology

SAVINI et al. (1971) reported the following results of a reproductive toxicity study: In rats it was not possible to separate the lethal effect on the embryo from the lethal effect on the mother. In rabbits, the quinine dose causing 50% of mortality of the fetus also killed several mothers. In dogs, the dose killing the embryos was 16–22 times less than the toxic dose for the adult dog. No macroscopic anomalies of the fetus were observed.

III. Human Tolerance

1. Acute Toxicity

The lethal dose of oral quinine for adults is between 2 and 8 g (range 1.5–20 g) as a single dose (CORBY et al. 1964). In 1- to 2-year-old children, quinine has produced fatalities at 1 g dosage (DEICHMAN and GERARDE 1969). Symptoms after high doses of quinine are nausea, vomiting, excitement, fever, confusion, amblyopia, delirium, syncope, respiratory arrest, and death. Quinine is a marked local irritant. When taken orally it may cause gastric pain, nausea, and vomiting. Subcutaneous or intramuscular injections of the drug are initially painful and sterile abscesses may result from local tissue damage. Intravenous administration may result in thrombosis of the injected vein from injury to the intima. Parenteral quinine is therefore reserved for cases of cerebral malaria, coma resulting from severe infection with *Plasmodium falciparum* (ROLLO 1980; SCHMIDT 1955). When quinine is administered rapidly by the intravenous route, approximately 0.2–0.4 mg/kg per second are suspected to produce arrhythmias, which can be fatal in some instances. This was concluded by LEVINE et al. (1973), who studied sudden deaths occurring in narcotic addicts. Amblyopia or blindness develops quickly, in most cases after an overdose of quinine. It is characterised by pallor of the optic disc, constriction of the retinal blood vessels, dilatation of the pupil and immobility of the iris. In most cases recovery is spontaneous, but slow. Treatment by blocking of the stellate ganglion increases the blood flow to the retina. This procedure was described as one possible method to be initiated as soon as the first visual disturbances are diagnosed (BANKES et al. 1972; VALMAN and WHITE 1977). Ototoxic effects have only rarely been reported. It is postulated that quinine produces a vasoconstriction with transient inner ear ischaemia (HAWKINS 1976) or it may have a direct effect on the spiral ganglion (HYBELS 1979).

Therapeutic doses of quinine have few effects on the central nervous system other than to cause feeble analgesia and antipyresis.

The actions of quinine on cardiac muscle are similar to those of quinidine (marked stimulatory action on the vagus centre and restoration of normal rhythm in arrhythmia and fibrillation) but less potent. On skeletal muscle, quinine increases the refractory period. This action is sometimes used in patients with myotonia or nocturnal cramps (ROLLO 1980).

High doses of quinine may induce abortion by stimulating contraction of the muscle of the gravid uterus (MCVIE 1979). Quinine also reaches the tissues of the fetus.

2. Side Effects at Normal Chemotherapeutic Dosage

When quinine is used at normal therapeutic doses, side effects may occur which consist of nausea, vomiting, tinnitus, quinine fever, and blackwater fever.

Drug-induced deafness was studied by a cooperative study group (ANONYMOUS 1973), who found one case of mild, transitory deafness amongst 312 patients receiving quinidine (900 mg daily for 5 days). This figure is quite low compared with deafness recorded after treatment with certain antibiotics (e.g. gentamycin, neomycin). Recently HALL (1974) reported manifestations of so-called quinine fever which occurred in 10% of white American soldiers who, suffering from malaria, were given a 10-day treatment schedule of quinine. The fever started after parasitaemia had been cleared on the 8th day, and subsided on the 13th day. This phenomenon rarely recurred in the same patient.

Fever episodes are also mentioned in a few cases after quinidine dosing, but with more evidence of an allergic mechanism than in the case of quinine. Rechallenge with quinidine immediately created a fever reaction (SAVRAN et al. 1975).

A most serious adverse reaction is the massive haemoglobinuria which may occur in patients infected with certain strains of *P. falciparum* (blackwater fever). This reaction is highly unpredictable and is neither related to the dose of quinine nor to the duration of treatment. It includes intravascular haemolysis resulting in acute anaemia, oliguria, uraemia, and frequently death. BEUTLER (1972) explained this phenomenon as a drug-dependent immune reaction of the so-called fuadine type. The mechanism involves serum antibodies (non-γ) which react with red blood cells only in the presence of the drug (e.g. fuadine, quinidine, quinine, phenacetin, sulphonamides). A different explanation is given by LASER et al. (1975), who suggest that haemolysis is induced by fatty acids normally bound to proteins in a stable complex, which is disrupted by quinine. In fact many cases of drug-induced, acute haemolysis in malarial patients are now considered to be due to a deficiency of glucose-6-phosphate dehydrogenase (see also Part I, Chap. 5, 15).

F. Deployment

I. Antimalarial Activity in Man

Quinine, administered at a maximum daily dose of 1.3–2 g (divided into three to four fractional doses) for 7–14 days normally cures malaria infection in man. In case of a serious attack of falciparum malaria, especially with coma, the first treatment given to the patient is a slow intravenous infusion of quinine until he regains consciousness and is able to take the drug orally.

II. Use of Quinine as an Antimalarial Agent

Quinine is considerably active against asexual blood forms of all human plasmodia but, used alone, it is not effective against exoerythrocytic forms or against mature gametocytes of *P. falciparum*. Quinine is, therefore, an effective suppressive agent, but has no prophylactic or radically curative properties. Because of the high rate of relapses following quinine used alone, and its inconveniently short half-life, quinine was more and more neglected until, in Southeast Asia approximately 10 years ago, multiple drug-resistant *P. falciparum* infections began to emerge which responded only to quinine. Now quinine is used once again for the treatment of malaria which other compounds fail to cure, mostly, however, not as a single drug but rather in combination with other antimalarials. The more important of these regimens have been reviewed by WHO (1973). Some drug combinations proposed re-

Table 4. Drug combinations with quinine used against chloroquine-resistant *P. falciparum* malaria

Drug regimen	Dosage/duration	References
Quinine +	540 mg every 8 h/3 days	HALL et al. (1975a)
sequential clindamycin	450 mg every 8 h/3 days	MILLER et al. (1974)
Quinine +	540 mg every 8 h/1–3 days	HALL et al. (1975b)
sequential sulfadoxine + pyrimethamine	1,000 mg + 75 mg/single dose	HALL et al. (1977)
Quinine +	1,920 mg daily/3 days	COLWELL et al. (1972)
sequential tetracycline	1,000 mg for 10 days	
Quinine +	2.0 g/four doses	HALL et al. (1977)
sequential mefloquine [a]	1.5 g/single dose [b]	

[a] Not commercially available
[b] May be split up into two to three doses

cently, by various authors are shown in Table 4. The combination of quinine with tetracyclines is advised (ANONYMOUS 1980) for the cases of treatment failure following therapy with combinations of quinine with sulphonamide and pyrimethamine.

G. Drug Resistance

I. Production of Resistance in Animals

Most early attempts to produce quinine-resistant plasmodial strains in animals using different techniques were not very successful (FINDLAY 1951). PETERS (1970) summarising the collected reports concluded that some malaria parasites seem to be innately resistant to quinine (e.g. *P. knowlesi, P. yoelii yoelii* 17X, *P. relictum* [German strain]); some species or strains have the ability to develop resistance (e.g., *P. relictum, P. gallinaceum, P. berghei*), whilst others are unable to do so (e.g., *P. cathemerium, P. cynomolgi, P. vivax*). Recently GLEW et al. (1978) succeeded in producing a markedly quinine-resistant strain of *P. falciparum* in *Aotus* monkeys by subcurative quinine therapy during six serial passages over 6 months.

Resistance to quinine was also found in association with resistance experimentally induced to chemically related compounds such as mefloquine (MERKLI and RICHLE 1980).

II. Resistance in Man

Plasmodium falciparum is known to show considerable differences in sensitivity to quinine in different parts of the world [see review by PETERS (1970)]. Strains which require high doses of quinine for successful treatment were found in South America and Southeast Asia. Sometimes a degree of quinine resistance in *P. falciparum* can be observed in connection with chloroquine resistance. Recent in vitro experiments and field trials (especially in Southeast Asia) confirm the suggestion that there is a tendency for quinine treatment schedules to have to be prolonged in order to obtain a satisfactory clinical effect (CHONGSUPHAJAISIDDHI et al. 1979; SUCHARIT and EAMSOBANA 1980). The dosage of quinine, however, should not exceed 2.0 g/day (~10 mg/litre plasma) since, otherwise, serious toxic effects of the drug must be expected. Worldwide in vitro drug-sensitivity test programmes initiated by WHO will, hopefully, provide in the near future more precise information on baseline levels of quinine sensitivity (or resistance). SUCHARIT et al. (1979) and SUCHARIT and EAMSOBANA (1980), for example, have reported recently on the situation in Thailand.

H. Conclusion

In spite of the fact that quinine has tended recently to be somewhat less active against *P. falciparum* infections than in the past (especially in Thailand), it has regained importance as an indispensable, rapidly acting, blood schizontocidal drug, under special precautions even applicable intravenously, especially when used in association with other antimalarials.

References

Anonymous (1973) Drug-induced deafness. JAMA 224:515–516

Anonymous (1980) Epidemiologic notes and reports: *Plasmodium falciparum* malaria contracted in Thailand resistant to chloroquine and sulphonamide-pyrimethamine. Morbidity and Mortality Weekly Report 29:493–495

Bankes JLK, Hayward JA, Jones MBS (1972) Quinine amblyopia treated with stellate ganglion block. Br Med J 4:85–86

Barrow SE, Taylor AA, Horning EC, Horning MG (1980) High-performance liquid chromatographic separation and isolation of quinidine and quinine metabolites in rat urine. J Chromatogr 181:219–226

Beermann B, Leander K, Lindström B (1976) The metabolism of quinidine in man: structure of the main metabolite. Acta Chem Scand [B] 30:465

Beutler E (1972) Drug-induced anemia. Fed Proc 31:141–146

Bigger JT, Hoffmann BF (1980) Antiarrhythmic drugs. In: Goodman LS, Gilman A (eds) The pharmacological basis of therapeutics, 6th edn. Macmillan, New York, pp 761–792

Brodie BB, Udenfriend S (1943) The estimation of quinine in human plasma with a note on the estimation of quinine. J Pharmacol Exp Ther 78:154–158

Brodie BB, Baer JE, Craig LC (1951) Metabolic products of the cinchona alkaloids in human urine. J Biol Chem 188:567–581

Brossi A, Uskoković M, Gutzwiller J, Krettli AU, Brener Z (1971) Antimalarial activity of natural, racemic and unnatural dihydroquinine, dihydroquinidine and their various racemic analogs in mice infected with *Plasmodium berghei*. Experientia 27:1100–1101

Brossi A, Uskoković M, Gutzwiller J, Krettli AU, Brener Z (1973) Antimalarial activity of racemic 3-epidihydroquinine, 3-epidihydroquinidine and their various racemic analogs in mice infected with *Plasmodium berghei*. Experientia 29:367–368

Brotherton J (1978) Biological assay of potential trichomonacides in vitro using a counter apparatus. Arzneimittelforsch 28:1665–1672

Caroll FI, Smith D, Wall ME, Moreland CG (1974) Carbon-13 magnetic resonance study. Structure of the metabolites of orally administered quinidine in humans. J Med Chem 17:985–987

Carroll FI, Philip A, Coleman MC (1976) Synthesis and stereochemistry of a metabolite resulting from the biotransformation of quinidine in man. Tet Lett (21):1757–1760

Carter G, van Dyke K (1972) Drug effects on phosphorylation of adenosine and its incorporation into nucleic acids of chloroquine sensitive and resistant erythrocyte-free malaria parasite. J Parasitol (Special Issue) 39:244–249

Chongsuphajaisiddhi T, Subchareon A, Puangpartk S, Harinasuta T (1979) Treatment of falciparum malaria in Thai children. Southeast Asian J Trop Med Public Health 10:132–137

Chou AC, Chevli R, Fitch CD (1980) Ferriprotoporphyrin IX fulfills the criteria for identification as the chloroquine receptors of malaria parasites. Biochemistry 19:1543–1549

Colwell EJ, Hickman RL, Kosakal S (1972) Tetracycline treatment of chloroquine-resistant falciparum malaria in Thailand. JAMA 220:684–686

Conrad KA, Molk BL, Chidsey CA (1977) Pharmacokinetic studies of quinidine in patients with arrhythmias. Circulation 55:1–7

Corby C, Dunnett N, Kimber KJ, Walls HJ (1964) Acute fatal quinine poisoning. In: Forensic immunology, medicine, pathology and toxicology (Proc 3rd Internat Meeting, London, April 16–24, 1963). Excerpta Medica Foundation, London, pp 118–119

Cramer G, Isaksson B (1973) Quantitative determination of quinidine in plasma. Scand J Clin Lab Invest 15:553–556

Davies EE, Warhurst DC, Peters W (1975) The chemotherapy of rodent malaria, XXI. Action of quinine and WR 122455 (a 9-phenanthrenemethanol) on the fine structure of *Plasmodium berghei* in mouse blood. Ann Trop Med Parasitol 69:147–153

Davidson MW, Griggs BG, Boykin DW, Wilson WD (1977) Molecular-structural effects involved in the interaction of quinolinemethanolamines with DNA. Implications for antimalarial action. J Med Chem 20:1117–1122

Deichman WB, Gerarde HW (1969) Toxicology of drugs and chemicals. Academic, New York, p 511

Drayer DE, Cook CE, Reidenberg MM (1976) Active quinidine metabolites. Clin Res 24:623A

Drayer DE, Lowenthal DT, Restivo KM, Schwartz A, Cook CE, Reidenberg MM (1978) Steady-state serum levels of quinidine and active metabolites in cardiac patients with varying degree of renal function. Clin Pharmacol Ther 24:31–39

Einheber A, Palmer DM, Aikawa M (1976) *Plasmodium berghei:* Phase contrast and electron microscopic evidence that certain antimalarials can both inhibit and reverse pigment clumping caused by chloroquine. Exp Parasitol 40:52–61

Findlay GM (1951) Recent advances in chemotherapy, 3rd edn, vol 2. Churchill J+A, London

Fischl V, Schlossberger H (1934) Handbuch der Chemotherapie. Fischers medizinische Buchhandlung, Leipzig, pp 140–223

Fitch CD (1972) Chloroquine resistance in malaria: drug binding and cross resistance patterns. J Parasitol (Special Issue) 39:265–271

Flaks B (1978) Effects of chronic oral dosing with quinine sulphate in the rat. Pathol Res Pract 163:373–377

Glew RH, Collins WE, Miller LH (1978) Selection of increased quinine resistance in *Plasmodium falciparum* in *Aotus* monkeys. Am J Trop Med Hyg 27:9–13

Guentert TW, Coates PE, Upton RA, Combs DL, Riegelman S (1979a) Determination of quinidine and its major metabolites by high-performance liquid chromatography. J Chromatogr 162:59–70

Guentert TW, Upton RA, Holford NHG, Riegelman S (1979b) Divergence in pharmacokinetic parameters of quinidine obtained by specific and nonspecific assay methods. J Pharmacokinet Biopharm 7:303–311

Guerra T (1977a) The introduction of cinchona in the treatment of malaria. Part 1. J Trop Med Hyg 80:112–118

Guerra T (1977b) The introduction of cinchona in the treatment of malaria. Part 2. J Trop Med Hyg 80:135–139

Hahn FE (1979) Quinine. In: Hahn FE (ed) Antibiotics, vol V, part 2. Springer, Berlin Heidelberg, New York, pp 353–362

Hall AP (1974) Quinine fever in falciparum malaria. Southeast Asian J Trop Med Public Health 5:413–416

Hall AP, Czerwinski AW, Madonia EC, Evensen KL (1973) Human plasma and urine quinine levels following tablets, capsules, and intravenous infusion. Clin Pharmacol Ther 14:580–585

Hall AP, Doberstyn EB, Nanakorn A, Sonkom P (1975a) Falciparum malaria semi-resistant to clindamycin. Br Med J 1975:12–14

Hall AP, Doberstyn EB, Mettaprakong V, Sonkom P (1975b) Falciparum malaria cured by quinine followed by sulfadoxine-pyrimethamine. Br Med J 1975:15–17

Hall AP, Doberstyn EB, Karnchanachetanee C, Samransamruajkit S, Laixuthai B, Pearlman E, Lampe RM, Miller CF, Phintuyothin P (1977) Sequential treatment with quinine and mefloquine or quinine and pyrimethamine-sulfadoxine for falciparum malaria. Br Med J 1:1626–1628

Hawkins JE Jr (1976) In: Keidel WD, Neff WD (eds) Clinical and special topics. Springer, New York Berlin Heidelberg, pp 707–748 (Handbook of sensory physiology, vol V/3)

Haznagy A (1976) Beitrag zur Bestimmung des Gesamtalkaloidgehaltes von Cortex Chinae. Pharmazie 31:713–715

Hiatt EP, Quinn GP (1945) The distribution of quinine, quinidine, cinchonine and cinchonidine in fluids and tissues of dogs. J Pharmacol Exp Ther 83:101–105

Hill J (1950) The schizonticidal effect of some antimalarials against *Plasmodium berghei.* Ann Trop Med Parasitol 44:291–297

Hill J (1963) Chemotherapy of malaria. Part 2. Antimalarial drugs. In: Schnitzer AJ, Hawking F (eds) Experimental chemotherapy, vol I. Academic, New York, pp 514–524

Hommel M, McColm AA, Trigg PI (1979) *Plasmodium knowlesi:* inhibition of invasion by pretreatment of erythrocytes with chloroquine and quinine. Ann Microbiol (Paris) 130(B):287–293

Hybels RL (1979) Drug toxicity of the inner ear. Med Clin North Am 63:309–319

Jearnpipatkul A, Panijpan B (1980) Molecular complexes of quinoline antimalarials with iron-porphyrin components of protease-digested methemoglobin. Chem-Biol Interact 33:83–90

Jearnpipatkul A, Govitrapong P, Yuthavong Y, Wilairat P, Panijpan B (1980) Binding of antimalarial drugs to hemozoin from *Plasmodium berghei*. Experientia 36:1063–1064

Jovanovic J, Remberg G, Ende M, Spiteller G (1976) Quinine-*N*-oxide – urinary component after the consumption of quinine beverages. Arch Toxicol 35:137–139

Karawya MS, Diab AM (1977) Colorimetric assay of quinine and quinidine in raw materials, formulations, and biological fluids. J Pharm Sci 66:1317–1319

Kelsey FE, Oldham FK, Geiling EMK (1943) Studies on antimalarial drugs. The distribution of quinine in the tissues of the fowl. J Pharmacol Exp Ther 78:314–319

Klayman DL, Griffin TS, Bower JD, Page SW (1973) Thiosulfuric acid analog of quinine as a potential antimalarial agent. J Med Chem 16:1042–1043

Laser H, Kemp P, Miller N, Lander D, Klein R (1975) Malaria, quinine, and red cell lysis. Parasitology 71:167–181

Leete E (1969) Biosynthesis of quinine and related alkaloids. Acc Chem Res 2:59–64

Levine LH, Hirsch CS, White LW (1973) Quinine cardiotoxicity: a mechanism for sudden death in narcotic addicts. J Forensic Sci 18:167–172

McVie JG (1979) Antimicrobial drugs. In: Girdwood RH (ed) Clinical pharmacology, 24th edn. Baillière Tindall, London, pp 69–157

Merkli B, Richle R (1980) Studies on the resistance to single and combined antimalarials in the *Plasmodium berghei* mouse model. Acta Trop (Basel) 37:228–231

Miller LH, Glew RH, Wyler DJ, Howard WA, Collins WE, Contacos PG, Neva FA (1974) Evaluation of clindamycin in combination with quinine against multidrug-resistant strains of *Plasmodium falciparum*. Am J Trop Med Hyg 23:565–569

Ochs HR, Greenblatt DJ, Woo E (1980) Clinical pharmacokinetics of quinidine. Clin Pharmacokinet 5:150–168

Palmer KH, Martin B, Baggett B, Wall ME (1969) The metabolic fate of orally administered quinidine gluconate in humans. Biochem Pharmacol 18:1845–1860

Pellegrino J, Katz N (1974) Experimental therapeutics on *Schistosoma mansoni*, IX. Activity of quinine and isomers. Rev Inst Med Trop Sao Paulo 16:301–304

Peters W (1970) Chemotherapy and drug resistance in malaria. Academic, London

Peters W, Portus JH, Robinson BL (1975) The chemotherapy of rodent malaria, XXII. The value of drug-resistant strains of *P. berghei* in screening for blood schizontocidal activity. Ann Trop Med Parasitol 69:155–171

Peters W, Howells RE, Portus J, Robinson BL, Thomas S, Warhurst DC (1977) The chemotherapy of rodent malaria, XXVII. Studies on mefloquine (WR 142490). Ann Trop Med Parasitol 71:408–418

Pettit GR, Gupta SK (1968) Structural biochemistry. Part VIII. 9-Amino-9-deoxy-cinchona alkaloids. J Chem Soc (C):1208–1213

Polet H, Barr C (1968) Chloroquine and dihydroquinine. In vitro studies of their antimalarial effect upon *Plasmodium knowlesi*. J Pharmacol Exp Ther 164:380–386

Pound NJ, Sears RW (1975) HSLC and TLC determination of quinidine and quinine and related alkaloids in pharmaceuticals. Can J Pharm Sci 10:122–126

Rollo IM (1980) Drugs used in the chemotherapy of malaria. In: Goodman LS, Gilman A (eds) The pharmacological basis of therapeutics, 6th edn. Macmillan, New York, pp 1038–1060

Saggers VH, Hariratnajothi N, Mc Lean AEM (1969) The effect of diet and phenobarbitone on quinine metabolism in the rat and in man. Biochem Pharmacol 19:499–503

Sainsbury M (1978) Quinoline alkaloids. In: Coffey S (ed) Rodd's chemistry of carbon compounds, 2nd ed, vol IV/G. Elsevier, Amsterdam, pp 225–246

Savini EC, Moulin MA, Herron MFJ (1971) Etude expérimentale des effets de la quinine sur le foetus de rat, de lapin, de chien. Therapie 26:563–574

Savran SV, Flamm MD Jr, Grant D (1975) Fever as a toxic reaction to quinidine. N Engl J Med 292:427

Schmidt LH (1955) Antimalarials. In: Manske RHF (ed) The alkaloids, chemistry and physiology, vol 5. Academic, New York, pp 141–161

Schmidt LH (1978a) *Plasmodium falciparum* and *Plasmodium vivax* infections in the owl monkey (*Aotus trivirgatus*) II. Responses to chloroquine, quinine, and pyrimethamine. Am J Trop Med Hyg 27:703–717
Schmidt LH, Crosby R, Rasco J, Vaughan D (1978b) Antimalarial activities of various 4-quinoline-methanols with special attention to WR 142,490 (mefloquine). Antimicrob Agents Chemother 13:1011–1030
Schroeder K (1913) Untersuchungen über einige Chininderivate. Arch Exper Path Pharmakol 72:361–386
Sherman JW (1976) The ribosome of the simian malaria *Plasmodium knowlesi*. V. A cell-free protein synthesizing system. Comp Biochem Physiol [B] 53:447–450
Stoll A, Jucker E (1953) China-Alkaloide. In: Foerst W (ed) Ullmanns Encyklopädie der technischen Chemie, 3rd edn, vol 3, Urban & Schwarzenberg, Munich, pp 210–222
Sucharit P, Suntharasamai P, Chintana T, Harinasuta T (1979) In vivo and in vitro studies of quinine sensitivity of *Plasmodium falciparum* in Thailand. Southeast Asian J Trop Med Public Health 10:138–141
Sucharit P, Eamsobana P (1980) In vitro response of *Plasmodium falciparum* in Thailand to antimalarial drugs. Ann Trop Med Parasitol 74:11–15
Sweeney TR, Strube RE (1979) Antimalarials. In: Wolf ME (ed) Burger's medicinal chemistry, 4th ed, Part II. Wiley, New York, pp 333–413
Thompson PE, Werbel LM (1972) Antimalarial agents. Academic, New York, pp 62–78
Toama MA (1980) *In vitro* synergism between tetracyclines and antimalarials. Chemotherapy 26:191–195
Trenholme GM, Williams RL, Rieckmann KH, Frischer H, Carson PE (1976) Quinine disposition during malaria and during induced fever. Clin Pharmacol Ther 19:459–467
Turner RB, Woodward RB (1953) The chemistry of the cinchona alkaloids. In: Manske RHF, Holmes HL (eds) The alkaloids, vol III. Academic, New York, pp 1–63
Ueda CT, Hirschfeld DS, Scheinman MM, Rowland M, Williamson BJ, Dzindzio BS (1976) Disposition kinetics of quinidine. Clin Pharmacol Ther 19:30–36
Uskoković MR, Grethe G (1973) The Cinchona alkaloids. In: Manske RHF (ed) The alkaloids, vol XIV. Academic, New York, pp 181–223
Valman HB, White DC (1977) Stellate block for quinine blindness in a child. Br Med J 1977:1065
Verpoorte R, Mulder-Krieger Th, Troost JJ, Baerheim Svendsen A (1980) Thin-layer chromatographic separation of cinchona alkaloids. J Chromatogr 184:79–96
Vetter RC (1936) Neuere Probleme der Chininaufbereitung. In: Festschrift E.C. Barell. F. Hoffmann-La Roche, Basel
Warhurst DC, Homewood CA, Peters W, Baggaley YC (1972) Pigment changes in *Plasmodium berghei* as indicators of activity and mode of action of antimalarial drugs. J Parasitol (Special Issue) 39:271–279
Warhurst DC, Thomas S (1975) Pharmacology of the malaria parasite – a study of dose-response relationships in chloroquine-induced autophagic vacuole formation in *Plasmodium berghei*. Biochem Pharmacol 24:2047–2056
Watabe T, Kiyonaga K (1972) The metabolic fate of quinine in rabbits. J Pharm Pharmacol 24:625–630
WHO Techn Rpt Series No 529 (1973) Chemotherapy of malaria and resistance to antimalarials. WHO, Geneva

CHAPTER 3

8-Aminoquinolines*

P. E. CARSON

A. Introduction

The role of the 8-aminoquinolines against malaria is currently focused on their activity as tissue schizontocides in the treatment and prophylaxis of vivax and ovale malaria. In addition they are gametocytocidal and sporontocidal and can prevent transmission of falciparum malaria. Of the two 8-aminoquinolines presently in use primaquine is the most generally available and quinocide, a structural isomer of primaquine, is used in the USSR. Although primaquine is the safest available 8-aminoquinoline it does have significant toxic effects, the best known being the induction of haemolytic anaemia in individuals with glucose-6-phosphate dehydrogenase (G6PD) deficiency. Furthermore, the radical cure of vivax and ovale malaria requires the administration of primaquine even in partially immune individuals over a period of at least several days. Nevertheless, because no other available tissue schizontocide is more effective or less toxic than primaquine there is a recognised need for investigations to differentiate the efficacy and the toxicity of primaquine as well as to discover new, less toxic, tissue schizontocides. Thus the Third Meeting of the Scientific Working Group on the Chemotherapy of Malaria of the World Health Organization held in Geneva, Switzerland in October 1980 was entirely devoted to the field of tissue schizontocidal drugs.

Despite this current focus on their tissue schizontocidal activity the development and studies of the 8-aminoquinolines have been of considerable importance to the advancement of medical science especially for their contributions in the fields of chemotherapy and human genetics. Moreover, the mechanisms of their antimalarial and haemolytic effects are still unknown and continued investigations of the 8-aminoquinolines remain important.

B. Chemistry

I. Introduction

Development of the 8-aminoquinolines appears to stem from 1891, when GUTTMAN and EHRLICH (1891) tested methylene blue against malaria, an event which is often considered to mark the advent of chemotherapy as we know it today.

Subsequently, methylene blue was modified by the addition of a dialkylaminoalkyl group, which was found to increase its antimalarial activity, and even-

* The author wishes to dedicate this chapter in memory of ALF S. ALFING, M.D. who has leader and mentor made this work posible

tually, after preparation of more than 12,000 compounds in Germany, pamaquine, a 6-methoxy-8-aminoquinoline, was announced in 1926 as the first synthetic antimalarial (ROEHL 1926; HORLEIN 1926). Publication of the structure was delayed until 1928, however (FARBENINDUSTRIE IG 1928). The exact sequence of events in the development of pamaquine (initially called plasmoquine or plasmochin) is not entirely clear. Documentation is to be found in the patent as well as the scientific literature. The most detailed and successful attempt at ferreting out this story is that provided by STECK (1972). The synthetic steps leading from methylene blue to pamaquine (which did not involve 12,000 compounds per se) were described by SCHULEMANN in 1932. Also valuable is the review provided by FLETCHER (1933), especially for documentation of the earliest clinical trials by SIOLI, MÜHLENS and others.

Until recently, when the Special Programme for Research and Training in Tropical Diseases was established under the auspices of the WHO, the incentives for development of antimalarial drugs have almost always been military and economic rather than humanitarian or social. Not surprisingly, therefore, it was not until World War II that there was another great surge in the testing and synthesis of new drugs. Ultimately, more then 13,000 compounds were listed in *A Survey of Antimalarial Drugs, 1941–1945* (WISELOGLE 1946). Of the more than 8,000 were taken off the shelves of drug and chemical manufactures. Subsequent to evaluation of the 13,000 compounds in avian malaria infections 93 were tested against *Plasmodium vivax* and *P. falciparum* infections of man (SCHMIDT, personal communication).

Although initially pamaquine as an 8-aminoquinoline had not been recognised as a member of a class of antimalarial drugs, in the course of the antimalarial drug development during World War II several hundred 8-aminoquinolines were prepared and screened for antimalarial activity against various avian malaria parasites. Toxicity was then studied in rats, dogs, and monkeys. Clinical units were also established to test potential antimalarial agents, including the 8-aminoquinolines, in human volunteers. The development and scope of this programme (which was second in size only to the Manhattan Project) is carefully but dramatically recounted in the survey edited by WISELOGLE (1946) and, when pertinent, certain aspects of the World War II Chemotherapy of Malaria Programme are alluded to in this chapter. [Other relevant reviews are those provided by SCHMIDT and COATNEY (1955) and THOMPSON and WERBEL (1972)].

II. Structure

For descriptive purposes the 8-aminoquinolines which have been of therapeutic interest may be considered as derivatives of 6-methoxy-8-aminoquinoline (Fig. 1). They are then classified according to the constitution of the aliphatic dialkylaminoalkyl group, which replaces one of the hydrogen atoms on the 8-amino nitrogen. The 8-aminoquinolines are further classified by the number of methylene groupings separating the terminal amino groups from the 8-amino nitrogen and by whether the terminal amino group is primary, secondary or tertiary. Variations both in antimalarial efficacy and toxicity are determined in large part by the nature of these aliphatic side chains.

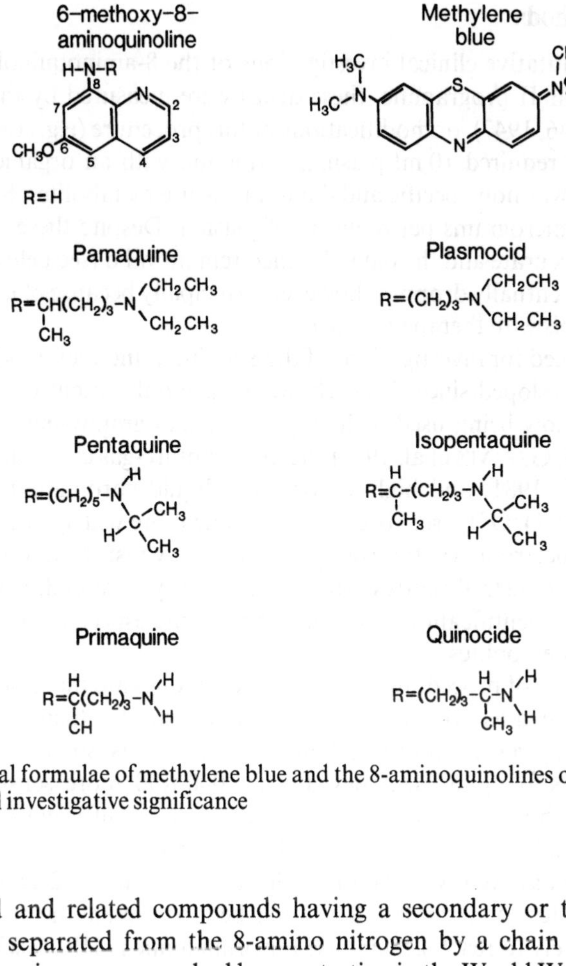

Fig. 1. Structural formulae of methylene blue and the 8-aminoquinolines of principal biological and clinical investigative significance

Plasmocid and related compounds having a secondary or tertiary terminal amino group separated from the 8-amino nitrogen by a chain of two or three methylene groupings never reached human testing in the World War II programme because of severe neurotoxicity (see below) [1].

Beginning with pamaquine the other 8-aminoquinolines shown in Fig. 1 all received extensive clinical testing as discussed in this chapter. They are characterised by having a side chain with a primary, secondary or tertiary terminal amino group separated from the 8-amino nitrogen by more than four methylene groupings. Primaquine and quinocide are structural isomers having a primary terminal amino group, pentaquine and isopentaquine are structural isomers having a secondary group and pamaquine (like plasmocid) has a tertiary group.

In addition to differences in biological and clinical effects associated with variation of the aliphatic side chains, recently published data indicate that administration of the *d* and *l* stereoisomers of primaquine may result in significantly different toxicity without alteration of efficacy (SCHMIDT et al. 1977 a).

1 Plasmocid had, however, received limited human testing as Fourneau 710, later called rhodoquine. Like pamaquine it was relatively ineffective against the blood forms of vivax and falciparum malaria. Acute toxicity was apparently fairly severe (FLETCHER 1933; SCHMIDT, personal communication). No data appear to be available on chronic or long-term toxicity

III. Assay Methods

During the quantitative clinical investigations of the 8-aminoquinolines initiated in the World War II programme, these drugs were measured by the methods of BRODIE et al. (1946, 1947), or modifications of this procedure (e.g. JONES et al. 1948 b). This method required 10 ml plasma, extraction with an organic solvent and diazotisation. It was non-specific and did not measure metabolites. Sensitivity was in the range of micrograms per millilitre of plasma. Despite these handicaps the procedure was accurate and the data obtained remain valid (see below). Use of the procedure was eventually dropped, however, principally because of lack of correlation of blood levels with therapeutic effect.

Despite the need for investigations of the 8-aminoquinolines, modern advances in technology developed since this early work have only recently been exploited. The techniques now being used include gas chromatography-mass spectrometry (BATY et al. 1975; GREAVES et al. 1979), electron capture-gas chromatography (RAJAGOPALAN et al. 1981) and high-performance liquid chromatography (HPLC) (CARSON et al. 1981). Of these, HPLC can be made more widely available than the others as mass spectrometry, for example, is relatively restricted to university and large medical or industrial centres. Mass spectrometry is needed, nevertheless, for investigation and identification of molecular structure especially of as yet unidentified unknown metabolites.

The advantages of procedures using these techniques are that not only can parent compounds such as primaquine be measured, but also their metabolites and other drugs when given concurrently. Sensitivity for at least some of these methods ranges as low as 10 ng/ml, i.e. they are a 1,000-fold more sensitive than the diazotisation method. For none of these methods have sufficient data been produced in biological systems to recommend or describe the exact procedure in this chapter, although active investigations indicate that within 1–2 years several, adequate, properly tested methods will be published. At present the procedure which appears most likely to reach general use for primaquine is HPLC with an electrochemical detection system. This is because only microlitre amounts of plasma are used, deproteinisation does not have to be absolutely complete, recoveries approach 100% and, unlike other methods, extraction, derivatisation and use of an internal standard are not required (NORA and PARKHURST, unpublished data).

C. Modes of Action

I. Introduction

Active investigation of the metabolism of the 8-aminoquinolines, especially primaquine, is once again being undertaken. The molecular mechanisms of action of these compounds are not yet known, however. Accordingly, the modes of action are characterised by their effects on various stages of the parasitic life cycles. This has resulted in their classification under the term "tissue schizontocides". This term is somewhat misleading because the 8-aminoquinolines are active against all stages of the parasite cycle in man and mosquito, even though the activity against the asexual erythrocytic forms is weak and clinically ineffective. Thus primaquine is the antimalarial agent for radical cure of those species of malaria which retain tissue stages and have true relapses, e.g. *P. vivax, P. ovale* of man and the simian malaria, *P. cynomolgi*. Primaquine is also a true causal prophylactic agent against the pre-erythrocytic forms of the four human species of malaria as well as against *P. cynomolgi*. In addition primaquine is sporontocidal and gametocytocidal, and can be used therefore to prevent the transmission of malaria including falciparum malaria.

II. Radical Cure and Prevention of Relapses; Deployment

From the time of announcement of pamaquine in 1926 as the first synthetic antimalarial, attention was naturally focused on its use for the treatment of clinical malaria. Recognition that pamaquine and subsequently developed 8-aminoquinolines would be most useful as tissue schizontocides and of little value for the treatment of acute attacks of clinical malaria, whether due to *P. vivax* or *P. falciparum*, was several years away. Toxic manifestations were quickly evident and the literature on curative regimens, not only for pamaquine but for all other 8-aminoquinolines, is inextricably tied to toxicity studies. Accordingly, even though toxicity is covered in Sect. E of this chapter, some aspects of toxicity as they pertain to therapeutic regimens, especially in people with glucose-6-phosphate dehydrogenase (G6PD) deficiency will necessarily be considered in this section.

Pamaquine was first provided under the trade name, Beprochin, subsequently changed to plasmoquine (sometimes plasmochin) by the manufacturers (I.G. Farbenindustrie in Germany) (James 1931 b; James et al. 1931). Early on clinicians who received the drug were not certain of its exact composition and some of their results may have differed considerably due to batch differences. Sinton et al. (1930) reported, for example, a significant increase in toxicity upon receiving a new batch of this drug during their pioneering studies.

By 1933 more than 600 articles had been published on plasmoquine and recognition that it was too toxic for general use was accepted. The Malaria Commission of the League of Nations in recommending restriction of its use did comment that the drug "will always remain remarkable" not only because it was the first effective synthetic antimalarial but also because "observation of its action on a particular stage of the malaria parasite" (the gametocytes – not the tissue stages!) led to change in the ideas and aims of malaria chemotherapy, i.e. recognition that chemotherapy would have to be directed against various stages of the parasitic life cycle rather than to development of a single agent which would cure all malaria (Malaria Commission 1933).

The generic name, pamaquine, did not come into use until development of the 8-aminoquinolines was again undertaken in the United States during and after World War II. This resulted from reawakened realisation that a drug was needed to prevent relapses of vivax malaria. The need was underscored because new suppressive drugs such as chloroquine and chloroguanide (proguanil, Paludrine) which were far more effective than mepacrine (atabrine, quinacrine) in eliminating the asexual blood forms still failed to prevent relapses of vivax malaria.

The previous data on pamaquine were reviewed in the context of radical cure and prevention of relapses in vivax malaria. Sinton's data (Sinton and Bird 1928; Sinton et al. 1930) were recognised to have demonstrated a significant success rate with pamaquine compared, for example, with that of quinine alone and an even better record with the combination of quinine and pamaquine. Additional supporting evidence from older British studies in India (JARVIS 1932; MANIFOLD 1931) and more recent studies on Mediterranean vivax malaria were also considered (KELLEHER and THOMPSON 1945). Review of studies which had failed showed that too little pamaquine or too short a regimen had been used. MOST et al. (1946) then compared quinine alone, mepacrine alone and a combined quinine-pamaquine regimen in three groups of military personnel naturally infected with vivax malaria (mostly of Southwest Pacific origin). The relapse rate in the group who received the combined regimen was only 11% compared with relapse rates of 89% for quinine alone and 84% for mepacrine alone. Their dramatic results considerably bolstered the decision to restudy pamaquine and develop new 8-aminoquinolines for additional study.

Accordingly, programmes for study not only of pamaquine but also of newly synthesised 8-aminoquinoline analogues were set up as described by WISELOGLE (1946).

At first pamaquine was restudied both to reassess its effectiveness and toxicity quantitatively and for standardisation in order to compare other compounds as they became available (BERLINER et al. 1948; CRAIGE et al. 1947a, b). Ultimately more than fifty 8-aminoquinolines were tested in man from 1944 onwards, primarily by ALVING and associates at the University of Chicago (ALVING et al. 1960, 1962). Most were soon eliminated either because of lack of efficacy or unacceptable toxicity. Pentaquine and isopentaquine proved less toxic and more effective than pamaquine but were superceded by primaquine (ALVING 1948; ALVING et al. 1948 a, b; ATCHLEY et al. 1948; RUHE et al. 1949; COOPER et al. 1953; EDGECOMB et al. 1950). The studies of SCHMIDT et al. (1982c) in rhesus monkeys with *P. cynomolgi* demonstrated a seven fold greater therapeutic index for primaquine than pamaquine, six fold greater than pentaquine and three fold greater than isopentaquine. This was soon borne out in human testing with a therapeutic index ten times better than pamaquine, and primaquine emerged in 1950 as the drug of choice for radical cure of vivax malaria (EDGECOMB et al. 1950).

In testing and developing primaquine most of the studies were conducted using the Chesson strain of vivax malaria (EHRMAN et al. 1945). This strain has long been known to be more difficult to cure than any other strain of vivax malaria thus far recognised. Hence it was reasoned, correctly, that infection with this strain in nonimmune volunteers would represent the most severe challenge to achieving radical cure. Thus the first therapeutic regimen of 30 mg primaquine/day for 14 days developed to cure Chesson vivax malaria would be a higher dose than that needed for the treatment of most strains of *P. vivax* infection. This has proven true and the present internationally accepted dosage schedule is 15 mg base/day for 14 days. This dosage schedule was principally worked out in extensive studies of Korean vivax malaria, but has been applied generally (ALVING et al. 1952; GARRISON et al. 1952; HANKEY et al. 1953; ALVING et al. 1953; JONES et al. 1953; DI LORENZO et al. 1953; COATNEY et al. 1953).

Several variations of this regimen have been used or proposed, based on various rationales and accumulated data. Some of the valid ones are as follows:

1. Either quinine or chloroquine is given together with primaquine. The rationale is that, because primaquine has little or no activity against the asexual blood forms, a drug which is active against these forms should be given to cure or control the clinical malaria during the radical curative therapy of the tissue stages with primaquine. Both quinine and chloroquine satisfy this function. Further studies with these drugs in rhesus monkeys (SCHMIDT 1981) and in man (ALVING et al. 1955) suggested that they also "potentiate" the action of primaquine when given concurrently, thus providing an important additional rationale for their use. [This is not "potentiation" in the sense used, e.g. in the context of sulphonamides and pyrimethamine, but rather an additive effect – Ed.]

In this context because mepacrine increases the toxicity of 8-aminoquinolines it is contraindicated for this purpose (ATCHLEY et al. 1948; EDGECOMB et al. 1950; ZUBROD et al. 1947; EARLE et al. 1948; MALARIA COMMISSION 1937). Proguanil, though not additionally toxic, proved unsatisfactory as well and, as it has been suggested, may even decrease the antimalarial activity of the 8-aminoquinolines; it is also not indicated for combined use with primaquine (ALVING et al. 1948 b; ATCHLEY et al. 1948; JONES et al. 1948 a).

The most likely candidate to replace chloroquine or quinine as a companion drug is mefloquine (RIECKMANN et al. 1974; TRENHOLME et al. 1975 b). This is a long-acting quinoline-methanol effective against the asexual blood forms both of chloroquine-resistant and chloroquine-sensitive *P. falciparum* as well as asexual stages of *P. vivax*. Human testing of the concurrent administration of primaquine and mefloquine either for "potentiation" or toxicity has not been reported, however, and use of this combination cannot be recommended as yet.

2. SCHMIDT et al. (1977b), after analysis of their data on several 8-aminoquinolines given to rhesus monkeys, proposed that radical cure of *P. cynomolgi* is a function of total dose (irrespective of time intervals). They also reviewed the therapeutic literature and extended this proposal to the therapy of *P. vivax*. In addition CLYDE and MCCARTHY (1977) cured 11 of 11 volunteers during their first attack after infection with Chesson strain *P. vivax* using 60 mg/day primaquine for 7 days (i.e. instead of 30 mg/day for 14 days). This concept is attractive and as pointed out by SCHMIDT "derives support from chemotherapeutic principles which are operative in the therapy of numerous infections and malignant diseases". One can speculate that this concept might be confirmed with single doses of 180 mg primaquine for strains of vivax malaria requiring only 15 mg/day for cure because single doses high enough to cure Chesson vivax malaria cannot be tolerated.

3. Intermittent regimens of chloroquine and primaquine given once a week were successfully developed by ALVING et al. (1960) initially to mitigate the haemolytic effect of primaquine in people with G6PD deficiency and therefore to allow relatively unsupervised use of primaquine in large populations. A regimen of once weekly doses of 300 mg chloroquine base and 45 mg primaquine base given for 8 weeks was actually more effective in preventing relapses of Chesson vivax malaria than 15 mg primaquine/day for 14 days. This schedule produced no evidence of clinically significant haemolytic anaemia in the black (GdA$^-$) G6PD-deficient individuals who were studied. [Coincidentally, this regimen or a variant of it using mefloquine instead of chloroquine is the one which RIECKMANN's data (RIECK-

MANN et al. 1968, 1969) (see Sect. C.IV) indicate would suffice to prevent transmission of falciparum malaria.]

This intermittent weekly regimen is also in accord with SCHMIDT's total dose concept, e.g. 45 mg once a week for 8 weeks is a total dose of 360 mg and 15 mg for 14 days is a total dose of 210 mg, a difference of 150 mg, which may account for the greater effectiveness of the weekly regimen.

In this context, however, the total dose concept must lead to extended rather than shortened regimens for those with G6PD deficiency. G6PD deficiency, an X-linked condition, occurs in approximately 200 to 300 million people of all races and, like the haemoglobinopathies, more than 100 molecular variants of G6PD have been reported. For practical clinical purposes, however, those affected may be divided into the GdA$^-$ and the GdB$^-$ variants. The GdA$^-$ variant occurs almost exclusively in people of African descent who have a less severe deficiency than people with the GdB$^-$ variant, usually identified as those of Mediterranean descent. Note should be made, however, that people from Southeast Asia and probably southern China may also have the same variant, or at least clinically as severe a deficiency (BEUTLER 1978; CARSON and FRISCHER 1966; CARSON 1960; CARSON et al. 1981) (see also Part I, Chap. 15).

As stated, blacks with the GdA$^-$ variant are not as severely affected as those with the GdB$^-$ variant. For example, doses of primaquine of 15 mg/day in healthy volunteers are tolerated with little or no evidence of haemolytic anaemia (although haemolysis can be demonstrated by laboratory tests, ALVING et al. 1960). However, as shown in Fig. 2, doses of 30 mg/day do induce a self-limited haemolytic anaemia, which is maximum in 8 or 9 days. It has also been thoroughly demonstrated that the severity of haemolysis in individuals with the GdA$^-$ variant is directly proportional to dose (KELLERMEYER et al. 1961, 1962). Thus, with respect to

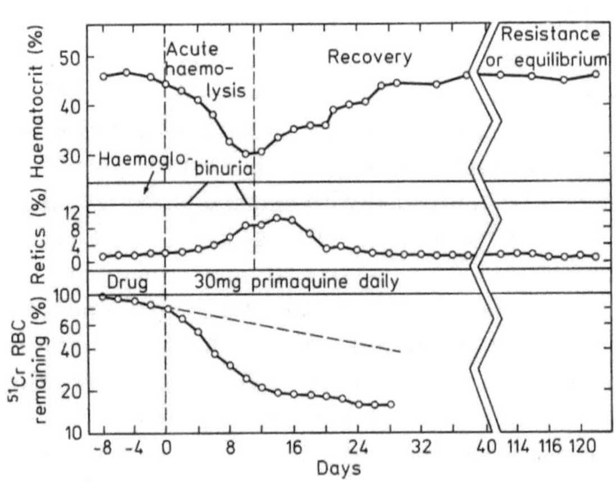

Fig. 2. Typical course of primaquine-induced hemolysis; composite data from three males with the GdA$^-$ variant of G6PD deficiency who received 30 mg primaquine daily. [Reprinted from ALVING et al. (1960).] Haemolysis is self-limited due to compensatory erythropoiesis. If, however, the dose of primaquine is increased a second haemolysis will ensue (KELLERMEYER et al. 1961). Haemolysis is not self-limited in individuals with the GdB$^-$ variant (SALVIDIO et al. 1967)

the total dose concept for cure of vivax malaria there are ample data to predict severe haemolytic anaemia in those with the GdA⁻ variant of G6PD deficiency on a dosage schedule of 60 mg/day for 7 days.

The predictions is much more ominous for those with the GdB⁻ variant in whom 30 mg/day cannot be tolerated and in whom primaquine-induced haemolysis is not self-limited (SALVIDIO et al. 1967). Furthermore, trial of the weekly intermittent regimen of 300 mg chloroquine and 45 mg primaquine in ten subjects with the GdB⁻ deficiency induced serious reactions even at half the weekly dose (ZIAI et al. 1967). On the other hand VIVONA et al. (1961) in a large-scale study in Korea found little evidence of serious reaction to this regimen. A Turkish soldier with G6PD deficiency had a normal haemogram after 4½ months on the weekly regimen. Nevertheless, under medical supervision small doses of primaquine (10–15 mg once weekly) over periods of many weeks sufficient to achieve the required total dose are all that can be recommended for patients with this severe, erythrocytic enzyme deficiency.

4. Individuals who have developed partial immunity to malaria are well known to require less antimalarial drug than non-immune individuals to suppress or cure their infection. Advantage of this can be taken to use either reduced dosages of 8-aminoquinolines, or shortened regimens, or both in such individuals. This concept is especially useful for large-scale field trials in endemic areas where 2 weeks of daily treatment is logistically difficult and sometimes impossible. Although many examples could be cited four will suffice: (a) COGGESHALL (COGGESHALL 1946; COGGESHALL and RICE 1949) reported that the dosage of pentaquine, 60 mg/day for 2 weeks, being used to treat returning veterans with long-standing infections, could be cut in half and still eradicate their infections. (b) THAELER et al. (1953), in a large-scale study among the Miskito Indians in Nicaragua, found 10 mg primaquine/day was as effective as 15 or 20 mg/day against recurrence of vivax malaria. (c) CEDILLOS et al. (1978) in a field evaluation in El Salvador reported that either a 5-day course of primaquine at 15 mg/day or a single 45-mg-dose regimen effectively reduced recurrence of parasite activity. (d) In retrospect, the dramatic results of MOST et al. (1946) (see above) in preventing relapses of vivax malaria with quinine and pamaquine were clearly a combined function of "potentiation" by quinine and partial immunity in their subjects, all of whom had had long-standing infections with one or several relapses. Their regimen of daily doses of 0.65 g quinine and 30 mg pamaquine for 14 days would be inadequate for treatment of non-immune individuals with initial attacks of vivax malaria (especially of the Chesson strain).

III. Causal Prophylaxis

The introductory statements seem to imply that the cellular biology of the malaria parasite is well understood. To infer this is, however, not yet valid. For example, in addition to the tissue schizonts first described in 1948 (SHORTT and GARNHAM 1948; HAWKING et al. 1948; SHORTT et al. 1948; SHORTT et al. 1949) another hepatic tissue form, the hypnozoite (KROTOSKI et al. 1980; KROTOSKI et al. 1982), has recently been discovered during a massive, sporozoite-induced infection of *P. cynomolgi* in a rhesus monkey. Even so, no pre-erythrocytic forms could be demonstrated prior to 48 h after sporozoite infection. Thus the changes and possibly the location of the sporozoites during the first 24 h or more after inoculation could not be ascertained. Moreover, the quantity of both tissue forms found at 48 h in hepatocytes of this monkey was small and not in accord with the size of the sporozoite inoculum until 7 or more days after the inoculation. Yet in *P. cynomolgi* the 8-aminoquinolines exert their causal prophylactic effect during the time period from just before sporozoite challenge through the 8th day after inoculation, i.e. through the period required for the differentiation of the sporozoites into tissue stages and the maturation of these prior to release of the trophozoites (the asexual blood forms) into the circulating blood.

In this context the studies of causal prophylaxis provide most revealing data concerning the tissue schizontocidal activity of the 8-aminoquinolines. These commenced with the classic protocol of JAMES, who reported (JAMES et al. 1931; James 1931 b) that pamaquine administered the day before, the day of and for 5 days[2] after inoculation of sporozoites by infected mosquitos into human volunteers completely protected them against either benign or malignant tertian malarial infection (i.e. either *P. vivax* or *P. falciparum*). Eventually, FELDMAN et al. (1946), JONES et al. (1948 b), and FAIRLEY (1947) completely or partially confirmed JAMES' work. Other studies have confirmed the validity of this regimen both in monkeys and in man for several 8-aminoquinolines against *P. cynomolgi, P. vivax* or *P. falciparum* (see below).

Although JAMES had empirically established the causal prophylactic activity of pamaquine, the biological justification for this regimen was only determined many years later by FAIRLEY (1945, 1947). He first demonstrated that massive subinoculation of blood (200 to 500 ml) from donors, either while infected mosquitos were biting or up to 60 min after the bites, could transmit malaria to non-immune recipients. Subsequent massive subinoculation from volunteers infected with vivax or falciparum malaria failed to transmit the infection until 192+ h after challenge with *P. vivax* sporozoites, and 144+ h after challenge with mosquitoes infected with *P. falciparum*. Additional studies showed that subinoculation of mixed infections did not alter these curiously specific prepatent periods for each species. ARNOLD et al. (1955) repeated the subinoculation experiments with *P. falciparum* and again found that blood drawn 144 h postinoculation failed to transmit the disease to non-immune recipients. Thus, prepatency is a true incubation period and the effect of 8-aminoquinolines or their metabolites given during this time must be on the developing tissue stages and not on the blood, i.e. erythrocytic forms of the malaria parasite.

Modifications of JAMES' protocol were then undertaken, in part to establish dose-response relationships not only for pamaquine but also for other 8-aminoquinolines, and in part to determine the optimal time of administration and susceptibility of the developing tissue (i.e. pre-erythrocytic) stages during the prepatent period. Results of certain of these studies led also to the still moot concept that a

2 Most investigators subsequently have described (and used) JAMES' regimen as extending for 6 days after challenge with sporozoites, instead of the 5 days described in his report. For the most part this has made no significant difference in interpretation of the results of various studies

metabolite of primaquine, rather than primaquine itself, exerts the antimalarial effect.

Especially during the periods 1946–1949 and 1972–1975 SCHMIDT and his associates (SCHMIDT 1982; SCHMIDT et al. 1982a, b, c, d) studied the effects of many potential antimalarial drugs on *P. cynomolgi* in rhesus monkeys. These data provided the "underpinning" for the studies in human volunteers with *P. vivax* and *P. falciparum* which established present therapeutic regimens, as well as the basis for many studies needed for improving therapy, for determining toxicity and for elucidating the mechanisms involved in drug-host-parasite relationships. Although these data are only now being published they are especially pertinent in the light of renewed investigations which have revealed new tissue forms such as the hypnozoite, and new methods for determining drug levels and metabolites and their cellular effects.

For example, during 1947–1949 SCHMIDT et al. (1982c) studied the causal prophylactic effect of isopentaquine and primaquine against *P. cynomolgi* in rhesus monkeys. The results indicate variable susceptibility of the parasite during prepatency, as well as differences between the two compounds in their causal prophylactic effects.

In sufficient dosage (though less than the maximum tolerated dose) both isopentaquine and primaquine when given the day before, the day of and for 8 days after inoculation completely prevented infection. Using less frequent dosages, e.g. either single or two dosages at various intervals, revealed that both isopentaquine and primaquine were also effective on the day of and the day after challenge. Isopentaquine gave poor protection, however, with schedules that covered days 2 to 5 after inoculation but was again protective on days 6 to 8. Primaquine in single doses was ineffective from days 2 to 8, although in two-dose schedules given 5 days apart protection could be demonstrated, e.g. for doses given on days 0 and 4 and on days 1 and 5 after challenge. No data correlating drug or metabolite levels at these times are available.

From these data the susceptibility of parasites to isopentaquine, primaquine and presumably other 8-aminoquinolines appears to be maximal in rhesus monkeys during the period immediately after challenge with sporozoites, exactly the time when identifiable tissue stages have not yet been seen. A second time of susceptibility at 6 to 8 days after challenge could be shown using isopentaquine, but not primaquine. At this time both hypnozoites and tissue schizonts are present. These data suggest that the prepatent tissue stages of *P. cynomolgi* have an initial period of susceptibility with an intervening period of resistance, followed by another period of susceptibility. Whether or not some tissue forms, e.g. the hypnozoite, but not others are differentially susceptible to the 8-aminoquinolines is still to be determined. (Neither is it known for sure whether the small hypnozoite is a precursor of the larger tissue schizont.)

In human infections hypnozoites have not yet been reported. Presumably, by analogy with *P. cynomolgi,* they will be found in *P. vivax* both during the prepatent period and as latent forms during periods of clinical remission between relapses. By contrast, as there are no latent tissue stages in *P. falciparum,* if there are hypnozoites in this species they will be found only during prepatency. Nevertheless, the 8-aminoquinolines have causal prophylactic activity against both species, although there are significant differences in their dose-response effects and times of susceptibility.

FELDMAN et al. (1946) reported complete protection by pamaquine in luetic patients using JAMES' regimen for both vivax and falciparum malaria. They stated that this regimen could be shortened to 3 days for *P. falciparum*. FAIRLEY's studies with pamaquine using 80 mg daily dosages were successful against falciparum but not vivax malaria (FAIRLEY 1947). JONES et al. (1948b) reported that pamaquine protected two out of five volunteers against the Chesson strain of vivax malaria. They also tested three other 8-aminoquinolines (including pentaquine). Using maximum tolerated dosages 15 of 21 volunteers were completely protected, with pamaquine being the least and pentaquine the most effective. Of the six volunteers who were not protected, alteration of the parasite by activity of the 8-aminoquinolines against the tissue stages was demonstrated in two ways: (a) cure of their infection was readily achieved by quinine or chloroquine, drugs which do not have activity against tissue forms, and (b) prepatency was significantly prolonged, an observation also noted by SCHMIDT in his studies of *P. cynomolgi*. In these studies not only was JAMES' schedule used but also shortened schedules, with drug given the day before, the day of and either on three or only two subsequent days. These schedules were equally effective, demonstrating (as in *P. cynomolgi*) increased susceptibility of the earliest tissue stages of *P. vivax* to the 8-aminoquinolines.

By 1950, primaquine (EDGECOMB et al. 1950) had emerged as the 8-aminoquinoline of choice and subsequent studies of these compounds have been conducted almost exclusively with primaquine[3] or related to primaquine, rather than to pamaquine, which had long been proven to be too toxic for general use.

In 1954 ARNOLD et al. (1954) reported that primaquine at dosages of 30 mg/day (using JAMES' regimen) was completely effective in preventing infection with the Chesson strain of vivax malaria and that doses as low as 10 and 15 mg/day were 70%–80% effective, a better capacity than pamaquine at doses of 31.5 and 90 mg/day.

ALVING et al. (1959) also compared the causal prophylactic effectiveness of primaquine against various other strains of *P. vivax*, demonstrating that, whereas 15 mg/day was only 60% effective against the Chesson strain (already known to require twice the dose necessary to cure other strains), this dose was 100% effective against the St. Elizabeth strain and against three strains of Malayan vivax malaria known as the Taiping, Pahang, and Kepong strains. In this report ALVING reiterated that therapeutic regimens of primaquine given after patency (even with the use of chloroquine to prevent clinical attacks) are almost completely ineffective in preventing relapses if terminated after only 7 days. He also reported the initial causal prophylactic studies against Chesson vivax malaria with single high doses of primaquine, e.g. 60, 120, and 180 mg given at various times before and after challenge with sporozoites. Expansion of these studies with single doses of primaquine then led to the concept that a metabolite of primaquine rather than the parent compound is responsible for its causal prophylactic, antimalarial activity.

As only some of the data obtained by ALVING and associates in these studies have been published (ALVING et al. 1959, 1962), in Table 1 all of the data obtained

3 All doses of primaquine (and other drugs if known) are expressed as the free base

Table 1. Summary of single-dose studies of causal prophylaxis with primaquine. The dosages indicated were administered in relation to the times of inoculation of sporozoites by the bite of ten *Anopheles quadrimaculatus* mosquitos infected with the Chesson strain of vivax malaria. (Data available for each male volunteer include age, height, weight, ethnic origin, infectivity of mosquitoes and length of prepatent period or follow-up in negative cases)

Time of administration	24 h before bite	18 h before bite	12 h before bite	4 h before bite	1 h after bite	12 h after bite	24 h after bite	48 h after bite	3 days after bite	5 days after bite	7 days after bite
180 mg primaquine base											
Number patent / Number treated	5/5	4/5	0/5	1/5	2/5	1/5	3/5	4/5	4/5	4/5	4/5
120 mg primaquine base											
Number patent / Number treated				0/5	0/1	1/2					
60 mg primaquine base											
Number patent / Number treated				9/10							

All untreated controls developed parasitaemia
Prepatent period in untreated controls: 10–14 days
Data compiled by R.D. Powell (1958–1962), University of Chicago-Army Malaria Research Project (unpublished)

on causal prophylaxis against Chesson vivax malaria provided by single doses of primaquine are summarised in one place for the first time. These data were obtained over a 5-year period, from 1958–1962 and, though incomplete, represent all that was (or could be) done. The results show that there is a dose-response effect, with the 60 mg dose being inadequate. Both 120 and 180 mg doses protected when given immediately before and up to 12 h after challenge with sporozoites. In the more extensive studies with doses of 180 mg, significant protection is provided from 12 h before through 12 h after challenge with sporozoites. Minimal protection is provided at 24 and 18 h before bite and at 24 h through 7 days after bite. Because it was thought that blood levels of primaquine (and pamaquine and other 8-aminoquinolines) disappear within 12 h after their administration, these data were interpreted to mean that a metabolite must be responsible for the antimalarial, i.e. causal prophylactic effect.

Definitive interpretation is, however, not yet possible. As described in Sect. D the new methods for determination of primaquine and (some of) its metabolites do confirm the virtual disappearance of primaquine from the blood by 24 h (not 12 h) after its administration. The new methods also reveal the rapid appearance of metabolites within an hour of the administration of primaquine, presumably (but not necessarily) via hepatic biotransformation. One of these metabolites can be measured in the blood for at least 120 h after administration of single doses of 90 or 120 mg (NORA et al., unpublished data). Therefore this metabolite may lack appreciable prophylactic effect against Chesson vivax malaria because protection is minimal with single doses of 180 mg given at 24 and 18 h before and from 24 to 72 h after bite by infected mosquitos when this metabolite would be easily measurable; the data are not necessarily inconsistent with activity of primaquine itself, which would be measurable during the period of maximum causal prophylactic effect.

However, as these data refer only to blood levels and the concentration and kinetics of primaquine and its metabolites in human liver cells and other organs is not known, the question of whether the antimalarial effect of primaquine is due to the parent compound or to its metabolites remains unanswered. These data do appear to confirm for Chesson vivax malaria that the early tissue stages of the malarial parasite after infection are more susceptible to the administration of primaquine than the later stages. The possibility that parasite susceptibility is also a function of total dose (as proposed for radical cure; see above) is enhanced as well.

These statements with respect to the interpretation of studies of causal prophylaxis with primaquine (and other 8-aminoquinolines) have applied to vivax malaria. The data for falciparum malaria are different. After repeating FAIRLEY's subinoculation experiments (FAIRLEY 1947) and JAMES' protocol using 30 mg primaquine/day, ARNOLD et al. (1955) reported the results of their causal prophylactic studies with a chloroquine-sensitive strain of *P. falciparum*, the Panama P-F-6 strain. The studies using JAMES' protocol with 30 mg primaquine/day completely protected recipients against challenge with sporozoites. Then single-dose studies at various dosages were conducted on the 1st, 3rd, and 5th days postinoculation. At 30 mg doses primaquine was 100% effective on the 1st day and 90% effective on the 3rd day; 15 mg was only 40% effective on the 1st day but 90% effective on the 3rd day; 10 mg was 20% effective on the 1st day but 40% effective on the 3rd day.

All three dosages as well as dosages of 45 mg were ineffective if administered on the 5th day. These data indicate maximum susceptibility of the prepatent tissue stages (for the days studied) at 3 days postinoculation, in marked contrast to the data obtained for vivax malaria which show decreased susceptibility by day 3.

POWELL and BREWER (1967) reported their causal prophylactic studies with a chloroquine-resistant strain of *P. falciparum* from Thailand. Using JAMES' regimen at dosages of 15, 30, and 45 mg, six of seven volunteers were protected; the unprotected volunteer had received the 15-mg daily dose. With single-dose studies using 45 mg primaquine, protection was only obtained when given the 1st day after challenge. This dose did not protect when given the day before, the day of, or on days 3 or 5 after challenge. These data are in contrast with those of ARNOLD et al. (1955), which showed maximum protection on day 3 rather than day 1, suggesting differential susceptibility to primaquine of developing tissue stages between these two strains of *P. falciparum*. These data for both strains of *P. falciparum* are also decidedly different from those obtained with the Chesson strain of *P. vivax*, for which no protection using single doses would be expected even with 45 mg on any day during prepatency.

In general, *P. falciparum* appears to be much more susceptible than *P. vivax* to the causal prophylactic action of 8-aminoquinolines.

Nevertheless, despite the considerable variability both in dose response and in the time of maximum susceptibility of tissue forms among the species and strains, the validity of JAMES' regimen using primaquine has been substantiated in every study, not only in the monkey but also in man, in many instances even at dosages as low as 15 mg/day. Thus the virtually unique efficacy of primaquine as a tissue schizontocide remains a most remarkable pharmacological phenomenon. However, without data on the tissue levels of primaquine and its metabolites and with incomplete knowledge of the cellular biology of the tissue stages of the various malaria parasites definitive conclusions concerning the exact mode of action of the 8-aminoquinolines remain frustratingly elusive more than 55 years after the development of pamaquine and 30 years after recognition of primaquine as the 8-aminoquinoline of choice for therapeutic use.

IV. Gametocytocidal and Sporontocidal Effects of Primaquine

The potential use of 8-aminoquinolines to prevent transmission of malaria was recognised early. SINTON and BIRD (1928) commented on the possible activity of pamaquine against the "crescents" (i.e. the gametocytes) with respect to statements by "the makers", the work of others and their own work. By 1933 the gametocytocidal properties of pamaquine were well recognised when, in fact, the MALARIA COMMISSION of the League of Nations (1933) recommended that the use of plasmoquine (pamaquine) "should be confined" to this purpose. The Commission also referred to the "paucity of observations", which is not surprising because the practical problems of performing definitive experiments when investigating malaria are nowhere more apparent than in those required to establish gametocytocidal and sporontocidal effects.

In 1931 JAMES (1931 a) plaintively and at length described the difficulties of maintaining the *Anopheles* mosquito and determining its infectivity, difficulties which persist to the present. In addition all who have attempted work in this area know that waves of gametocytes in sufficient numbers for infecting mosquitoes do not appear in every volunteer. Furthermore, the normal delay in their appearance means that the volunteer carrier will have become partially immune and will also have received suppressive drugs. This, however, is ultimately an advantage if sufficient immunity is achieved so that drugs can be tested for their gametocytocidal and sporontocidal properties without concomitant use of other suppressive or curative drugs which would obscure the results. In any case, the simultaneous availability of healthy mosquitoes and a partially immune carrier with sufficient gametocytes who does not require suppressive therapy is rare.

These technical obstacles were again mentioned by ARNOLD et al. (1955). Nevertheless, by the late 1950s and early 1960s the sporontocidal and gametocytocidal effects of primaquine against falciparum malaria were well known (JEFFERY et al. 1956; YOUNG 1959; BURGESS and BRAY 1961; GUNDERS 1961; RAFFAELE and CARRESCIA 1962; JEFFERY et al. 1963). The elegant, carefully conducted experiments of RIECKMANN et al. (1968, 1969) best serve to describe these effects.

These workers studied both a chloroquine-resistant, Malayan (Camp.), and a chloroquine-sensitive, Uganda I, strain of *P. falciparum*. Anopheline mosquitoes were fed on volunteers infected with one or the other of these strains of *P. falciparum* after the appearance of gametocytes which were quantitated by daily counts of peripheral blood smears. Single doses of 15, 30 or 45 mg primaquine were then administered and new batches of mosquitoes were again fed on the volunteers at various times after receiving the drug. Gametocyte counts were continued while evidence that the mosquitoes had become infected was determined by following the development of oocysts and sporozoites by dissection and microscopic examination. In addition, various batches of such infected mosquitoes were allowed to bite non-infected, non-immune volunteers to determine if their sporozoites were truly infective for the human host. Among the significant results obtained were the following:

1. Gametocytes were infective for mosquitoes before and for 3–6 h after the administration of 45 mg primaquine. By 9–12 h, microscopically visible morphological changes, together with decrease in size of both oocysts and sporozoites, could be demonstrated and the mosquitoes were already non-infective for the human host. These effects were found for both strains of *P. falciparum* studied although occurring somewhat later for the chloroquine-sensitive strain. Doses of 15 mg were less effective and gave more variable results but were also clearly sporontocidal.

2. Within 2–3 days after the administration of 30 or 45 mg primaquine the gametocytes markedly decreased or disappeared. They increased again within a few days though never to previous levels. They became reinfective in approximately 7–14 days if primaquine was not readministered. Results even with 15 mg were definite though less dramatic and, again, were less in the chloroquine-sensitive than in the resistant strain.

From these results the occurrence of the sporontocidal effects within hours after administration of primaquine and well before the decrease in circulating gametocytes deserves special emphasis. Whether or not morphological changes in the gametocytes could be demonstrated prior to their decrease after single doses of primaquine was not reported. Such studies would be possible using the techniques of KASS et al. (1971a, b) for concentrating gametocytes with subsequent electron microscopic study. As with the studies of causal prophylaxis, these data do not demonstrate whether the effects are due to primaquine or to a metabolite.

In endemic areas the administration of 30–45 mg primaquine once a week to adults (with appropriate paediatric doses for children) would be necessary (and would serve) to prevent transmission of falciparum malaria. If given in combination with a long-acting blood schizontocide such as mefloquine to prevent further development of gametocytes, such a regimen could be limited in time as well[4].

V. Summary of Modes of Action

The 8-aminoquinolines are active against all stages of the life cycle of the malaria parasite except for clinically ineffective activity (i.e. activity at doses fully tolerated by the host) against the asexual blood forms in the simian species, *P. cynomolgi*, and the four human species, *P. vivax*, *P. falciparum*, *P. ovale*, and *P. malariae*. Primaquine is the current prototype in most common use. Although the life cycle of the malaria parasite for each of these species is well characterised, the cellular (and molecular) biology of each of the exoerythrocytic and sexual parasite stages is largely unknown and poorly understood. The presently available data demonstrate that each stage of the parasite during its life cycle is differentially susceptible to primaquine or one or another of its metabolites. There are, furthermore, distinct differences in the susceptibility of the parasite to the 8-aminoquinolines even during the analogous parasitic stage, not only among species but also among different strains of each species. Whether or not there is a final, common molecular mechanism of action of primaquine or its metabolites against the malaria parasite at whatever stage in whatever species or strain is undetermined. In all experimental work in malaria great care must be used to distinguish each effect until full knowledge is attained. This means that studies of radical cure with prevention of relapses, causal prophylaxis, and sporontocidal and gametocytocidal effects must, for the present, be considered separately from each other even for the same antimalarial drug. Scientific investigators and clinicians must remain alert to these differences at all times during their studies and treatment of this most widespread infectious disease.

---

4 These studies, incidentally, provide some of the clearest and most unequivocal data available in the entire literature on the differential effects of antimalarial drugs on falciparum malaria showing:

1. The lack of effect of primaquine against the asexual parasites of either the chloroquine-resistant Malayan strain or the chloroquine-sensitive Ugandan strain
2. The lack of effect of chloroquine against the asexual parasites of the chloroquine-resistant Malayan strain and its immediate effect on the asexual parasites of the chloroquine-sensitive Ugandan strain
3. The efficacy of tetracycline against the asexual parasites of the Malayan strain
4. The lack of effect of chloroquine on gametocytes of either strain and the lack of effect of tetracycline against the gametocytes of the Malayan strain. (Tetracycline was not used against the Ugandan strain in these studies)

D. Pharmacokinetics and Metabolism

During the reinvestigation of primaquine initiated in the World War II Chemotherapy of Malaria Programme in the United States, studies of the pharmacokinetics and metabolism of the 8-aminoquinolines depended on the diazotisation procedure of BRODIE and UDENFRIEND et al. (1946, 1947) (Sect. B.III). Since these procedures measured the parent compounds and did not distinguish metabolites, only limited data could be obtained. Nevertheless, much significant work was done which remains valid and forms the basis for renewed investigations using new technology that are now under way in several laboratories.

With respect to blood levels of the parent drug, e.g. whether pamaquine, pentaquine or primaquine, the results were remarkably similar (ZUBROD et al. 1947; CRAIGE et al. 1947a; BERLINER et al. 1948; EARLE et al. 1948; ALVING et al. 1948a, b; ATCHLEY et al. 1948; EDGECOMB et al. 1950; CLAYMAN et al. 1952). Absorption was rapid, usually peaking by 3 h after oral administration. Disappearance was also rapid, apparently being complete after dosages of 30–60 mg in 12 h or less by these methods, which were sensitive in the range of micrograms per millilitre. Urinary excretion was in the range of less than 1%–3% of administered drug/24 h. Faecal excretion was not measured as it was shown, at least for pamaquine, to be impossible to do because "the compound is rapidly destroyed when incubated at 37 °C in a suspension of feces" (ZUBROD et al. 1947). Additional studies with pamaquine included intramuscular injection in four patients. Comparison of single oral and intramuscular doses of the drug showed that "the peak concentration is higher and is reached earlier after intramuscular injection. Yet, at the end of 3 h, the concentration is approximately the same, regardless of route of administration" (ZUBROD et al. 1947).

After a 15-min intravenous infusion of 20 mg pamaquine, only 5%–6% could be accounted for in the blood. "Such a disappearance cannot be accounted for by metabolism and excretion and must represent localization" (ZUBROD et al. 1947).

In patients receiving daily dosages of these drugs there was a three- to four-fold variation in mean plasma concentrations and, from time to time, individuals with ten times greater blood levels than others receiving the same dosage. The rate of disappearance from the blood did not always correlate with the blood levels. Furthermore, correlation with therapeutic effect, i.e. cure of first attacks and relapses of vivax malaria, was so poor that eventually blood determinations (except for special studies) were discontinued. The lack of correlation of blood levels with therapeutic effect was taken as evidence that the antimalarial activity might be due to a metabolite. If, however, the concept of total dose is considered, this lack of correlation might be irrelevant as only tissue concentrations would be expected to correlate. Recent studies of primaquine by new methods essentially have confirmed the early work showing rapid absorption and virtual elimination of this compound from the blood in 24 h (CARSON et al. 1981; GREAVES et al. 1979, 1980a, b). These studies are all in early phases, however, and considerably more data are needed.

Unless the patient is in remission the 8-aminoquinolines must be given in combination with drugs which suppress or eliminate the asexual blood forms in order to minimise or prevent the clinical manifestations of malaria. Consequently, the effect of concurrent administration of other antimalarial drugs on the kinetics and metabolism of the 8-aminoquinolines is of practical as well as experimental importance. The available data for quinine and chloroquine suggest that they do not markedly change the blood levels of the 8-aminoquinolines although what effect they have on metabolism or tissue distribution is not yet known. Because they do not have tissue schizontocidal activity *per se* but do "potentiate" the efficacy of primaquine, it will be significant to elucidate their effects, if any, on the metabolism of the 8-aminoquinolines.

In contrast to quinine and chloroquine, mepacrine given concurrently with pamaquine caused a marked increase in plasma levels of the 8-aminoquinoline without change in the expected levels of mepacrine. This effect was observed even when pamaquine was given as long as 3 months after the last dose of mepacrine (ZUBROD et al. 1947). When given with pamaquine and pentaquine this drug was associated with significantly increased methaemoglobinaemia and toxicity (ZUBROD et al. 1947; CRAIGE et al. 1947 a; ATCHLEY et al. 1949). Whether the mechanism of these phenomena was due to change in metabolism or of distribution of the 8-aminoquinolines was not determined.

Proguanil given concurrently with pentaquine also raised the plasma level of the 8-aminoquinoline without apparent increase in toxicity of methaemoglobin formation. Therapeutic effect was not enhanced, however (ALVING et al. 1948 b; JONES et al. 1948 a).

Despite the historical and current emphasis on metabolite formation and tissue distribution with respect to antimalarial activity, toxicity, and haemolytic effect, relatively few data are available. Various metabolic degradation schemes and structure-activity relationships have been reviewed and proposed (ALVING et al. 1962; THOMPSON and WERBEL 1972; SMITH 1956; STROTHER et al. 1981). The consensus of these schemes has been to postulate relative stability of the quinoline nucleus with conversion of the 6-methoxy group to a 6-hydroxy derivative, followed by formation of the 5,6-dihydroxy derivative in turn converted to a 5,6-quinolinequinone. The latter two compounds would have clinical activity, e.g. causing methaemoglobinaemia and an antimalarial effect. Human data on formation of these compounds are unavailable and relatively few animal studies have been reported.

ZUBROD et al. (1947) reported that blood and tissue levels in the dog 3 h after administration of 10 mg/kg pamaquine showed maximum localisation in the liver and lung, 28 and 20 times the blood level respectively, with concentrations in the brain and heart approximately ten and five times greater than the blood level.

JOSEPHSON and his colleagues reported identification of the 5,6-quinolinequinone derivative of pamaquine in chicken droppings (JOSEPHSON et al. 1951 a, b).

HUGHES and SCHMIDT (1950) reported studies on the metabolism of various 8-aminoquinolines in rhesus monkeys. They also found peak values of the parent drugs as early as 2 h after either intramuscular or oral administration and rapid elimination from the blood. Because they found large amounts of alkali-soluble, ethylene dichloride-insoluble substances they inferred that a significant proportion of metabolic products could be acidic in nature, a prediction confirmed 32 years later (see below).

SMITH (1956) reported his unique studies on the metabolism of ^{14}C-labelled pentaquine in the rhesus monkey. Two separate compounds were used, one labelled on the 6-methoxy group and one on the 2-position of the terminal isopropyl group (of the aliphatic side chain). Although the rapidity of metabolism was confirmed, quite different results were obtained with respect to the two labels. Three radioactive metabolites from the 6-methoxy label and six from the side chain label were detected. His data showed that the 6-methoxy group was "cleared with extreme rapidity, while the terminal isopropyl group is more resistant to oxidation".

Ryer (1971), using 6-O-methyl-[^{3}H]primaquine in rats, again confirmed rapid metabolism with the greatest concentration in the liver. In a more extensive study Holbrook et al. (1981), also using the tritium-labelled primaquine in rats, found lung to have a greater concentration than liver. Attempts to isolate ^{3}H-labelled quinoline metabolites were unsuccessful.

Strother et al. (1981) reported their studies in dogs using primaquine labelled with tritium in the ring system. They confirmed rapid elimination from the body and utilised modern technology to reveal several metabolites including the 6-hydroxy derivative. They studied model metabolites which rapidly formed methaemoglobin in human G6PD-deficient erythrocytes and in dog erythrocytes to an even greater extent. Incubation of primaquine with a mouse liver microsomal system (containing an NADPH generating system) also produced active methaemoglobin-forming products. These results essentially confirm those of Fraser and Vesell (1968), who also showed increased induction of mechanical fragility in G6PD-deficient cells exposed to putative metabolites.

Studies in man are again being undertaken using newer technology. Baty et al. (1975) using gas chromatography-mass spectrometry reported that 6-methoxy-8-aminoquinoline is a metabolite of primaquine found both in blood and urine. Confirmation of this from other laboratories or by other methods has not yet been forthcoming, however.

Carson et al. (1981) using an HPLC assay with an ultraviolet detection system reported the rapid appearance of three metabolites after ingestion of single doses of 90–120 mg primaquine. Two metabolites were found in blood; one of these but not the other was found in urine as well. In addition a urinary metabolite (not found in the blood) was also demonstrated. One of the metabolites in blood persists for up to 52 h, whereas the other persists for at least 120 h (Nora and Parkhurst, unpublished data). The shorter-lived blood metabolite and the urinary metabolite are as yet unidentified. In a collaborative effort with McChesney, Parkhurst and Nora (1982, unpublished data) have tentatively identified the long-lasting metabolite as a carboxyl derivative with the carboxyl group replacing the terminal amino group on the aliphatic side chain. This compound has not been proposed in previous metabolic schemes although the possibility of such a compound was predicted by Hughes and Schmidt (1950).

Clearly, the renewed studies on primaquine and its pharmacokinetics and metabolism are still in their infancy and much more work is required.

E. Toxicity

I. Introduction

From the outset of human trials of pamaquine against malaria in 1926, serious toxicity was soon recognised. By 1929 Sinton et al. (1930) and many others were to recommend that it should not be used except under close medical supervision. SINTON's extensive reviews (SINTON and BIRD 1928; SINTON et al. 1930) as well as the review by the Malaria Commission of the League of Nations (MALARIA COMMISSION 1933) more than suffice to provide an overall clinical picture of the problems encountered. These included anorexia, epigastric pain, nausea, vomiting, diarrhoea, abdominal cramps, cyanosis, methaemoglobinaemia, albuminuria, haemoglobinuria, jaundice, depression, weakness, and collapse.

Although the recommendation to restrict the use of pamaquine reached by SINTON and many others summarised in the report of the MALARIA COMMISSION can be stated in retrospect as logical, based on an overall analysis of the clinical data, the situation was in fact confusing and controversial for several years[5]. Analysis was further confounded because the manifestations of malaria, especially malignant tertian malaria, are themselves protean. Many workers who used pamaquine claimed little or no toxicity and excellent therapeutic results; others claimed almost exactly the opposite and several deaths were attributed to its use. These matters of opinion appear on an objective basis to have been related to batch and possibly formulation differences of the drug itself, to use of greatly varying dosage schedules with and without concomitant drugs, to the species (and strains) of malaria studied and to the many different populations from which the patients were drawn.

It remained for the World War II Malaria Chemotherapy Programme in the United States with the renewed studies of pamaquine and the large-scale synthesis and development of 8-aminoquinolines to initiate a rational, sufficiently broad programme from which basic studies of toxicity have emerged.

From the results of this programme, toxicity of the 8-aminoquinolines may be discussed most clearly from four aspects, (a) specific neurotoxicity of the plasmocid type (precluding human trial of this class of 8-aminoquinolines), (b) general clinical toxicity of the pamaquine type, (c) induction of haemolytic anaemia in genetically predisposed individuals, especially those with G6PD deficiency, and (d) structural and stereoisomerism.

II. Neurotoxicity

The 8-aminoquinolines in lethal and toxic sublethal doses in various animal studies cause pathological changes in all organ systems including the central nervous system (WISELOGLE 1946). There are significant differences, however, which appear to be related primarily to the structure of the aliphatic side chain. The most striking of these is the specific neurotoxicity of plasmocid and related compounds (see Sect. B.II and Fig. 1). Plasmocid in rhesus monkeys was found to cause severe, irreversible, brain damage that was extraordinarily selective for brain stem nuclei, especially III, IV, VI, and VIII (WISELOGLE 1946; SCHMIDT and SCHMIDT 1949a). This work was confirmed (RICHTER 1949; SCHMIDT and SCHMIDT 1949b; LYLE and SCHMIDT 1962) and comparative studies were also made with pamaquine, penta-

5 Many of the more than 600 papers published by 1933 are either unavailable or to be found only in major university or specialised libraries. Attention of the reader is called therefore to the annual volumes of the *Tropical Diseases Bulletin* (specially from 1927 to 1933) in which the worldwide literature on malaria including all the trials with plasmoquine (pamaquine) is abstracted

quine, isopentaquine, and primaquine (SCHMIDT and SCHMIDT 1951). In studies with lethal doses of these four compounds, neurotoxicity was most marked with pentaquine, which primarily affected the dorsal motor nucleus as well as other areas of the brain stem. In sublethal, reversible intoxication the neuronal damage of these four compounds was "low grade", i.e. not comparable to the plasmocid type of specific neurotoxicity. Eventually the plasmocid effect was again confirmed (SIPE et al. 1973) with electron microscopic studies which revealed that "the most conspicuous and the earliest discernible lesion" in the rhesus monkey is degeneration of neuronal mitochondria in the large multipolar neurons of the selectively targeted nuclei of the brain stem and diencephalon. In view of modern receptor theory further work might reveal molecules of similar configuration which are specifically related to normal function of these brain stem nuclei.

III. General Toxicity of the Pamaquine Type

The basic studies on toxicity of pamaquine and newly synthesised 8-aminoquinolines were conducted principally in rats, dogs, and monkeys. In addition to revealing the plasmocid type of toxicity these studies demonstrated that lethal doses of pamaquine and related compounds affected all organ systems, with hepatotoxicity being perhaps the most prominent feature. The toxic effects of sublethal doses, however, were reversible and were primarily gastrointestinal and haematological (WISELOGLE 1946). Human trial confirmed the latter effects with additional variations from compound to compound (BREWER et al. 1961). Disappearance of toxic manifestations on stopping the drug, i.e. reversibility of toxicity, was demonstrated repeatedly.

General symptoms were headache, anorexia, nausea, vomiting, and diarrhoea but the most prominent symptom was epigastric discomfort, often progressing to severe pain and tenderness with retrosternal radiation (CLAYMAN et al. 1952; BREWER et al. 1961; CRAIGE et al. 1947b; ATCHLEY et al. 1948). Although ingestion of drug with meals alleviated symptoms, studies of gastric acidity showed no deviations from normal (CLAYMAN et al. 1952). Drug fever was not uncommon (ATCHLEY 1948). Both leucocytosis and neutropenia occurred, the former more with primaquine (EDGECOMB et al. 1950; CLAYMAN et al. 1952) and the latter more with pamaquine and pentaquine (CLAYMAN et al. 1952; BREWER et al. 1961; CRAIGE et al. 1947b; ATCHLEY et al. 1948). Electrocardiograms sometimes showed reversible T-wave changes (CLAYMAN et al. 1952; CRAIGE et al. 1947b). In studies with pentaquine three subjects developed postural hypotension which persisted for several months (CRAIGE et al. 1947b). Otherwise toxic manifestations were rapidly reversible on stopping the drug.

Cyanosis was frequently observed primarily related to methaemoglobinaemia (BREWER et al. 1961; CRAIGE et al. 1947a, b; ATCHLEY et al. 1948; ALVING et al. 1948a, b; EARLE et al. 1948; EDGECOMB et al. 1950; JONES et al. 1953; ZUBROD et al. 1947). The appearance of cyanosis was not usually associated with any symptoms per se although methaemoglobinaemia correlated better with general toxicity than blood levels of the parent drug. Pamaquine, pentaquine, isopentaquine, and primaquine all caused methaemoglobinaemia usually only at high doses, i.e. 60 mg or more/day with considerable interindividual variability. Methaemoglobin levels were usually less than 5 g% and levels greater than 12 g% were rare. Observations which still need further investigation, especially in the light of new knowledge and technology include:

1. The finding that methaemoglobinaemia induced by pamaquine and pentaquine was markedly increased during simultaneous administration of mepacrine (and for pamaquine, at least, long after mepacrine had been stopped) (ZUBROD et al. 1947; EARLE et al. 1948; ATCHLEY et al. 1948).

2. The observation that the administration of pentaquine results in a striking diminution of the arterial and venous oxygen saturation of the blood, even after taking into account the lowering of the oxygen-carrying capacity of haemoglobin contributed by combined anaemia and methaemoglobinaemia (CRAIGE et al. 1947 b). (These observations were made before the relationship between 2,3-diphosphoglycerate (2,3DPG) and haemoglobin and its oxygen-carrying capacity were known.)

3. The finding that methaemoglobinaemia at all doses was greater with primaquine than pamaquine, and that quinine could diminish the methaemoglobinaemia induced by primaquine (EDGECOMB et al. 1950; CLAYMAN et al. 1952), and pentaquine (CRAIGE et al. 1947 b) but not that induced by pamaquine (JONES et al. 1948 b; CLAYMAN et al. 1952).

Neither the mechanisms by which mepacrine increases the methaemoglobinaemia induced by pentaquine, or quinine decreases the methaemoglobinaemia induced by primaquine have been elucidated even though the mechanisms for reduction of methaemoglobin, once formed in the human erythrocyte, are now known to be mediated enzymatically (SCHWARTZ and JAFFE 1978). Two specific enzyme activities are involved. Normally methaemoglobin is reduced to haemoglobin by NADH methaemoglobin diaphorase, whose activity is sufficent to reduce the small amounts of methaemoglobin constantly being formed in the circulation, but insufficient to completely overcome the oxidising capacity of compounds such as the 8-aminoquinolines. Homozygous recessive individuals with deficient enzyme activity have constant (non-drug induced) methaemoglobinaemia. Heterozygous individuals have intermediate activity sufficient to prevent methaemoglobinaemia ordinarily but considerably less than normal capacity to withstand the effects of oxidant drugs. Such individuals therefore develop methaemoglobinaemia even with small doses of drugs like primaquine. This was documented, for example, by COHEN et al. (1968) in six American military personnel who became cyanotic on the weekly prophylactic regimen of chloroquine and primaquine used in Southeast Asia during the Vietnam conflict. Studies of the erythrocytes of these individuals not only confirmed decreased enzymatic activity but administration of small amounts of primaquine (and other agents) reinduced methaemoglobinaemia. In addition studies of family members revealed several who were presumably heterozygous for this enzyme deficiency. To what extent persons heterozygous for this condition account for the large interindividual variability observed with respect to methaemoglobinaemia induced by administration of the 8-aminoquinolines is unknown. Conservative calculation suggests an incidence (for heterozygosity) of 1 in 200 and the actual incidence may be greater.

The second enzyme which reduces methaemoglobin in human erythrocytes is NADPH methaemoglobin reductase. To be effective this enzyme must be invoked by addition of an electron exchanger such as methylene blue or ascorbate. In vivo, the administration of methylene blue as an antidote for toxic methaemoglobinaemia was known long before elucidation of this enzymatic activity (Goodman and Gilman 1941). During the studies with primaquine in which concurrent administration of quinine reduced the methaemoglobinaemia induced by primaquine, methylene blue was also tested (Edgecomb et al. 1950; Clayman et al. 1952). This compound was even more effective than quinine, as would be predicted both clinically and biochemically. Presumably the mechanism for quinine protection is different from that of methylene blue as quinine is not haemolytic in G6PD-deficient individuals, whereas methylene blue is. Quinine instead may alter the metabolism of primaquine so that methaemoglobin formation is diminished, whereas methylene blue acts by invoking activity of NADPH methaemoglobin reductase in normal, non-G6PD-deficient individuals.

In this context attention must be given to the requirement of this enzyme for its coenzyme, NADPH. As provision of this coenzyme requires an intact hexose monophosphate shunt for which G6PD activity is the initial step (Fig. 3 and see below), its activity in G6PD-deficient erythrocytes cannot be invoked by methylene blue and indeed methylene blue administered in vivo induces haemolysis in G6PD-deficient individuals (Alving et al. 1962; Brewer and Tarlov 1961). The consequent failure of methaemoglobin reductive capacity via this enzyme activity forms the basis for Brewer's methaemoglobin reduction test (Brewer et al. 1960, 1962 a, b) for G6PD deficiency in which normal erythrocytes in the presence of glucose and methylene blue readily reduce methaemoglobin whereas G6PD-deficient erythrocytes do not.

IV. Primaquine-Induced Haemolytic Anaemia, G6PD Deficiency and Malaria

Haemoglobinuria and haemolytic anaemia were among the toxic reactions attributed to pamaquine during the first years of its use. Realisation that this occurred only in certain susceptible individuals, however, was gradual. During and in the years immediately after the World War II Chemotherapy of Malaria Programme, clinical investigation of this complication became a focus of interest. Earle et al. (1948) in 1947 recorded seven cases of haemolytic anaemia in their renewed studies of pamaquine. Alving and associates established that the general toxicity of primaquine at therapeutic dosages was minimal but that its unsupervised use had one remaining limitation, the induction of acute haemolytic anaemia first observed among male black volunteers (Hockwald et al. 1952).

In the subsequent, now classic, studies by Alving et al. primaquine-induced haemolytic anaemia was shown to be an intrinsic erythrocytic defect (Dern et al. 1953, 1954) associated with formation of Heinz bodies (Beutler et al. 1954a, 1955 a), a function of red-cell age (Beutler et al. 1954b) and a manifestation of multiple-drug sensitivity (Dern et al. 1955, reprinted 1981; Frischer and Carson 1981). A lower than normal level of reduced glutathione (GSH) was found in the erythrocytes of affected individuals (Beutler et al. 1955b). The GSH itself was found to be unstable both in vitro and in vivo (Beutler et al. 1954a, 1955a; Flanagan et al. 1955, 1958; Beutler 1957).

Studies were then undertaken of the recently discovered enzyme, glutathione reductase (GSSG-R), which promptly led, in 1956, to the discovery of G6PD deficiency (CARSON et al. 1956; CARSON 1960)[6]. This condition was then recognised to underlie susceptibility to favism (CROSBY 1956; SANSONE and SEGNI 1957), the fulminating haemolysis associated with ingestion of fava (broad) beans, known since ancient history in the Mediterranean basin. Together with investigations of many populations around the world, G6PD deficiency was eventually revealed to occur in people of all races whose ethnic origins were from endemic malarious regions of the world. The attractive hypothesis followed that this genetic polymorphism protects against malaria as proposed for the sickle-cell gene. Adequate proof for this hypothesis has yet to be adduced, however.

The prevalence and variability of G6PD deficiency has been described in conjunction with the therapeutic regimens of primaquine (Sect. C.II). In this context it should be understood, nevertheless, that affected individuals are normally healthy (CARSON and FRISCHER 1966; CARSON et al. 1981). They do have a decreased erythrocyte life span (BREWER et al. 1961 b), which is not clinically significant. When stressed, however, not only by certain drugs but also during serious intercurrent illnesses, such as acute hepatitis, pneumonia, diabetic acidoses, etc., spontaneous non-drug-induced haemolysis may be precipitated (CARSON and FRISCHER 1966). In addition some affected individuals suffer from chronic, non-spherocytic, haemolytic anaemia (KIRKMAN et al. 1964). Thus although many drugs induce haemolytic anaemia in G6PD-deficient individuals, there are also certain conditions and variations of the deficiency that result in non-drug-induced haemolysis. Moreover, the shortened red-cell life span also suggests that endogenous factors constantly affect red-cell integrity even in the absence of drugs or stresses associated with intercurrent illness.

In addition to G6PD deficiency several other genetically determined conditions have subsequently been found to result in predisposition of affected individuals to haemolysis of the primaquine type (CARSON and FRISCHER 1966; CARSON et al. 1981; CARSON 1968). These are listed in Table 2 and fall into two classes: Enzyme deficiencies of the metabolic system that protects the erythrocyte against oxidant stress, and molecular variants of haemoglobins that are susceptible to oxidant stress. Thus oxidant stress may be considered as the integrating factor involved in erythrocytic susceptibility to haemolysis among those with these genetically determined conditions. The present working hypothesis is that in this erythrocytic biological system the oxidant stress is ultimately hydrogen peroxide formed either di-

---

6 The biological and clinical ramifications consequent to the discovery of G6PD deficiency have been considerable (BEUTLER 1978; CARSON and FRISCHER 1966; FRISCHER and CARSON 1981) but are beyond the scope of this chapter. In addition to the considerations given in this chapter, these include development of the field of haemolytic enzymopathies, contributions to the understanding and use of X-linkage both in cell and population genetics, and development of the field of pharmacogenetics. Sufficient data have also been reported which indicate that (a) further investigation of the whole body metabolism of glucose in G6PD deficiency and related conditions would be productive (CARSON et al. 1963; EPPES et al. 1966, 1969; CARSON 1970) and (b) erythrocytic membrane-cytoplasmic interactions are significant and need further exploration (CARSON et al. 1959, 1963, 1966; CARSON and TARLOV 1962; AJMAR et al. 1968; CARSON 1970; FRISCHER et al. 1973 c)

Table 2. Genetic conditions known to be associated with susceptibility to clinical drug-induced haemolysis

Enzyme deficiencies [a]	Haemoglobins [b, c]
G6PD	Hb Zurich
6-PGD	Hb Buschwick
GSH synthetase	Hb Torino
GSSG reductase	Hb Rush
GSH peroxidase	

[a] See CARSON and FRISCHER (1966)
[b] See LEHMANN and KYNOCH (1976)
[c] Hb E and Hb H demonstrate sulphhydryl instability and are unstable to dichlorophenolindophenol (FRISCHER and BOWMAN 1975). (See also Part I, Chap. 15)

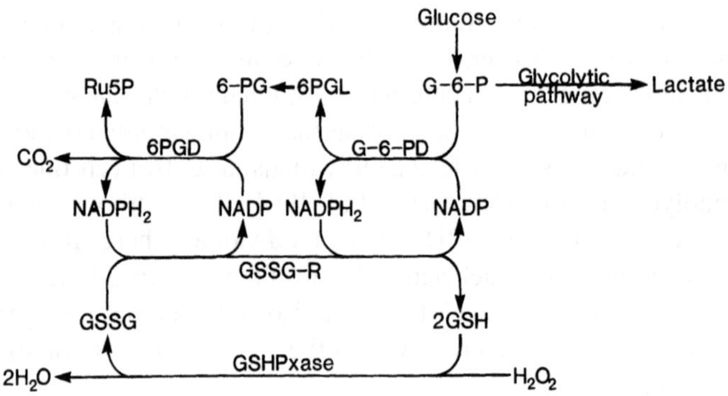

Fig. 3. Enzymatic pathway of glucose oxidation in the human erythrocyte. G6P, glucose-6-phosphate; G6PD, G6P dehydrogenase; 6PG, 6-phosphogluconate; 6PGD, 6-PG dehydrogenase; 6PGL, 6-PG lactone; Ru5P, ribulose-5-phosphate; NADP, oxidised nicotinic adenine dinucleotide phosphate; $NADPH_2$, reduced NADP; GSSG, oxidised glutathione; GSSG-R, glutathione reductase; GSH, reduced glutathione; GSHPxase, glutathione peroxidase

rectly by haemolytic drugs, for example, or indirectly by oxygen radicals which may be converted to hydrogen peroxide via the superoxide dismutase reaction. It is now generally accepted that hydrogen peroxide is detoxified by the glutathione peroxidase reaction and not by catalase despite its high activity in human erythrocytes (BEUTLER 1978; FRISCHER et al. 1968; CARSON and FRISCHER 1966; COHEN and HOCHSTEIN 1963).

In this context the integrity of the biochemical pathways depicted in Fig. 3 is necessary for defence of the human erythrocyte against oxidant stress. In this scheme the erythrocyte normally oxidises only about 10% of the total glucose available while about 90% is utilised via the non-oxidative, glycolytic pathway (MURPHY 1960). When stressed by substances such as methylene blue, ascorbic acid or primaquine, the oxidative system is activated and there is manifold increase of O_2 consumption and CO_2 production. With impairment of the system, e.g. by

G6PD deficiency, CO_2 production fails and the haemolytic sequence can proceed (CARSON et al. 1981; CARSON and FRISCHER 1966).

The exact haemolytic sequence of events has been controversial, especially with respect to the relative roles of the NADP/NADPH and GSSG/GSH systems. In addition KIRKMAN and his associates (KIRKMAN et al. 1980; WILSON et al. 1980) have shown that intact G6PD-deficient erythrocytes are far lessable to withstand stress than would be expected from studies of haemolysates of these cells, a phenomenon which he has called "intracellular restraint". Furthermore, the glutathione instability observed in intact G6PD-deficient erythrocytes both in vitro and in vivo (see below) does not occur in G6PD-deficient haemolysates (CARSON 1968).

In this context we have utilised erythrocytes made GSSG-R deficient by treatment with BCNU [1,3-bis(2-chloroethyl)-*l*-nitrosourea] to compare their CO_2 production with normal and G6PD-deficient erythrocytes. The data obtained revealed two mechanisms for activation of glucose oxidation in human erythrocytes (CARSON et al. 1981). One mechanism, exemplified by methylene blue, operates via the NADP/NADPH system; the other, exemplified by ascorbic acid, operates via the GSSG/GSH system. The latter mechanism is apparently due to formation of H_2O_2, which, when generated by other means such as by xanthine oxidase, also operates via the GSSG/GSH system. [It is also of interest that in intact erythrocytes exposed to H_2O_2 the NAD associated with the NADH methaemoglobin diaphorase is removed (FRISCHER et al. 1973c).]

Classification of drugs by their mechanism of activation of glucose oxidation has been initiated and, in addition to those which act by either one or the other mechanism, several have been found, including primaquine, which are intermediate, i.e. operate via both mechanisms. In addition to extrinsic factors such as drugs, intrinsic factors in plasma and serum exist (as yet unidentified) which can activate glucose oxidation by either mechanism (CARSON et al. 1981).

Several interpretations and possible consequences can be postulated from these considerations with respect to haemolysis and to malaria. Among these are:

1. In G6PD deficiency all compounds which activate glucose oxidation in the human erythrocyte are potentially haemolytic (if not detoxified when administered) regardless of their mechanism of activation. This is because G6PD is the initial reaction in the oxidative system; its deficiency results in failure of the entire system and the cell becomes vulnerable to oxidative haemolysis.

2. Extremely severe GSSG-R deficiency and deficiency of other elements of the GSSG/GSH system will also render the cell susceptible to oxidative haemolysis. GSSG-R deficiency contributes to oxidative haemolysis in vivo (FRISCHER and AHMAD 1977), and favism has not only been reported in GSSG-R deficiency (LOOS et al. 1976) but also in GSH synthetase deficiency (PRINS et al. 1966). This suggests that favism occurs by attack on the GSSG/GSH system. The dosages of methylene blue sufficient to induce haemolysis in GSSG-R deficiency compared with the dosages which cause haemolysis in G6PD deficiency will need to be tested, however.

3. The haemolytic potential of ascorbic acid has not been elucidated even for G6PD deficiency except, perhaps, in massive doses (CAMPBELL et al. 1975). Both *l*-ascorbic and *d*-ascorbic acid generate H_2O_2, and both stimulate CO_2 production in human red-cell incubation systems. As only *l*-ascorbic acid is antiscorbutic its rapid tissue and cellular metabolism may mitigate its potential haemolytic effect.

This potential effect therefore can only be tested with *d*-ascorbic acid (which is not antiscorbutic nor thought to be of biological significance).

4. In G6PD-deficient erythrocytes failure of the NADP/NADPH system necessarily results in failure of the GSSG/GSH system. This allows direct attack by either extrinsic or intrinsic compounds which generate oxygen radicals, H_2O_2 or other peroxides. Thus, the haemolytic activity of methylene blue may be indirect by allowing sufficient accumulation of endogenous substances capable of generating enough H_2O_2 to damage or destroy the red-cell. Similarly, spontaneous non-drug-induced haemolytic anaemia occurring during intercurrent diseases in G6PD-deficient individuals may be induced by increased levels of endogenous substances capable of activating glucose oxidation, either because of increased synthesis or decreased inhibition of their formation.

In this context we have recently demonstrated plasma and serum factors which, in red-cell incubation systems, stimulate glucose oxidation and enhance the activation induced by methylene blue, ascorbic acid and primaquine (CARSON et al. 1981). At least one of these factors (found in serum) is dialysable and heat stable but has not yet been identified (HOHL and CARSON 1982, unpublished data). These considerations are entirely in accord with KIRKMAN's concept of intracellular restraint which suggests that low concentrations of these intrinsic substances might suffice to induce haemolysis.

5. Because one of the major goals in current investigations is to determine whether the antimalarial and haemolytic mechanisms of primaquine are different, the antimalarial activity of primaquine can now be reconsidered. Restudy of the antimalarial activity of methylene blue did reveal that it, like primaquine, acts against the (late) exoerythrocytic stages of the parasite, i.e. as a tissue schizontocide (ALVING et al. 1962; APPEL 1917; LJACHOWETZKY 1924, 1927; PITSCHUGIN 1925; VOROBIEW 1927). There is also evidence suggesting that methylene blue is gametocytocidal (VOROBIEW 1927; THOMSON 1912). Thus the mechanism for the antiparasitic activity of primaquine and methylene blue may be the same. Accordingly, the data indicating retention by primaquine of the methylene blue type of activation of glucose oxidation in GSSG-R-deficient erythrocytes suggests but does not prove that its antimalarial activity may be associated with the NADP/NADPH rather than the GSSG/GSH system. Unfortunately, the same reservation applies to this speculation as to the studies on causal prophylaxis, namely that there may be no carry-over of these erythrocytic mechanisms in the tissues. Moreover, the proven differentiation of the antimalarial and haemolytic activity of dapsone (MCNAMARA et al. 1966) is not necessarily analogous because the antimalarial activity of dapsone is against the asexual blood forms, not the tissue stages.

In addition, despite current dogma, these and previously presented data do not yet prove that a metabolite of primaquine rather than primaquine itself is the actual antiparasitic agent. By contrast the haemolytic effect of primaquine continues likely to be a metabolite, both because of the delay in onset of haemolysis after its administration (given its rapid disappearance from the blood) and because of the considerably greater oxidative activity of postulated metabolites. Furthermore, evidence obtained in this laboratory suggests also that erythrocytic glucose oxidation can be increased 24 h after ingestion of single doses of 90–120 mg primaquine, although little or no primaquine can be demonstrated in the serum or red-cells at this time (CARSON et al. 1981). Neither have we been able to confirm that serum or plasma after ingestion of primaquine have increased capacity to stimulate erythrocytic glucose oxidation. Therefore the possibility that primaquine somehow induces an endogenous factor in the haemolytic sequence cannot be ruled out and differentiation of the antimalarial and haemolytic mechanisms of primaquine continues to be a viable investigative goal.

6. While investigations of this nature offer promise for avoidance of the induction of haemolytic anaemia, practical considerations dictate that epidemiological surveys for G6PD deficiency and nutritional status could be of considerable importance. FRISCHER et al. (1973b) have developed a simple visual test useful in field studies which simultaneously identifies G6PD, GSSG-R, and 6-PGD deficiencies. If desired, the test can be made quantitative by use of a small, inexpensive, battery-operated spectrophotometer. Although genetic deficiency of GSSG-R is extremely rare, decreased activity is associated with malnutrition and riboflavin deficiency. In surveys using this test significantly decreased GSSG-R activity was found in populations in Iran, Ethiopia, and South Vietnam (FRISCHER et al. 1973a) and led to the discovery of the specific inhibition of glutathione reductase by BCNU (FRISCHER 1977; FRISCHER and AHMAD 1977). Thus this test can be used not only to ascertain G6PD deficiency but nutritional status as well.

The test utilises the non-enzymatic reduction of 2,6-dichlorophenolindophenol (DCIP). FRISCHER and BOWMAN (1975) have also developed an equally simple test using DCIP which identifies oxidatively unstable haemoglobins. The most prevalent of these is HbE, which occurs in 30 million or more people in Southeast Asia. Combined use of both tests is entirely feasible. Thus epidemiological surveys in preparation for malaria eradication programmes, for example, could be facilitated with these practical tests evolved from basic research.

V. Isomerism

The role of isomerism in toxicity of the 8-aminoquinolines has received minimal attention. In his review STECK (1972) noted consideration of the possibility that variable isomeric contamination of pamaquine might contribute to toxicity but this was essentially discounted. There are two differences in toxicity among isomers of primaquine, however, which deserve consideration and comment:

1. SCHMIDT et al. (1977a) reported their studies of the comparative curative antimalarial activities and toxicities of primaquine and its *d* and *l* isomers in mice and rhesus monkeys. Primaquine as supplied is the racemate. EINHEBER (as reported by SCHMIDT) compared the acute oral toxicities of the *d* and *l* isomers in mice and found that *d*-primaquine was at least four times as toxic as *l*-primaquine. SCHMIDT and co-workers confirmed these findings in mice but also studied the toxicities of these compounds in rhesus monkeys and found exactly the opposite relationship, i.e. the subacute toxicity of *l*-primaquine is between three and five times that of *d*-primaquine and at least twice that of primaquine. The capacity of all three compounds to effect cure of sporozoite-induced infections of *P. cynomolgi* was, however, essentially identical. By analogy to most other studies with the 8-aminoquinolines the simian rather than the murine results would be more likely to carry-over to human trials. Unfortunately, no studies could be made for haemo-

lytic potential as there are no animal models of G6PD deficiency. (Some tentative predictions could be made for these compounds, however, by comparative studies of glucose oxidation in the red-cell incubation systems.)

Any significant decrease even in gastrointestinal toxicity by use of *d*-primaquine would appear to be well worthwhile. Whether or not the equivalent antimalarial activity demonstrated for *P. cynomolgi* would carry over to *P. vivax* in human infections seems likely but must be tested.

2. Quinocide is an isomer of primaquine with the methyl group on the aliphatic side chain displaced from the 1-position to the 4-position (Fig. 1). This compound was among those synthesised in 1949 during the World War II Chemotherapy of Malaria programme in the United States. It was also synthesised in 1956 in the USSR where it is used with apparently satisfactory therapeutic effect (Alving et al. 1962; Brewer et al. 1961 a). These investigators found that quinocide was more haemolytic than primaquine in G6PD-deficient subjects and caused considerably more gastrointestinal distress. They did not obtain sufficient data to compare its therapeutic index with pamaquine or primaquine, although in two volunteers it appeared to be less effective than primaquine.

These two examples once again demonstrate that even minimal molecular variation between two drugs can be pharmacologically significant.

F. Drug Resistance

In biology there are few "absolutes" and the definition of "true" as opposed to "relative" drug resistance is not always clear. Presumably selection, genetically, of a malaria parasite which is in no way affected by an antimalarial drug (at any biologically possible dose) would represent "true" drug resistance. While this may have happened in a few instances, discussion of most examples and observations refers to "relative" drug resistance.

The phenomenon of drug resistance to the 8-aminoquinolines is, of course, a special aspect of the general subject which with respect to malaria is covered elsewhere in this book. Peters (1970) in his exhaustive compilation of this subject included a review both of experimentally induced resistance to the 8-aminoquinolines in animal species and of the relatively few data on human species.

Drug resistance is also clearly a function of the drug-host-parasite relationship (Powell et al. 1966) as particularly affected by genetic and metabolic factors and for the 8-aminoquinolines must once again be considered according to the various modes of action against the different stages of the parasitic life cycle.

With respect to radical cure and prevention of relapses the relative resistance of Chesson vivax malaria to primaquine was discussed in Sect. C.I. This relative resistance and presumably that of other Southwest Pacific strains of vivax malaria was soon recognised during World War II and still pertains. In this context selection of malaria parasites resistant to various antimalarial drugs is well known and frequently documented (Peters 1970). The widespread emergence of chloroquine-resistant falciparum malaria is perhaps the most important example. To date, however, despite anticipation on general principles, selection of strains of malaria more resistant to primaquine than Chesson vivax malaria has either not occurred or has not spread in sufficient numbers to be of consequence.

ARNOLD et al. (1961) attempted to select a substrain of Chesson vivax malaria resistant to primaquine by use of suboptimal doses and serial passage by subinoculation in volunteers. These were studies therefore of the already weak activity of primaquine against the asexual blood forms. They did, in fact, succeed after 36 sequential subinoculations in demonstrating asexual blood forms with significantly increased resistance to primaquine. Although gametocytes which emerged during these studies were infective to mosquitoes, the apparently viable sporozoites failed to infect human hosts; hence whether these parasites were resistant to primaquine during other stages of their life cycle in man was never determined.

In assessing drug resistance, host factors must be differentiated from parasite factors. A few instances of unusually high blood levels of 8-aminoquinolines without therapeutic effect have been observed (for example, see above). Mistaken attribution of drug resistance to the parasite instead of the host is not uncommon. In the experimental setting this can be worked out as, for example, with apparent resistance to the antimalarial activity of sulphalene (TRENHOLME et al. 1975 a).

Other factors must also be considered in assessing parasite resistance to drugs. The weak efficacy of the 8-aminoquinolines against the asexual blood forms may be due to relative drug resistance of the parasite during this stage of the life cycle. On the other hand, the relative lack of effect may be due to failure of the drug (or its antimalarial metabolite) to reach the parasite. Such possibility apparently does not pertain during the tissue stages. The studies on causal prophylaxis (Sect. C.III) certainly demonstrate not only the effectiveness of primaquine but also the considerable variability in susceptibility of the parasite to this drug at various times of development among different species and strains. While construing these observations as examples of relative drug resistance is not incorrect, they do underscore the need for continuing investigation of the metabolism of the 8-aminoquinolines and the molecular and cellular biology of the malaria parasite.

References

Ajmar F, Scharrer B, Hashimoto F, Carson PE (1968) Interrelation of stromal NAD(P)ase and human erythrocytic 6-phosphogluconic dehydrogenase. Proc Natl Acad Sci USA 59:538–545

Alving AS (1948) Pentaquine (SN-13,276) and isopentaquine (SN-13,274), therapeutic agents effective in reducing relapse rate in vivax malaria. Proc of the fourth intl cong on trop med and malaria, Washington, DC, May 1948. Vol I, pp 734–741. Available from: Department of State, Washington

Alving AS, Arnold J, Hockwald RS, Clayman CB, Dern RJ, Beutler E, Flanagan CL (1955) Potentiation of the curative action of primaquine in vivax malaria by quinine and chloroquine. J Lab Clin Med 46:301–306

Alving AS, Arnold J, Robinson DH (1952) Status of primaquine. 1. Mass therapy of subclinical vivax malaria with primaquine. JAMA 149:1558–1570

Alving AS, Craige B Jr, Jones R Jr, Whorton CM, Pullman TN, Eichelberger L (1948 b) Pentaquine (SN-13,276), a therapeutic agent effective in reducing the relapse rate in vivax malaria. J Clin Invest 27:25–33

Alving AS, Hankey DD, Coatney GR, Jones R Jr, Coker WG, Garrison PL, Donovan WN (1953) Korean vivax malaria. II. Curative treatment with pamaquine and primaquine. Am J Trop Med Hyg 2:970–976

Alving AS, Johnson CF, Tarlow AR, Brewer GJ, Kellermeyer RW, Carson PE (1960) Mitigation of the hemolytic effect of primaquine and enhancement of its action against exoerythrocytic forms of the Chesson strain of *Plasmodium vivax* by intermittent regimes of drug administration. Bull WHO 22:621–631

Alving AS, Powell RD, Brewer GJ, Arnold JD (1962) Malaria, 8-aminoquinolines and haemolysis. In: Goodwin LG and Nimmo-Smith RH (eds) Drugs, parasites, and hosts, pp 83–94. Churchill, London

Alving AS, Pullman TN, Craige B Jr, Jones R Jr, Whorton CM, Eichelberger L (1948a) The clinical trial of eighteen analogues of pamaquine (plasmochin) in vivax malaria (Chesson strain). J Clin Invest 27:34–35

Alving AS, Rucker K, Flanagan CL, Carson PE, Schrier SL, Kellermeyer RW, Tarlov AR (1959) Obervations on primaquine in the prophylaxis and cure of vivax malaria. Proc of the sixth internl congresses on trop med and malaria, Lisbon Sept 1958. vol 7, pp 203–209. Instituto de Medicina Tropical, Lisbon, Anais Inst Med Trop 16:Suppl II

Appel L (1917) Zur Behandlung der Malaria mit Methylenblau und Salvarsan. Dtsch Med Wochenschr 43:1359–1360

Arnold J, Alving AS, Clayman CB, Hockwald RS (1961) Induced primaquine resistance in vivax malaria. Trans R Soc Trop Med Hyg 55:345–350

Arnold J, Alving AS, Hockwald RS, Clayman CB, Dern RJ, Beutler E, Jeffery GM (1954) The effect of continuous and intermittent primaquine therapy on the relapse rate of Chesson strain vivax malaria. J Lab Clin Med 43:429–438

Arnold J, Alving AS, Hockwald RS, Clayman CB, Dern RJ, Beutler E, Flanagan CL, Jeffery GM (1955) The antimalarial action of primaquine against the blood and tissue stages of falciparum malaria (Panama, P-F-6 strain). J Lab Clin Med 43:391–397

Atchley JA, Yount EH, Husted JR, Pullman TN, Alving AS, Eichelberger L (1948) Reactions observed during treatment with pentaquine, administered with quinacrine (atabrine), metachloridine (SN-11,437), and with sulfadiazine. J Nat Mal Soc 7:118–124

Baty JD, Price-Evans DA, Robinson PA (1975) The identification of 6-methoxy 8-aminoquinoline as a metabolite of primaquine in man. Biomed Mass Spectrom 2:304–306

Berliner RW, Earle DP Jr, Taggart JV, Welch WJ, Zubrod CG, Knowlton P, Atchley JA, Shannon JA (1948) Studies on the chemotherapy of the human malarias. VII. The antimalarial activity of pamaquine. J Clin Invest (Suppl) 27:108–113

Beutler E (1957) The glutathione instability of drug-sensitive red cells. J Lab Clin Med 49:84–95

Beutler E (1978) Glucose-6-phosphate dehydrogenase deficiency. In: Stanbury JB, Wyngaarden JB, Predrickson DS (eds) The metabolic basis of inherited disease, 4th edn. McGraw-Hill, New York, pp 1430–1451

Beutler E, Dern RJ, Alving AS (1954a) The hemolytic effect of primaquine. III. A study of primaquine-sensitive erythrocytes. J Lab Clin Med 44:177–184

Beutler E, Dern RJ, Alving AS (1954b) The hemolytic effect of primaquine. IV. The relationship of cell age to hemolysis. J Lab Clin Med 44:439–442

Beutler E, Dern RJ, Alving AS (1955a) The hemolytic effect of primaquine. VI. An *in vitro* test for sensitivity of erythrocytes to primaquine. J Lab Clin Med 45:40–50

Beutler E, Dern RJ, Flanagan CL, Alving AS (1955b) The hemolytic effect of primaquine. VII. Biochemical studies of drug-sensitive erythrocytes. J Lab Clin Med 45:286–295

Brewer GJ, Tarlov AR, Alving AS (1960) Methaemoglobin reduction test. A new, simple, *in vitro* test for identifying primaquine-sensitivity. Bull WHO 22:633–640

Brewer GJ, Tarlov AR, Alving AS (1961a) The toxicity of the 8-aminoquinoline antimalarial drugs. Bull Nat Soc Ind Mal Mosq Dis 9:331–351

Brewer GJ, Tarlov AR, Alving AS (1962a) The methemoglobin reduction test for primaquine-type sensitivity of erythrocytes. A simplified procedure for detecting a specific hypersusceptibility to drug hemolysis. JAMA 180:386–388

Brewer GJ, Tarlov AR (1961) Studies on the mechanism of primaquine-type hemolysis: the effect of methylene blue. Clin Res 9:65

Brewer GJ, Tarlov AR, Kellermeyer RW (1961b) The hemolytic effect of primaquine. XII. Shortened erythrocyte life span in primaquine-sensitive male Negroes in the absence of drug administration. J Lab Clin Med 58:217–224

Brewer GJ, Tarlov AR, Kellermeyer RW, Alving AS (1962b) The hemolytic effect of primaquine. XV. Role of methemoglobin. J Lab Clin Med 59:905–917

Brodie BB, Udenfriend S, Taggart JV (1946) Analysis of basic organic compounds in biological tissues: 4. Coupling with diazonium salts. Fed Proc 5:125–126

Brodie BB, Udenfriend S, Taggart JV (1947) The estimation of basic organic compounds in biological fluids. IV. Estimation by coupling with diazonium salts. J Biol Chem 168:327

Burgess RW, Bray RS (1961) The effect of a single dose of primaquine on the gametocytes, gametogony, and sporogony of *Laverania falciparum*. Bull WHO 24:451–456

Campbell GD Jr, Steinberg MH, Bower JD (1975) Ascorbic acid induced hemolysis in glucose-6-phosphate dehydrogenase deficiency. Ann Intern Med 82:810

Carson PE (1960) Glucose-6-phosphate dehydrogenase deficiency in hemolytic anemia. Fed Proc 19:995–1006

Carson PE (1968) Hemolysis due to inherited erythrocyte enzyme deficiencies. In: Conference on pharmacogenetics. Ann NY Acad Sci 151:765–776

Carson PE (1970) Clinical metabolic and molecular consequences of disorders of the pentose phosphate pathway. International symposium on pharmacogenetics, Royal Society of Medicine (1969) Proc R Soc Med 63:175–176

Carson, PE, Ajmar F, Hashimoto F, Bowman JE (1966) Electrophoretic demonstration of stromal effects on haemolysate glucose-6-phosphate dehydrogenase and 6-phosphogluconic dehydrogenase. Nature 210:813–815

Carson PE, Flanagan CL, Ickes CE, Alving AS (1956) Enzymatic deficiency in primaquine-sensitive erythrocytes. Science 124:484–485

Carson PE, Frischer H (1966) Glucose-6-phosphate dehydrogenase deficiency and related disorders of the pentose phosphate pathway. Am J Med 41:744–761

Carson PE, Hohl R, Nora MV, Parkhurst GW, Ahmad T, Scanlan S, Frischer H (1981) Toxicology of the 8-aminoquinolines and genetic factors associated with their toxicity in man. Bull WHO 59:427–437

Carson PE, Okita GT, Frischer H, Hirasa J, Long WK, Brewer GJ (1963) Patterns of hemolytic susceptibility and metabolism. Proc 9th congr Europ Soc Haemat, Lisbon 1963, pp 655–665. Karger, Basel

Carson PE, Schrier SL, Kellermeyer RW (1959) Glucose-6-phosphate dehydrogenase and human erythrocytes: characteristics of glucose-6-phosphate dehydrogenase from normal and primaquine-sensitive erythrocytes. Nature 184:1291–1293

Carson PE, Tarlov AR (1962) Biochemistry of hemolysis. Ann Rev Med 13:105–126

Cedillos RA, Warren M, Jeffery GM (1978) Field evaluation of primaquine in the control of *Plasmodium vivax*. Am J Trop Med Hyg 27:466–472

Clayman CB, Arnold J, Hockwold RS, Yount EH, Edgcomb JH, Alving AS (1952) Toxicity of primaquine in Caucasians. JAMA 149:1563–1568

Clyde DF, McCarthy VC (1977) Brief communications. Radical cure of Chesson strain vivax malaria in man by 7, not 14 days of treatment with primaquine. Am J Trop Med Hyg 26:562–563

Coatney GR, Alving AS, Jones R Jr, Hankey DD, Robinson DH, Garison PL, Coker WG, Donovan WN, DiLorenzo A, Marx RL, Simmons IH (1953) Korean vivax malaria. V. Cure of the infection by primaquine administered during long-term latency. Am J Trop Med Hyg 2:985–988

Coggeshall LT, Rice FA, Yount ER Jr (1948) The cure of recurrent vivax malaria and status of immunity thereafter. Proc fourth intl congresses of trop med and mal. Washington DC May 1948. vol I, pp 749–755. Available from: Department of State, Washington

Coggeshall LT, Rice FA (1949) Cure of chronic vivax malaria with pentaquine. JAMA 139:437–439

Cohen G, Hochstein P (1963) Gluthathione peroxidase: the primary agent for the elimination of hydrogen peroxide in erythrocytes. Biochemistry 2:1420–1428

Cohen RJ, Sachs JR, Wicker DJ, Conrad ME (1968) Methemoglobinemia provoked by malarial chemoprophylaxis in Vietnam. N Engl J Med 279:1127–1131

Cooper WC, Myatt AV, Hernandez T, Jeffery GM, Coatney GR (1953) Studies in human malaria. XXXI. Comparison of primaquine, isopentaquine, SN-3883, and pamaquine as curative agents against Chesson strain vivax malaria. Am J Trop Med Hyg 2:949–957

Craige B Jr, Eichelberger L, Jones R Jr, Alving AS, Pullman TN, Whorton CM (1947b) The toxicity of large doses of pentaquine (SN-13,276), a new antimalarial drug. J Clin Invest 27:17–24

Craige B Jr, Jones R Jr, Whorton CM, Pullman TN, Alving AS, Eichelberger L (1947a) Clinical standardization of pamaquine (plasmochin) in mosquito-induced vivax malaria, Chesson strain. A preliminary report. Am J Trop Med 27:309–315

Crosby WH (1956) Newsletter. Favism in Sardinia. Blood 11:91

Dern RJ, Beutler E, Alving AS (1954) Clinical and experimental. The hemolytic effect of primaquine. The natural course of the hemolytic anemia and the mechanism of its self-limited character. J Lab Clin Med 44:171–176

Dern RJ, Beutler E, Alving AS (1955) The hemolytic effect of primaquine. V. Primaquine sensitivity as a manifestation of a multiple drug sensitivity. J Lab Clin Med 45:30–39; reprinted (1981) J Lab Clin Med 97:750–759

Dern RJ, Weinstein IM, LeRoy GV, Talmage DW, Alving AS (1953) The hemolytic effect of primaquine. I. The localization of the drug-induced hemolytic defect in primaquine-sensitive individuals. J Lab Clin Med 43:303–309

DiLorenzo A, Marx RL, Alving AS, Jones R Jr (1953) Korean vivax malaria. IV. Curative effect of 15 milligrams of primaquine daily for 7 days. Am J Trop Med Hyg 2:983–984

Earle DP Jr, Bigelow FS, Zubrod CG, Kane CA (1948) Studies on the chemotherapy of the human malarias. IX. Effect of pamaquine on the blood cells of man. J Clin Invest (Suppl) 27:121–129

Edgecomb JH, Arnold J, Yount EH Jr, Alving AS, Eichelberger L (1950) Primaquine, SN-13,272, a new curative agent in vivax malaria: A preliminary report. J Nat Mal Soc 9:285–292

Eppes RB, Brewer CJ, DeGowin RL, McNamara JV, Flanagan CL, Schrier SL, Tarlov AR, Powell RD, Carson PE (1966) Oral glucose tolerance in Negro men deficient in glucose-6-phosphate dehydrogenase. N Engl J Med 275:855–861

Eppes RB, Lawrence AM, McNamara JV, Powell RD, Carson PE (1969) Intravenous glucose tolerance in Negro men deficient in glucose-6-phosphate dehydrogenase. N Engl J Med 281:60–63

Ehrman FC, Ellis JM, Young MD (1945) *Plasmodium vivax* Chesson strain. Science 101:377

Fairley NH (1945) Chemotherapeutic suppression and prophylaxis in malaria. An experimental investigation undertaken by medical research teams in Australia. Trans R Soc Trop Med Hyg 38:311–355

Fairley NH (1947) Sidelights on malaria in man obtained by subinoculation experiments. Trans R Soc Trop Med Hyg 40:621–676

Farbenindustrie IG (1928) Redaktionelle Notiz. Archiv für Schiffs- und Tropen-Hygiene 32:382

Feldman HA, Packer H, Murphy FD, Watson RB (1946) Pamaquine naphthoate as a prophylactic for malarial infections. The American Association of Immunologists. Thirtieth annual meeting. Fed Proc 5:244

Flanagan CL, Beutler E, Dern RJ, Alving AS (1955) Biochemical changes in erythrocytes during hemolysis induced by aniline derivatives. J Lab Clin Med 46:814

Flanagan CL, Schrier SL, Carson PE, Alving AS (1958) The hemolytic effect of primaquine. VIII. The effect of drug administration on parameters of primaquine sensitivity. J Lab Clin Med 51:600–608

Fletcher W (1933) New drugs in the treatment of malaria. Trop Dis Bull 30:193–202

Fraser IM, Vesell ES (1968) Effects of metabolites of primaquine and acetanilid on normal and glucose-6-phosphate dehydrogenase deficient erythrocytes. J Pharmacol Exp Ther 162:155–165

Frischer H (1977) Erythrocytic glutathione reductase deficiency in a hospital population in the United States. Am J Hematol 2:327–344

Frischer H, Ahmad T (1977) Severe generalized glutathione reductase deficiency after antitumor chemotherapy with BCNU [1,3-bis(chlorethyl)-l-nitrosourea]. J Lab Clin Med 89:1080–1091

Frischer H, Carson PE (1981) Multiple gene interactions in pharmacogenetics. J Lab Clin Med 97:760–763

Frischer H, Bowman JE (1975) Hemoglobin E, an oxidatively unstable mutation. J Lab Clin Med 85:531–539

Frischer H, Bowman JE, Carson PE, Rieckmann KH, Willerson D Jr, Colwell EJ (1973 a) Erythrocytic glutathione reductase, glucose-6-phosphate dehydrogenase and 6-phosphogluconic dehydrogenase deficiencies in populations of the USA, South Vietnam, Iran, and Ethiopia. J Lab Clin Med 81:603–612

Frischer H, Carson PE, Bowman JE, Rieckmann KH (1973 b) Visual test for erythrocytic glucose-6-phosphate dehydrogenase, 6-phosphogluconic dehydrogenase, and glutathione reductase deficiencies. J Lab Clin Med 81:613–624

Frischer H, McNamara J, Rieckmann KH, Stockert T, Powell RD, Carson PE (1968) H_2O_2 effects on intracellular enzymes and glutathione; activation of glutathione reductase. Clin Res 16:303

Frischer H, Nelson R, Noyes C, Carson PE, Bowman JE, Rieckmann KH, Ajmar F (1973 c) NAD(P)-glycohydrolase deficiency in human erythrocytes and alteration of cytosol NADH-methemoglobin diaphorase by membrane NAD-glycohydrolase activity. Proc Natl Acad Sci USA 70:2406–2410

Garrison PL, Hankey DD, Coker WG, Donovan WM, Jastranski B, Coatney GR, Alving AS, Jones R Jr (1952) Cure of Korean vivax malaria with pamaquine and primaquine. JAMA 149:1562–1563

Goodman L, Gilman A (1941) Methylene blue. Cyanosis. In: The pharmacological basis of therapeutics, 1st edn. MacMillan, New York, pp 868–870, 1031–1033

Greaves J, Evans DAP, Gilles HM, Fletcher KA, Bunnag D, Harinasuta T (1980 b) Plasma kinetics and urinary excretion of primaquine in man. Br J Clin Pharmacol 10:399–405

Greaves J, Evans DAP, Fletcher KA (1980 a) Urinary primaquine excretion and red cell methaemoglobin levels in man following a primaquine: chloroquine regimen. Br J Clin Pharmacol 10:293–295

Greaves J, Price-Evans DA, Gilles HM, Baty JD (1979) A selected ion monitoring assay for primaquine in plasma and urine. Biomed Mass Spectrom 6:109–112

Gunders AE (1961) The effect of a single dose of pyrimethamine and primaquine in combination upon gametocytes and sporogony of *Laverania falcipara* (*Plasmodium falciparum*) in Liberia. Bull WHO 24:650–653

Guttman P, Ehrlich P (1981) Über die Wirkung des Methylenblau bei Malaria. Berl Klin Wochenschr 28:953–956

Hankey DD, Jones R Jr, Coatney GR, Alving AS, Coker WG, Garrison PL, Donovan WN (1953) Korean vivax malaria. I. Natural history and response to chloroquine. Am J Trop Med Hyg 2:958–969

Hawking F, Perry WLM, Thurston JP (1948) Tissue forms of a malaria parasite, *Plasmodium cynomolgi*. Lancet 1:783–789

Hockwald RS, Arnold J, Clayman CB, Alving AS (1952) 4. Toxicity of primaquine in negroes. JAMA 149:1568–1570

Holbrook DJ Jr, Griffin JB, Fowler L, Gibson BR (1981) Tissue distribution of primaquine in the rat. Pharmacology 22:330–336

Horlein (1926) Über die chemischen Grundlagen und die Entwicklungs-Geschichte des Plasmochins. Archiv für Schiffs- und Tropen-Hygiene 30 (Suppl 1–3):305–310

Hughes HB, Schmidt LH (1950) Metabolism of various 8-aminoquinolines in rhesus monkey. Proc Soc Exp Biol Med 73:581–585

James SP (1931 a) Some general results of a study of induced malaria in England. Trans R Soc Trop Med Hyg 24:477–525

James SP (1931 b) On the prevention of malaria with plasmoquine. Lancet:341–345

James SP, Nicol WD, Shute PG (1931) A drug which prevents malaria. Lancet:1248–1249

Jarvis OD (1932) Further researches into the treatment of chronic B.T. malaria with plasmoquine and quinine. Indian J Med Res 20:627, and J R Army Med Corps 59:190

Jeffery GM, Collins WE, Skinner JC (1963) Antimalarial drug trials on a multi-resistant strain of *Plasmodium falciparum*. Am J Trop Med Hyg 12:844–850

Jeffery GM, Wolcott GB, Young MD, Williams D Jr (1952) Exoerythrocytic stages of *Plasmodium falciparum*. Am J Trop Med Hyg 1:917–926

Jeffery GM, Young MD, Eyles DE (1956) The treatment of *Plasmodium falciparum* infection with chloroquine, with a note on infectivity to mosquitoes of primaquine- and pyrimethamine-treated cases. Am J Hyg 64:1–11

Jones R Jr, Craige B Jr, Alving AS, Whorton MC, Pullman TN, Eichelberger L (1948 b) A study of the prophylactic effectiveness of several 8-aminoquinolines in sporozoite-induced vivax malaria (Chesson strain). J Clin Invest (Suppl) 27:6–11

Jones R Jr, Pullman TN, Whorton CM, Craige B Jr, Alving AS, Eichelberger L (1948 a) The therapeutic effectiveness of large doses of paludrine in acute attacks of sporozoite-induced vivax malaria (Chesson strain). J Clin Invest 27:51–55

Jones R Jr, Jackson LS, DiLorenzo A, Marx RL, Levy BL, Kenney EC, Gilbert M, Johnston MN, Alving AS (1953) Korean vivax malaria. III. Curative effect and toxicity of primaquine in doses from 10 to 30 mg daily. Am J Trop Med Hyg 2:977–982

Josephson ES, Greenberg J, Taylor DJ, Bami HL (1951 a) A metabolite of pamaquine from chickens. J Pharmacol Exp Ther 103:7–9

Josephson ES, Taylor DJ, Greenberg J, Amar PR (1951 b) A metabolic intermediate of pamaquine for chickens. Proc Soc Exp Biol Med 96:700–703

Kass L, Willerson D Jr, Rieckmann KH, Carson PE, Becker RP (1971 a) *Plasmodium falciparum* gametocytes. Electron microscopic observations on material obtained by a new method. Am Soc Trop Med Hyg 20:187–194

Kass L, Willerson D Jr, Rieckmann KH, Carson PE (1971 b) Blastoid transformation of lymphocytes in falciparum malaria. Am Soc Trop Med Hyg 20:195–198

Kelleher MFH, Thompson K (1945) Treatment of malaria. Lancet 2:217

Kellermeyer RW, Tarlov AR, Brewer GJ, Carson PE, Alving AS (1962) Hemolytic effect of therapeutic drugs. Clinical considerations of the primaquine-type hemolysis. JAMA 180:388–394

Kellermeyer RW, Tarlov AR, Schrier SL, Carson PE, Alving AS (1961) The hemolytic effect of primaquine. XIII. Gradient susceptibility to hemolysis of primaquine-sensitive erythrocytes. J Lab Clin Med 58:225–233

Kirkman HN, Rosenthal IM, Simon ER, Carson PE (1964) "Chicago I" type of glucose-6-phosphate dehydrogenase in congenital hemolytic disease. J Lab Clin Med 63:715–725

Kirkman HN, Wilson WG, Clemons EH (1980) Regulations of glucose-6-phosphate dehydrogenase. I. Intact red cells. J Lab Clin Med 95:876–887

Krotoski WA, Garnham PCC, Bray RS, Krotoski DM, Killick-Kendrick R, Draper CC, Targett GAT, Guy MW (1982) Observations on early and late post-sporozoite tissue stages in primate malaria. I. Discovery of a new latent form of *Plasmodium cynomolgi* (the hypnozoite), and failure to detect hepatic forms within the first 24 h after infection. Am J Trop Med Hyg 31:24–35

Krotoski WA, Krotoski DM, Garnham PCC, Bray RS, Killick-Kendrick R, Draper CC, Targett GAT, Guy MW (1980) Relapse in primate malaria: discovery of two populations of exoerythrocytic stages. Preliminary note. Br Med J (Jan):153–154

Lehmann H, Kynoch PAM (1976) Human hemoglobin variants and their characteristics. Elsevier, Amsterdam

Ljachowetzky AM (1924) Combined treatment of malaria by intravenous injections of methylene-blue and neosalvarsan. Russian J Trop Med 2:3–10

Ljachowetzky AM (1927) Treatment of chronic malaria. Russian J Trop Med 5:202–204

Loos H, Roos D, Weening R (1976) Familial deficiency of glutathione reductase in human blood cells. Blood 48:53–62

Lyle DJ, Schmidt IG (1962) The selective effect of drugs upon nuclei of the oculogyric system. Am J Opthalmol 54:706–716

Manifold JA (1931) Report on trial of plasmoquine and quinine in treatment of of benign tertian malaria. J R Army Med Corp 56:321, 410

Malaria Commission (1933) Third General Report Therapeutics of Malaria. I. General aims. In: League of Nations. Bull WHO 2:185–285

Malaria Commission (1937) Fourth General Report. The treatment of malaria. In: League of Nations. Bull WHO 6:1011–1012

McNamara JV, Eppes RB, Powell RD, Carson PE (1966) The effects of para-aminobenzoic acid on the hemolytic effects of 4,4′-diaminodiphenylsulfone. Milit Med 131:1057–1060

Most H, Kane CA, Lavietes PH, London IM, Schroeder FE, Hayman JM (1946) Combined quinine-plasmochin treatment of vivax malaria: effect on relapse rate. Am J Med Sci 212:550–560

Murphy JR (1960) Erythrocyte metabolism. II. Glucose metabolism and pathways. J Lab Clin Med 55:286–302

Peters W (1970) Experimental drug resistance II 8-aminoquinolines and other compounds. Pamaquine. Quinine, mepacrine, 8-aminoquinolines and hydroxynaphthalenes. Primaquine, quinine, mepacrine, 8-aminoquinolines, and hydroxynaphthalenes. WIN 5037; 6-methoxy-8-(5-propylaminoamylamino) quinoline phosphate. In: Chemotherapy and drug resistance in malaria. Academic, London, pp 286, 449, 453

Pitschugin PI (1925) Das Methylenblau bei Behandlung von Malaria bei Kindern. Jahrb f Kinderheilkunde 108 (5–6):347–353

Powell RD, Brewer GJ (1967) Effects of pyrimethamine, chlorguanide, and primaquine against exoerythrocytic forms of a strain of chloroquine-resistant *Plasmodium falciparum* from Thailand. Am J Trop Med Hyg 16:693–698

Powell RD, Brewer GJ, DeGowin RL, Carson PE (1966) Effects of glucose-6-phosphate dehydrogenase deficiency upon the host and upon host-drug-malaria parasite interactions. Milit Med 131:1039–1056

Prins HK, Oort M, Loos JA, Zurcher C, Beckers T (1966) Congenital non-spherocytic hemolytic anemia, associated with glutathione deficiency of the erythrocytes. Blood 27:145

Raffaele G, Carrescia PM (1961) Efficacia dosi di sintesi Azione della primachina. Riv Malar 41:51–59

Rajagopalan TG, Anjaneyulu B, Shanbag VD, Grewal RS (1981) Electron-capture gas chromatographic assay for primaquine in blood. J Chromatogr 224:265–273

Rieckmann KH, McNamara JV, Frischer H, Stockert TA, Carson PE, Powell RD (1968) Gametocytocidal and sporontocidal effects of primaquine and of sulfadiazine with pyrimethamine in a chloroquine-resistant strain of *Plasmodium falciparum*. Bull WHO 38:625–632

Rieckmann KH, McNamara JV, Kass L, Powell RD (1969) Gametocytocidal and sporontocidal effects of primaquine upon two strains of *Plasmodium falciparum*. Milit Med 134:802–819

Rieckmann KH, Trenholme GM, Williams RL, Carson PE, Frischer H, Desjardins RE (1974) Prophylactic activity of mefloquine hydrochloride (WR 142490) in drug-resistant malaria. Bull WHO 51:375–377

Richter RB (1949) The effect of certain quinoline compounds upon the nervous system of monkeys. J Neuropathol Exp Neurol 8:155–169

Roehl (1926) Die Wirkung des Plasmochins auf die Vogel Malaria. Naturwissenschaften 14:1156–1159

Ruhe DS, Cooper WC, Coatney GR, Josephson ES (1949) Studies in human malaria XV. The therapeutic action of pamaquine (Plasmochin) against St. Elizabeth strain vivax malaria. Am J Hyg 49:367–373

Ryer HF (1971) The distribution, excretion and retention of primaquine-o-methyl-^{3}H-diphosphate following oral administration to rats. Fed Proc 30:335

Salvidio E, Pannacciulli I, Tizianello A, Ajmar (1967) Nature of hemolytic crises and the fate of G-6-PD deficient, drug-damaged erythrocytes in Sardinians. N Engl J Med 276:1339–1344

Sansone G, Segni G (1957) Sensitivity to broad beans. Lancet 2:295

Schmidt IG, Schmidt LH (1949a) Neurotoxicity of the 8-aminoquinolines. I. Lesions in the central nervous system of the rhesus monkey induced by administration of plasmocid J Neuropathol Exp Neurol 7:368–393

Schmidt IG, Schmidt LH (1949b) Neurotoxicity of the 8-aminoquinolines. II. Reactions of various experimental animals to plasmocid. J Comp Neurol 91:337–367

Schmidt IG, Schmidt LH (1951) Neurotoxicity of the 8-aminoquinolines. III. The effects of pentaquine, isopentaquine, primaquine, and pamaquine on the central nervous system of the rhesus monkey. J Neuropathol Exp Neurol 10:231–256

Schmidt LH (1981) Comparative efficacies of quinine and chloroquine as companions to primaquine in a curative drug regimen. Am J Trop Med Hyg 30:20–25

Schmidt LH (1982) *Plasmodium cynomolgi* infections in the rhesus monkey. Background of studies. Am J Trop Med Hyg 31: Part 2, pp 609–611

Schmidt LH, Alexander S, Allen L, Rasco J (1977 a) Comparison of the curative antimalarial activities and toxicities of primaquine and its *d* and *l* isomers. Antimicrob Agents Chemother 12:51–60

Schmidt LH, Coatney GR (1955) Review of investigations in malaria chemotherapy (USA) 1946 to 1954. Am J Trop Med Hyg 4:203–216

Schmidt LH, Fradkin R, Genther CS, Hughes HB (1982 c) III. Delineation of the potentials of primaquine as a radical curative and prophylactic drug. Am J Trop Med Hyg 31:666–680

Schmidt LH, Fradkin R, Genther CS, Rossan R, Squires W (1982 a) I. The characteristics of untreated sporozoite-induced and trophozoite-induced infections. Am J Trop Med Hyg 31:612–645

Schmidt LH, Fradkin R, Genther CS, Rossan R, Squires W (1982 b) II. Responses of sporozoite-induced and trophozoite-induced infections to standard antimalarial drugs. Am J Trop Med Hyg 31:646–665

Schmidt LH, Fradkin R, Vaughan D, Rasco J (1977 b) Radical cure of infections with *Plasmodium cynomolgi*: A function of total 8-aminoquinoline dose. Am J Trop Med Hyg 26:1116–1128

Schmidt LH, Genther CS, Rosan RN (1982d) IV. Acquisition of *Anopheles quadrimaculatus* infected with the M strain and *Anopheles freeborni* infected with the M, B, or Ro strain. Am J Trop Med Hyg 31:681–698

Schulemann W (1932) Synthetic anti-malarial preparations. Proc Roy Soc Med 25:897–905

Schwartz JM, Jaffe ER (1978) Hereditary methemoglobinemia with deficiency of NADH dehydrogenase. In: Stanbury JB, Wyngaarden JB, Fredrickson DS (eds) The metabolic basis of inherited disease, 4th edn. McGraw-Hill, New York, p 1430

Shortt HE, Fairley NH, Covell G, Shute PG, Garnham PCC (1949) The pre-erythrocytic stage of *Plasmodium falciparum*. Trans R Soc Trop Med Hyg 44:405–419

Shortt HE, Garnham PCC (1948) Demonstration of a persisting exoerythrocytic cycle in *Plasmodium cynomolgi* and its bearing on the production of relapses. Br Med J 1:1225–1232

Shortt HE, Garnham PCC, Covell G, Shute PG (1948) The pre-erythrocytic stage of human malaria, *Plasmodium vivax*. Br Med J 1:1547

Sinton JA, Bird W (1928) Studies in malaria, with special reference to treatment. Part IX. Plasmoquine in the treatment of malaria. Indian J Med Res 16:159–177

Sinton JA, Smith S, Pottinger D (1930) Studies in malaria, with special reference to treatment. Part XII. Further researches into the treatment of chronic benign tertian malaria with plasmoquine and quinine. Indian J Med Res 17:793–814

Sipe JC, Vick NA, Schulman S, Fernandez C (1973) Plasmocid encephalopathy in the rhesus monkey: a study of selective vulnerability. J Neuropathol Exp Neurol 32:446–457

Smith CC (1956) Metabolism of pentaquine in the rhesus monkey. J Pharmacol 116:67–76

Steck EA (1972) Pamaquine. In: The chemotherapy of protozoan diseases. vol III, sect 4–5, pp 23, 147–23, 151. Division of medicinal chemistry, Walter Reed Army Institute of Research, Washington

Strother A, Fraser IM, Allahyari R, Tilton BE (1981) Metabolism of 8-aminoquinoline antimalarial agents. Bull WHO 59:413–425

Thaeler AD Jr, Arnold J, Alving AS (1953) A clinical study of primaquine (SN-13,272) in the treatment of malaria among the Miskito Indians of Nicaragua. Am J Trop Med Hyg 2:989–999

Thompson PE, Werbel LM (1972) 8-Aminoquinolines. In: Antimalarial agents, chemistry and pharmacology. Medicinal chemistry, vol 12. Academic, New York, p 101

Thomson D (1912) The destruction of crescents: conclusions regarding the prevention of malaria by the administration of quinine. Ann Trop Med Parasitol 6:223–230
Trenholme GM, Williams RL, Frischer H, Carson PE, Rieckmann KH (1975a) Host failure in treatment of malaria with sulfalene and pyrimethamine. Ann Intern Med 82:219–223
Trenholme GM, Williams RL, Desjardins RE, Canfield CJ, Carson PE, Frischer H, Rieckmann KH (1975b) Mefloquine in the treatment of human malaria. Science 190:792–795
Vivona S, Brewer GJ, Conrad M, Alving AS (1961) The concurrent weekly administration of chloroquine and primaquine for the prevention of Korean vivax malaria. Bull WHO 25:267–269
Vorobiew (1927) Appel's method for the treatment of malaria. Russ J Trop Med 5:406–414
Wilson W, Kirkman HN, Clemons EH (1980) Regulation of glucose-6-phosphate dehydrogenase. II. Resealed red cell ghosts. J Lab Clin Med 95:888–896
Wiselogle FY (ed) (1946) A survey of antimalarial drugs 1941–1945, vol I. Edwards Brothers, Ann Arbor, pp 1–536
Young MD (1959) The effect of small doses of primaquine upon malarial infections. Indian J Malar 13:69–74
Ziai M, Amirhakim GH, Reinhold JG, Tabatabaee M, Gettner M, Bowman JE (1967) Malaria prophylaxis and treatment in G-6-PD deficiency. An observation on the toxicity of primaquine and chloroquine. Clin Pediatr (Phila) 6:242–243
Zubrod CG, Kennedy TJ, Shannon JA (1947) Studies on the chemotherapy of the human malarias. VIII. The physiological disposition of pamaquine. J Clin Invest 27:114–120

CHAPTER 4

Sulphonamides and Sulphones

H. J. SCHOLER, R. LEIMER, and R. RICHLE

A. Introduction

This chapter is focused on the sulphonamides and sulphones[1] which are in current use as antimalarial drugs (mostly in combination with pyrimethamine). These are, mainly, the sulphonamides sulfamonomethoxine, sulfadoxine and sulfalene, the sulphone dapsone and, to some extent, also the derivatives of dapsone, diformyldapsone and acedapsone. Only the properties of the single drugs are discussed. (For those of the combinations with pyrimethamine and other inhibitors of dihydrofolic acid reductase, see this part, Chap. 6.) The sulphonamide probably best known, sulfadiazine, is included in most paragraphs as a reference, although it is not considered an antimalarial.

B. Chemistry

I. Structure

1. Sulphonamides

The sulphonamides are derivatives of sulphanilamide, which is the amide of sulphanilic acid (4-aminobenzene sulphonic acid). The individual drugs are characterised by a specific substituent, R, at the amido nitrogen of sulphanilamide which is commonly referred to as N^1, whereas their amino nitrogen referred to as N^4 must be free (unsubstituted). In many of the sulphonamides in current use as antibacterial drugs and in all those used as antimalarials, R is a six-membered aromatic ring (a pyrimidine or a pyrazine) with one or two methoxy groups (Table 1).

2. Sulphones

The sulphones used in chemotherapy – mainly in leprosy and, secondarily, in malaria – are bis (4-aminophenyl) sulphone (dapsone) and a few derivatives thereof, mostly with two equal substitutents $R_1 = R_2$ at the two amino groups. The most important drugs are dapsone itself, and its bis-formyl and bis-acetyl derivatives which essentially act as chemical slow releasers of the parent compound (Table 2).

---

1 It is customary in Great Britain to use "ph" in spelling the words "sulphonamide", "sulphone", etc. The spellings "sulfonamide" and "sulfone" are used in the United States and many other countries, and have been adopted for the spelling of individual compounds, e.g. as "International Nonproprietary Names (INN)" by the World Health Organization. [Eds.]

Table 1. Chemical structure of sulphonamides

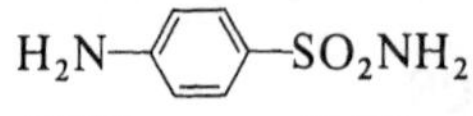
Sulphanilamide
("N^4") ("N^1")

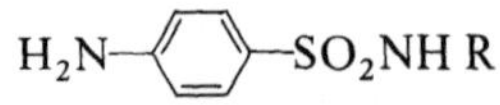

R:

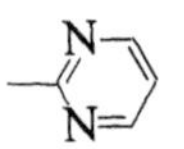
MW 250.28; MP 252–256 °C
N^1-2-Pyrimidinylsulphanilamide
=2-Sulphanilamidopyrimidine
Generic name: *sulfadiazine*

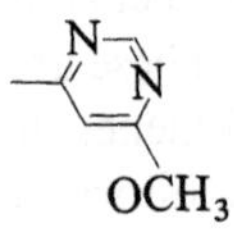
MW 280.32; MP 203–205 °C
N^1-(6-Methoxy-4-pyrimidinyl) sulphanilamide
=4-Sulphanilamido-6-methoxypyrimidine
=4-Methoxy-6-sulphanilamidopyrimidine
Generic name: *sulfamonomethoxine*

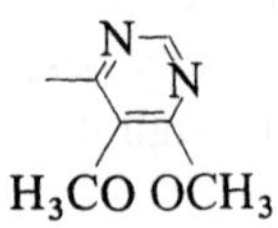
MW 310.34; MP 190–194 °C
N^1-(5, 6-Dimethoxy-4-pyrimidinyl) sulphanilamide
=4-Sulphanilamido-5,6-dimethoxypyrimidine
=4,5-Dimethoxy-6-sulphanilamidopyrimidine
Generic names: *sulfadoxine* (sulformethoxine, sulforthomidine)

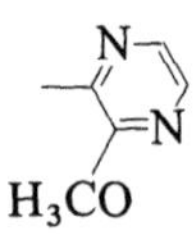
MW 280.32; MP 176 °C
N^1-(3-Methoxy-2-pyrazinyl) sulphanilamide
=2-Sulphanilamido-3-methoxypyrazine
=2-Methoxy-3-sulphanilamidopyrazine
Generic names: *sulfalene* (sulfamethoxypyrazine, sulfamethopyrazine)

Table 2. Chemical structure of sulphones

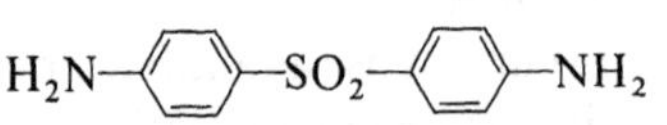
MW 248.30 MP 178–180.5 °C
Bis (4-aminophenyl) sulphone
=4,4′-Sulphonyldianiline
=4,4′-Diaminodiphenylsulphone
Generic names: *dapsone* (DDS, diaphenylsulphone)

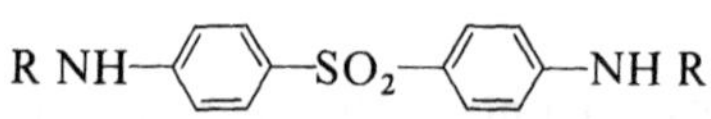

R=

—CH O
MW 304.3 MP 267–270 °C
Bis (4-formamidophenyl) sulphone
=4′4‴-Sulphonylbis (formanilide)
=4,4′-Diformyldiaminodiphenyl sulphone
Generic name: *diformyldapsone* (DFD)

$—COCH_3$
MW 332.39 MP 289–292 °C
Bis (4-acetamidophenyl) sulphone
=4′4‴-Sulphonylbis (acetanilide)
=4,4′-Diacetyldiaminodiphenyl sulphone
Generic name: *acedapsone* (DADDS)

Table 3. pK_a values and water solubility of sulphonamides (intact drugs and N^4-acetyl-metabolites) and sulphones

Name	Intact drug			N^4-acetyl metabolite		
	pK_a	Water solubility (mg/litre)		pK_a	Water solubility (mg/litre)	
		Basal[a]	At various pHs		Basal[a]	At various pHs
Sulfadiazine	6.52[b] 6.4[c]	121[c]	pH 5 : 127[c] pH 6 : 177 pH 7 : 678 pH 8 : 5,694	6.34[b] 5.9[c]	174[c]	pH 5 : 198[c] pH 6 : 416 pH 7 : 2,595 pH 8 :24,400
Sulfamono-methoxine	5.94[b]	–	pH 7.4: 267[d]	–	–	pH 7.4: 900[d]
Sulfadoxine	6.15[e] 5.8[a]	165[c]	pH 5 : 210[e] pH 6 : 480 pH 7 : 3,350 pH 8 : 5,120	5.51[b]	127[c]	pH 5 : 227[e] pH 6 : 1,050 pH 7 : 9,500 pH 8 :80,600
Sulfalene		575[c]	pH 5 : 604[c] pH 6 : 858 pH 7 : 3,400 pH 8 :28,800	5.9[f]	110[c]	pH 5 : 147[c] pH 6 : 488 pH 7 : 3,893 pH 8 :37,949
	pK_b		At unspecified pH:			
Dapsone	13.0[g]		14[h]			
Diformyldapsone	–		6–12[i]			
Acedapsone	–		0.3[h]			

[a] Basal solubility (according to KREBS and SPEAKMAN 1945) of the non-ionised portion
[b] RIEDER 1963
[c] KRÜGER-THIEMER and BÜNGER 1965 (determined potentiometrically)
[d] BRIDGES et al. 1969
[e] BÖHNI et al. 1969
[f] KRÜGER-THIEMER et al. 1969
[g] ORZECH et al. 1976
[h] ANAND 1979
[i] SONNTAG et al. 1972b (determined in saline)

II. Physicochemical Properties

Tables 1 and 2 also show the melting points of the sulphonamides and sulphones. For the sulphonamides and their main N^4-acetyl derivatives, solubilities at various pHs and the pKa values are indicated in Table 3.

III. Assay Methods

1. Sulphonamides (for details, see REEVES et al. 1978; GILPIN 1979)

The traditional techniques are based on the reaction of BRATTON and MARSHALL (1939) by which the free N^4-amino group is diazotised with nitrite and assayed *col-*

orimetrically after coupling with a chromogen, commonly *N-1*-naphthyl-ethylene diamine. The sensitivity limit is around 1 mg/litre. By acid hydrolysis, possible substituents at the N^4-amino group are split off, so that the respective derivatives can also be diazotised and assayed. Usually, the samples are assayed in two sets, the first without hydrolysis, yielding the directly reacting, free sulphonamide (i.e. the sulphonamide with free N^4-amino group), and the second with previous hydrolysis yielding the total sulphonamide. In blood, where N^1-substituted metabolites (which also give a positive Bratton and Marshall reaction) are rare, and the N^4-acetyl metabolite is, practically, the only derivative substituted in position 4, the free sulphonamide portion is usually regarded as the intact (unmetabolised) drug and the difference between the total and free sulphonamide as the N^4-acetyl metabolite. ["Total" and "free" sulphonamide in the present sense must not be confused with the portion in the plasma water (not bound to protein) and the "total" sulphonamide comprising both the protein-bound and unbound portion.]

When applied to urine, this simple estimation is unreliable, particularly with respect to the concentration of intact drug, due to the fact that metabolites with free N^4-amino group are more prevalent, particularly the N^1-glucuronides. The latter even occur in blood at rates up to a small percentage. For a separate determination of the glucuronides, the samples are extracted with ethyl acetate or di-isopropyl ether, the unchanged drug and N^4-acetate passing into the solvent phase and the glucuronides remaining in the aqueous phase (RIEDER 1972, 1976).

The Bratton and Marshall technique is applicable to both whole blood and plasma (serum). The sulphonamides and their metabolites are stable against the usual, initial deproteinisation with trichloracetic acid. By this procedure both the unbound and protein-bound portions are estimated since the latter are released from the protein. Non-protein-bound sulphonamide can be assayed alone by using an initial step such as ultrafiltration or equilibrum dialysis (SCHOLTAN and SCHMIDT 1962).

During the past few years, high-performance liquid chromatography (HPLC) and gas chromatography have been applied to the assay of the sulphonamides, offering the advantage of simultaneous determination of the unchanged drugs and their metabolites, and of the inhibitors of dihydrofolic acid reductase used in combination (e.g. BYE and LAND 1977; COBB and HILL 1977; VREE et al. 1978; VERGIN and BISHOP 1980; BONINI et al. 1981).

2. Sulphones

a) Dapsone (for details see ORZECH et al. 1976)

Colorimetry with Bratton and Marshall's diazotisation method is, in principle, applicable but does not distinguish between dapsone and its metabolites which still have one free amino group. A different colorimetric method based on the formation of a Schiff base between dapsone and 4-dimethyl-aminobenzaldehyde is specific for the intact compound (LEVY and HIGGINS 1966).

With *fluorometry*, dapsone and its metabolite in plasma, *N*-mono-acetyl dapsone, can be measured separately in the same extract, and after a different extraction, also *N*-diacetyldapsone (=acedapsone) (GLAZKO et al. 1968; PETERS et al. 1970a).

Separate determination of dapsone, *N*-monoacetyldapsone and *N*-diacetyldapsone was also accomplished with *microbore column chromatography* (GORDON and PETERS 1970). Extreme sensitivity (threshold <1 μg/ml) was achieved with this technique by the use of a fluorometric detector (MURRAY et al. 1975). More recently, a very rapid though somewhat less sensitive HPLC method was described for the simultaneous assay of dapsone and *N*-monoacetyldapsone (CARR et al. 1978).

The main urinary metabolites, dapsone-*N*-glucuronide, N^1-monoacetyldapsone-N^2-glucuronide, and dapsone sulphamate, are characterised by the fact that the glucuronides are converted into dapsone and *N*-monoacetyl dapsone, respectively, by weak hydrolysis, whereas strong hydrolysis is required for the formation of dapsone from the sulphamate (PETERS et al. 1970a; GELBER et al. 1971).

b) Diformyldapsone

Diformyldapsone and its metabolites, *N*-monoformyldapsone, *N*-monoacetyldapsone and dapsone, are determined by selective hydrolysis and subsequent colorimetry according to Bratton and Marshall (VOGH et al. 1972).

c) Acedapsone

The fluorometric and chromatographic assay methods for acedapsone (=*N*-diacetyldapsone) were mentioned above (GLAZKO et al. 1968; PETERS et al. 1970a; GORDON and PETERS 1970; MURRAY et al. 1975).

C. Mode of Action

I. Bacteria

The antibacterial activity of the sulphonamides was explained by antagonism against *p*-amino benzoic acid (PABA), brought about by structure analogy of sulphanilamide to PABA (WOODS 1940). First evidence of sulphonamide inhibition of bacterial folic acid biosynthesis was reported by MILLER (1944). The commonly accepted view that the bacteriostatic action of sulphonamides is antagonised competitively by PABA and non-competitively by folic acid was established by LAMPEN and JONES (1946, 1947). Inhibition of dihydropteroate synthetase (the enzyme combining 2-amino-4-hydroxy-6-hydroxymethyl-7,8-dihydropteridine diphosphate with PABA to form dihydropteroic acid) in cell-free bacterial extracts was demonstrated by SHIOTA (1959) and BROWN et al. (1961). An analogous mechanism of action has been suggested for the sulphones based on the observation that their action on bacteria was equally antagonised by PABA (LEVADITI 1941; DONOVICK et al. 1952). Present knowledge on the inhibition of folic acid biosynthesis by both sulphonamides and sulphones was recently reviewed by ANAND (1979); some still unresolved questions were discussed by EDWARDS (1980).

II. Plasmodia

The mode of action of the sulphonamides and sulphones against plasmodia is considered analogous. For the sulphonamides (sulphanilamides) this was supported by the finding of antagonism of PABA to the antimalarial effect on *Plasmodium gallinaceum* as early as in 1942 (MAIER and RILEY) and for the sulphones (dapsone) in 1963 (BISHOP). This antagonism to both sulphonamides and sulphones was found to be competitive (ROLLO 1955; BISHOP 1963), and for the sulphonamides the same was confirmed in *P. berghei* (THURSTON 1954). In *P. gallinaceum*, seemingly competitive (ROLLO 1955) or non-competitive antagonism (BISHOP 1963) to sulphonamides and sulphones, respectively, was also obtained with folic acid; however, higher doses were required than with PABA (ROLLO 1955). It was suggested that the antagonism of folic acid may only be due to release of PABA in the host, and the fact that folinic acid was still less antagonistic than folic acid (*P. gallinaceum*) was explained by less PABA release (GOODWIN and ROLLO 1955). No antagonism to sulphonamides was observed with folinic acid in *P. berghei* (THURSTON 1954).

PABA is an essential, exogenous growth factor for both *P. berghei* (JACOBS 1964) and *P. falciparum* (KRETSCHMAR 1966). The suppressive ("chemotherapeutic") effect of milk diet on *P. berghei* (MAEGRAITH et al. 1952) has been explained by its extremely low PABA content as first suggested by HAWKING (1953). Folic acid or foline acid did not replace PABA as growth factor (*P. berghei* in mice, JACOBS 1964). JERUSALEM and KRETSCHMAR (1967) suggested that plasmodial growth would not only be determined by the PABA content of the diet, but also by the availability of PABA to the erythrocytes. The concentration of acetylated PABA (which is inactive as growth factor) was found to be lower in rat erythrocytes parasitised with *P. berghei* than in unparasitised erythrocytes, so that inhibition of acetylation of PABA may be a selective factor for parasitic survival (CENEDELLA et al. 1969). No study exists on the possible influence of sulphonamides and sulphones on PABA uptake and acetylation in erythrocytes. Evidence was reported for an accumulation of sulphones (dapsone) at the surface of rat erythrocytes, leading to reduced uptake of glucose in the erythrocytes and inhibited glucose consumption by intraerythrocytic *P. berghei* (CENEDELLA and JARRELL 1970). Thus, altered permeability of the erythrocytic membrane (which is also suggested by the haemolytic side effects of the sulphones) may account for an additional "indirect" mechanism of action on the intraerythrocytic schizonts, which is independent from the effect on PABA utilisation and folic acid biosynthesis by the parasite.

III. Stages of Plasmodia Influenced

The sulphonamides and sulphones in principle act on all the multiplying stages in the life cycle of the plasmodia. In a number of models with non-human Plasmodium species, activity has been demonstrated on both the tissue and blood schizonts in the vertebrate host as well as on sporogony in the insect vector. Activity on the exoerythrocytic stages (tissue schizonts and sporogony) was generally better with the sulphonamides than with the sulphones (see Sect. F. I). In the human plasmodia, however, evidence of activity is restricted for both the sulphonamides and the sulphones to the blood schizonts (PETERS 1970, 1971c). On the gametocytes, which do not multiply, the sulphonamides and sulphones were found entirely inactive in any of the plasmodia tested.

D. Human Pharmacokinetics and Metabolism

I. Sulphonamides

1. Bioavailability

Of most of the sulphonamides, and of all those dealt with in this chapter, absorption after oral administration is considered complete. This has been proven for sulfadoxine (GLADTKE 1965) and sulfalene (DOST and GLADTKE 1969) by the finding of equal areas under the plasma concentration curves after oral and intravenous administration.

2. Concentration in Plasma

Maximum concentrations in plasma are produced 3–6 h after the oral dose. Typical maximum and/or steady-state concentrations are indicated in Table 4. These figures refer to the unchanged "total" sulphonamides, i.e. to both their protein-bound and unbound portions. In addition to the unchanged compounds, the plasma also contains metabolites, mainly the N^4-acetyl derivatives, which are all inactive antimicrobially. In the sulphonamides treated here, the concentration of these metabolites in plasma usually is less than 10% of the unchanged compounds (Table 4). The significance of variables in the metabolic rate will be discussed below.

3. Protein Binding

Most of the sulphonamides present in the plasma are extensively *bound to the proteins,* mainly to albumin. The extent of protein binding is specific for the individual sulphonamides, but also depends on their concentration in the plasma and, further, on the concentration and quality of albumin. The percentages given in Table 4 refer to chemotherapeutically significant sulphonamide concentrations and normal albuminaemia. Only the unbound portion (often expressed as "concentration in the plasma water") is commonly considered antimicrobially active (KRÜGER-THIEMER et al. 1965) and essentially determines glomerular filtration and distribution in other body compartments. [In typical cases, the concentration in the plasma water of sulfadoxine was 7% (BÜNGER 1967) and that of sulfalene 24% (HERTING et al. 1965) of the total plasma concentration; due to the, relatively, lowest protein binding, the percentage is around 50% in sulfadiazine (BÜNGER 1967).] Protein binding of sulphonamides (in most of the observations sulfadiazine) was found reduced in *hypoalbuminaemia* associated with malnutrition (SHASTRI and KRISHNASWAMY, 1979) or chronic liver disease (BOOBIS and BRODIE 1977; WALLACE and BRODIE 1976) and that which normally occurs in neonates (WALLACE 1976). In spite of normal or only slightly decreased albumin levels, protein binding is also reduced in patients with uraemia, probably due to altered albumin composition (ANDREASEN 1973; BOOBIS 1977). Furthermore, the sulphonamides may be partially displaced from their protein binding by other drugs with still higher affinity to plasma albumin, such as phenylbutazone, or they may inversely displace other drugs such as tolbutamide, or bilirubin in neonates with jaundice (KABINS 1972; ANTON 1973; see also Sect. E.I.e).

Table 4. Pharmacokinetic characteristics of sulphonamides and sulphones in man. Legend see opposite page

Name	Typical plasma conc. mg/litre[a] (D = adult oral dose in mg)	Binding to plasma albumin	Mean plasma half-lives[h], (numb. of individ.)	Apparent distribution volume litres/kg	Conc. in CSF in % of plasma conc.	% metabolites in plasma			% metabolites in urine			
Sulfadiazine	~30 (D 2 × 800/day[b] 80 (D 400)[c] 80 (D 400)[c] 30–40 (4 h after D 1,000 i.v.)[d]	38%–49%[e] 54%[f]	16 (17)[g] 10 (8)[d] 13 (6)[b] 18 (6)[f]	0.36[d]	50%[h]	Unchanged compound 80%–90%	N^4-acetate 10%–20%[c]		Unchanged cpd. 60%	N^4-acetate 30%	N^1-glucuronide[g] 10%	
Sulfamonomethoxine	160 (D 2,000)[i]	65%–93%[e] 80%[j]	30[e]		16%[k]				Unchanged cpd. 18%	N^4-acetate 65%	N^1-glucuronide 8%	sulphate 6%
Sulfadoxine	100–200 (D 1,000–2,000)[m] 30–130 (D initial 200, then 1,500 weekly)[n]	91.5%[m] 93%[n]	135 (8)[m] 123 (8)[n] 179 (101)[m] 195 (6)[p]	0.125[o] 0.15[n]	9.3%[n] 25%[m] 21–56%[q]	Unchanged cpd. ~95%	N^4-acetate 3%–5%	N^4- <3%[m]	Unchanged cpd. 30% 23% 56%	N^4-acetate 60% 64% 29%	N^1-glucuronide 10% 13% –	sulphate –[g] –[m] 9%[l]
Sulfalene	50–100 (D initial 1,000, then 500 daily)[r] 150–300 (D initial 2,000, then 1,500 daily)[s]	68%[t] 77%[r]	65 (23)[s] 67 (4)[t]	0.237[t]	31%[r]	Unchanged cpd. ~91%	N^4-acetate 9%[r]		Unchanged cpd. 10%	N^4-acetate 72%	N^1-glucuronide[g] 18%	
Dapsone	1.2–1.5 (D 100)[u] 3.5–4 (D 300)[v]	81.5%[w] 75%–78%[x] (monoacetyl-dapsone 97%–100%)[x]	21 (5)[u] 30 (7)[y] 29 (39)[z] [monoacetyl-dapsone 30.5 (35)]	~1.0 estimated after[u,v]		Unchanged cpd. slow 50% rapid 17% acetylators	Mono-acetate 50%[A] 87%		20% unchanged compound 20% glucuronide 1.5% monoacetate 1.5% monoacetate glucur.[A] 57% sulphamate			
Diformyl-dapsone	2.9 (D 1,600)[B] (mostly dapsone)		24–36 (6)[B] (mostly dapsone)			>90% dapsone <10% monoformyl-[B] and diformyldapsone			31%–71% free amines[B]			
Acedapsone	0.04–0.06 (D 300 i.m.) (mostly dapsone 225 i.m.) and mono-acetyldapsone[u,c]		43 d[u] 46 d[D] (cf. text)			Unchanged cpd. – 10%	Monoacetyl-dapsone 50% 40%	Dapsone 50%[E] 50%				

4. Plasma Half-life

The mean plasma half-lives found with the four drugs in adults and children over 4 years old are listed in Table 4. Considerable interindividual differences are met with a given drug [e.g. in 17 individuals receiving sulfadiazine the mean was 16 h, but the range was from 9.7–24.5 h, and in eight individuals receiving sulfadoxine the mean was 123 h, but the range was from 78.7–200 h (KRÜGER-THIEMER and BÜNGER 1965)]. In addition, even intraindividual differences occur. Since the elimination of the sulphonamides from plasma is mainly a function of renal excretion of the unchanged drugs and their metabolites, most of the variables in plasma half-life are to be explained by the variables in renal excretion and will be discussed below. The important divergence consistently found in *young* infants should, however, be mentioned here. During the 1st month of life, the plasma half-life of sulphonamides is definitely *longer* than in adults (KRAUER et al. 1968); with sulfalene, e.g. it was up to four times longer (DOST and GLADTKE 1969). The sulphonamides are generally considered contraindicated in neonates (cf. Sect. E. I.1.e.).

Plasma half-life must, of course, be taken into account with the dosage schedules used for *repeated administration* of the various sulphonamides. The principle probably most widely accepted is to administer a certain, equal individual dose (D) at a dose interval which is similar to the half-life. [As a first, "loading" dose, the double quantity (2D) may be given]. Thus, the preferred dose intervals for sulfadiazine, sulfamonomethoxine, sulfalene and sulfadoxine are 12 h, 24 h, approximately 3 days and 7 days, respectively. An alternative schedule is a loading dose followed by daily maintenance doses which, for the long-acting sulphonamides, are substantially smaller, e.g. one-fourth of the loading dose in the case of sulfalene (KRÜGER-THIEMER et al. 1969) and even less in the case of sulfadoxine (BÜNGER 1967).

5. Volume of Distribution

The apparent volumes of distribution of the sulphonamides dealt with here are indicated in Table 4. As a general rule, they are inversely correlated with the extent

[a] Maxima or steady-state means
[b] REEVES et al. (1979)
[c] GOTH (1978)
[d] OHNHAUS and SPRING (1975)
[e] RIEDER (1963)
[f] SHASTRI and KRISHNASWAMY (1979)
[g] KRÜGER-THIEMER et al. (1965)
[h] FORTH et al. (1977)
[i] MATVEEVA (1979)
[j] NEUGODOVA et al. (1977)
[k] PADEISKAYA et al. (1972)
[l] BRIDGES et al. (1969)
[m] BÖHNI et al. (1969)
[n] BÜNGER (1967)
[o] PORTWICH and BÜNGER (1964)
[p] PECK et al. (1975) (sulfadoxine together with pyrimethamine)
[q] CHAPTAL et al. (1966)
[r] HERTING et al. (1965)
[s] KRÜGER-THIEMER et al. (1969)
[t] WIEGAND et al. (1965)
[u] GLAZKO et al. (1968)
[v] GOODWIN and SPARELL (1969)
[w] AFFRIME and REIDENBERG (1973)
[x] BIGGS and LEVY (1971)
[y] AHMAD and ROGERS (1980)
[z] PETERS et al. (1972)
[A] GELBER et al. (1971)
[B] SONNTAG et al. (1972a)
[C] GOSS et al. (1975)
[D] PETERS et al. (1977)
[E] CHANG et al. (1969)

of plasma protein binding. When calculated for only the unbound sulphonamide portion in the plasma, this particular "V_{dis} plasma water" is definitely greater [in the case of sulfalene, V_{dis} was 0.237 and "V_{dis} plasma water" 0.73 (WIEGAND et al. 1965)].

6. Uptake in Erythrocytes

Only a few data exist on the concentration of sulphonamides in the erythrocytes in spite of the obvious interest of this parameter for antimalarials against the blood schizonts. In two volunteers receiving 2 g sulfalene orally (together with 50 mg pyrimethamine), the concentrations of the unchanged sulphonamide in the erythrocytes measured 8–120 h after the dose were, on average, 32% and 41%, respectively, of the concomitant (total) concentrations in the plasma (TRENHOLME et al. 1975). Of sulfadiazine, sulfamonomethoxine and sulfadoxine the concentrations in human erythrocytes determined by BERNEIS and BOGUTH (1976) were 1.15, 1.25 and 1.0 times, respectively, the concentrations in the surrounding aqueous medium; the sulphonamides present in the erythrocytes were partially bound to haemoglobin, but this binding proved to be much less extensive than the binding to plasma albumin; the distribution to plasma albumin, plasma water, erythrocyte water and haemoglobin was 55%, 31%, 11% and 3%, respectively in the case of sulfadiazine, and 84%, 11%, 3.5%, and 1.5% in the case of sulfamonomethoxine.

7. Passage into CSF

The concentrations of the four sulphonamides in CSF are listed in Table 4 as percentages of the concomitant (total) plasma levels. The considerable range from one individual to the other (between 9.3% and 56% in the case of sulfadoxine) is only partially to be explained by the presence of meningitis (CHAPTAL et al. 1966; BÖHNI et al. 1969). As shown by HERTING et al. (1965) for sulfalene, the fractional concentrations of "free" drug (not bound to protein) are equal in plasma and in CSF. In view of the relatively great portion of "free" drug, even the lower concentrations in CSF are probably adequate chemotherapeutically.

8. Passage into Milk

The concentration of sulphonamides in human milk is generally estimated at 5% –15% of the concomitant plasma level (OTTEN et al. 1975). This was confirmed for sulfadoxine, where the percentage was 5%–25% (BÖHNI et al. 1969).

9. Transplacental Passage

The sulphonamides readily pass through the placenta. This is desirable in view of the possible risk of fetal malaria, but must also be considered a possible fetotoxic risk (see below). The plasma concentrations in the cord blood of neonates are, generally, nearly as high as in the maternal plasma (RUMLER et al. 1970). The percentage found with sulfadiazine was 50%–90% (MANDELL and SANDE 1980) and with sulfadoxine 70%–100% (BÖHNI et al. 1969).

10. Biliary and Faecal Excretion

The sulphonamides also pass into the bile with concentrations ranging from 20% to 80% of the concomitant concentrations in plasma (sulfadoxine: STAUBER and PUXKANDL 1966; BÖHNI et al. 1969, sulfalene: HERTING et al. 1965; CALABI et al. 1973). However, biliary excretion was estimated at less than 10% of the dose (BÖHNI et al. 1969; CALABI et al. 1973). Total excretion of sulfadoxine with the faeces was found to be only 8.4% of the oral dose (BÖHNI et al. 1969).

11. Renal Excretion and Its Influence on Plasma Half-life

a) Total Renal Clearance of the Unchanged and Metabolised Compounds

Renal excretion is by far the most important route of elimination of the sulphonamides; 90% or even more of the oral doses are generally recovered in the urine, either as the unchanged compound or metabolites (OTTEN et al. 1975). Total renal clearance is inversely correlated with plasma half-life, e.g. with the "ultra-long" acting sulfadoxine, it was found to be as small as 0.92 ml/min (at a concomitant inulin clearance of 103 ml/min; PORTWICH and BÜTTNER 1964), and in another study 0.6–2.3 ml/min (REBER et al. 1964). As an important feature the metabolites, particularly the N^4-acetyl and N^1-glucuronyl derivatives, generally are excreted at a higher rate than the unchanged drug. In the case of sulfadoxine total renal clearance of the unchanged compound was 0.4–1.2 ml/min, but of the N^4-acetyl and N^1-glucuronyl derivatives it was 11–56 and 7–18 ml/min, respectively (REBER et al. 1964). This is why the concentration of the metabolites is consistently higher in the urine than in plasma (Table 4). [For a complete list of the urinary metabolites see REIMERDES and THUMIN (1970)].

The principal mechanisms of renal excretion of unchanged sulphonamides and their metabolites are glomerular filtration, tubular reabsorption and, less important or perhaps less known, tubular secretion. The efficiency of all these mechanisms is specific to each drug. Sulfadoxine, for example, distinguishes itself by an extremely high rate of tubular reabsorption (PORTWICH and BÜTTNER 1964). On the other hand, each of the mechanisms is affected by certain variables leading to changes in the total renal clearance of a given drug and, as a consequence of this, to the inter- and intraindividual variation in the half-life mentioned earlier.

b) Glomerular Filtration; Impact of Renal Insufficiency and Protein Binding

Glomerular filtration of the compounds is, of course, impaired when there exists any *renal insufficiency* characterised by reduced creatinine or inulin clearance. The plasma half-life of sulfadiazine was 22 h during anuria, compared with 10 h during normal kidney function (OHNHAUS and SPRING 1975). With endogenous creatinine clearance values of 60 ml/min, 20 ml/min and zero, the sulfadiazine dosage should be reduced by 25%, 50% and 60%–65%, respectively (DETTLI 1974; WAGNER 1975). With the "ultra-long" acting sulfadoxine, on the other hand, no reduction of the (normally small) urinary excretion was observed at creatinine clearance values between 10 and 20 ml/min (BÖHNI et al. 1969).

Since only the unbound portions are ultrafiltrated, glomerular filtration of the sulphonamides and their metabolites is increased in association with *reduced plasma protein binding* of any origin (see above), resulting in shorter half-lives e.g. in undernourished individuals with 2.8% plasma albumin and 40% protein binding of sulfadiazine, the half-life of this drug was 12 h compared with 18 h in well-nourished control people with 4.1% serum albumin and 54% protein binding (SHASTRI and KRISHNASWAMY 1979). The shorter half-life should indeed impair the chemotherapeutic efficacy of a given dosage schedule; however, this is at least partially compensated for by the fact that the unbound portion of the drug, which is responsible for antimicrobial activity (KRÜGER-THIEMER et al. 1965), is greater with reduced protein binding.

c) Tubular Reabsorption; Influence of Urinary pH, Circadian Rhythm and Age

As a general rule, tubular reabsorption of weak electrolytes depends on their dissociation, and is most extensive for the undissociated molecules (so-called *non-ionic diffusion*). Since most of the sulphonamides behave as weak acids the relative amount of non-ionised molecules is the greatest when the pH of the urine is equal or inferior to the pKa of the compound in question, but is very much diminished when the pH is above the pKa (DETTLI and SPRING 1966); at the same time solubility is changing as indicated in Table 3. The pKa values of the sulphonamides considered as antimalarials range between 5.8 and 6.5 (see Table 3). Consequently, reabsorption is more extensive, total excretion smaller and half-life longer at urinary pHs 5.8–6.5 and less, than at pHs which are above this level. The impact of the composition of the diet is obvious. It is, furthermore, a well-established fact that the pH of human urine is lower during sleep than in the waking state. This explains a *diurnal cycle* of the speed of renal excretion and of the half-life of sulphonamides. With sulfasymazin (pKa 5.5) this intraindividual difference of the half-live was threefold (DETTLI and SPRING 1966), whereas with sulfadiazine (pKa 6.4) it was only small (11.4 h at night and 9.0 h during the day) though still significant statistically (OHNHAUS and SPRING 1975).

The definitely longer half-life of the sulphonamides to be taken into account for the *neonate and for infants less than 1 month old* (see above, p. 131) was partially explained by the longer sleeping time during the age in question, leading to longer periods of urinary acidosis (DETTLI and SPRING 1966). It was further explained by lacking or very weak acetylation in the neonate (DOST and GLADTKE 1969). Half-life becomes, on the contrary, *shorter* than in adults during the *months 2–12* as shown for sulfalene (approximately 45 h compared with 65 h; DOST and GLADTKE 1969) and sulfadoxine (approximately 95 h compared with 130–180; GLADTKE 1965), the adult half-life being gradually reached by the 1st to 4th year (KRAUER et al. 1968; DOST and GLADTKE 1969). The reasons for this transient shortening are unknown.

In addition to "non-ionic diffusion", there is evidence for an *active mechanism of tubular reabsorption* working also with ionised molecules. This was confirmed for sulfadoxine where extensive reabsorption was found to be maintained even at very high urinary pH (PORTWICH and BÜTTNER 1964). A substantial role for active reabsorption mechanisms (which are independent from the variables affecting non-ionic diffusion) can be postulated for the long-acting sulphonamides in general.

d) Tubular Secretion and Other Mechanisms of Preferential Excretion of the Metabolites

Tubular secretion was invoked for the N^4-acetyl and N^1-glucuronyl derivatives of the sulphonamides to explain the preferential urinary excretion of these metabolites (REBER et al. 1974; OTTEN et al. 1975). Other but still partial explanations of the latter fact are: (a) Due to lower protein binding (RIEDER 1963) glomerular filtration of the N^1-glucuronides must be relatively extensive [protein binding of the N^4-acetyl metabolite is generally as high as that of the unchanged sulphonamide (RIEDER 1963)]; (b) tubular reabsorption of the metabolites is less than that of the unchanged drug; in the case of sulfadoxine, the tubular reabsorption rates calculated for the intact molecule, the N^4-acetate and the N^1-glucuronide were 91%–98%, 88% and 70%–89%, respectively (BÖHNI et al. 1969); lower "non-ionic" diffusion of the N^4-acetate can also be expected from its comparatively low pKa (Table 3).

e) Genetic Differences in N^4-Acetylation

The potential impact of the metabolic rate of the sulphonamides on urinary excretion and plasma half-life is all the more interesting as genetically fixed interindividual differences exist in the acetylation capacity for sulphonamides and other drugs (EVANS et al. 1960); it must also be kept in mind that the N^4-acetate of the sulphonamides is inactive antimicrobially. The distinction between the "slow" and "rapid" acetylator phenotype is routinely performed with a single oral dose of the "short-acting" sulphonamide, sulfamethazine (= sulfadimidine), of which around 20% is found acetylated in the plasma of "slow acetylators" but as much as 60% –80% in the plasma of "rapid acetylators" (EVANS 1969). However, no such differences have ever been observed with the "long-acting" sulphonamides. With sulfalene, the mean percentage of the N^4-acetate in plasma was 7.7% in "slow" and 13.8% in (very typical) "rapid acetylators" (WILLIAMS et al. 1975); a statistically significant difference in the mean plasma half-life of sulfalene was indeed found between healthy volunteers of the "slow" and "rapid" phenotype (83 vs 56 h) but this difference was no longer apparent when the same volunteers were infected with *P. falciparum* (WILLIAMS et al. 1978). There was no distinct correlation between the acetylator phenotype and the chemotherapeutic response to sulfalene in the volunteers with experimental malaria (WILLIAMS et al. 1975, 1978). The occasional chemotherapeutic failures were also not to be explained by low levels of unchanged sulfalene in the plasma or erythrocytes nor by drug resistance of the parasite, but they were attributed to a "host factor" of unknown nature (TRENHOLME et al. 1975; WILLIAMS et al. 1978).

II. Sulphones

1. Dapsone

a) Principal Pharmacokinetic Characteristics

Absorption after oral administration is considered fairly complete in view of the 70%–80% urinary recovery of the drug including metabolites (CHATTERJEE and PODDAR 1957; ELLARD 1966; GLAZKO et al. 1968). The *maximum concentrations in plasma* which are produced 3–6 h after the oral doses are relatively low (in the order of 1–5 mg/litre with the doses used in chemotherapy; see Table 4), indicating an apparent volume of distribution of, roughly, 0.5–1.0 litre/kg. *Protein binding* of the unchanged compound in plasma is usually 70%–80% (BIGGS and LEVY 1971). Markedly decreased protein binding was observed in patients with hepatic cirrhosis (AFFRIME and REIDENBERG 1973). The *plasma half-lives* reported in the literature range between 21 and 30 h (Table 4). Dapsone was found to be concentrated on the membrane of rat erythrocytes (CENEDELLA and JARRELL 1970). Concentrations are greater than in plasma, or are maintained for longer periods, in liver, kidney, muscle and skin; lepromatous skin is said to contain more drug than normal skin (MEYERS et al. 1980). The penetration of dapsone into peripheral nerves observed in dogs and sheep (ALLEN 1975) is of interest in view of the polyneuritic side effects (see below). No data were found on CSF levels. Bile-fistula monkeys excreted 15% –19% in the bile, and their dapsone plasma half-lives were shorter than in normal animals, suggesting enterohepatic recirculation (GLAZKO et al. 1969). No data were found on the sulphone content of human faeces. *Urinary excretion,* which is certainly the main route of elimination, was inhibited by probenecid leading to higher dapsone plasma levels (GOODWIN and SPARELL 1969). This effect of probenecid suggests that tubular secretion plays a significant role in the excretion of the sulphones. Dapsone passes into human milk as indicated by its finding in the urine of breast-fed infants from mothers taking the drug (MARTINDALE 1972).

b) Metabolism

The principal metabolites of dapsone in man are mono-*N*-acetyl-dapsone (MADDS), which is mainly found in plasma, and the acid-labile dapsone glucuronide as well as the more stable dapsone sulphamate, which are the main urinary metabolites (BUSHBY 1967; GELBER et al. 1971) [see Table 4; for a complete list of the metabolites see ORZECH et al. (1976)].

The portion of MADDS in human plasma is extremely dependent on the acetylator phenotype (PETERS et al. 1970b), the dapsone/MADDS ratio being around 1.0 in "slow" and around 0.2 in "rapid acetylators" (GELBER et al. 1971; LAMMINTAUSTA et al. 1979). The practical significance of this difference is not fully understood. By virtue of its one free amino group MADDS is still active antimicrobially, as observed in bacteria (PAYNE et al. 1953; GUPTA et al. 1955). On the other hand, binding of MADDS to the plasma proteins is extremely strong (97%–100%), i.e. ten times as strong as the binding of DDS (BIGGS and LEVY 1971; RILEY and LEVY 1973). This explains a low glomerular filtration rate and the low urinary concentrations of MADDS and its *N*-glucuronide found even in "rapid acetylators" (GELBER et al. 1971; see Table 4). Since in the plasma there is a balance between acetylation and deacetylation (GLAZKO et al. 1968) MADDS should act as a "reservoir" for dapsone. However, urinary excretion of dapsone and its analogues was indistinguishable in "rapid" and "slow acetylators" (GELBER et al. 1971), and the difference in dapsone plasma half-life was small [29 h in "rapid" vs 28 h in "slow acetylators"; the half-life of MADDS was 30 and 31 h, respectively (PETERS et al. 1972)]. Chemotherapeutic response of leprosy to treatment with dapsone was indistinguishable in "slow" and "rapid acetylators" (ELLARD et al. 1972). On the other hand, development of dapsone resistance was observed more often in "rapid" than in "slow" acetylators (J. H. PETERS 1974). The response of leprosy also to acedapsone did not differ between the two acetylator phenotypes (PETERS et al. 1977). No comparative study exists on the role of metabolism in the response of malaria to the sulphones.

2. Diformyldapsone

For lack of a free amino group this compound is inactive antimicrobially, but is rapidly converted into the active metabolites, monoformyldapsone and, mainly, dapsone, the latter accounting for more than 90% of the radioactivity in plasma after oral administration of radiolabelled diformyldapsone to volunteers. Not surprisingly, the plasma half-life of total (unchanged and metabolised) drug did not differ much from the half-life of dapsone (SONNTAG et al. 1972a; see Table 4). Probably due to extremely low solubility in water, absorption is incomplete and relatively irregular. Based on the comparative study of the urine and expired air from volunteers after oral administration of [^{14}C]- and [^{35}S]-diformyldapsone, total absorption was estimated at only 13% of the dose on the average, with an individual range between 7% and 25%; around 20% of the absorbed portion was attributed to biliary excretion (MAREN et al. 1970; SONNTAG et al. 1972a). This is the reason why the dosage of diformyldapsone must be higher than that of dapsone.

3. Acedapsone

This drug is analogous to diformyldapsone in becoming active only by the formation of its metabolites with one or two free amino group(s), monoacetyldapsone and dapsone itself (CHANG et al. 1969). In contrast to all other sulphonamides and sulphones, which normally are taken orally, acedapsone must be injected intramuscularly in an oily suspension. Its release from the injection site is extremely slow, but any portion released is rapidly metabolised to the above-mentioned active compounds, the concentrations of which in the plasma are small (in the order of only 0.05 mg/litre after a single i.m. dose of 200–300 mg; see Table 4) but very long lasting. The apparent plasma "half-life" of the metabolites (which, of course, far more reflects the slow release from the intramuscular depot than postdistributive elimination strictly speaking) proved to be as long as 6–7 weeks (GLAZKO et al. 1968; PETERS et al. 1977). The plasma concentrations of monoacetyldapsone and dapsone are fairly equal, and the two metabolites were first believed to account for all the drug present in plasma (CHANG et al. 1969). Only by using more sensitive assay methods could acedapsone also be detected in a proportion of about 10% of total drug (MURRAY et al. 1973; PETERS et al. 1977). The acetylator phenotype was found to have but little influence on the proportion of acetylated dapsone in plasma after the administration of acedapsone (43% in "rapid" vs 35% in "slow acetylators") and no influence at all on the apparent "half-life" of dapsone and acetylated dapsone (MURRAY et al. 1973; PETERS et al. 1977).

E. Toxicity

I. Sulphonamides

1. Side Effects in Human Chemotherapy

a) Gastrointestinal

Troubles such as upper abdominal pain, nausea, vomiting (sometimes associated with headache) were recorded quite rarely with the sulphonamides dealt with in this chapter; e.g. with sulfadoxine in only one out of 400 cases (McGUINNESS 1969), none out of 424 (BECKERMANN 1964) and in 2% of an unspecified number of patients (PINES 1967). In children treated with sulfalene for malaria, vomiting though occasionally occurring (REY et al. 1968; STOREY et al. 1973) was far less frequent than with chloroquine, and this was considered a definite advantage for the sulphonamide.

b) Renal

Crystalluria potentially leading to anuria used to be a major risk of therapy with the older sulphonamides (APPEL and NEU 1977), but became quite rare with the development of drugs with better solubility of the unchanged compound and the N^4-acetate even at low urinary pH. The rare incidents observed with sulfadiazine all occurred as a consequence of definite overdosage or when fluid intake and/or alkalisation of the urine were inadequate (DORFMAN and SMITH 1970; CRAFT et al. 1977). The risk is practically non-existent with the long-acting sulphonamides used for malaria, thanks to good solubility parameters and to the small quantities which are excreted per day (KRÜGER-THIEMER and BÜNGER 1965). For example, with sulfadoxine, maximum urinary excretion per day is in the order of 10% of a dose (during the first 24 h after the dose; BÖHNI et al. 1969); after a very high dose of, e.g. 2,500 mg, the urine contains not more than 250 mg unchanged drug and metabolites/day; even on the assumption of a very small urine volume and low pH, the pertinent concentrations are still below the saturation threshold (see Table 3). As a matter of fact, no published report exists on crystalluria observed with sulfamonomethoxine, sulfadoxine or sulfalene.

c) Haematological

Haemolytic anaemia occurred with some of the older sulphonamides, though less frequently than with the sulphones. With sulfadiazine the incidence was estimated at 0.05% (MANDELL and SANDE 1980). To the reviewer's knowledge, no instance was recorded with sulfamonomethoxine, sulfadoxine, sulfadoxine or sulfalene, even in patients with glucose-6-phosphate dehydrogenase (G6PD) deficiency (sulfadoxine: HARINASUTA et al. 1967; LAING 1968a, b; CHIN et al. 1966; LEWIS and PONNAMPALAM 1975; PEARLMAN et al. 1977; sulfalene: WILLERSON et al. 1974; most of the patients were receiving the sulphonamides in combination with pyrimethamine). With sulfalene, the absence of a haemolytic effect on blood from G6PD-deficient individuals was also shown in vitro (FLATZ et al. 1970).
Leucopenia (mostly neutropenia) has been infrequent with the newer sulphonamides and, as a rule, mild and easily reversible. The figures on the incidence vary

considerably from one author to another, probably because of differences in the definition of leucopenia and in the frequency of haemograms. With sulfadoxine, no instance was recorded in 4,160 cases (AGUIRRE 1967), one instance each in 424 and 400 patients, respectively (BECKERMANN 1964; MCGUINNESS 1969) but seven instances in 74 patients (BERGMANN et al. 1963). Only one of the cases was grave (agranulocytosis with 900 leucocytes/cmm) and was associated with an allergotoxic skin reaction of the Stevens-Johnson type (BERGMANN et al. 1963).

d) Skin

Among the side effects still occurring with the newer, long-acting sulphonamides, skin reactions are, relatively, the most frequent and potentially most serious. Their incidence is difficult to indicate in view of the dose relationship to be discussed below, but probably is in the order of 0.5%–1%, including all forms, at medium dosage of the sulphonamides (FORTH et al. 1977; for sulfadoxine see AGUIRRE 1967; BECKERMANN 1964; BERGMANN et al. 1963; an exceptionally high rate with several grave incidents was observed by TAYLOR 1968). They often develop around the 10th day of chemotherapy. Since even at the highest dosages they only affect relatively few individuals – who run the risk of becoming affected again at repeated exposure – an individual "idiosyncrasy" is obvious and commonly interpreted as hypersensitivity. Photosensitisation seems to play a role in some cases, and pictures resembling periarteritis nodosa have occasionally been recorded (LEHR 1972). On the other hand, the definite dose relationship in frequency and even more in severity suggests a toxic component. Therefore the reactions are commonly referred to as "allergotoxic".

A great variety of reactions exist, from mild, transient forms such as rashes, pruritus, urticarias, papular and vesiculous exanthemas to severe, bullous or exfoliative forms (Stevens-Johnson syndrome and Lyell syndrome, respectively). These often involve also the mucous membranes including the conjunctiva and may lead to death and, at recovery, to permanent scars of the skin or eyes (BERGOEND et al. 1968; HURIEZ et al. 1972; TAYLOR 1968). The Lyell syndrome (also referred to as toxic epidermal necrosis) is considered as even graver than the Stevens-Johnson syndrome (also referred to as erythema exsudativum multiforme grave); however, a distinction between the two syndromes has not been made by all authors, and the picture can obviously be intermediate. When they do occur, the severe forms (Stevens-Johnson and Lyell syndrome taken together) have a mortality rate of 10%–20%.

The relative frequency of the severe forms obviously depends on the sulphonamide dosage, but has always been much lower than that of the mild forms. The highest proportion reported was one severe form per 16 cases with skin reactions of any form, and was observed in Fes, Morocco, with the highest dosage of sulfadoxine used during the prophylactic mass campaign against epidemic meningitis, which will be discussed below [FAUCON et al. (1970); in the individuals in question, the incidence of all skin reactions, including the mild and moderate forms, was 1.6% and that of the severe forms alone, 0.1%]. With medium doses, the proportion of severe forms has been generally still lower, and with the low sulphonamide doses used for malaria (mostly in combination with pyrimethamine) the risk was considered to be extremely small (BRUCE-CHWATT 1968). For recent observations on severe skin reactions see HORNSTEIN and RUPRECHT (1982) N Eng J M 307:1529 and OLSEN (1982) Lancet 2:994.

Both the Stevens-Johnson and Lyell syndrome also occur with other drugs such as sulphones (CATALANO 1971), antibiotics, anti-inflammatory and analgetic agents (HURIEZ et al. 1972). They have been observed with almost any of the sulphonamides, e.g. cases following the use of sulfalene were described by NOLA et al. (1969) and HURIEZ et al. (1972). It is difficult to decide whether any individual sulphonamide is more risky than another.

An unique experience exists with *sulfadoxine* from the prophylactic mass campaign against epidemic meningitis in Morocco, 1966–1967. High doses were used (individual adult dose 2,500 mg) once or repeatedly at weekly intervals. In the whole of Morocco, the number of individuals receiving sulfadoxine prophylaxis was 109158. Of these 1,002 (0.92%) developed skin reactions of any form and severity; in 78 individuals (0.07%) the reaction was severe (Steven-Johnson or Lyell syndrome) and there were 11 deaths (0.010%) (BERGOEND et al. 1968; HURIEZ et al. 1972). The incidence of both skin reactions (of any form) and deaths was different from one region of Morocco to another. This was obviously correlated with the different number of the sulfadoxine doses (250 mg each for adults) administered in the various provinces of the country (BERGOEND et al. 1968). In the provinces where only a single dose was given (36,673 individuals) the incidence of all skin reactions was only 0.013% and there was no death (<0.003%). In the province with two doses (600 individuals) the overall incidence of skin reaction was 0.33 still with no death, whereas in those with normally three to four doses (10,567 individuals) the incidence of skin reactions rose to 0.87%, and one case (0.0095%) was fatal. In the provinces (including the province of Fes) where the normal treatment schedule was up to 12 doses (61,318 individuals), the incidence of overall skin reactions was the highest, 1.4%, and there were ten deaths (0.016%). The experience from the province of Fes was the subject of the above-mentioned special study (FAUCON et al. 1970): 31,957 individuals, 1.6% skin reactions of any form, 0.10% severe forms (Steven-Johnson or Lyell syndrome) and 0.019% deaths (ten cases).

e) Drug Interactions; Kernicterus

The drug interactions occurring with the sulphonamides are to be explained by competitive binding to the plasma proteins and partial displacement of the sulphonamide and/or the other drug. The increased proportion of the unbound compound(s) in the plasma may result in higher activity and toxicity of either the sulphonamide or the other drug, or of both, depending on the binding affinity and concentration of the components. Phenylbutazone is a potent displacer of the sulphonamides, whereas tolbutamide, metothrexate and the coumarins (warfarin, dicumarol) are rather displaced by the sulphonamides (KABINS 1972; ANTON 1973). These drugs should not be used concomitantly, or only with care.

Various drugs including the sulphonamides can displace bilirubin from its albumin binding with subsequent increase of the free bilirubin in plasma and of the binding of bilirubin to tissues (ODELL 1959). Premature neonates are predisposed to kernicterus since they tend to exhibit (a) high concentrations of total bilirubin in plasma, (b) low binding capacity of plasma albumin and (c) low tissue pH, which greatly increases the bilirubin tissue binding (WENNBERG et al. 1979) leading to cell damage (NELSON et al. 1974), particularly of the neurons of the basal brain nuclei (German: *Kerne*). Kernicterus can occur in such infants without the administration of any displacing drug as exemplified by a recent series of more than 30 cases (TURKEL et al. 1980). However, in a single but well-documented study the incidence of kernicterus was significantly higher in premature neonates receiving a sulphonamide (sulfisoxazole) at high dosage i.v. than in those receiving a different antibacterial regimen (SILVERMAN et al. 1956). As a consequence of this finding, the sulphonamides were considered contraindicated for premature neonates, and this contraindication was generally extended to all infants during the first 2 weeks of life and even to all mothers during the last 2 weeks of pregnancy. To be exact, no observation has come to the reviewers' knowledge where the administration of a sulphonamide to the mother has been followed by kernicterus in the newborn. No instance of kernicterus was recorded in a controlled study of the children of a series of mothers receiving sulphadiazine during the entire period of pregnancy for prophylaxis of rheumatic fever (BASKIN et al. 1980).

2. Animals Tolerance: Teratogenicity Experiments

Teratogenicity experiments (and, in the case of dapsone, an isolated study on carcinogenicity) are the only animal tolerance studies discussed in this chapter; it was felt that in view of the very vast experience with the tolerance and side effects of the sulphonamides (and sulphones) in man, the ordinary animal data, e.g. on LD_{50} and chronic toxicity, would be of too little interest.

Dental anomalies were observed in newborn mice and rats when their mothers were fed during the whole gestation period with a diet containing 0.025% of sulfamoprine (=4,6-dimethoxy-2-sulfanilamidopyrimidine) (GREEN 1963; PAGET and THORPE 1964). This sulphonamide was consequently withdrawn from the market. [In various reviews, e.g. those of SHEPARD (1976) and WILLIAMS (1974) sulfamoprim was erroneously referred to as sulfadimethoxine = 2,6-dimethoxy-4-sulfanilamido-pyrimidine or sulfamethazine = 4,6-dimethyl-2-sulfanilamido-pyrimidine.]

The teratogenicity of sulfamoprine has remained an isolated finding. It was reproduced by BERTAZZOLI et al. (1965) and SCHÄRER (1964, unpublished); however, with sulfalene, sulfadimethoxine and sulfadoxine, which were tested comparatively by the same authors, no teratogenicity was observed (Schärer's findings with sulfadoxine are included in BÖHNI et al. 1969). The innocuous daily doses of sulfalene, sulfadimethoxine and sulfadoxine administered to the mothers were in the order of 100–160 mg/kg.

When administering the high daily doses of 500 or 1,000 mg/kg to rats and/or mice during days 9–14 of gestation, KATO and KITAGAWA (1973) found cleft palates with the following sulphonamides: sulfamonomethoxine, sulfadimethoxine, sulfamethoxypyridazine, sulfamethomidine, sulfisoxazole and sulfadiazine [the percentage of malformed fetuses decreased in this range of the drugs from 80% (sulfamonomethoxine) to 7% (sulfadiazine)]. No cleft palates were observed with sulfisomidine and sulfanilamide. The teratogenic effect of sulfadimethoxine was titrated. With daily doses of 1,000, 500, 300 and 100 mg/kg, the percentage of rat fetuses with cleft palates was 55%, 21%, 2% and zero, respectively.

No evidence exists of any teratogenicity of sulphonamides in man (SMITHELLS 1966; FICKENTSCHER 1978).

II. Sulphones

1. Side Effects in Man

a) Haematological

The three groups of haematological side effects (methaemoglobinaemia, haemolytic anaemia and agranulocytosis) are significant in that they occurred with the relatively low doses of the sulphones used for leprosy and malaria, whereas the side effects on the other organ systems, such as the peripheral nerves and liver (see below), were mainly or exclusively observed with the higher doses used in the sulphone treatment of dermatitis herpetiformis, severe acne and similar skin disorders.

α) Methaemoglobinaemia. With 400 mg dapsone administered in four doses over a period of 48 h, methaemoglobinaemia (8%) and Heinz bodies appeared from 36 h after the first dose (HJELM and DE VERDIER 1965). Up to 22% of methaemoglobin was observed in patients with normal G6PD receiving dapsone in daily doses of 300 mg/kg for leprosy (DEGOWIN et al. 1966b). With a dosage schedule routinely used for malaria prophylaxis in the US army in Vietnam, 25 mg dapsone daily combined with 300 mg chloroquine and 45 mg primaquine once weekly, significant methaemoblobinaemia was produced in five out of eight volunteers whether they were G6PD deficient or not (WILLERSON et al. 1972). An analogous observation was made with diformyldapsone at a daily dosage of 200 mg combined with the weekly administration of chloroquine and primaquine; since diformyldapsone alone did not cause methaemoglobin formation at a definitely higher dosage, a synergism between the sulphone and chloroquine-primaquine was suggested (CLYDE et al. 1970b). No correlation was found between methaemoglobinaemia and haemolytic anaemia (to be discussed in the next paragraph) although they often occurred in the same individual (DEGOWIN 1967; WILLERSON et al. 1972).

A close dose relationship of both methaemoglobinaemia and haemolysis was found by MANFREDI et al. (1979) in patients receiving dapsone for dermatitis herpetiformis. Extremely high methaemoglobinaemia, sometimes exceeding 60% and presenting the picture of extreme cyanosis, was observed in instances of dapsone poisoning in children or in definitely overdosed dermatitis herpetiformis patients; these cases usually showed also severe haemolysis (COOKE 1970; SHELLEY and GOLDWEIN 1976; ELONEN et al. 1979; SCHVARTSMAN 1979).

It was suggested by HJELM and DE VERDIER (1965) that a metabolite, dapsone-monohydroxylamine, would be responsible for methaemoglobin formation. This hypothesis was supported by CUCINELL et al. (1972) as well as GLADER and CONRAD (1973), who were able to produce the hydroxylamine derivative from dapsone incubated with rat liver microsomes, and to prove that this compound has high potency in forming methaemoglobin in vitro. However, dapsone hydroxylamine was not found as a metabolite in patients developing methaemoglobinaemia (GLADER and CONRAD 1973).

β) Haemolytic Anaemia. The first case of dapsone-induced haemolytic anaemia was described by RAMANUJAM and SMITH (1951) in a leprosy patient receiving dapsone in daily doses increasing from 100–300 mg. The daily doses of dapsone considered safe were 100 mg in G6PD-normal and 50 mg in G6PD-deficient subjects (DEGOWIN et al. 1965). However, haemolysis as indicated by prompt fall of the haematocrit values was found with the US army schedule for malaria prophylaxis, 25 mg dapsone daily plus chloroquine and primaquine weekly, in G6PD-deficient but not in G6PD-normal American blacks (EPPES et al. 1967). In some of the G6PD-deficient individuals treated according to this schedule, haemolysis was quite marked (CHERNOF 1967). A synergism of dapsone and primaquine in the production of haemolysis was suggested all the more as haemolysis was also observed with primaquine alone, in the presence of G6PD deficiency, although at a higher dosage (FISHER et al. 1970). Production of both haemolysis and methaemoglobinaemia and increase of these effects by chloroquine and primaquine administered concomitantly was observed with diformyldapsone (CUCINELL et al. 1974).

As for methaemoglobin formation, the (still hypothetical) hydroxylamine metabolite of dapsone was also held to be responsible for haemolysis. Dapsone monohydroxylamine was found to deplete glutathione in human erythrocytes deficient in G6PD (GLADER and CONRAD 1973). HALMEKOSKI et al. (1976) succeeded in detecting the hydroxylamine in the plasma of one out of eight patients receiving 100 mg dapsone daily for dermatitis herpetiformis. However, no correlation with haemolytic side effects was found, and in vitro, the authors found equally strong haemolytic effects with dapsone and monoacetyldapsone as with the hydroxylamine derivative.

γ) Agranulocytosis. Probably the first instance of agranulocytosis caused by dapsone was recorded in a dermatitis herpetiformis patient receiving the drug in daily doses increasing from 50–125 mg (MCKENNA and CHALMERS 1958). Another instance was observed in a patient with severe acne treated with three times 100 mg dapsone every week (FIRKIN and MARIANI 1977).

More alarming was the series of 16 cases occurring with only 25 mg dapsone/day in US soldiers in Vietnam. The soldiers had received the regular dapsone malaria prophylaxis, either alone or in combination with chloroquine and primaquine, for 3 weeks to 3 months; eight of the cases were fatal (OGNIBENE 1970; CATALANO 1971; JOPLINS and OGNIBENE 1972). Neutropenia developing into a "pseudoleukaemic" picture had been observed in another soldier still earlier (JONES and CARDAMONE 1968). These incidents led to the limitation of dapsone for malaria prophylaxis in the US army (OGNIBENE 1970). Under malaria prophylaxis with dapsone, 25 mg daily combined with proguanil (Paludrine) 200 mg daily, three cases of agranulocytosis (with no fatality) were also recorded in soldiers of the New Zealand and Australian troops in Vietnam; dapsone was considered the inducing agent (STICKLAND and HURDLE 1970; SMITHURST et al. 1971).

b) Peripheral Neuropathy

The cases reported were virtually restricted to dermatological patients (with dermatitis herpetiformis, etc.) receiving dapsone in high doses and for long periods (SAQUETON et al. 1969; HUBLER and SOLOMON 1972; RAPOPORT and GUSS 1972; WYATT and STEVENS 1972; VIVIER and FOWLER 1974; EPSTEIN and BOHM 1976; GEHLMANN et al. 1977; KOLLER et al. 1977; HELANDER and PARTANEN 1978). Most of the cases presented as polyneuritis with muscular weakness in the upper and/or lower extremity. Biopsies proved that axonal degeneration of the nerves was present (VIVIER and FOWLER 1974; GEHLMANN et al. 1977; HELANDER and PARTANEN 1978). Optical atrophy developed in a young man with imaginary leprosy after having taken 600 mg dapsone daily for 10 days (HOMEIDA et al. 1980).

c) Miscellaneous Side Effects

Hepatotoxicity (elevated liver enzymes, icterus) was observed in a total of seven patients treated with high doses of dapsone for dermatological disorders (MILLIKAN and HARRELL 1970; GOETTE 1977; STONE and GOODWIN 1978). Again in dermatitis herpetiformis patients receiving dapsone at high dosage, severe hypoalbuminaemia developed (KINGHAM et al. 1979; YOUNG and MARKS 1979).

d) Anti-Inflammatory Effects

Dapsone showed an anti-inflammatory effect in a variety of animal models (GEMMELL et al. 1977). The anti-inflammatory properties of dapsone probably explain the usefulness of this drug in the management of dermatitis herpetiformis (SCHUPPLI 1968) and of other severe skin diseases including pemphigus (PIAMPHONGSANT 1976).

2. Teratogenicity and Carcinogenicity Experiments in Animals

The only reference on any sulphone found in SHEPARD's catalogue of teratogenic agents (1976) was a rat study on 2-sulphamoyl-4,4′-diamino-diphenylsulphone (SDDS) published in Japanese (ASANO et al. 1975). The citation in SHEPARD (1976) is as follows: "Asano et al. gave pregnant rats up to 4,00 mg/kg of SDDS from day 9 until 14 of gestation and found no significant increase in fetal defects. Post-natal studies were negative".

In a recent carcinogenicity study, daily oral doses of 100 mg/kg dapsone were administered to mice and rats of both sexes five times weekly over 2 years. The incidence of tumours was equal in the treated animals to that observed in untreated controls, with the exception of fibrosarcomas and angiosarcomas of the spleen which (related to severe splenic fibrosis) only ocurred in male rats receiving the drug. In separate groups of rats which were treated with dapsone together with benzopyrene, there was no evidence that the well-known carcinogenicity of the latter would be enhanced by the sulphone (GRICIUTE and TOMATIS 1980).

F. Chemotherapy in Experimental Models

I. Activity Against Non-Human Plasmodia

1. Introduction

The first papers on sulphonamides in experimental malaria were published as early as 1938 by two groups of authors, COGGESHALL (1938) and CHOPRA and DAS GUPTA (1938) who described activity of sulphanilamide and soluseptazine, respectively, against *Plasmodium knowlesi* in rhesus monkeys. The activity of sulphones (promine, acedapsone) was detected in 1941 by COGGESHALL et al. (1941), who used rhesus monkeys infected with *P. cynomolgi*. The avian plasmodia, *P. cathemeriums P. lophurae* (COGGESHALL 1938), *P. relictum* and *P. nucleophilum* (MANWELL et al. 1941), were first found not to respond to sulphonamides (sulphanilamide, sulphanilyl sulphanilate, sulphapyridine), but some years later, in 1944, both the sulphonamides (e.g. sulfadiazine) and sulphones (dapsone) proved definitely active against *P. gallinaceum* in chicks (COATNEY and COOPER 1944; COGGESHALL et al. 1944; FREIRE and PARAENSE 1944). The inactivity against the other avian plasmodia previously used was partially explained by the lower and more transient concentrations of the drugs in the serum of the respective host animals, canaries and ducks (MARSHALL et al. 1942; MARSHALL 1945). High activity of sulphonamides such as sulfadiazine against the rodent plasmodium *P. berghei* was observed by HILL (1950) shortly after the description of this new species by VINCKE and LIPS (1948).

The following discussion is limited essentially to experience with the antimalarial sulphonamides (sulfamonomethoxine, sulfadoxine, sulfalene; sulfadiazine is included as a reference compound) and sulphones (dapsone, diformyldapsone, acedapsone) in infections with *P. gallinaceum*, *P. berghei* (and related rodent plasmodia), *P. knowlesi* and *P. cynomolgi*. Blood schizontocidal activity will be discussed in the first place since only this effect of the sulphonamides and sulphones has been unequivocally confirmed with human plasmodia in man. Activity on the tissue schizonts and on the sporogony cycle will be considered briefly, essentially using the example of the rodent plasmodia.

For more details, the reader is referred to the following reviews: CURD (1943) (early experience with monkey plasmodia and the various avian species); GOODWIN and ROLLO (1955), DAVEY (1963); HILL (1963, 1966); ROLLO (1964); HERRERO (1967); PETERS (1970); RICHARDS (1970); THOMPSON and WERBEL (1972) (with structure-activity relationships); PINDER (1973).

2. Blood Schizontocidal Action

a) Methods of Evaluation

With all techniques, blood containing an appropriate number of erythrocytes parasitised with the plasmodia is taken from donor hosts and is injected into new hosts receiving the drugs to be tested, and parasitaemia developing in these treated hosts is compared with the parasitaemia in untreated controls (for a recent review of standard procedures, see PETERS 1980).

The following two methods were used for the comparative testing of sulphonamides and sulphones listed in Tables 7 and 8:

α) "4-Day" Suppressive Test with P. berghei *in Mice* (PETERS 1970). Together with the "Rane test" (RANE and RANE 1973) this is probably the most commonly used screening technique for antimalarials. Mice of a standardised weight or age are infected i.p. or i.v. with approximately 10^7 parasitised erythrocytes to produce at least 30% parasitemia in the untreated controls 4 days after the infection. (Such heavily infected controls will die 6–7 days after the infection.) To randomised groups of infected mice, the drugs are administered at suitable dose levels (e.g. 1,3,10 and 30 mg/kg) once daily for four consecutive days, from Day 0 (the day of infection) until Day 3. On Day 4 blood smears are taken from all treated mice and

Table 5. Blood schizontocidal activity[a] of the antimalarial sulphonamides and sulphones[b] against representative species of non-human plasmodia in birds, rodents, and monkeys

Plasmodium gallinaceum (in chicks)			
Freire and Paraense (1944)	SZ[c]	Greenberg and Richeson (1950)	SZ[d]
Brackett et al. (1945)	SZ	Thurston (1953a)	SZ
Marshall (1945)	SZ	Greenberg (1954)	SZ[d]
Brackett and Waletzky (1946)	SZ[c]	Rollo (1955)	SZ[d]
Davey (1946a)	SZ[c]	Taylor and Greenberg (1955)	SZ
Wiselogle (1946)	SZ[c]	Ramakrishnan et al. (1962)	DDS[c]
Greenberg et al. (1948)	SZ	Basu et al. (1964)	DDS[d]
Cantrell et al. (1949)	SZ[c]	Richards (1966)	SZ, SO, DDS[d]
Greenberg (1949)	SZ[d]	Benazet and Werner (1967)	SZ, SO, SL
Plasmodium berghei and related species[e] (mostly in mice, exceptionally in rats)			
Hill (1950)	SZ	Richards (1968)[f]	DFD
Thurston (1950)	SZ, DDS	Schneider (1968)	SZ, DDS
Baldi and della Rocca (1951)	DDS	Aviado (1969)	SZ, SO, SL, DDS, DFD, ACD
Mudrow-Reichenow (1951)	SZ, DDS	Aviado et al. (1969)	SO, SL[d]
Ramakrishnan et al. (1951)	SZ	Ott (1969) (*P. chabaudi*)	DDS
Rollo (1951)	SZ	Fink and Kretschmar (1970) (*P. vinckei*)	SZ
Thurston (1951)	SZ	Richards (1970)	SZ, SO, SL, DDS[d]
Thurston (1953a)	SZ	Yoshinaga et al. (1970)	
Fabiani and Orfila (1954)	SZ	Peters (1971a)	SZ, SO[d]
Elslager and Worth (1965)	ACD	Peters (1971b)	SL[d]
Peters (1965a, b)	SZ, DDS	Popoff et al. (1971)	DDS, DFD, ACD
Thompson et al. (1965a)	DDS,	Thompson and Werbel (1972)	SZ, SO, SL, DDS, DFD, ACD
Waitz et al. (1965)	ACD	Loev et al. (1973)	DDS, ACD
Hawking (1966)	SZ	Peters et al. (1975b)	SZ, SM, SO, SL, DDS, DFD
Peters (1966)	SZ, DDS	Korolkovas et al. (1978)	DDS
Richards (1966)	SZ, SO, DDS[d]	Rane and Kinnamon (1979)	SZ, DDS[c]
Aviado (1967)	SO, DDS, DFD		
Benazet and Werner (1967)	SZ, SO, SL		
Most et al. (1967)	DDS[c]		
Peters (1967b) (*P. chabaudi*)	SZ, DDS		
Thompson (1967)	DDS, ACD		
Thompson et al. (1967)	SZ, DDS		
Aldighieri et al. (1968)	SL[d]		
Krettli and Brener (1968)	SZ, SO		
Marubini et al. (1968)	SL[d]		
Peters (1968)	SZ, SO[d]		
Plasmodium knowlesi (in rhesus monkeys)			
Coggeshall et al. (1941)	SZ, ACD	Singh et al. (1952b)	SZ
Coggeshall and Maier (1941)	SZ	Ray and Nair (1955)	SZ
Richardson et al. (1946)	SZ	Ramakrishnan et al. (1962)	DDS
Wiselogle (1946)	SZ	Rothe et al. (1969)	SL[d]
Plasmodium cynomolgi (in rhesus monkeys)			
Wiselogle (1946)	SZ	Basu et al. (1964)	DDS[d]
Hawking and Thurston (1951)	SZ	Thompson et al. (1965c)	ACD[d]
McFadzean (1951)	SZ	Thompson (1967)	DDS, ACD
Singh et al. (1956)	SZ	Davidson et al. (1976)	SZ, SL, DDS, DFD
Basu and Prakash (1962)	SZ, DDS		
Ramakrishnan et al. (1962)	DDS	Schmidt et al. (1977)	SZ[d]

the untreated controls to determine the doses of the drugs reducing parasitaemia by a certain percentage. The most usual parameters are the 50% and 90% effective doses (ED_{50} and ED_{90}), i.e. the doses (administered four times) reducing parasitaemia by 50% and 90%, respectively.

β) Test with P. cynomolgi *in Rhesus Monkeys* (DAVIDSON et al. 1976). Young rhesus monkeys (*Macaca mulatta*) are infected i.v. with 5×10^8 erythrocytes parasitised with schizonts (trophozoites) of *P. cynomolgi* taken from donor monkeys. Untreated controls regularly develop parasitaemia for many weeks. Groups of the infected animals are given the drugs orally (via nasogastric tube) at suitable dose levels (e.g. 100, 31.6, 10 mg/kg etc.) once daily for seven consecutive days, starting on Day 0 (the day of infection). Blood smears are examined daily to Day 14, and then every 2nd day. Red-cell counts are also made so that the total count of parasites/mm^3 of blood can be calculated. Animals which become parasite-positive are killed on Day 30, while negative monkeys are splenectomised. The latter are then examined for 30 more days to detect subpatent parasitaemia. Animals remaining parasite-negative after splenectomy are considered cured. The different degrees of transient suppression of parasitaemia are judged as indicated in the footnote to Table 8.

γ) Impact of the Diet. For antimalarial tests in general, and particularly those with sulphonamides and sulphones, the choice of the diet given to the host animals is important. As outlined in Sect. C. II, the diet must not be free of PABA, since the latter is required by the plasmodia as an essential, exogenous growth factor. On the other hand, since PABA is a competitive antagonist to the action of the sulphonamides and sulphones, any excessive supply must be avoided. Unfortunately, the assay of the PABA content in animal food is difficult and the exact optimum unknown. All that one can do is to use always the same diet, whose reasonable and constant PABA content is continuously "bioassayed" by the proof of reproducible activity of standard doses of the sulphonamides or sulphones. In most tests with *P. berghei*, reproducibility was found satisfactory, e.g. with the following commercial pelleted diets: "Altromin-R" in Germany (KRETSCHMAR 1965), "Oxoid modified mouse diet 41 B" in England (PETERS 1980) and "Nafag-Reindiät Nr. 909 (900) PAB 45" in our own experiments in Switzerland. The PABA content of the last-mentioned diet is indicated by the producer to be 45 mg/kg.

b) Survey of Experimental Data

Published experience on blood schizontocidal activity of selected, antimalarial sulphonamides and sulphones is listed in Table 5 according to the plasmodial species

---

[a] With a single exception (acedapsone in rats infected with *P. berghei*, THOMPSON 1967) the drugs were found active at any degree at the doses used by the authors

[b] Names of the drugs abbreviated with: SM, sulfamonomethoxine; SO, sulfadoxine; SL, sulfalene; DDS, dapsone; DFD, diformyldapsone; ACD, acedapsone; reference sulphonamide; SZ, sulfadiazine

[c] Also tested and found active against the tissue schizonts

[d] Also found potentiated in combination with an inhibitor of dihydrofolic acid reductase (mostly pyrimethamine, more rarely trimethoprim, proguanil or cycloguanil pamoate)

[e] The species other than *P. berghei* are indicated in parenthesis

[f] Cited in RICHARDS (1970)

Table 6. Comparative response of *Plasmodium berghei* (in mice) and *P. gallinaceum* (in chicks) to sulphonamides and dapsone alone and in combination with pyrimethamine (blood schizontocidal activity; from RICHARDS 1966)

Sulphonamides (sulphone)	Alone		In combination with pyrimethamine [b]	
	P. berghei	*P. gallinaceum*	*P. berghei* S[c]+P	*P. gallinaceum* S+P
Sulfadiazine	0.2[a]	3.0	0.02+0.0125	0.125+0.0015
Sulfadoxine	1.0	20.0	0.1 +0.0125	2.6 +0.004
Sulfa-dimethoxine	1.0	14.0	0.1 +0.0125	1.5 +0.0034
Dapsone	0.6	100	0.06+0.018	12.5 +0.004

[a] The figures indicate ED_{50} values in milligrams per kilogram per os (daily doses, administered on seven consecutive days, producing 50% reduction of parasitaemia compared with untreated controls)
[b] ED_{50} of pyrimethamine alone was 0.15 mg/kg per day in *P. berghei* and 0.03 mg/kg per day in *P. gallinaceum*
[c] S, dose of the sulphonamide (sulphone); P, dose of pyrimethamine administered in combination

(*P. gallinaceum, P. berghei, P. knowlesi, P. cynomolgi*) and the authors (in chronological order). With the single exception mentioned in the footnote the drugs were found to inhibit or reduce parasitaemia to some degree, at the doses used by the authors. In view of the enormous differences in the techniques and parameters used by the various authors we refrained from specifying the active doses [For reviews indicating such doses see DAVEY (1963), HILL (1963, 1966) and AVIADO (1969)]. A more quantitative comparison of activities will be attempted in the following paragraph on the basis of selected models.

It can, nevertheless, be stated that the schizontocidal activity of sulphonamides and sulphones is generally better in mammalian than in avian plasmodia. This is exemplified by data from *P. berghei* (mammalian) and *P. gallinaceum* (avian) which were obtained by a single author (RICHARDS 1966) and are, therefore, to be compared quite well. In the experience of this author, the different response held true when the sulphonamides and dapsone were administered alone or in synergistic mixtures with pyrimethamine, although the latter when given alone was more active in *P. gallinaceum* than in *P. berghei* (Table 6). Furthermore, it is a general rule that, among the mammalian plasmodia, rodent species are virtually all highly susceptible (*P. chabaudi* was found to be even more susceptible than *P. berghei*; PETERS 1967b), whereas the susceptibility of the monkey plasmodia differs from high (*P. knowlesi*) to only moderate (*P. cynomolgi*); *P. inui* is probably the least susceptible (COGGESHALL and MAIER 1941; COGGESHALL et al. 1941). As mentioned above, *P. gallinaceum* in chicks is relatively the most susceptible among the avian plasmodia, perhaps partially due to poorer bioavailability of the sulphonamides and sulphones in the hosts (canaries, ducks) that harbour the other species such as *P. cathemerium* and *P. lophurae*.

Table 7. Comparative blood schizontocidal activity of sulphonamides and sulphones against *P. berghei* in mice [4-day tests or similar procedures; see PETERS (1970, 1980)]

Compound	Effective doses in mg/kg per day according to different authors (parameter in parenthesis)							
	(ED_{50}[a] p.o.)	(ED_{50}[b] s.c.)	(ED_{75}[c] s.c.)	(ED_{90}[d] p.o.)	(ED_{98}[e] i.p.)	(ED_{99}[f] p.o.)	(ED_{50}[g] p.o.)	(ED_{50}[h] p.o.)
Sulfadiazine	0.2	0.01	0.06	0.05	0.3	0.18	0.4	3.0
Sulfamonomethoxine	–	0.03	–	–	–	–	–	0.5
Sulfadoxine	1.0	0.13[i]	–	–	–	–	0.22	2.5
Sulfalene	–	0.07	–	–	–	–	–	2.6
Sulfadimethoxine	1.0	2.0	–	–	–	–	0.5	5.0
Sulfamethoxazole	1.0	–	–	–	–	–	–	> 30.0
Dapsone	0.6	0.10	0.9	–	–	0.05	–	3.0
Diformyldapsone	–	0.20	–	–	–	–	–	5.0
Diacetyldapsone	–	–	–	–	–	–	–	2.5

[a] RICHARDS (1966)
[b] PETERS et al. (1975b)
[c] THOMPSON et al. (1967)
[d] HILL (1950)
[e] HAWKING (1966)
[f] THURSTON (1950), cit. PETERS (1970)
[g] KRETTLI and BRENER (1968)
[h] RICHLE (unpublished results)
[i] The ED_{50} of sulfadoxine found by PETERS (1965a) was 0.04 mg/kg

c) Comparative Activity in Selected Models

α) Plasmodium berghei in Mice. Table 7 presents a collection of those results from mouse experiments with *P. berghei* which (a) were all obtained with a "4-day test" (or a very similar procedure) and (b) provide comparative, quantitative data on the activity of the main, antimalarial sulphonamides and sulphones dealt with in this chapter. With most of these antimalarials, the doses found active were low, usually a very few milligrams per kilogram or less, whereas with other sulphonamides which are not known as antimalarials (sulfadimethoxine and sulfamethoxazole are included in the table as examples) they were higher. However, a great range of active doses exists within the group of the antimalarials.

This is most striking when one compares the figures in the horizontal line of the table, i.e. those reported for the same compound by different authors. With sulfadiazine and dapsone (on which we found the greatest number of data), for example, the extremes of the effective doses differ by the factors of 300 (from 0.01 up to 3 mg/kg and 60 (from 0.05 up to 3 mg/kg), respectively. This variation is only partially explained by differences in the route of administration (per os, s.c. or i.p.) and of the parameters (ED_{50}, ED_{80}, ED_{90}, etc.) but probably more so by differences in the strains of both the parasite and the murine host and, last but not least, by differences in the diet.

More reliability should be expected from comparison in the vertical line, i.e. from the activity found with different drugs by the same authors, who obviously used the same parameter, strain of parasite and host, diet, etc. It is, however, still surprising that the order of activity found by different authors for the individual drugs was not identical. For instance, in the experience of PETERS et al. (1975b) (second column of the table) the order was as follows (from the most to the least active): sulfadiazine, sulfamonomethoxine, sulfalene, dapsone, sulfadoxine, diformyldapsone, whereas in our own experience (last column of the table) it was: sulfamonomethoxine, sulfadoxine, sulfalene, sulfadiazine and dapsone (*ex aequo*), diformyldapsone. [Acedapsone is not included for lack of data from PETERS et al. (1975b)].

It can be concluded that the *P. berghei*-mouse model is appropriate to identify the antimalarially active sulphonamides and sulphones, whereas its value for distinguishing the degrees of potency among the active members of these classes of drugs is less evident. Marked differences of the active doses must be taken into account from one laboratory to another.

β) Plasmodium cynomolgi in Rhesus Monkeys. Table 8 shows the results from the above-mentioned *P. cynomolgi* model which were obtained by DAVIDSON et al. (1976) with four of the antimalarial sulphonamides and sulphones dealt with in this chapter, sulfadiazine, sulfalene, dapsone and diformyldapsone and, in addition, with sulfadimethoxine which is not used as an antimalarial drug. Sulfamonomethoxine, sulfadoxine and acedapsone were not included in the comparative testing. All compounds proved to be clearly active. Marked differences in the degree of activity were encountered among the individual animals receiving identical doses of the same drug (this is particularly evident for the "curative" doses), making it impossible to determine the exact end points. The following conclusions seem, nervertheless, permitted. Sulfadimethoxine is

Table 8. Comparative blood schizontocidal activity of sulphonamides and sulphones against *P. cynomolgi* in rhesus monkeys (DAVIDSON et al. 1976)

Compound	Doses in mg/kg per day producing antimalarial effects [a]							
	316	100	31.6	10.0	3.16	1.0	0.316	0.1
Sulfadiazine		C	MS	MS	MS	MS	MS	SS
		MS	MS	MS	MS	MS	MS	I
Sulfalene							C	
		C	MS	MS	MS	MS	MS	MS
		C	MS	MS	MS	MS	MS	I
							SS	
Sulfadimethoxine		MS	MS	MS	I	SS		
		MS	SS	SS	I	I		
Dapsone			C	C				
			MS	CS	MS	MS	MS	
			CS	MS	MS	MS	MS	
			MS	MS				
Diformyldapsone			C					
	C	C	MS	MS	MS	MS		
	CS	MS	MS	MS	MS	MS		
			MS					

[a] I, ineffective – course of parasitaemia similar to that in placebo-treated controls; SS, slight suppression – parasitaemia temporarily below 1,000 mm^3; MS, marked suppression – parasites absent for at least two successive days; recrudescence before D+30; CS, complete suppression – parasitaemia became negative but reappeared after splenectomy; C, curative – parasitaemia became negative and remained so up to at least 30 days after splenectomy. Each symbol represents one animal

clearly less active than the drugs used as antimalarials. No "cures" were obtained with this compound, and the doses from 3.16 mg/kg downwards were virtually inactive. With all the four other compounds, at least individual "cures" were recorded at the higher doses in the order of 10–100 mg/kg administered on seven consecutive days, and doses as low as 0.316 mg/kg were still definitely suppressive. Dapsone showed a tendency to produce "cures" at three to ten times lower doses than the other three "curative" compounds. Accepting this as a real difference one could argue that, thanks to their better tolerance, the other compounds, particularly the sulphonamides, can nevertheless be administered at a correspondingly higher dosage than dapsone.

When considering the relatively high and frequent doses necessary to produce the higher degree of activity, particularly "cures", one must take into account that *P. cynomolgi* is among the monkey plasmodia that show a relatively poor susceptibility to the sulphonamides and sulphones (see Sect. F. I. 2). In the generally more susceptible *P. knowlesi*, sulfalene proved "curative" at a daily dosage of only 0.5 mg/kg given for 7 days (ROTHE et al. 1969). Unfortunately, no comparative data are available on the activity of the other antimalarial sulphonamides and sulphones in the *P. knowlesi* model.

3. Tissue Schizontocidal Activity

a) Methods of Evaluation (for details see PETERS 1980)

The target organisms are the pre-erythrocytic schizonts developing in the reticuloendothelial (avian plasmodia) or liver parenchyma cells (mammalian plasmodia) of the vertebrate host during the prepatent period of the disease, i.e. between the infection with sporozoites from the insect vector and the appearance of parasitaemia. The drugs must be administered only during the prepatent period. Activity is evaluated either indirectly by a delay or non-appearance of parasitaemia (in *P. gallinaceum* also by non-appearance of the secondary exoerythrocytic forms) or, more exceptionally, directly by the finding of a reduced number of tissue schizonts in smears or sections from the appropriate organ, e.g. the liver, of the host. With the indirect method, one must make sure by appropriate controls that the delay or non-appearance of parasitaemia is not due to a residual activity of the drug on the early generations of blood schizonts. The exclusion of this possibility is of spezial importance with slowly eliminated ("long-acting") drugs tested on *P. berghei* since the prepatent period is only about 48 h in this parasite. Drugs completely preventing the patency of the disease by virtue of their action on the pre-erythrocytic tissue schizonts are referred to as "causal prophylactic agents".

b) Survey of Data

α) Monkey Plasmodia and *P. gallinaceum*. In 1938 sulphanilamide and sulphanilyl sulphanilate were claimed by COGGESHALL to act on *P. knowlesi* in the rhesus monkey not only therapeutically but also prophylactically but there is, retrospectively, little evidence of true "causal prophylaxis". Interestingly enough, a definite though incomplete action of sulfadiazine in tissue schizonts was later proven in *P. cynomolgi* (HAWKING and THURSTON 1952), the blood schizonts of which are generally less susceptible than those of *P. knowlesi*.

True "causal prophylactic" activity of sulphonamides including sulfadiazine was first demonstrated in the *P. gallinaceum* model in 1944 by three groups of authors (FREIRE and PARAENSE 1944; COATNEY and COOPER 1944; COGGESHALL et al. 1944) and was extensively confirmed during the subsequent years. In Table 5 the papers describing tissue schizontocidal activity of sulfadiazine, in addition to the effect on the blood schizonts, are indicated by *Footnote c*. Additional reports just on (always successful) "causal prophylaxis" with sulfadiazine in *P. gallinaceum* were those of DAVEY (1946b), ENGLISH et al. (1946) and SINGH et al. (1952a). The doses of sulfadiazine eradicating the pre-erythrocytic tissue schizonts of *P. gallinaceum* were somewhat higher than those clearing parasitaemia (BRACKETT and WALETZKY 1946) but of a similar order of magnitude (range 20–100 mg/kg administered twice daily, as reviewed by HILL 1963). However, even larger doses of the drug were usually not sufficient to eradicate the secondary exoerythrocytic forms when the treatment was started beyond the prepatent period (DAVEY 1946b; FINDLAY 1951). No experience seems to exist with any of the newer antimalarial sulphonamides in the prophylactic *P. gallinaceum* model.

At a dosage of 60 mg/kg daily the sulphone dapsone had no effect on the pre-erythrocytic tissue schizonts of *P. gallinaceum* (RAMAKRISHNAN et al. 1962).

Table 9. Tissue schizontocidal and sporontocidal activity[a] of antimalarial sulphonamides and sulphones[b] against *P. berghei* or *P. yoelii* in the rodent host and in the insect vector, respectively

Effects on	
Tissue schizonts in mice (exceptionally[c] in rats)[d]	Sporogony in *Anopheles stephensi*[e]
MOST et al. (1967) DDS[f] (*P. berghei*)	RAMKARAN and PETERS (1969) SO[g] (*P. berghei*)
GREGORY and PETERS (1970) SZ, DDS (*P. yoelii*)	
VINCKE (1970) SO[g] (*P. berghei*)	
FINK (1972) SZ (*P. yoelii*)	
FINK (1974) SZ, SO, DDS (*P. yoelii*)	VINCKE (1970) SO[g] (*P. berghei*)
HILL (1975) SO, ACD (*P. berghei*)	
MOST and MONTUORI (1975) SO, DDS (*P. berghei*)	
PETERS et al. (1975a) SZ, SM, SO (*P. yoelii nigeriensis*)	PETERS and RAMKARAN (1980) SO (*P. berghei* and *P. yoelii*)
RANE and KINNAMON (1979) SZ, DDS (*P. berghei*)	

[a] The drugs were found active at any degree at the doses or concentrations used by authors with the following exceptions: DDS (MOST et al. 1967) and DFD (PETERS et al. 1975a) inactive against tissue schizonts in mice; sulfadoxine and DDS at best marginally active against tissue schizonts in rats (MOST and MONTUORI 1967)
[b] Names of the drugs abbreviated as in Table 5
[c] Both rats and mice were used by VINCKE (1970) and MOST and MONTUORI (1975)
[d] Evaluated indirectly from non-appearance of parasitaemia in sporozoite-infected animals treated prophylactically during the prepatent period (repository drug action on parasitaemia excluded by controls), and by VINCKE (1970) and MOST and MONTUORI (1975) also directly from reduction of schizonts in liver sections
[e] Inhibition of oocyst formation in the mosquitoes receiving the drug directly in sucrose solution (RAMKARAN and PETERS 1969; PETERS and RAMKARAN 1980) or indirectly by sucking blood from mice to which the drug was administered before (VINCKE 1970; PETERS and RAMKARAN 1980)
[f] Also tested and found active against the blood schizonts
[g] Also found potentiated in combination with an inhibitor of dihydrofolic acid reductase (pyrimethamine)

β) Rodent Plasmodia. A survey of all pertinent published experiments known to the reviewers is given in Table 9, *left part,* and a comparison of the effective doses determined by three authors with different species or varieties (*P. berghei, P. yoelii yoelii, P. yoelii nigeriensis*) is presented in Table 10. With the exception of diformyldapsone (which was indeed administered at a low dosage) all drugs tested, namely sulfadiazine, sulfamonomethoxine, sulfadoxine and dapsone, exhibited

Table 10. Comparative tissue schizontocidal activity of antimalarial sulphonamides and sulphones against rodent plasmodia

Drugs	FINK (1974) *P. yoelii yoelii* (mice)[a] ED_{50} (mg/kg)	PETERS et al. (1975b) *P. yoelii nigeriensis* (mice)[b] ED_{99} (mg/kg)	VINCKE (1970) *P. berghei* (mice)[c] ED_{90} (mg/kg)	(rats) ED_{90} (Mg/kg)
Sulfadiazine	30 (15–60)	30 –60		
Sulfamono-methoxine		0.3– 1.0		
Sulfadoxine	84 (60–118)	3 –10	100 (S alone) S+P[d] 5+0.2	75 (S alone) S+P[d] 10+0.1
Dapsone	20 (13–32)	3 –10		
Diformyldapsone		> 1.0		

[a] Single i.p. dose of the drugs 2–4 h after i.v. infection with sporozoites; ED_{50} (author: CPD_{50}) preventing parasitaemia in 50% of the animals (with the 95% confidence limits calculated by the author)
[b] Single s.c. dose of the drugs 3 h after i.v. infection with sporozoites; ED_{99} (authors: minimum fully effective dose = MFED) preventing parasitaemia in all animals
[c] Two oral (or, with similar results, i.p.) doses of the drugs on the day before, and the day of, the i.v. infection with sporozoites; ED_{90} (estimated by the reviewers from the author's data) preventing parasitaemia (mouse experiments) or producing negative liver sections (rat experiments) in virtually all animals
[d] Synergism when sulfadoxine (S) was given in combination with pyrimethamine (P); the ED_{90} of pyrimethamine alone was approximately 10 mg/kg in mice and 20 mg/kg in rats

definite "causal prophylactic" activity, although somewhat higher doses were usually required than for blood schizontocidal activity (Table 7). It must indeed be taken into account that in the tests for blood schizontocidal activity, the doses were administered four times (Table 7), but only once in most of the tests for tissue schizontocidal activity ("causal prophylaxis"). The variation observed with the "causal prophylactic" doses of sulfadoxine (3–100 mg/kg) may reflect a different susceptibility of the plasmodial lines in question. A marked synergism was observed by one author (VINCKE 1970), with combinations of sulfadoxine plus pyrimethamine (Table 10).

4. Sporontocidal Activity

a) Methods of Evaluation (see PETERS 1980)

Starved mosquitoes (species of *Anopheles*, mostly *A. stephensi*, in the case of *P. gallinaceum* also *Aedes aegypti*) are allowed to feed on host animals, the blood of which contains mature, male and female gametocytes of a transmissible plasmodial strain. Subsequent sporogony is checked either by counting the oocysts grown around the midgut after an appropriate period or, less usually, by inoculating new host animals with homogenates prepared from the insects at the time when the sporozoites are normally mature. Inhibition of sporogony is indicated by a reduced number of well-developed oocysts or by a failure to infect new hosts. [The sulphonamides and sulphones lack any inhibitory effect on the gametocytes; see HERRERO (1967), PETERS (1970).] The drugs are fed to the mosquitoes either directly in sucrose solution, or indirectly by administering them to the host animals before the blood meal.

b) Survey of Data

α) Monkey Plasmodia and *P. gallinaceum*. The only pertinent experience with a simian *Plasmodium* is a note by GERBERG (1971) that sulfadiazine was sporontocidal in *Anopheles stephensi* when fed to the latter at a concentration of 0.1% in sucrose solution.

Sporontocidal activity of a sulphonamide was first observed by TERZIAN (1947) with *P. gallinaceum* in *Aedes aegypti*. Concentrations of 0.01%–0.1% of sulfadiazine added to the nutrient sucrose solution given to this insect were partially to fully effective. A similar efficacy of sulfadiazine on *P. gallinaceum* was confirmed in a different vector, *Anopheles quadrimaculatus*. It was also observed that the sulphonamide had no killing effect on the gametocytes or ookinetes, but acted only when the oocysts began to grow (TERZIAN et al. 1949). Depending on the vector species and the concentration of the drug, TERZIAN (1950) even noted an increase in the number of younger oocyst stages [for a critical account of Terzians's misunderstandable title, *The sulfonamides as factors in increasing susceptibility to parasitic invasion,* see PETERS (1970)]. In 1971, Gerberg confirmed the schizontocidal activity of 0.1% of sulfadiazine in the *P. gallinaceum*/*Ae. aegypti* system. On the other hand, no sporontocidal activity against *P. gallinaceum* in *Ae. aegypti* was observed with the sulphone dapsone, when the insects were fed on chicks receiving the drug at a single dose of 120 mg/kg (RAMAKRISHNAN et al. 1962) or even of 300 mg/kg (RAMAKRISHNAN et al. 1963). However, sporogony was completely inhibited with 210 mg/kg dapsone administered to the chicks in combination with only 0.028 mg/kg pyrimethamine; since pyrimethamine alone was not active at doses of less than 2 mg/kg, this was evidence of marked synergism (RAMAKRISHNAN et al. 1963).

β) Rodent Plasmodia. The experiments with rodent plasmodia are listed in the *right part* of Table 9. When fed to *Anopheles stephensi* in their nutrient sucrose solution, 0.03% of sulfadoxine produced a 50% reduction of the number of mature oocysts of *P. berghei*. Only about one-tenth of this concentration of sulfadoxine was required for the same effect when pyrimethamine was added to the nutrient at the minute concentration of around 10^{-6}%. Since pyrimethamine alone was 50% effective at a concentration of $6 \cdot 10^{-5}$%, this was consistent with a marked synergism (RAMKARAN and PETERS 1969). >99% reduction of the oocyst number was obtained with 0.5% of sulfadoxine alone (PETERS and RAMKARAN 1980) and with 0.01% and $7.3 \cdot 10^{-6}$%, respectively, of the combination of sulfadoxine and pyrimethamine (RAMKARAN and PETERS 1969).

When *A. stephensi* was infected with a blood meal from mice previously receiving sulfadoxine at single i.p. or oral doses of 15 and 10 mg/kg, respectively, a significant inhibition of oocyst formation was observed with *P. berghei* (VINCKE 1970) and *P. yoelii yoelii* (PETERS and RAMKARAN 1980).

In experiments with sulphonamides and the insect vectors, it must be taken into account that the drugs may kill the insects when the concentrations or doses are too high. The concentrations of sulfadoxine, for example, in the nutrient sucrose solution killing 50% of the insects was 0.3% for *Aedes aegypti* and 0.08% for *Anopheles stephensi*. Mice had to receive i.p. doses as high as 1,000 and 680 mg/kg sulfadoxine to kill 50% of *Ae. aegypti* and *A. stephensi*, respectively, that fed on their blood. Sulfadiazine was less toxic to the insects (BEESLEY and PETERS 1968).

II. Activity on Human Plasmodia in Monkeys and in Insect Vectors

1. Blood Schizontocidal Activity on *P. falciparum* and *P. vivax* in the Owl Monkey, Aotus trivirgatus

Published information is limited to data on sulfadiazine when administered to monkeys at a maximum dosage of 20–80 mg/kg daily for seven consecutive days. This drug was only 30%–40% curative on infections with two strains of *P. falciparum* and one strain of *P. vivax*, and even less so (about 10% cures) on infection with a third strain *P. falciparum* (SCHMIDT 1979). The cure rate was increased up to 67% or more when 20 mg/kg sulfadiazine was administered together with 2.5 mg/kg pyrimethamine (experiment with one strain *P. falciparum*) and 20 or 5 mg/kg sulfadiazine together with 0.625 mg/kg pyrimethamine (experiment with *P. vivax*); this was considered as evidence of synergism, since the corresponding doses of pyrimethamine alone were definitely less effective (SCHMIDT et al. 1977). Quite low doses of sulfadoxine alone (1.25 mg/kg) significantly reduced parasitaemia without being curative (SCHMIDT 1979). This experience is probably not representative for the normal response of *P. falciparum* and *P. vivax* to sulphonamides, since the strains used showed a certain degree of resistance to pyrimethamine and perhaps also other antimalarials.

2. Activity on the Sporogony of *P. falciparum* and *P. vivax* in Anopheles Species

Sulfadiazine fed to *Anopheles quadrimaculatus* at a concentration of 0.1% inhibited oocyst formation of *P. falciparum* in 80% of the insects (TERZIAN and WEATHERSBY 1949). Fed at the same concentration the drug was without effect on the sporogony of *P. vivax* in *A. quadrimaculatus* and *A. stephensi* (TERZIAN et al. 1968). In 1971, GERBERG confirmed that sulfadiazine fed in the nutrient solution at a concentration of 0.1% had a sporontocidal activity on *P. falciparum* in *A. stephensi*.

Data on the effect of sulphonamides or sulphones administered to human gametocyte carriers on the sporogony in mosquitoes which had fed on blood from these subjects are few and conflicting (for a critical account, see PETERS 1970). The available information is limited to *P. falciparum* (mostly in *A. gambiae*). Sulfadoxine and dapsone administered at doses of 1,000 mg and 200 mg, respectively, had no effect on sporogony (LAING 1965 b), but no oocysts were found in the insects fed from some gametocyte carriers receiving 500 mg sulfadoxine together with 6.25 or 12.5 mg pyrimethamine, or 100 mg dapsone plus 6.25 mg pyrimethamine (LAING 1968 b). Such isolated observations are difficult to evaluate since the infectivity of a single blood meal remains unknown. In *A. stephensi* fed on one human volunteer presenting *P. falciparum* gametocytaemia and receiving a combination of sulfadiazine (500 mg three times daily) plus pyrimethamine (50 mg daily) oocyst formation was, if at all, only marginally reduced (RIECKMANN et al. 1968). The particular strain of *P. falciparum* was chloroquine resistant, but was not known to have been previously exposed to sulphonamides or sulphones (no mention is made by the authors of its previous exposure to pyrimethamine).

G. Development in Man

I. Sulphonamides

DÍAZ DE LEÓN (1937) was the first who claimed to have obtained a clinical cure with a sulphonamide in human malaria. In his historic paper the successful treatment of 15 cases of *P. vivax* malaria with Rubiazol (6-carboxy-4-sulphamido-2′-4′diaminoazobenzene) is reported. In the same year HILL and GOODWIN (1937) published their experience with Prontosil for curative treatment of *Plasmodium falciparum* malaria. Ninety-three patients were treated with intramuscular injections of 10 ml Prontosil soluble every 12 h. After four injections marked improvement occurred, no relapses and no adverse reactions being recorded. Also in 1937, VAN DER WIELEN reported on the curative effect of Prontosil album in blood-induced *P. malariae* infections in two patients with dementia paralytica.

Over the following years a number of papers reporting the use of, and varying success with, sulphonamides in the treatment of human malaria were published, for instance by DÍAZ DE LEÓN (1938, 1940); NIVEN (1938); HALL (1938); PAKENHAM-WALSH and OXON (1938); SORLEY and CURRIE (1938); CHOPRA (1939); FARINAUD and ELICHE (1939); MENK and MOHR (1939); SINTON et al. (1939); COGGESHALL et al. (1941).

For a further 10 years i.e. until 1950, there still existed considerable interest in the use of sulphonamides in malaria. This is reflected by some important clinical trials such as those by FAIRLEY (1945) with sulfadiazine, sulfamerazine and sulfamethazine, by FINDLAY et al. (1946) with sulfadiazine, sulfathiazole, sulfamethazine and succinylsulfathiazole, and by COATNEY et al. (1947 a, b) with sulfadiazine and sulfapyrazine.

However, with the advent of more reliable synthetic antimalarials of other chemical types in the early 1950s, chemotherapeutic work in malaria with the relatively short-acting sulphonamides available at that time was reduced to research of more academic interest. Excellent reviews on the early trials with sulphonamides in malaria were made by CURD (1943), FINDLAY (1951) and HILL (1963).

The development of longer-acting sulphonamides for antibacterial chemotherapy, which started with the introduction of sulfamethoxypyridazine in 1956, revitalised interest in the use of this group of drugs in malaria. Clinical work with the long-acting sulphonamides in the field of malaria was reviewed by HERRERO (1967), RICHARDS (1970) and PINDER (1973).

Besides sulfadiazine, which has been widely tested in human malaria, this review deals with the long-acting sulphonamides sulfadoxine and sulfalene. These two sulphonamides are (in combination with pyrimethamine) in wide clinical use for treatment of malaria. This is also true for sulfamonomethoxine.

Table 11. Sulfadiazine in curative treatment of malaria

Country Subjects	Parasite and mode of infection	Treatment schedule (dose in mg)	No. of cases			Average duration to clearance (days) of		Reference
			Treated	Cleared (%)	Recru-descence (%)	Asexual parasitaemia	Fever	
Panama	*P. falciparum*	6,000 SD (1st day) + 4,000 SD (days 2–6)	5	3		1–2	1–3	COGGESHALL et al. 1941
	P. vivax	As above	7	7		2–5	2–3	
	P. malariae	As above	1	1		2	2	
	Naturally acquired							
West Africa European troops	*P. falciparum* Naturally acquired	6,000 SD (1st day) 4,000 SD (daily for further 5 days)	18	16	–	2.4	2.5	FINDLAY et al. 1946
		STZ (as SD)	18	17	–	2.6	2	
		SMZ (as SD)	40	37	–	2.6	2.3	
		SCS (1,800 daily for 6 days)	10	7	–	3.3	3	
		SP (as SD)	20	17	–	4.2	4	
		SM (as SD)	20	16	–	2.8	3.6	
The Gambia African infants and small children semi-immune	*P. falciparum* and/or	500 SD (single dose)	14	1	–	Not indicated		HURLY 1959
	P. malariae	1,000 SD (single dose)	9	0	–	Not indicated		
	P. ovale Naturally acquired	100 mg/kg P (single dose)	11	2		Not indicated		
		500 SD + 100 mg/kg P (single dose)	7	7		Within 3 days		
		250 SD + 10 mg/kg P (single dose)	14	14		Within 3 days		

United States Non-immune volunteers	*P. falciparum* Malaysian III, Malaysian IV, Thailand II, South Vietn. I Experimental (blood-induced) infection	500 SD (every 6 h, 5 days)	1	1	1	5	5	Chin et al. 1966
		500 SD (every 6 h, 5 days) + 50 P (single dose) for further sulphonamides see Table 3	4	4	2	3.7	4.2	
United States Non-immune and partially immune volunteers	*P. falciparum* Malay. (Camp) strain	500 SD (every 6 h, 2 days)	2	1	1	Not indicated		Powell et al. 1967
	Thailand (JHK) strain	500 SD (every 6 h, 5 days)	2	2	2	Not indicated		
	Vietn. (CV) strain (blood-induced or mosquito-induced infect.)	500 SD (every 6 h, 5 days) + 50 P (daily, 3 days)	12	12	1	2–5	4–6	
United States Semi- and non-immune volunteers	*P. falciparum* Vietn. (Marks) strain Experimental (blood-induced) infection	500 SD (every 6 h for 5 days) (see also Table 5, sulfalene)	3	1		Not indicated		Willerson et al. 1974

SD, Sulfadiazine; STZ, sulfathiazole; SMZ, sulfamethazine; SCS, succinylsulfathiazole; SM, sulfamerazine; SL, sulfalene; SP, sulfapyrazine; P, pyrimethamine.
Underlined numbers refer to studies with individual compounds; other numbers refer to comparative studies with various combinations (e.g. with pyrimethamine or primaquine)

1. Sulfadiazine

a) Curative Potential (see Table 11, compilation of trials)

The curative effect of sulfadiazine in *P. falciparum* malaria was investigated for the first time by COGGESHALL et al. in 1941. Of five patients three were cured, with clearance of parasitaemia in 1–2 days and defervescence within 1–3 days. FINDLAY et al (1946) investigated the therapeutic effect off several sulphonamides, including sulfadiazine (for details see Table 11) in acute cases of *P. falciparum* malaria in European troops in West Africa. Sulfadiazine (6 g on the 1st day plus 4 g daily for a further 5 days) as well as the other sulphonamides tested had a slight effect in controlling infection, but were far inferior to mepacrine and quinine.

HURLY (1959), who treated African infants and children in The Gambia, observed a reduction of the density of parasitaemia in all cases given 0.5 or 1.0 g of the drug, but in only one case out of 23 who were given sulfadiazine alone was the infection eradicated. However administered in combination with pyrimethamine, sulfadiazine was fully effective against asexual forms of *P. falciparum, P. malariae* and *P. ovale*.

In volunteers infected with various drug-resistant strains CHIN et al. (1966) as well as POWELL et al. (1967) achieved only poor efficacy within sulfadiazine alone (and with other sulphonamides, see Table 13). When combined with pyrimethamine, sulfadoxine and sulfamethoxypyridazine were superior to sulfadiazine.

WILLERSON et al. (1974), too, reported on the results of chemotherapeutic studies with sulfadiazine (and sulfalene, see also Table 15) in volunteers infected with a multiresistant strain of *P. falciparum* (Vietnam Marks). Two non-immune subjects received 500 mg sulfadoxine every 6 h for 5 days. Both had only an insufficient response to therapy. One additional, partially immune subject was cured.

P. vivax and *P. malariae*. COGGESHALL et al. (1941) reported on the successful treatment of seven cases of *P. vivax* malaria and of one case of quartan malaria with sulfadiazine (6 g the 1st day and 4 g daily for the next 5 days). Fever disappeared within 2–3 days and clearance of asexual parasitaemia was obtained within 2–5 days.

JOHNSON (1943; quoted by FINDLAY et al. 1946) used sulfadiazine in blood-induced infections with *P. malariae* (13 cases) and *P. vivax* (one case). Fever and parasites disappeared, but three patients had relapses which were controlled by a further course of the drug.

In a trial with African children eight pure *P. malariae* cases, six mixed *P. malariae* and *P. falciparum* infections and one mixed *P. falciparum* and *P. ovale* infection responded well to combined treatment with single doses of sulfadiazine (250 and 500 mg) and pyrimethamine (10 and 100 mg) (HURLY 1959).

b) Suppressive Potential (see Table 12, compilation of trials)

P. falciparum. The suppressive action of sulfadiazine, sulfamerazine and sulfamethazine was investigated in non-immune volunteers by FAIRLEY (1945). At a dosage of 1 g daily, started on the day before or on the day of exposure to the mosquitoes and given for 24–30 days, these drugs were found to suppress 20, and to cure 17 out of 21 mosquito-transmitted *P. falciparum* infections. Similar results were obtained in blood-induced malaria.

COATNEY et al. (1947a, b) tested sulfadiazine and sulfapyrazine as protective agents against mosquito-induced *P. falciparum* (McLendon strain) in trials involving 74 treated and 36 control subjects (non-immune volunteers). Sulfadiazine, in dosages at the upper limit of tolerance (12 g/day), continued for 46 h after exposure, did not act as a causal prophylactic, although the prepatent and incubation periods were doubled. Four grams of sulfadiazine daily for 6 days after exposure, or 2 g daily for 5 or 10 days, likewise produced only a delay of patent infection. However, 4 g sulfadiazine daily for 11 days after exposure prevented infection in four of five subjects, and 4 g daily for 42 days permanently protected all of ten subjects. Two grams daily for the same period protected nine of ten subjects and 1 g eight of nine, while 0.5 g daily protected three of five subjects from patent parasitaemia and clinical attacks. Half a gram of sulfapyrazine daily for 42 days after exposure gave results similar to those with the same dosage of sulfadiazine.

P. vivax. Sulfadiazine as well as sulfamerazine and sulfamethazine given in daily doses of 1 g for 24 days, failed in mosquito- and blood-induced *P. vivax* infections; all 48 volunteers developed overt malaria while taking the drug or shortly after cessation of its administration (FAIRLEY 1945).

COATNEY et al. (1947b) described trials in which sulfadiazine, in dosages up to 3 g daily for 6 weeks after exposure, failed to prevent or to eradicate infections with the St. Elisabeth strain of *P. vivax*. When plasma concentrations above 5 mg/100 ml were maintained, however, the drug was definitely suppressive, delaying attacks of malaria until the cessation of treatment, and in four of five subjects it induced prolonged latency, so that parasitaemia did not appear until 9–11 months after exposure. On lower dosage regimens (2 and 1 g daily for 6 weeks) the majority of subjects developed clinical episodes while receiving treatment. Parasitaemia also appeared despite suppressive treatment with sulfapyrazine in dosages of 0.5 and 1 g daily for 6 weeks.

c) Effect on Gametocytes

In his curative trial with sulfadiazine and pyrimethamine HURLY (1959) found that the gametocytes of *P. falciparum* and/or *P. malariae* persisted in the blood of several children, but their infectivity was not determined. Occurrence or persistence of gametocytes of *P. falciparum* after the administration of sulfadiazine was also observed by POWELL et al. (1967).

2. Sulfamonomethoxine

a) Curative Potential

P. falciparum. In 1970, YOSHINAGA et al. reported on the efficacy of sulfamonomethoxine in curative treatment of *P. falciparum* and of mixed *P. falciparum* and *P. vivax* infections in Kenya. Two hundred and twelve patients were treated with total doses from 1–9 g, administered within 2–4 days. Patients receiving an initial dosage larger than 20 mg/kg were cured, but those who were treated with an initial dosage of less than 20 mg/kg did not respond. Sulfamonomethoxine

Table 12. Sulfadiazine in suppressive treatment of malaria

Country Subjects	Parasite and mode of infection	Treatment schedule			No. of sub-jects	Positive blood films		Reference
		Dose (mg)	Adminis-tration	Duration		%	Found after	
Australia Non-immune volunteers	*P. falciparum* Mosquito-induced infection (ten infective bites over 7 days)	1,000 SD or 1,000 SM or 1,000 SMZ	Daily	30 days (starting at 1st day of bite)	21	19	3–9 days after end of treatment	FAIRLEY (1945)
	P. falciparum Blood-induced infection	1,000 SD or 1,000 SM or 1,000 SMZ	Daily	24 days (starting on day before infection)	24	17	During or shortly after end of treatment	
	P. vivax Mosquito-induced infection (20–23 infective bites over 7 days)	1,000 SD or 1,000 SM or 1,000 SMZ	Daily	24 days (starting 1–2 days before exposure)	24	100	During or shortly after end of treatment	
	P. vivax Blood-induced infection	1,000 SD or 1,000 SM or 1,000 SMZ	Daily	24 days (starting on day before infection)	24	100	During or shortly after end of treatment	

United States Non-immune volunteers	*P. falciparum* McLendon strain Mosquito-induced infection (interrupted bite technique)	12,000 SD	Daily	2 days (starting at day before bites or 2 h after bites)	15	93	Coatney et al. (1947a)
		4,000 SD	Daily	8, 14, 42 days (starting 2–3 days before bites or 2 h after bites)	20	30	
		2,000 SD	Daily	10, 15, 45, 50 days (starting 2–4 days before bites)	20	55	
		1,000 SD	Daily	45 days (starting 2 days before bites)	9	11	
		500 SP	Daily	45 days (starting 2 days before bites)	10	50	
United States Non-immune volunteers	*P. vivax* St. Elisabeth strain, Mosquito-induced infection	3,000 SD	Daily	44 days (starting 2 days before bites)	10	100	Coatney et al. (1947b)
		2,000 SD	Daily	Same as above	5	100	
		1,000 SD	Daily	Same as above	5	100	
		500 or 1,000 SP	Daily	Same as above	10	100	

SD, sulfadiazine; SM, sulfamerazine; SMZ, sulfamethazine; SP, sulfapyrazine
Underlined numbers refer to studies with individual compounds; other numbers refer to comparative studies with various combinations (e.g. with pyrimethamine or primaquine)

Table 13. Sulfadoxine in curative treatment of malaria

Country Subjects	Parasite and mode of infection	Treatment schedule (doses in mg)	No. of cases			Average duration to clearance (days) of		Reference
			Treated	Cleared (%)	Recrudescence (%)	Asexual parasitaemia	Fever	
Tanzania Semi-immune Bantu Africans	*P. falciparum* Naturally acquired	250–1,000 S	25	22 (88)	–	2.6–3	1.8	LAING (1965c)
United States Non-immune volunteers	*P. falciparum* Malaysian III, Malaysian IV, Thailand II, South Vietn. I Experimental (blood-induced) infection	1,000 S (single dose)	4	3	1	4.3	6	CHIN et al. (1966)
		1,000 S + 50 P (single dose)	24	23 (96)	2	3.3	3.8	
		500 SD (every 6 h, 5 days)	1	1	1	5	5	
		500 SD (every 6 h, 5 days) + 50 P (single dose)	4	4	2	3.7	4.2	
		2,000 SMP (1st day) + 1,000 SMP (once daily, 6 days)	2	2	1	4	3.5	
		1,000 SMP (1st day) + 500 SMP (once daily, 4 days) plus 50 P (single dose)	8	8	3	3.1	3.7	
Thailand Semi-immune Thais	*P. falciparum* Chloroquine-resistant, naturally acquired	1,000–1,500 S (single dose)	18	11 (61)	2 (11)	5.7	2.6	HARINASUTA et al. (1967)
		1,000 S (single dose) + 1,500 C (2-day treatment)	13	11 (85)	0	4	1.4	
		250 S + 25–50 P (single dose)	15	11 (73)	3 (20)	4.2	2.4	
		1,000 S + 50 P (single dose)	19	17 (89)	2 (11)	2.9	1.1	

Malaysia Semi-immune Malays (adults and school-children)	*P. falciparum* Naturally acquired	1,000 S (single dose)	9	8 (89)	–	3.1	2.1	Laing (1968b)
		200–1,000 S + 12.5–50 P (single dose)	49	44 (90)	–	2.3	2	
		600–2,580 C (1–3 days)	36	25 (69)	–	2.7	1.4	
	P. vivax Naturally acquired	1,000 S (single dose)	13	7 (54)	–	3.0	1.6	
		200–500 S + 25–50 P (single dose)	14	12 (86)	–	2.4	2	
		600–1,700 C (1–3 days)	13	13 (100)	–	1.2	0.7	
United States Non-immune volunteers	*P. vivax* Chesson strain, Experimental (blood-induced) infection	2,000 S (single dose)	4	4	4	Not indicated		Martin and Arnold 1969a
		1,000 SL (single dose)	3	3	3	Not indicated		
		100 DDS (daily for 10 days)	5	5	5	Not indicated		
		1,000 SL + 500 TMP						
		Single dose	12	12	5	2.5	1.2	
		Two doses (every 3rd day)	1	1	0	Not indicated		
		Three doses (every 3rd day)	8	8	0	Not indicated		
The Gambia Semi-immune local people Mostly children (6 months–12 years)	*P. falciparum* Naturally acquired	250–1,000 S (single dose)	18	14 (74)	–	1–6	2.0	Laing 1970
		25–50 S (single dose)	15	10 (67)	–	2–6	1.9	
		0.2–2 mg/kg S + 0.01–0.1 mg/kgP (single dose)	68	67 (98)	–	1–3	1.5	
		5–25 DDS (single dose)	18	10 (55)	–	1–6		

S, sulfadoxine; SD, sulfadiazine; SDM, sulfadimethoxine; SL, sulfalene; SMP, sulfamethoxypyridazine; C, chloroquine; P, pyrimethamine; DDS, dapsone; TMP, trimethoprim

Underlined numbers refer to studies with individual compounds; other numbers refer to comparative studies with various combinations (e.g. with pyrimethamine or primaquine)

proved effective also in cases where no clearance of parasitaemia had been obtained by a previous treatment course with chloroquine.

The schizontocidal and radical curative activities of sulfamonomethoxine were also studied by RAMOS and CABRERA (1972) in the Philippines. Thirty-six subjects with asymptomatic *P. falciparum* infection were treated with the drug, seven at a total dosage of 80 mg/kg, given in 3 days, and 29 at 100 mg/kg, given in 4 days. All were radically cured of their infection. Of 29 cases of *P. falciparum,* infections presenting RI grade of chloroquine resistance and one of the RII grade treated with 80 or 100 mg/kg, 28 were radically cured whereas 2 patients receiving the lower dosage exhibited recrudescence and RII response, respectively.

P. vivax. Of 48 cases of *P. vivax* infection, who received 80 mg/kg, 21 were radically cured, while of seven cases treated with 100 mg/kg only one was cured (RAMOS and CABRERA 1972).

b) Suppressive Potential

P. falciparum and/or *P. vivax*. The suppressive potential of sulfamonomethoxine was also studied in the Philippines by CABRERA and RAMOS (1972). One gram of the drug was administered in a single weekly dose for eight consecutive weeks to 127 subjects who were all negative for plasmodia before the start of suppressive treatment. Of the 127 subjects given prophylaxis, 13 (10.2%) became positive for malaria parasites. Nine of these were *P. falciparum* and four were *P. vivax* infections. The early appearance of *P. falciparum* (four subjects were positive at the end of the 1st week and another four subjects after the 2nd week) was attributed by the investigators to the possible existence of the infection in the exoerythrocytic stage of development prior to the start of suppressive treatment.

c) Effect on Gametocytes

RAMOS and CABRERA (1972) claimed that sulfamonomethoxine would have no effect on the gametocytes of *P. falciparum* but good activity on those of *P. vivax*. The latter finding was never confirmed by other authors.

3. Sulfadoxine

The first clinical trials to prove a substantial curative and suppressive effect of this long-acting sulphonamide in human malaria were performed by LAING (1964, 1965 c) in Tanzania. The favourable results obtained by LAING were confirmed by further studies in both naturally acquired and experimentally induced malaria.

a) Curative potential

P. falciparum. Trials to assess the curative effect of sulfadoxine, mainly in comparison with combinations with pyrimethamine, have been carried out in naturally acquired infections in East and West Africa (Tanzania, The Gambia) and in Southeast Asia (Malaysia, Thailand). Furthermore, one study in volunteers experimentally infected with different strains of *P. falciparum* was made in the United States. The results of these studies are compiled in Table 13.

In Tanzania 25 Bantu Africans were treated for acute falciparum malaria with single doses ranging from 250 mg in young children to 1 g in adults. Except for three patients, classified as failures because of slow response, asexual parasitaemia subsided within 2.6–3 days and fever within 1.8 days (LAING 1965c). In Thailand HARINASUTA et al. (1967) found that sulfadoxine in a single dose of 1,000 or 1,500 mg cured 11 of 18 patients suffering from chloroquine-resistant *P. falciparum* malaria, but the clinical response was slower than after a single dose of 1,000 mg sulfadoxine plus 50 mg pyrimethamine. Similar results were obtained by LAING (1968 b) in Malaysia. Sulfadoxine alone in a single dose of 1,000 mg proved an effective but slow schizontocide in *P. falciparum* infections. In this trial, too, a faster parasitological and clinical response was observed with combinations of sulfadoxine and pyrimethamine.

In a hospital trial in The Gambia, also performed by LAING (1970), 18 patients were treated with a single, 250- to 1,000-mg dose of sulfadoxine. Six were cured within 3 days, eight responded more slowly (3–6 days) and four were failures. Fifteen other patients were given subtherapeutic doses of sulfadoxine (25–50 mg). Even with this small dosage there was an appreciable schizontocidal effect, ten patients being cleared of asexual parasitaemia within a week. However, the best results were again achieved with combinations of sulfadoxine (or dapsone) and pyrimethamine, indicating strong potentiation.

CHIN et al. (1966) reported on the evaluation of sulfadoxine, sulfamethoxypyridazine and sulfadiazine, alone or combined with pyrimethamine, against blood-induced infections with different drug-resistant strains of *P. falciparum*. The number of volunteers was too small to determine the relative merits of each sulphonamide when used alone, but the results indicate that all three sulphonamides exerted antimalarial activity. When combined with pyrimethamine, sulfadoxine and sulfamethoxypyridazine were superior to sulfadiazine and, of the regimens tested, 1,000 mg sulfadoxine given together with 50 mg pyrimethamine as a single oral dose showed the most promise for successful treatment of the multi-drug-resistant falciparum malarias.

P. vivax. Contrary to *P. falciparum* infections, where sulfadoxine proved to be an effective though slow schizontocide, its efficacy in *P. vivax* malaria seems to be less satisfactory. LAING (1968 b), who treated 13 patients in Malaysia with single doses of 1,000 mg, found a slow response in nearly every patient and five failures were noted. The results were much better when sulfadoxine was used in combination with pyrimethamine but were still inferior to those obtained with chloroquine.

Poor results with sulfadoxine as well as with sulfalene and dapsone were obtained also by MARTIN and ARNOLD (1969 a) in volunteers with blood-induced infections of the Chesson strain of *P. vivax*. The parasites were completely refractory to dapsone (1,000 mg daily for 10 days). The two sulphonamides, given in a single dose of 2,000 mg (sulfadoxine) or 1,000 mg (sulfalene), were capable of completely suppressing parasitaemia but neither effected a radical cure.

b) Suppressive Potential

P. falciparum. The various suppressive trials, all performed in Africa, are compiled in Table 14.

Table 14. Sulfadoxine in suppressive treatment of malaria

Country Subjects	Parasite and mode of infection	Treatment schedule			No. of subjects	Positive blood films		Reference
		Dose (mg)	Adminis-tration	Duration		%	Found after	
Tanzania Schoolchildren, semi-immune	*P. falciparum* Pyrimethamine-resistant Naturally acquired infection	(1) 500 S+25 P	Weekly	6 weeks	191	0	6 weeks	LAING (1964)
		(2) 500 S	Weekly	6 weeks	200	0	6 weeks	
		(3) 25 P	Weekly	6 weeks	192	26	6 weeks	
Nigeria Schoolchildren, semi-immune	*P. falciparum* *P. malariae* Naturally acquired	(1) 500 S	Weekly	4 weeks	195	0.5 *P.f.*	4 weeks	SHUTE and DOWLING (1966)
						0 *P.m.*	4 weeks	
		(2) 500 S	Single dose		233	2 *P.f.*	4 weeks	
						0 *P.m.*	4 weeks	
		(3) 300 C	Single dose		222	16 *P.f.*	4 weeks	
						0 *P.m.*	4 weeks	
		(4) Control group	Untreated		78	77 *P.f.*	4 weeks	
						13 *P.m.*	4 weeks	
Tanzania Schoolchildren, semi-immune	*P. falciparum* Pyrimethamine-resistant Naturally acquired infection *P. ovale*	(1) 500 S+25 P	Weekly	6 weeks	156	0	6 weeks	LAING (1968a)
		(2) 25 P	Weekly	6 weeks	72	35	6 weeks	
		(3) 500 S	Weekly	6 weeks	134	1.5	6 weeks	
		(4) 150 C	Weekly	6 weeks	155	3	6 weeks	
		(1) 12.5 P	Weekly	8 weeks	112	14	8 weeks	
		(2) 250 S	Weekly	8 weeks	118	1.7	8 weeks	
		(3) 150 C	Weekly	8 weeks	152	0	8 weeks	
		(1) 125 S	Single dose		126	0.8 *P.o.*	7 days	
		(2) 100 S	Single dose		37	3 *P.f.*	7 days	
						8 *P.o.*	7 days	
		(3) 75 S	Single dose		36	3 *P.f.*	7 days	
		(4) 50 S	Single dose		35	3 *P.f.*	7 days	
						3 *P.o.*	7 days	
		(5) 25 S	Single dose		33	9 *P.f.*	7 days	

Tanzania	*P. falciparum*				*Day 7*	*Day 14*	*Day 21*	
Schoolchildren,	(*P. malariae,*	(1) 62.5 S	Single dose	51	7.8	18	60.4	CLYDE (1967)
semi-immune	*P. vivax,*	(2) 125 S	Single dose	89	1.1	2.4	22.7	
	P. ovale)	(3) 250 S	Single dose	123	0	0.8	9.7	
		(4) 500 S	Single dose	76	1.3	1.3	8.2	
		(1) 62.5 SDM	Single dose	61	14.8	30.7	67.2	
		(2) 125 SDM	Single dose	120	1.7	2.6	32.2	
		(3) 250 SDM	Single dose	131	0	2.3	13.2	
		(1) 62.5 SMP	Single dose	49	10.2	39.1	77.1	
		(2) 125 SMP	Single dose	66	3.0	15.2	45.6	
		(3) 250 SMP	Single dose	115	0	4.4	18.2	
		(1) 50 DDS	Single dose	54	3.7	9.8	67.3	
		(2) 100 DDS	Single dose	114	0	3.5	16.5	
		(3) 200 DDS	Single dose	143	0	0.7	11.5	

S, sulfadoxine; SDM, sulfadimethoxine; SMP, sulfamethoxypyridazine; C, chloroquine; P, pyrimethamine; DDS, dapsone; TMP, trimethoprim

The results of a field trial with sulfadoxine in Tanzanian school children were reported by LAING (1964). All children had previously received 25 mg pyrimethamine weekly for 2 months in order to eliminate the drug-sensitive parasites. After this period 27% still showed asexual parasitaemia (*P. falciparum*). Suppressive treatment was then continued for 6 weeks with weekly doses of (a) sulfadoxine alone (500 mg) or (b) sulfadoxine plus pyrimethamine (25 mg) or (c) pyrimethamine alone as before. Examination after 6 weeks showed that asexual parasitaemia had disappeared in the two groups received sulfadoxine alone or in combination, whereas in the third group receiving pyrimethamine alone the percentage of the children with parasitaemia was still 26%.

The duration of the suppressive effect of a single dose of 500 mg sulfadoxine against infections with *P. falciparum* was found to be longer than that of a single dose of chloroquine (300 mg) in Nigerian school children (SHUTE and DOWLING 1966). In this trial, too, a good suppressive effect was obtained with 500 mg sulfadoxine once a week.

Sulfadoxine in weekly doses of 500 mg and 250 mg and in a single test in weekly doses of 125 mg (5 mg/kg) was, again by LAING (1968a), found successful in suppressing malaria, including pyrimethamine-resistant falciparum malaria in asymptomatic Bantu school children normally exhibiting parasitaemia at a percentage of 60%–70%.

Another field trial in Tanzanian schoolchildren was performed by CLYDE (1967). Sulfadoxine, sulfadimethoxine and sulfamethoxypyridazine in single doses of 250 mg and dapsone in a single dose of 200 mg cleared asexual parasitaemia, whereas lower doses were less effective. Blood schizonts remained absent for about 12 days after treatment with sulfadoxine and dapsone, and for a shorter period after treatment with the other two compounds.

P. malariae and *P. ovale*. According to SHUTE and DOWLING (1966) the action of sulfadoxine against infections with *P. malariae* appeared to be slower than that of chloroquine. Five infections were detected at the end of the 1st week among 195 children treated with 500 mg of the former drug, while in 222 children treated with 300 mg of the latter no infection became apparent. However, CLYDE (1967) found that single doses of 125, 250 and 500 mg sulfadoxine cleared asexual parasitaemia of *P. malariae* and of *P. ovale* within 7 days, and that after this treatment the blood schizonts remained absent for about 12 days.

During his field and therapeutic trials it was noted by LAING (1968a) that *P. ovale* was somewhat refractory to sulfadoxine alone but sensitive to combinations with pyrimethamine; *P. malariae* appeared to be sensitive to sulfadoxine alone in the two cases treated by this author.

c) Effects on Gametocytes and Sporogony

Gametocytes of *P. falciparum* appeared to be unaffected by sulfadoxine (LAING 1965a, 1965c), and mosquitoes (*Anopheles gambiae*) fed on a patient treated with 1,000 mg had normally developing oocysts or sporozoites. Sulfadoxine, therefore, was considered to have no sporontocidal action against *P. falciparum*.

SHUTE and DOWLING (1966), too, found that 500 mg sulfadoxine given either as a single dose or once weekly for 4 weeks had no recognisable gametocytocidal effect on *P. falciparum* and *P. malariae*. A rise of the gametocyte count of *P. falci-*

parum was observed by HARINASUTA et al. (1967) in 15 of 18 patients after a single dose of 1,000–1,500 mg and gametocytes did not disappear before an average treatment period of 28 days.

In curative treatment of vivax malaria with single doses of 1,000 mg sulfadoxine the gametocytes were usually present after the clearance of the schizonts (LAING 1968 b).

4. Sulfalene

a) Curative Potential

P. falciparum. With the exception of two hospital trials in Somalia the curative potential of sulfalene was only investigated in experimental infections in mostly non-immune volunteers (see Table 15).

The first trial demonstrating the schizontocidal action of sulfalene on *P. falciparum* was performed by BARUFFA (1966) in Somalia. Treatment of acute falciparum malaria with 1.5–2.5 g of the compound administered weekly for 2–18 weeks resulted in clearance of asexual parasitaemia in all 27 patients within 1–5 days. No relapses occurred in patients followed up for long periods. A similarly favourable result was obtained by MAZZONI (1967), who, again in Somalia, treated 55 patients for 2–7 weeks with weekly doses of 2.5 g (adult dose) or 40 mg/kg (children).

MARTIN and ARNOLD (1968) found sulfalene to be very effective against a chloroquine-pyrimethamine-resistant strain of *P. falciparum* (Camp strain). Seven volunteers were all cured when 1 g was given as a single dose. However, against a strain of *P. falciparum* sensitive to all common antimalarial drugs (Uganda I strain), sulfalene was not as satisfactory; it cured only two of five infected volunteers who had received 1 g and three of six who were given 2.5 g. In both *P. falciparum* strains the speed of action was slow. The clearance of parasites was slower than with quinine. In a further trial with volunteers MARTIN and ARNOLD (1969b) demonstrated that the sensitivity of the Uganda I strain to sulfalene increased considerably after resistance to pyrimethamine was induced. Nine of 11 infected volunteers were cured by a single dose of 1 g. In the opinion of the authors this confirms the hypothesis that the sulphonamide sensitivity of a strain depends on whether or not it synthesises its own folic acid.

In contrast to the good result obtained by MARTIN and ARNOLD (1969 b) in pyrimethamine-resistant *P. falciparum* malaria, CLYDE et al. (1971 b) achieved only a poor curative effect in volunteers infected with pyrimethamine-resistant strains. Doses of 0.25 g or 1 g sulfalene were administered to 33 infected volunteers, 14 of whom, all infected with pyrimethamine-resistant strains, were not cured.

WILLERSON et al. (1974) reported on the results of chemotherapeutic studies in volunteers infected with a multiresistant strain of *P. falciparum* from Vietnam (Marks strain). Sulfalene in a single dose of 1 g was given to three non-immune volunteers and two partially immune subjects. Radical cure was achieved in four of the five subjects, but clearance of fever and clinical symptoms was slow in the non-immune persons (6 days). Clearance of asexual parasites occurred after 1–6 days (mean 2.5 days). In this trial radical cure in non-immune volunteers was most often achieved with combined drug regimens, including trimethoprim and sulfalene (five

Table 15. Sulfalene in curative treatment of malaria

Country Subjects	Parasite and mode of infection	Treatment schedule (dose in mg)	No. of cases			Average duration to clearance (days) of		Reference
			Treated	Cleared (%)	Recrudescence (%)	Asexual parasitaemia	Fever	
Somalia Somalia patients (adults and children)	*P. falciparum* Naturally acquired	1,500–2,000–2,500 SL (once weekly for 2–18 weeks)	27	27	0	1.9	1.6	BARUFFA (1966)
Somalia Somali patients (adults and children)	*P. falciparum* Naturally acquired	2,500 SL (adults) 40 mg/kg (children) (once weekly for 2–7 weeks)	55	55	0	Not indicated	1–4	MAZZONI (1967)
United States Non-immune volunteers	*P. falciparum* Uganda I strain	1,000–2,500 SL (within 12 h)	11	11	6	6–8.4	3–4	MARTIN and ARNOLD (1968)
	Camp strain Experimental (blood-induced) infection	1,000 SL (single dose)	7	7		4	3.4	
United States Non-immune volunteers	*P. falciparum* Camp strain	1,000 SL (single dose)	9	9	0	Not indicated	Not indicated	MARTIN and ARNOLD (1969b)
	Uganda I strain	1,000–2,500 SL	11	11	6	6–8.4	3–4	
	Uganda I (P-resistant)	1,000 SL (single dose)	11	11	2	3	1.4	
United States Non-immune volunteers	*P. vivax* Chesson strain Experimental (blood-induced infection)	1,000 SL (single dose)	3	3	3	Not indicated	Not indicated	MARTIN and ARNOLD (1969a)

United States Non-immune volunteers	*P. falciparum* McLendon, Man. Tay. Poo. Smith,	250 SL (single dose)	11	6	3	4.2	Not indicated	CLYDE et al. (1971b)
	Brai-strain Experimental (blood-induced) infection	1,000 SL (single dose)	22	13	6	4	Not indicated	
United States Semi- and non-immune volunteers	*P. falciparum* Vietn. (Marks) strain	<u>1,000 SL</u> (single dose)	<u>5</u>	<u>5</u>	<u>1</u>	<u>2.5</u>	6	WILLERSON et al. (1974)
	Experimental (blood-induced) infection	500 SD (every 6 h for 5 days)	3	1		Not indicated	Not indicated	
United States Non-immune volunteers	*P. falciparum* Vietn. (Marks) strain Experimental (mosquito- or blood-induced infection	1,000 SL (single dose)	8	4	3	5.5	3.5	R.L. WILLIAMS et al. (1978)

SL, sulfalene; SD, sulfadiazine; P, pyrimethamine.
Underlined numbers refer to studies with individual compounds; other numbers refer to comparative studies with various combinations (e.g. with pyrimethamine or primaquine)

of seven volunteers), quinine and tetracycline (five of five volunteers) or quinine and sulfalene (two of two volunteers).

WILLIAMS et al. (1978) found in eight volunteers infected with the Vietnam Marks strain of *P. falciparum* that the acetylator phenotype (rapid or slow acetylators) did not influence the therapeutic response to sulfalene or to the combination of sulfalene plus pyrimethamine. Three of the four individuals who were not cured by 1 or 2 g sulfalene or by 2 g sulfalene plus 50 mg pyrimethamine were slow acetylators. In view of these findings a yet unidentified host factor which determines the therapeutic response to these agents was postulated by the authors.

P. vivax. In three volunteers with blood-induced infections of *P. vivax* (Chesson strain) 1 g sulfalene was capable of completely suppressing the parasitaemia but no radical cure was achieved (MARTIN and ARNOLD 1969 a) and in all three volunteers recrudescence occurred.

b) Suppressive Potential (see Table 16, compilation of trials)

P. falciparum. The only trial with mass treatment, in which sulfalene was given at 2-weekly intervals for 5 months to symptomless carriers of *P. falciparum* and/or *P. malariae*, was carried out by MICHEL (1968) in a holoendemic area in Senegal. Four groups, each of about 100 children aged 1–14 years, were treated according to the following regimens: sulfalene 125–500 mg, sulfalene plus 6.2–25 mg pyrimethamine, chloroquine 20 mg/kg, and placebo. Sulfalene alone was found to have little effect on the incidence of parasitaemia, which only fell from 87.8% to 41.1%. The combination with pyrimethamine reduced the percentage from 75.2% to 13.2% and chloroquine reduced it from 75.8% to 14.5%.

CLYDE et al. (1971 a) studied the prophylactic activity of antimalarial drugs (sulfalene with chloroquine and primaquine; chloroquine with primaquine; pyrimethamine; diformyldapsone with chloroquine and primaquine) in non-immune volunteers exposed to mosquitoes infected with two chloroquine-resistant strains of *P. falciparum* from Vietnam. Sulfalene, 200 or 250 mg weekly with chloroquine (300 mg) and primaquine (45 mg), suppressed both these strains as did diformyldapsone (100–800 mg) with chloroquine and primaquine.

Infections with Other Plasmodia. There are no reports on the suppressive action of sulfalene alone on infections caused by *P. vivax* or *P. ovale*. In his field trial in Senegal MICHEL (1968) found complete suppression of *P. malariae* parasitaemia with sulfalene alone as well as with sulfalene plus pyrimethamine and with chloroquine.

c) Effect on Gametocytes

BARUFFA (1966) generally found gametocytes of *P. falciparum* when treatment with sulfalene (1.5–2.5 g) was started more than 2 days after the onset of signs and symptoms of malaria. This finding was confirmed in a similar study performed by MAZZONI (1967). During his suppressive trial MICHEL (1968) observed a decrease of *P. malariae* gametocytes after 4 months of bi-weekly treatment with 125, 250 or 500 mg sulfalene.

Table 16. Sulfalene in suppressive treatment of malaria

Country Subjects	Parasite and mode of infection	Treatment schedule: Dose (mg)	Treatment schedule: Administration	Treatment schedule: Duration	No. of subjects	Positive blood films: %	Positive blood films: Found after	Reference
Senegal Children aged 1–14 years in a holoendemic area	*P. falciparum* *P. malariae* Naturally acquired infection	125–250–500 SL	Bi-weekly	5 months	102	41.1	5 months	MICHEL 1968
		125–250–500 SL + 6.2–12.5–25 P			121	13.2		
		20 mg/kg C			137	14.5		
		Placebo			112	91.9		
United States Non-immune volunteers	*P. falciparum* Smith strain and Bray strain (C-resistant) Experimental (mosquito-induced) infection	200–250 SL + 300 C + 45 PQ	Weekly (starting on day before challenge)	8 weeks	6	0	8 weeks	CLYDE et al. 1971a

SL, sulfalene; P, pyrimethamine; C, chloroquine; PQ, primaquine
Underlined numbers refer to studies with individual compounds; other numbers refer to comparative studies with various combinations (e.g. with pyrimethamine or primaquine)

II. Sulphones

Dapsone was first tested for antimalarial activity in the form of the sodium didextrose sulphonate (Promin) by COGGESHALL et al. (1941). It was found to be as effective as sulphanilamide and its derivatives against *P. knowlesi, P. cynomolgi* and *P. inui* infections in monkeys, but no effect on *P. cathemerium* infections in canaries could be demonstrated. The treatment of 17 acutely ill patients with vivax and falciparum malaria revealed a definite effect on naturally acquired human malaria infections. Further evidence of the antimalarial activity of dapsone was provided in patients treated for leprosy (LEIKER 1956, and TARABINI 1958, quoted by ARCHIBALD and ROSS 1960). In 1960 ARCHIBALD and ROSS suggested on the basis of clinical trials in West Africa that the suitability of dapsone as a malaria prophylactic should be more thoroughly investigated.

Several derivatives of dapsone (2-sulphamoyl-4,4′-diaminophenyl-sulphone = SDDS; diformyldapsone; acedapsone) have also been tested for antimalarial activity, but only dapsone (in the form of a fixed combination with pyrimethamine) is still in clinical use for prophylactic purposes.

1. Dapsone

a) Curative Potential (see Table 17, compilation of trials)

P. falciparum. In early clinical studies (ARCHIBALD and ROSS 1960) 200 mg single doses of dapsone showed considerable activity in clearing the blood of *P. falciparum* schizonts in Nigerian school children. However, the substance was much slower in its action than chloroquine and, in contrast to the latter, was only poorly active in clearing asexual parasitaemia of *P. malariae*. These results confirmed earlier reports from leprosariums according to which dapsone reduced the rate of malarial infections in treated lepers compared with those treated with other antileprotic drugs (LEIKER 1956; TARABINI 1958, quoted in ARCHIBALD and ROSS 1960).

In Tanzania, LAING (1965 b) found single doses of 200 mg (and proportionally less for children under 12 years) to be curative in 33 of 40 semi-immune Africans suffering from acute *P. falciparum* malaria.

The effectiveness of dapsone against a chloroquine-resistant strain of *P. falciparum* (Malayan Camp) was investigated in six volunteers (two with blood-induced and four with mosquito-induced infections) by DEGOWIN et al. (1966 a). The administration of 100 mg daily for 5 days, even when supplemented by administration of 1,620 mg quinine base daily for the first 2 days of treatment with dapsone, did not consistently effect radical cure nor rapid termination of acute attacks in non-immune individuals.

LAING (1970) treated 18 patients (mostly children) suffering from slight to moderate *P. falciparum* infections in West Africa with small single doses of dapsone (5–25 mg); ten showed parasite clearance within a week but there were eight failures.

P. malariae and *P. vivax*. Dapsone was found to be poorly effective in clearing asexual parasitaemia of *P. malariae* (ARCHIBALD and ROSS 1960), only one out of three patients being cleared. LAING et al. (1974) reported on an acute attack of quartan malaria in a leprosy patient taking 300 mg dapsone twice weekly in whom

Table 17. Dapsone (DDS) in curative treatment of malaria

Country Subjects	Parasite and mode of infection	Treatment schedule (dose in mg)	No. of cases			Average duration to clearance (days) of		Reference
			Treated	Cleared (%)	Recrudescence (%)	Asexual parasitaemia	Fever	
Nigeria Nigerian schoolchildren	*P. falciparum* *P. malariae* Naturally acquired infection	200 DDS (single dose) 300 C (single dose)	17 *P.f.* 3 *P.m.* 16 *P.f.* 3 *P.m.*	17 *P.f* 1 *P.m.* 16 *P.f.* 1 *P.m.*		2–4 4 2–3 2–3	– – – –	ARCHIBALD and ROSS (1960)
Tanzania Semi-immune Bantu Africans	*P. falciparum* Naturally acquired infection	50–200 DDS (single dose)	40	35 (87)	2	3.2	2.4	LAING (1965b)
United States Non- or partially immune volunteers	*P. falciparum* Malayan (Camp) strain and Vietnam (V) strain, chloroquine resistant; (two blood-induced and four mosquito-induced infections)	100 DDS (daily, for 5 days)	1	1	1	4	2	DEGOWIN et al. (1966a)
		1,000 DDS (in 3 days)	1	1	0	3	7	
		100 DDS (daily for 5 days) + 3,240 QU (in 2 days)	4	4	1	2.7	4.2	
United States Non-immune volunteers	*P. vivax* Chesson strain (blood-induced infection)	100 DDS (daily for 10 days)	5	0	5	Not indicated		MARTIN and ARNOLD (1969a)
The Gambia Semi-immune local people (mostly children)	*P. falciparum* Naturally acquired	5–25 DDS (single dose)	18	10 (55)	–	1–6	–	LAING 1970
Malaysia Leprosy patient	*P. malariae* Naturally acquired	300 DDS (twice weekly)	1					LAING et al. (1974)

DDS, dapsone; QU, quinine; SL, sulfalene; S, sulfadoxine
Underlined numbers refer to studies with individual compounds; other numbers refer to comparative studies with various combinations (e.g. with pyrimethamine or primaquine)

Table 18. Dapsone (DDS) in suppressive treatment of malaria

Country Subjects	Parasite and mode of infection	Treatment schedule: Dose (mg)	Treatment schedule: Adminis-tration	Treatment schedule: Duration	No. of subjects	Positive blood films: %	Positive blood films: Found after	Reference
United States Non-immune volunteers	*P. falciparum* Malayan (Camp) and Vietnam (CV) strain (mosquito-induced infection)	5 DDS	Daily	32 days (starting on day −1)	1	100	–	DEGOWIN et al. (1966)
		10 DDS			1	100	–	
		15 DDS			1	0	–	
		25 DDS			13	15	–	
		50 DDS			13	15		
		50 DDS	Daily	8 days (starting on day −1)	2	100	–	
		100 DDS	Daily		3	100		
Tanzania Schoolchildren (semi-immune)	*P. falciparum* (P. malariae, P. vivax, P. ovale) Naturally acquired infection		Single dose			Day 7	Day 14 / Day 21	CLYDE (1967)
		50 DDS			54	3.7	9.8 / 67.3	
		100 DDS			114	0	3.5 / 16.5	
		200 DDS			143	0	0.7 / 11.5	
United States Non-immune volunteers	*P. falciparum* Malayan (Camp) strain, mosquito-induced infect.	25 DDS plus 300 C plus 45 PQ	Daily / Weekly / Weekly	Started 4–8 weeks before exposure, continued till 4–6 weeks after exposure	10	10	40 days after exposure	EPPES et al. (1967)
	Vietnam (CV) strain, mosquito-induced infect.				9	0	40 days after exposure	

Vietnam American soldiers	*P. falciparum* Naturally acquired	25 DDS or placebo plus 300 C plus 45 PQ	Daily Weekly Weekly	Not indicated	Of 117 cases of malaria 47 were found in the DDS group and 70 in the control group receiving placebo			Joy et al. (1969b)
Vietnam American soldiers	*P. falciparum* Naturally acquired	25 DDS plus 300 C plus 45 PQ	Daily Weekly Weekly	2 months	Malaria attack rate of a brigade taking DDS in addition to C and PQ was 10% of the attack rates found in soldiers taking only C plus PQ			Joy et al. (1969a)
United States Non- or partially immune volunteers	*P. falciparum* Malaya Tay strain Mosquito-induced infection	25 DDS plus 300 C	Daily Weekly	8 weeks (starting on day of exposure)	16	0	–	Clyde (1971c)
United States Non-immune volunteers	*P. falciparum* Vietnam (Marks) strain	25 DDS plus 300 C	Daily Weekly	4–8 weeks (starting on day before exposure)	8	25	–	Willerson et al. (1972)
	Mosquito-induced infection	25 DDS plus 300 C plus 45 PQ	Daily Weekly Weekly	4–8 weeks (starting on day before exposure)	8	12.5		–

DDS, dapsone; C, chloroquine; PQ, primaquine
Underlined numbers refer to studies with individual compounds; other numbers refer to comparative studies with various combinations (e.g. with pyrimethamine or primaquine)

spectrofluorometric examination showed a comparatively high plasma concentration of dapsone (1.64 mg/litre).

In *P. vivax* malaria, too, dapsone appeared to be unsatisfactory. According to MARTIN and ARNOLD (1969a) the parasites (Chesson strain) were completely refractory to the drug (100 mg daily for 10 days) and parasitaemia even increased during therapy. RIECKMANN et al. (1968, as quoted by LAING et al. 1974) found dapsone to be useless against a New Guinea strain of *P. vivax*.

b) Suppressive Potential (see Table 18, compilation of trials)

P. falciparum. DEGOWIN et al. (1966a) showed that relatively small doses of dapsone (25 or 50 mg daily, beginning 1 day before exposure and continued for 30 days after exposure) prevented patency of infections in 22 of 26 volunteers exposed to mosquitoes infected with the Malayan Camp or Vietnam CV strain of *P. falciparum*. However, 50 or 100 mg daily administered only during the period of pre-erythrocytic schizogony (from the day before until the 6th day after exposure) did not prevent patency of infections with the Malayan Camp strain. Thus, a causal prophylactic effect could be excluded.

In a field trial in Tanzanian schoolchildren CLYDE (1967) obtained clearance of *P. falciparum* parasitaemia with single doses of 200 mg dapsone, while single doses of 50 and 100 mg were less effective. Under the conditions of continuous reinfection the parasite-free period was around 12 days after the 200-mg dose. In the same trial a similar effect was obtained with sulfadoxine, sulfadimethoxine and sulfamethoxypyridazine in single doses of 250 mg.

The protective effect of dapsone was studied by EPPES et al. (1967) in mosquito-induced infections of volunteers with two chloroquine-resistant *P. falciparum* strains (Malayan Camp and Vietnam CV). The incidence of parasitaemia was only slightly reduced by concurrent weekly administration of chloroquine and primaquine with no dapsone. However, 25 mg dapsone administered once daily in addition to the weekly doses of chloroquine and primaquine proved highly effective. All 19 subjects receiving the triple combination were protected against patency, and in 18 a permanent "suppressive cure" was achieved. In one volunteer parasitaemia was detected 10 days after the last dose of medication.

In a field trial carried out by JOY et al. (1969b), 25 mg dapsone daily were added to the conventional weekly chloroquine-primaquine schedule administered to US soldiers in Vietnam. A similar number of soldiers received the weekly doses of chloroquine and primaquine plus placebo to be taken daily. Of 117 cases of malaria found among the soldiers who took their tablets regularly, 47 were found in the dapsone group and 70 in the placebo group.

In a further field trial JOY et al. (1969a) administered 25 mg dapsone daily in addition to the once weekly chloroquine-primaquine schedule for a period of 2 months to soldiers of a US brigade operating in a malarial area of Vietnam. The malaria attack rate in this brigade was 10% of the attack rates found in other, identically exposed units not taking dapsone.

In a prophylactic trial (CLYDE et al. 1971c) 16 volunteers exposed to *A. stephensi* mosquitoes heavily infected with a chloroquine-resistant *P. falciparum* strain were given 25 mg dapsone daily in addition to 300 mg chloroquine (base) weekly for 2 months. None of the subjects developed malaria during the course of treatment nor during the 8-week follow-up period.

The suppressive effect of the combination of dapsone (25 mg) daily with chloroquine (300 mg) and primaquine (45 mg) once weekly on chloroquine-resistant *P. falciparum* malaria (Vietnam Marks strain) was also tested by WILLERSON et al. (1972). Of the eight volunteers receiving this combination seven were protected while of another eight volunteers receiving only dapsone plus chloroquine, six were protected.

c) Effects on Gametocytes and Sporogony

Gametocytes of *P. falciparum* were not affected by a single dose of 200 mg dapsone (ARCHIBALD and ROSS 1960) and the drug had no sporontocidal properties against *P. falciparum* (LAING 1965 b).

2. Diformyldapsone

a) Curative Potential (see Table 19, compilation of trials)

P. falciparum. Diformyldapsone was designed as an oral repository drug. According to CLYDE et al (1970 a) it had an antimalarial activity similar to, but more prolonged than, dapsone. Single doses of 200–2,000 mg diformyldapsone, with or without trimethoprim, were given to volunteers suffering from mosquito-induced *P. falciparum* infection (Uganda I, Thailand Man, Malaya Poo and Malaya Tay strains). Asexual parasitaemia was not cleared in 8 of 23 treated episodes. In the remaining 15 episodes parasitaemia was cleared on average within 4.5 days and fever in 5.2 days. Recrudescence occurred among these cases from 7 to 25 days after treatment. When diformyldapsone was given with trimethoprim, more rapid clearance of asexual parasitaemia occurred, but 11 of 20 cases showed recrudescence.

P. vivax. No studies for assessment of the curative potential of diformyldapsone in infections with *P. vivax, P. malariae* or *P. ovale* were found in the literature.

b) Suppressive Potential (see Table 19, compilation of trials)

P. falciparum. The prophylactic efficacy of diformyldapsone was assessed by CLYDE et al. (1970 a, 1971 c) and by WILLERSON et al. (1972) in non-immune volunteers with mosquito-induced *P. falciparum* infections (chloroquine-sensitive and chloroquine-resistant strains). Eight hundred to 2,000 mg of the drug given once weekly for 2 months, commencing within 4 days from exposure to heavily infected mosquitoes, protected four of six volunteers, and 100–1,600 mg combined with 300 mg chloroquine and 45 mg primaquine protected 93 of 99 volunteers (CLYDE et al. 1970 a). However, unacceptably high levels of methaemoglobinaemia were observed with the triple combination.

In their second study on *P. falciparum* infections, CLYDE et al. (1971 c) found diformyldapsone given weekly alone or with chloroquine as effective as dapsone given daily with chloroquine weekly. This finding was confirmed in 1972 by WILLERSON et al.

Table 19. Acedapsone (DADDS) and diformyl-diamino-diphenyl-sulfone (DFD) in suppressive treatment of malaria

Country Subjects	Parasite and mode of infection	Treatment schedule			No. of subjects	Positive blood films				Reference
		Dose (mg)	Administration	Duration		%	Found on			
Tanzania School-children (semi-immune)	*P. falciparum* *P. malariae* (naturally acquired infection)	6.9 DADDS per kg	i.m.	Single dose	60	Before 58	Day 15 5	Day 30 17	Day 60 25	LAING et al. (1966)
		10.8 CGP per kg	i.m.	Single dose	60	40	0	5	8	
		12.9 DADDS plus 12.9 CGP per kg	i.m.	Single dose	60	38	0	2	2	
New Guinea Village inhabitants, adults and children (semi-immune)	*P. falciparum* *P. vivax* *P. malariae* (naturally acquired infection)	90–150–225 DADDS	i.m.	Single dose	210	Before *P.f.* 20.5 *P.v.* 18.6 *P.m.* 10.9	Day 60 2.4 15.7	Day 90 12.8 25.2	Day 120 28.1 30.0	RIECKMANN (1967)
		140–280–350 CGP plus 10/kg ADQU	i.m. oral	Single dose	192	*P.f.* 20.3 *P.v.* 16.1 *P.m.* 2.1	1.6 1.6	14.6 8.3	37.0 14.6	
		90–150–250 DADDS plus 94–15–225 CGP	i.m.	Single dose	200	*P.f.* 20.5 *P.v.* 15.5 *P.m.* 3.5	0 0	3 4.5	14 14	
United States Non-immune volunteers	*P. falciparum* Uganda I, Thailand Man., Malaya Poo., Malaya Tay strain (mosquito-induced infection)	400 DFD 800 DFD	2 single doses	Day 0, Day +6	2 2	100 100	Day 11–12 Day 11–12			CLYDE et al. (1970a)
		800 DFD	Weekly	8 weeks	2	0				
		1,200 DFD			2	100				
		2,000 DFD			2	100				
		100–1,600 DFD plus 300 C plus 45 PQ	Weekly	8 weeks	99	6				

United States Non-immune volunteers	*P. falciparum* Thailand Man.	400 DFD	Weekly	8 weeks	4	25	Day 15	CLYDE et al. (1971c)
		800 DFD			4	0	–	
	Malaya Thai Vietnam Smith (mosquito-induced infection)	400 DFD plus 300 C	Weekly	8 weeks	14	7	Day 13	
		800 DFD plus 300 C	Weekly	8 weeks	19	5	Day 12	
	P. vivax Chesson strain (mosquito-induced infection)	400 DFD	Weekly	8 weeks	7	60	Day 13 to 16	
		800 DFD			2	50	Day 65	
United States Non-immune volunteers	*P. falciparum* Vietnam (Marks) strain (mosquito-induced infection)	400 DFD plus 300 C	Weekly	1 or 2 months	8	37.5	During (one case) or 7–8 days after completion of medication	WILLERSON et al. (1972)
Thailand Semi-immune village inhabitants	*P. falciparum* *P. vivax* Naturally acquired infection	400 DFD	Weekly	26 weeks	117	22 *P.f.* 24 *P.v.*		PEARLMAN et al. (1975)
		200 DFD plus 12.5 P			118	14 *P.f.* 14 *P.v.*		
		25 P			118	54 *P.f.* 54 *P.v.*		
		100 DDS plus 12.5 P			123	10 *P.f.* 14 *P.v.*		
		Placebo			117	62 *P.f.*		

CGP, cycloguanil pamoate; ADQU, amodiaquine; C, chloroquine; PQ, primaquine; DDS, dapsone; P, pyrimethamine
Underlined numbers refer to studies with individual compounds; other numbers refer to comparative studies with various combinations (e.g. with pyrimethamine or primaquine)

A chemosuppressive field trial with diformyldapsone alone and in combination with pyrimethamine was performed by PEARLMAN et al. (1975) in an area of Thailand with chloroquine-resistant *P. falciparum* malaria. Diformyldapsone alone, in a weekly dose of 400 mg given for 26 weeks, was only moderately effective (see Table 19), whereas the combination of diformyldapsone (200 mg) plus pyrimethamine (12.5 mg) provided an effective chemosuppression against both *P. falciparum* and *P. vivax* parasitaemia. However, this combination was not more efficacious than dapsone (100 mg) plus pyrimethamine.

P. vivax. Four hundred or 800 mg diformyldapsone once weekly was administered for 2 months to nine volunteers challenged with the Chesson strain of *P. vivax* (CLYDE et al. 1971c). Parasitaemia broke through early in the prophylactic treatment in four of the subjects, and in a further subject a delayed primary attack was observed 12 days after the treatment was discontinued.

Only a moderate suppressive effect of diformyldapsone on *P. vivax* parasitaemia was observed also by PEARLMAN et al. (1975) in a field trial on Thai villagers (see Table 19).

c) Effects on Gametocytes and Sporogony

CLYDE et al. (1970a) did not find any gametocytocidal or sporontocidal activity in his trial with diformyldapsone in volunteers infected with various strains of *P. falciparum*.

3. Acedapsone

Acedapsone was developed as an alternative or adjunctive repository drug to cycloguanil pamoate. The substance alone, administered in a single intramuscular dose of 6.9 mg/kg to Tanzanian schoolchildren, was effective in clearing patent infections with *P. falciparum* and *P. malariae* (see Table 19) but acted more slowly than cycloguanil pamoate or a combination of acedapsone and cycloguanil pamoate (LAING et al. 1966).

An indefinite and short-lived effect of acedapsone alone (single dose of 90, 150 or 225 mg) against *P. vivax* infections was found by RIECKMANN (1967) in a comparative study conducted in a malarious area of New Guinea (for more detailed results see Table 19).

H. Drug Resistance

I. Experimental Resistance in Non-Human Plasmodia

1. Methods for the Production of Resistant Lines (for details, see PETERS 1980)

a) Increasing Drug Pressure

With this most commonly employed method, the plasmodia are passaged repeatedly (e.g. weekly) through the host animals, which are kept under treatment with a given drug. At each of the passages the dose of the drug must be definitely inhibitory to the plasmodia, but must still allow some multiplication, in order to ensure transmission to new host animals. With increasing resistance of the parasites, the dose must be increased step by step until the plateau of maximum resistance is reached. The factor by which the ultimate dose of the drug still allowing multiplication of the plasmodia is greater than the first which was just subinhibitory when the experiment was started is called the resistance factor. Another, homologous definition of the resistance factor is: "Dose subinhibitory to the resistant line of the parasite divided by the dose subinhibitory to the parent strain of the parasite from which the resistant line was derived."

b) Relapse Technique

The principle of this method is to treat the infected host animals with a single large dose of the drug, to wait for parasitaemia to recrudesce and then to passage the parasite into new hosts. When the latter have developed a reasonably high level of parasitaemia, they receive the same high drug dose as the first hosts and, as soon as they again show parasitaemia, their blood is used for a further passage. The procedure is repeated (with or without increasing the dose of the drug), and the degree of the resistance of the parasite to the given drug is checked periodically by comparing its susceptibility with that of the parent strain in a standard chemotherapeutic experiment, e.g. the "4-day test" in the case of *P. berghei*. The resistance factor is then determined as a certain end point (e.g. ED_{50}) observed with the resistant line divided by that observed with the parent strain.

2. General Characterisation of the Resistant Lines

Besides the above-mentioned resistance factor, the following characters are the most interesting and will be discussed in the following paragraph with respect to the sulphonamides and sulphones: (a) the number of passages required to achieve a given resistance factor; (b) the stability or instability of the resistance, i.e. whether or not it was retained during further passages of the strain without drug pressure; (c) the susceptibility or cross-resistance to other antimalarials of the lines made resistant to sulphonamides and sulphones; and (d) the inverse picture, i.e. whether plasmodial lines made resistant to other antimalarials are susceptible or cross-resistant to the sulphonamides and sulphones. For a more detailed account of the additional characters and problems still pending (e.g. those of the different genetic and biochemical patterns of the resistance, partially depending on the method by which it was produced) the reader is referred to PETERS (1970, 1980).

A useful parameter of cross-resistance is the "index of resistance" (= I) applied by PETERS et al. (1975b) to the various resistant lines of *P. berghei* that they investigated in the "4-day suppressive test" in mice. The I_{90} is calculated as the ED_{90} found with the resistant line divided by the ED_{90} found with the corresponding, sensitive parent strain (see Table 21). The "index of resistance" is directly comparable with the resistance factor; when the two figures, e.g., are equal, the line is just as resistant to the other antimalarial as to the first to which is made resistant.

3. Selected Characters of Resistant Lines

a) Resistance Factors and Passages Required

Resistance of sulphonamides and sulphones can be produced with relative ease. BISHOP and BIRKETT (1948) were successful with the first attempt they made with sulfadiazine on *P. gallinaceum*. Using the method of increasing drug pressure, 30–40 passages were required to achieve resistance factors of around 30 × to sulfadiazine with *P. gallinaceum* (BISHOP and MCCONNACHIE 1948), and of 100 × or more to sulfadiazine (THURSTON 1953 b, KRISHNASWAMI et al. 1954) and dapsone (THOMPSON et al. 1965 b) in the case of *P. berghei* (see Table 19). The upper limit of the resistance factor was often determined by the maximum tolerance of the drug to the host animal. Since the tolerance of the sulphonamides is generally better, their resistance factors tend to be greater than those of the sulphones. For example, the resistance factor of only 20 × observed with dapsone and *P. cynomolgi* (RAMAKRISHNAN et al. 1962) was limited by the relatively poor susceptibility of this *Plasmodium* species on one hand and, on the other, by the toxicity of the sulphone to the monkeys. With respect to both the degree of resistance and the speed of its development, there nevertheless also exist true differences from one experiment to another which may be due to the occurrence and selection of genetically different resistant mutants. Very exceptionally the attempts to produce resistance to sulphonamides or sulphones have even failed (e.g. with sulfadiazine in *P. gallinaceum;* MCCONNACHIE 1951).

b) Stability of Resistance

Resistance was, in most of the instances, retained when the parasites were passaged through new hosts without further drug pressure (*P. gallinaceum* resistant to sulfadiazine: BISHOP and MCCONNACHIE 1948; *P. berghei* resistant to sulphanilamide: HAWKING 1966; or to sulfadiazine: THURSTON 1953 b; KRISHNASWAMI et al. 1954). The resistance of *P. gallinaceum* to sulfadiazine was also shown to be stable after passage through the insect vector and to extend to the exoerythrocytic schizonts (BISHOP and MCCONNACHIE 1948). With a line of *P. berghei* made resistant to dapsone, some decrease of resistance was observed during the passages through untreated rodent hosts (THOMPSON et al. 1967). This partial loss of resistance is probably not to be generalised but rather reflect a particular property of the resistant mutant in question. In the line of *P. cynomolgi* made resistant to dapsone by RAMAKRISHNAN et al. (1962) resistance was obviously stable.

c) Cross-resistance of Sulphonamide and Sulphone-resistant Plasmodia to Other Antimalarials

Based on representative observations from the literature, a general depiction of the cross-resistance pattern of plasmodia made resistant to sulphonamides and sulphones is attempted in the *upper part* to Table 20, classifying the response to the other antimalarials into the categories proposed by PETERS (1967 a): *S*, sensitive; *SS*, "hypersensitive"; *R*, moderately resistant; *RR*, very resistant. It is clearly evident that the lines resistant to sulphonamides and sulphones generally remain sensitive to chloroquine, primaquine, mepacrine and quinine. A great variety of responses has, however, been documented to proguanil (cycloguanil) and especially to pyrimethamine, ranging from normally sensitive to highly cross-resistant. The lines made resistant to a given sulphonamide were usually found to be to some degree cross-resistant to other sulphonamides and to sulphones and, vice versa, the lines made resistant to a sulphone were cross-resistant to other sulphones and to sulphonamides. As a single exception a line of *P. berghei* made resistant to sulphanilamide was still sensitive to dapsone (Kazim and Dutta 1980). It must, however, be taken into account that the resistance factor of this particular line to sulphanilamide itself was only 8×. (See also the considerable range of the degree of cross-resistance among individual sulphonamides documented in Table 21).

4. Cross-resistance to Sulphonamides and Sulphones of Plasmodia Resistant to Other Antimalarials

This pattern is depicted, again in the simplified manner adopted from Peters (1967 a), in the two first columns of the *lower part* of Table 20. As a general rule, the plasmodia made resistant to other antimalarials proved to be still normally sensitive to the sulphonamides and sulphones. This is particularly true for the parasites resistant to pyrimethamine, cycloguanil, chloroquine and mepacrine; some of them were even found to be slightly hypersensitive. With plasmodia resistant to proguanil either sensitivity or slight cross-resistance to sulphonamides was noted (*P. gallinaceum*, Bishop and McConnachie 1948). Depending on the individual sulphonamide and sulphone tested, either sensitivity or (moderate) cross-resistance was also encountered with *P. berghei* made resistant to primaquine (Peters et al. 1975 b; see also Table 21).

The generally normal activity of the sulphonamides and sulphones against plasmodia resistant to other antimalarials is confirmed in more detail by the response to individual sulphonamides and sulphones observed by Peters et al. (1975 b) in chemotherapeutic mouse experiments with *P. berghei* lines resistant to pyrimethamine, cycloguanil, chloroquine and primaquine, and by Richards (1966) and Krettli and Brener (1968) with lines of the same species resistant to chloroquine (Table 21, *columns on the right*). The indices of resistance of less than 1.0×, which mainly occurred with the lines resistant to pyrimethamine and chloroquine, indicate slight hypersensitivity to the sulphonamides and sulphones in question. The indices of resistance greater than 1.0× must be compared with the resistance factors of the lines to the antimalarial to which each one had been made resistant. With the extremely high resistance factors of the pyrimethamine- and cycloguanil-resistant lines (109× and >140×, respectively) and of the chloroquine-resistant RC line (194×), the indices of resistance of up to about 10× occurring in the experiments with some of the individual sulphonamides may still be regarded as evidence of "sensitivity". However, in the case of the primaquine-resistant line, quite low indices of resistance are considered to prove some cross-resistance, since the resistance factor of the line to primaquine itself was only 14.5×. The differences in the response of this line to the individual drugs were remarkable.

The difference in the response to different sulphonamide and sulphone drugs was even more pronounced in the experiments performed by Peters et al. (1975 b) with the sulphonamide-resistant line (see the *enclosed column* in Table 21, *left part*). The resistance factor of this line to sulfaphenazole to which it had been made resistant, was 196×. Cross-resistance of a correspondingly high degree only occurred with sulfamonomethoxine, diformyl-dapsone and, perhaps, sulfadoxine, whereas with dapsone and, mainly, sulfadiazine and sulfalene, cross-resistance was surprisingly low. (With indices of resistance of less than 10×, the line should even be regarded as "sensitive" to sulfadiazine and sulfalene according to the criteria we

Table 20. Patterns of cross-resistance and sensitivity in experimentally induced drug resistance of various *Plasmodium* species[a]

Strain made resistant to:	Plasmodium species[b]	Authors	Sulphonamide	Sulphone	Pyrimethamine	Proguanil Cycloguanil	Chloroquine	Primaquine (8-aminoquinoline)	Mepacrine	Quinine
Sulphonamides and sulphones										
Sulfadiazine	*P.g.*	d	10× [c] 32×			R				
Sulfadiazine	*P.b.*	e	4×		S	R				
Sulfadiazine	*P.b.*	f	100×		RR	R–RR	S		S	S
Sulfadiazine	*P.b.*	g	300×		S					
Sulfaphenazole	*P.b.*	h	70×	RR	S		S	S	S	S
Sulfanilamide	*P.b.*	i	8×	S	S		S	S	S	
Dapsone	*P.g.*	k	RR	≫ 4× [c]	R	R				
Dapsone	*P.b.*	l		185×	(R)					
Dapsone	*P.b.*	m	R	80×	R	R	S	S	S	S
Dapsone	*P.c.*	n	R	20×	S	S	S			
Pyrimethamine	*P.g.*	k	S	S	200× [c]					
Pyrimethamine	*P.b.*	h	S	S	250×	R	S	S		S
Proguanil	*P.g.*	d	S–R			various factors				
Proguanil	*P.g.*	o	S	S		> 25× [c]				
Cycloguanil	*P.b.*	h	S	S	S–(R)	> 140× [c]	S	S	S	S
Chloroquine	*P.b.*	p	S	S	S		20×	S	R	
Chloroquine	*P.b.*	q	S	S	S	S	60× [c]	R	RR	R
Primaquine	*P.b.*	h	S–(R)	(R)	S	R	S	14.5× [c]	S	S
Mepacrine	*P.b.*	m	SS	S	S	SS	R	S	60× [c]	R

[a] Presentation adopted from PETERS 1967a: S, normally sensitive; SS, hypersensitive; R, resistant; RR, highly resistant
[b] Abbreviations: *P.g., Plasmodium gallinaceum; P.b., P. berghei; P.c., P. cynomolgi*
[c] The degrees of resistance of the resistant lines to the parent compounds are indicated with the resistance factors
[d] BISHOP and MCCONNACHIE (1948)
[e] ROLLO (1951)
[f] THURSTON (1953b)
[g] KRISHNASWAMI et al. (1954)
[h] PETERS et al. (1975b)
[i] KAZIM and DUTTA (1980)
[k] BISHOP (1965)
[l] THOMPSON et al. (1965b)
[m] PETERS (1966)
[n] RAMAKRISHNAN et al. (1962)
[o] RICHARDS (1966)
[p] HAWKING and GAMMAGE (1962)
[q] PETERS (1965a)

Table 21. Comparative response of drug-resistant *P. berghei* to individual sulphonamides and sulphones in chemotherapeutic experiments in the mouse[a]

Sulphonamides and sulphones used for the chemotherapeutic challenge	Activity on the normally sensitive parent strains (mg/kg)		Indices of resistance[b] observed with the lines made resistant to					
			Sulfa-phenazole (196×)[c]	Pyrimeth-amine (109×)[c]	Cyclo-guanil (>140×)[c]	Chloroquine		Prima-quine (14.5×)[c]
	ED_{50}	ED_{90}				NS-line (4.3×)[c]	RC-line (194×)[c]	
[d] Sulfadiazine	0.01	0.30	7.3	–[e]	0.8	0.3	1.3	0.2
Sulfamonomethoxine	0.03	0.10	200	0.5	2.6	0.5	16.7	3.1
Sulfadoxine	0.13	1.60	> 62	0.5	3.8	–	0.5	1.5
Sulfalene	0.07	0.19	4.2	3.7	1.8	–	4.2	> 5.3
Dapsone	0.1	0.4	38	–	1.2	0.2	0.7	11.0
Diformyldapsone	0.2	0.7	>130	0.4	5.9	0.4	1.2	3.4
						(>12×)[g]		
[e] Sulfadiazine	0.2	–	–	–	–	1.0		–
Sulfadoxine	1.0	–	–	–	–	1.0		–
Dapsone	0.6	–	–	–	–	1.0		–
						(20×)[g]		
[f] Sulfadiazine	0.4	0.95	–	–	–	0.6		–
Sulfadoxine	0.22	1.15	–	–	–	0.6		–

[a] 4-day suppressive tests (PETERS 1970, 1980) or similar techniques

[b] Calculated according to PETERS et al. (1975b):

$$I_{90} = \frac{ED_{90} \text{ with resistant line}}{ED_{90} \text{ with sensitive parent strain}}$$

For the results from RICHARDS (1966) I_{50} was calculated analogously from the ED_{50} values, since this author did not determine ED_{90}

[c] Resistance factor

[d] PETERS et al. (1975b)

[e] RICHARDS (1966)

[f] KRETTLI and BRENER (1968)

[g] Only one chloroquine-resistant line was used

stipulated before.) These data suggest that some mechanism(s) of resistance to sulphonamides displayed by the plasmodia may differ depending on the individual compound. We are indeed ignorant of the mechanism(s) in question. Perhaps a barrier built up by the plasmodia to the uptake of a given sulphonamide or sulphone drug could still be passed through by another. Once more, is must also be kept in mind that the experience made with the sulphonamide-resistant mutant selected by PETERS et al. (1975b) may not necessarily apply to other mutants.

II. Resistance to Sulphonamides and Sulphones in Human Plasmodia

Strictly speaking, resistance to sulphonamides or sulphones has not been observed with human plasmodia. This is, however, explained by the fact that there has been only very limited use of sulphonamides or sulphones as single drugs in human malaria. For many years these drugs were almost exclusively used in combination with an inhibitor of dihydrofolate reductase, mainly pyrimethamine, which, in various experiments performed with non-human plasmodia, had been shown to delay the development of resistance to both the sulphonamide or sulphone and the pyrimethamine component (see, e.g. PETERS 1974). In some parts of the world, particularly in Southeast Asia and Brazil, there is, however, increasing evidence of the emergence of *P. falciparum* strains resistant to sulphone (dapsone) plus pyrimethamine (VERDRAEGER 1970) and more recently, also to sulphonamide (sulfadoxine) plus pyrimethamine (BUNNAG et al. 1980; DESOUZA 1980). There is, of course, little doubt that the plasmodia resistant to the combination also are resistant to the sulphone and sulphonamide alone.

A certain percentage of treatment failures (and of breakthroughs during prophylaxis) has occurred since the first use of the combinations of the sulphones and sulphonamides with pyrimethamine. The fact that treatment failures are not necessarily consistent with drug resistance was proven e.g. by CLYDE (1972) and WILLIAMS et al. (1978). When *P. falciparum* was transferred from volunteers in whom treatment with sulfalene had failed into new volunteers, the latter were curable with normal doses of this same drug. The above-mentioned evidence of true resistance to the combination was based on the observation of a definite increase in the percentage of drug failures in given areas and/or the necessity of administering the drugs at a higher dosage to achieve the same results as in earlier periods.

For the formal proof of resistance of human plasmodia to the combinations in question and, particularly, to their sulphonamide and sulphone components, a suitable method is still required to determine the sensitivity of the parasites to these drugs in vitro.

J. Role of Sulphonamides and Sulphones as Antimalarials

The significant antimalarial properties of the sulphonamides and sulphones are as follows. They exert activity against all actively dividing stages in the life cycle of the plasmodia, but only their blood schizontocidal action has been firmly established in human malaria. Among the human plasmodia *P. falciparum* is the most susceptible, whereas *P. vivax* is less so. Most importantly, the sulphonamides and sulphones retain their full activity against plasmodia which have become resistant to virtually any other antimalarials including chloroquine. As another outstanding quality they act synergistically with the antifolic antimalarials, pyrimethamine and proguanil.

For many years, the sulphonamides and sulphones have no longer been used alone for malaria but exclusively in combination with an inhibitor of dihydrofolic acid reductase, mainly pyrimethamine. By virtue of the above-mentioned properties of the sulphonamide or sulphone component, these combinations have become important chemotherapeutics against chloroquine-resistant falciparum malaria. They have also proved to be useful for suppressive treatment and prophylaxis in countries where chloroquine resistance occurs.

The presently preferred sulphonamide components are the "long-acting" compounds dealt with in this chapter, the biological half-life of which is not too different from that of pyrimethamine. The preferred sulphone is dapsone. It is difficult to say to what extent the antimalarial activity of the combinations containing the sulphonamides may be better documented than that of the combinations containing dapsone. At the relatively low doses used in the combination with pyrimethamine, tolerance of both the sulphonamides and sulphones has been quite good, and the severe side-effects known to occur with these drugs (Stevens-Johnson or Lyell syndrome with the sulphonamides and agranulocytosis with dapsone) were recorded but rarely.

The synergistic combinations of sulphonamides or sulphones with pyrimethamine indeed also offer the advantage of a delay in the development of resistance of the plasmodia to any of the components. Recently, however, resistance even to these combinations has emerged in some areas of Asia and South America, unfortunately in those with the highest incidence of chloroquine resistance. In the future, the synergistic combinations of sulphonamides or sulphones with pyrimethamine, which may be regarded as single drugs in this context, should be combined more and more with other antimalarials such as quinine or mefloquine.

References

Affrime M, Reidenberg MM (1973) The binding of drugs to plasma from patients with cirrhosis. Pharmacologist 15:207

Aguirre M (1967) Application clinique des sulfamides, appareil respiratoire. Proc 5th int congr chemother, Vienna 1967, vol 3, pp 243–246

Ahmad RA, Rogers HJ (1980) Plasma and salivary pharmacokinetics of dapsone estimated by a thin layer chromatographic method. Eur J Clin Pharmacol 17:129–133

Aldighieri J, Dupoux R, Quilici M, Sautet J (1968) Action de la kelfizine associée à la pyriméthamine sur les affections à *Plasmodium berghei* chez la souris blanche. Bull Soc Pathol Exot Filiales 61:765–768

Allen BW (1975) The penetration of dapsone, rifampicin, isoniazid and pyrazinamide into peripheral nerves. Br J Pharmacol 55:151–155

Anand N (1979) Sulfonamides and sulfones. In: Wolff E (ed). Burger's medicinal chemistry, 4th edn part 2. Wiley, New York pp 1–40

Andreasen F (1973) Protein binding of drugs in plasma from patients with acute renal failure. Acta Pharmacol Toxicol 32:417–429

Anton AH (1973) Increasing activity of sulfonamides with displacing agents: A review. Ann NY Acad Sci 226:273–292
Appel GB, Neu HC (1977) The nephrotoxicity of antimicrobial agents, III. Engl J Med 296:784–787
Archibald MM, Ross CM (1960) A preliminary report on the effect of diaminodiphenyl sulphone on malaria in Northern Nigeria. J Trop Med Hyg 63:25–27
Asano Y, Susami M, Ariyuki F, Higaki K (1975) The effects of administration of 2-sulfamoyl-4,4-diaminodiphenylsulfone (SDDS) on rat fetuses (in Japanese). Oyo Yakuri 9:695–707
Aviado DM (1967) Pathologic physiology and chemotherapy of *Plasmodium berghei.* I. Suppression of parasitemia by sulfones and sulfonamides in mice. Exp Parasitol 20:88–97
Aviado DM (1969) Chemotherapy of *Plasmodium berghei* including bibliography on *Plasmodium berghei.* Exp Parasitol 25:399–482
Aviado DM, Singh G, Berkley R (1969) Pharmacology of new antimalarial drugs sulfonamides and trimethoprim. Chemotherapy 14:37–53
Baldi A, della Rocca L (1951) Sulla terapia dell'infezione da *Plasmodium berghei* nel topo. Riv Malariologia 30:173–194
Baruffa G (1966) Clinical trials in *Plasmodium falciparum* malaria with a long-acting sulphonamide. Trans R. Soc Trop Med Hyg 60:222–224
Baskin CG, Law S, Wenger NK (1980) Sulfadiazine rheumatic fever prophylaxis during pregnancy: Does it increase the risk of kernicterus in the newborn? Cardiology 65:222–225
Basu PC, Prakash S (1962) The course of parasitaemia of *Plasmodium cynomolgi bastianelli* in *Macaca mulatta* monkeys: its sensitivity to different antimalarials. Indian J Malaria 16:321–326
Basu PC, Singh NN, Singh N (1964) Potentiation of activity of diaphenylsulfone and pyrimethamine against *Plasmodium gallinaceum* and *P. cynomolgi bastianelli.* Bull WHO 31:699–705
Beckermann F (1964) Klinische Erfahrungen mit einem neuen Langzeitsulfonamid bei schweren bakteriell bedingten Krankheiten In: Kümmerle HP, Preziosi P (eds) Proceedings 3rd int congr chemotherapy, Stuttgart 1963. Thieme, Stuttgart
Beesley WN, Peters W (1968) The chemotherapy of rodent malaria, VI. The action of some sulphonamides alone or with folic reductase inhibitors against malaria vectors and parasites, part 1: introduction and anti-vector studies. Ann Trop Med Parasitol 62:288–294
Benazet F, Werner GH (1967) Activité du sulfalène (para-aminobenzène sulfamido-2-methoxy-3-pyrazine) sur le paludisme expérimental des animaux de laboratoire. WHO/Mal/67:630 (Cyclostyled report) WHO, Geneva
Bergmann M, Zauger J, Hieger W (1963) Klinische Erfahrungen bei der Behandlung von Harnwegsinfektionen mit dem Langzeitsulfonamid Ro 4-4393. Z Urol Nephrol 56:141–148
Bergoend H, Löffler A, Amar R, Maleville J (1968) Réactions cutanées survenues au cours de la prophylaxie de masse de la méningite cérébro-spinale par un sulfamide long-retard (à propos de 997 cas). Ann Dermatol Syphiligr 95:481–490
Berneis K, Boguth W (1976) Distribution of sulfonamides and sulfonamide potentiators between red blood cells, proteins and aqueous phases of the blood of different species. Chemotherapy 22:390–409
Bertazzoli C, Chieli T, Grandi M (1965) Absence of tooth malformation in offspring of rats treated with a long-acting sulfonamide. Experientia 21:151–152
Biggs JT, Levy L (1971) Binding of dapsone and monoacetyldapsone by human plasma proteins. Proc Soc Exp Biol Med 137:692–695
Bishop A (1963) Some recent developments in the problem of drug resistance in malaria. Parasitology 53:10
Bishop A (1965) Resistance to diamino-diphenylsulphone in *Plasmodium gallinaceum.* Parasitology 55:407–414
Bishop A, Birkett B (1948) Drug resistance in *Plasmodium gallinaceum,* and the persistence of paludrine resistance after mosquito transmission. Parasitology 39:125–137

Bishop A, McConnachie EW (1948) Resistance to sulfadiazine and "Paludrine" in the malaria parasite of the fowl (*P. gallinaceum*). Nature 162:541–543

Böhni E, Fust B, Rieder J, Schaerer G, Havas L (1969) Comparative toxicological, chemotherapeutic and pharmacokinetic studies with sulphormethoxine and other sulphonamides in animals and man. Chemotherapy 14:195–226

Bonini M, Mokofio F, Barazi S (1981) Contribution au dosage de quatre antipaludéens, chloroquine, quinine, pyriméthamine et sulfadoxine, seuls et en mélange dans les milieux biologiques. J Chromatogr 224:332–337

Boobis SW (1977) Alteration of plasma albumin in relation to decreased drug binding in uremia. Clin Pharmacol Ther 22:147–153

Boobis SW, Brodie MJ (1977) The effect of chronic alcohol ingestion and alcoholic liver disease on drug-protein binding. Br J Pharmacol 4:629

Brackett S, Waletzky E (1946) The inability of drugs with both causal prophylactic and suppressive action to cure established infections with avian malaria. J Parasitol [Suppl] 32:8–9

Brackett S, Waletzki E, Baker M (1945) The rate of action of sulfadiazine and quinine on the malarial parasite *Plasmodium gallinaceum*. J Pharmacol 84:254

Bratton AC, Marshall EK (1939) A new coupling component for sulfanilamide determination. J Biol Chem 128:537–550

Bridges JW, Kibby MR, Walker SR, Williams RT (1969) Structure and species as factors affecting the metabolism of some methoxy-6-sulphanilamido-pyrimidines. Biochem J 111:167–172

Brown GM, Weisman RA, Molnar DA (1961) The biosynthesis of folic acid. J Biol Chem 236:2534–2543

Bruce-Chwatt LJ (1968) Treatment of malaria JAMA 205:186–187

Bunnag D, Harinasuta T, Suntharasamai P, Migasena S, Charoenlarp P, Viravan C, Puangpartk S, Vanijanond S, Riganti M (1980) Monitoring of antimalarial drugs in the treatment of acute falciparum malaria. 10th Int cong trop med malaria, Manila 1980, Abstract No. 453

Bünger P (1967) Die Pharmakokinetik des Fanasils. In: Mossner G, Thomssen R (eds) Infektionskrankheiten, 4. Int Kongr Infektionskrankh, München 1966, Schattauer, Stuttgart, pp 855–868

Bushby SM (1967) Metabolism of the sulfones. Int J Lep 35:572–579

Bye A, Land GJ (1977) Gas-liquid chromatographic determination of sulfadiazine and its main metabolite in human plasma and urine. J Chromatogr 139:181–185

Cabrera BD, Ramos OL (1972) The causal prophylactic activity of 4-methoxy-6-sulfanilamidopyrimidine monohydrate (sulfamonomethoxine: DJ 1550) against malaria infections in Palawan, Philippines. Southeast Asian J Trop Med Public Health 3:501–504

Calabi V, Vannini E, Farina N (1973) Farmacocinetica della sulfametopirazina: Eliminazione biliare. Farmaco [Prat] 28:585–595

Cantrell W, Kelsey FE, Gerling EMK (1949) Sulfonamide blood levels in prophylactic trials against *Plasmodium gallinaceum*. J Infect Dis 84:32

Carr K, Oates JA, Nies AS, Woosley RL (1978) Simultaneous analysis of dapsone and monoacetyldapsone employing high performance liquid chromatography: a rapid method for determination of acetylator phenotype. Br J Clin Pharmacol 6:421–427

Catalano PM (1971) Dapsone agranulocytosis. Arch Dermatol 104:675

Cenedella RJ, Jarrell JJ (1970) Suggested new mechanisms of antimalarial action for DDS involving inhibition of glucose utilization by the intraerythrocytic parasite. Am J Trop Med Hyg 19:592–598

Cenedella RJ, Marens LK, Van Dyke K, Saxe LH (1969) Acetylation in vitro of para-aminobenzoic acid by unparasitized and *Plasmodium berghei* parasitized rat reticulocytes. Exp Parasitol 25:142–145

Chang T, Chang SF, Baukema J, Savory A, Dill WA (1969) Metabolic disposition of dapsone. Fed Proc 28:289

Chaptal J, Huguet R, Jean R, Blanc P, Dumas R (1966) Diffusion hémo-meningée d'un sulfamide retard: la sulfanilamido-4-diméthoxy-5,6-pyrimidine. J Méd Montpellier 1:55–65

Chatterjee KR, Poddar RK (1957) Radioactive tracer studies on uptake of diaminodiphenyl-sulphone by leprosy patients. Proc Soc Exp Biol Med 94:122–125
Chernof D (1967) Dapsone-induced hemolysis in G6PD deficiency. JAMA 201:554–556
Chin W, Contacos PG, Coatney GR, King HK (1966) The evaluation of sulfonamides, alone or in combination with pyrimethamine, in the treatment of multiresistant falciparum malaria. Am J Trop Med Hyg 15:823–829
Chopra RN (1939) M & B. 693 in Indian strains of malaria. Indian Med Gaz 74:658–660
Chopra RN, Das Gupta BM (1938) A note on the therapeutic efficiency of soluseptazine in simian malaria (*P. knowlesi*). Indian Med Gaz 73:395
Clyde DF (1967) Antimalarial effect of diaphenylsulfone and three sulfonamides among semi-immune Africans. Am J Trop Med Hyg 16:7–10
Clyde DF (1972) Responsibility for failure of sulphonamides in falciparum malaria: host or parasite? Trans R Soc Trop Med Hyg 66:806–807
Clyde DF, Rebert CC, McCarthy VC, Dawkins AT, Cucinell SA (1970a) Diformyldiaminodiphenyl sulfone (DFD) as an antimalarial in man. Milit Med 135:527–536
Clyde DF, Rebert CC, DuPont HL, Cucinell SA (1970b) Metabolic effects of the antimalarial diformyldiphenyl sulfone in man. Fed Proc 29:808
Clyde DF, Miller RM, Music SI, McCarthy VC (1971a) Prophylactic and sporontocidal treatment of chloroquine-resistant *Plasmodium falciparum* from Vietnam. Am J Trop Med Hyg 20:1–5
Clyde DF, Miller RM, Schwartz AR, Levine MM (1971b) Treatment of falciparum malaria with sulfalene and trimethoprim. Am J Trop Med Hyg 20:804–810
Clyde DF, Rebert CC, McCarthy VC, Miller RM (1971c) Prophylaxis of malaria in man using the sulfones DFD and DDS alone and with chloroquine. Milit Med 136:836–841
Coatney GR, Cooper WC (1944) The prophylactic effect of sulfadiazine and sulfaguanidine against mosquito-borne *Plasmodium gallinaceum* infection in the domestic fowl. Public Health Rep 59:1455–1458
Coatney GR, Cooper WC, Young MD, McLendon SB (1947a) Studies in human malaria. I. The protective action of sulfadiazine and sulfapyrazine against sporozoite-induced falciparum malaria. Am J Hyg 46:84–104
Coatney GR, Cooper WC, Young MD, Burgess RW, Smarr RG (1947b) Studies in human malaria. II. The suppressive action of sulfadiazine and sulfapyrazine against sporozoite-induced vivax malaria. Am J Hyg 46:105–117
Cobb PH, Hill GT (1977) High-performance liquid chromatography of some sulfonamides. J Chromatogr 123:444–447
Coggeshall LT (1938) Prophylactic and therapeutic effect of sulfonamide compounds in experimental malaria. Proc Soc Exp Biol 38:768–773
Coggeshall LT, Maier J (1941) Determination of the activity of various drugs against the malaria parasite. J Infect Dis 69:108–113
Coggeshall LT, Maier J, Best CA (1941) The effectiveness of two new types of chemotherapeutic agents in malaria (promine and sulfadiazine). JAMA 117:1077–1081
Coggeshall LT, Porter RJ, Laird RL (1944) Prophylactic and curative effects of certain sulfonamide compounds on exoerythrocytic stages in *Plasmodium gallinaceum* malaria. Proc Soc Exp Biol Med 57:286–292
Cooke TJL (1970) Dapsone poisoning. Med J Aust 23:1158–1159
Craft AW, Brocklebank JT, Jackson RH (1977) Acute renal failure and hypoglycemia due to sulphadiazine poisoning. Postgrad Med J 53:103–104
Cucinell SA, Israili ZH, Dayton PG (1972) Microsomal *N*-oxidation of dapsone as a cause of methemoglobin formation in human red cells. Am J Trop Med Hyg 21:322–331
Cucinell SA, Rebert C, Clyde D (1974) Clinical pharmacology of diformyldapsone. J Clin Pharmacol 14:51–57
Curd FHS (1943) The activity of drugs in the malaria of man, monkeys and birds. Ann Trop Med Parasitol 37:115–143
Davey DG (1946a) The use of avian malaria for the discovery of drugs effective in the treatment and prevention of human malaria. I. Drugs for clinical treatment and clinical prophylaxis. Ann Trop Med Parasitol 40:52–73

Davey DG (1946b) The use of avian malaria for the discovery of drugs effective in the treatment and prevention of human malaria. II. Drugs for causal prophylaxis and radical cure or the chemotherapy of exoerythrocytic forms. Ann Trop Med Parasitol 40:453–471

Davey DG (1963) Chemotherapy of malaria. I. Biological basis of testing methods. In: Schnitzer RJ, Hawking F (eds). Experimental chemotherapy. Academic, New York, pp 487–511

Davidson DE, Johnson DO, Tanticharoenyos P, Hickman RL, Kinnamon KE (1976) Evaluating new antimalarial drugs against trophozoite-induced *Plasmodium cynomolgi* malaria in rhesus monkeys. Am J Trop Med Hyg 25:26–33

DeGowin RL (1967) A review of therapeutic and hemolytic effects of dapsone. Arch Intern Med 120:242–248

DeGowin RL, Eppes RB, Powell RD, Carson PE (1965) Studies on sulfone-induced hemolysis. Clin Res 13:270

DeGowin RL, Eppes RB, Carson PE, Powell RD (1966a) The effects of diaphenyl sulfone (DDS) against chloroquine-resistant *Plasmodium falciparum*. Bull WHO 34:671–681

DeGowin RL, Eppes RB, Carson PE, Powell RD (1966b) The hemolytic effects of diaphenylsulfone (DDS) in normal subjects and in those with glucose-6-phosphate-dehydrogenase deficiency. Bull WHO 35:165–179

DeSouza JM (1980) Actual chloroquine, sulfadoxine-pyrimethamine association response in an intense malarial area of transmission (Paragominas, Pará State, Brazil). 10th Int congr trop med malaria, Manila 1980, Abstr. No. 431

Dettli L (1974) Dosage adjustment of chemotherapeutic agents in patients with kidney disease. In: Daikos GK (ed). Progress in chemotherapy, vol 1 Antibacterial chemotherapy. Hellenic Society of Chemotherapy Athens, pp 719–721

Dettli L, Spring P (1966) Diurnal variations in the elimination rate of a sulfonamide in man. Helv Med Acta 33:291–306

Díaz de León A (1937) Primeros casos de paludismo tratados por un derivado de la sulfanilamida. Bol Of Sanit Panam 16:1039–1040

Díaz de León A (1938) Las sulfanilamidas en el tratamiento del paludismo. Medicina (B Aires) 18:89–90

Díaz de León A (1940) El paludismo y su tratamiento intravenoso por las sulfanilamidas. Medicina (B Aires) 20:551–558

Donovick R, Bayan A, Hamre D (1952) The reversal of the activity of antituberculous compounds in vitro. Am Rev Respir Dis 66:219–227

Dorfman LE, Smith JP (1970) Sulfonamide crystalluria, a forgotten disease. J Urol 104:482–483

Dost FH, Gladtke E (1969) Pharmakokinetik des 2-Sulfanilamido-3-methoxy-pyrazins beim Kind (Elimination, enterale Absorption, Verteilung und Dosierung). Arzneimittelforsch 19:1304–1307

Edwards D (1980) Antimicrobial drug action. Macmillan, London

Ellard GA (1966) Absorption, metabolism and excretion of di(*p*-aminophenyl)sulphone (dapsone) and di(*p*-aminophenyl)sulphoxide in man. Br J Pharmacol 26:212–217

Ellard GA, Gammon PT, Helmy HS, Rees RJW (1972) Dapsone acetylation and the treatment of leprosy. Nature 239:159–160

Elonen E, Neuvonen PJ, Halmekoski J, Mattila MJ (1979) Acute dapsone intoxication: a case with prolonged symptoms. Clin Toxicol 14:79–85

Elslager EF, Worth DF (1965) Repository antimalarial drugs: *N,N'*-diacetyl-4,4'-diaminodiphenylsulphone and related 4-acylaminodiphenylsulphones. Nature 206:630–631

English JP, Clark JH, Clapp JW, Seeger D, Ebel RH (1946) Studies in chemotherapy. XIII. Antimalarials. Halogenated sulfanilamidoheterocycles. J Am Chem Soc 68:453–458

Eppes RB, McNamara JV, Degowin RL, Carson PE, Powell RD (1967) Chloroquine-resistant *Plasmodium falciparum:* protective and hemolytic effects of 4,4'-diamino-diphenyl sulfone (DDS) administered daily together with weekly chloroquine and primaquine. Milit Med 132:163–175

Epstein FW, Bohm W (1976) Dapsone-induced peripheral neuropathy. Arch Dermatol 112:1761–1762

Evans DAP (1969) An improved and simplified method of detecting the acetylator phenotype. J Med Genet 6:405–407
Evans DAP, Manley KA, McKusick VA (1960) Genetic control of isoniazid metabolism in man. Br Med J 2:485–491
Fabiani G, Orfila J (1954) Action d'un traitement sulfamidé sur le paludisme expérimental de la souris blanche. C R Soc Biol (Paris) 148:1390–1392
Fairley NH (1945) Chemotherapeutic suppression and prophylaxis in malaria. Trans R Soc Trop Med Hyg 38:311–365
Farinaud E, Eliche J (1939) Nouvelles observations sur le traitement du paludisme par les dérivés de la sulfonamide. Bull Soc Path Exot Filiales 32:674–681
Faucon R, Zannetti P, Jardel JP, Alary JC (1970) La méningite cérébrospinale à Fes à 1966–1967. Méd Trop (Mars) 30:599–623
Fickentscher K (1978) Zum Problem der Teratogenität von Arzneimitteln. Pharmazie 2:151–155
Findlay GM (1951) Recent advances in chemotherapy, vol II. Churchill, London
Findlay GM, Maegraith BG, Markson JL, Holden JR (1946) Investigations in the chemotherapy of malaria in West Africa. Ann Trop Med Parasitol 40:358–367
Fink E (1972) Kausalprophylaktische Wirkung von Standard-Malariamitteln bei der Nagetiermalaria (*Plasmodium berghei yoelii*). Z Tropenmed Parasitol 23:35–47
Fink E (1974) Assessment of causal prophylactic activity in *Plasmodium berghei* and its value for the development of new antimalarial drugs. Bull WHO 50:203–232
Fink E, Kretschmar W (1970) Chemotherapeutische Wirkung von Standard-Malariamitteln in einem vereinfachten Prüfverfahren an der *Plasmodium vinckei*-Infektion der NMRI-Maus. Z Tropenmed Parasitol 21:167–181
Firkin FC, Mariani AF (1977) Agranulocytosis due to dapsone. Med J Aust 2:250–251
Fisher GU, Gordon MP, Lobel HA, Runcik K (1970) Malaria in soldiers returning from Vietnam. Epidemiologic, therapeutic and clinical studies. Am J Trop Med Hyg 19:27–39
Flatz G, Voss B, Voss S (1970) Zur Anwendung von Sulfamethoxypyrazin bei Personen mit Mangel der Glucose-6-phosphat-Dehydrogenase der Erythrocyten. Klin Wochenschr 48:88–91
Forth W, Henschler D, Rummel W (1977) Allgemeine und spezielle Pharmakologie und Toxikologie, 2nd edn Bibliograph, Munich
Freire AS, Paraense WL (1944) The prophylactic and curative action of sulfadiazine (2-sulfanilamide-pyrimidine), sulfapyridine (2-sulfanilamide-pyridine) and sulfanilamide (*p*-aminobenzo-sulfonamide) on erythro- and exoerythrocytic cycles of *Plasmodium gallinaceum* (Therapeutic and parasitological aspects). Rev Bras Biol 4:27–48
Gehlmann LK, Koller WC, Malkinson FD (1977) Dapsone-induced neuropathy. Arch Dermatol 113:845–846
Gelber R, Peters JH, Gordon GR, Glazko AJ, Levy L (1971) The polymorphic acetylation of dapsone in man. Clin Pharmacol Ther 12:225–238
Gemmell DM, Lewis AJ, Stimson WH (1977) Studies on the anti-inflammatory properties of dapsone in a variety of animal models Br J Pharmacol 61:508–509
Gerberg EJ (1971) Evaluation of antimalarial compounds in mosquito test systems. Trans R Soc Trop Med Hyg 65:358–363
Gilpin RK (1979) Pharmaceuticals and related drugs. Anal Chem 51:257R–287R
Glader BE, Conrad ME (1973) Hemolysis by diphenylsulphones: Comparative effects of DDS and hydroxylamine-DDS. J Lab Clin Med 81:267–272
Gladtke E (1965) Ein Sulfanilamid mit extrem langsamer Elimination. Elimination, Verteilung, Dosierung und enterale Absorption von 4-Sulfanilamido-5,6-dimethoxypyrimidin beim Kind. Klin Wochenschr 43:1332–1334
Glazko AJ, Dill WA, Montalbo RG, Holmes E (1968) A new analytical procedure for dapsone. Am J Trop Med Hyg 17:465–473
Glazko AJ, Chang T, Baukema J, Chang SF, Savory A, Dill WA (1969) Central role of MADDS in the metabolism of DDS. Int J Lep 37:462–463
Goette DK (1977) Dapsone-induced hepatic changes. Arch Dermatol 113:1616–1617
Goodwin CS, Sparell G (1969) Inhibition of dapsone excretion by probenecid. Lancet 2:884–885

Goodwin LG, Rollo IM (1955) The chemotherapy of malaria, piroplasmosis, trypanosomiasis, and leishmaniasis. In: Hutner SH, Lwoff A (eds). Biochemistry and physiology of protozoa, vol 2, Academic, New York, pp 225–251

Gordon GR, Peters JH (1970) Microbore column chromatography of 4,4′-diaminodiphenyl sulfone and its acetylated derivatives. J Chromatogr 47:269–271

Goss AR, Hargrave JC, Curnow DH (1975) Serum sulphone levels in leprosy patients being treated with acedapsone. Clin Exp Pharmacol Physiol 2:86–87

Goth A (1978) Medical pharmacology, 9th edn, Mosby, St. Louis

Green KG (1963) "Bimez" and teratogenic action. Br Med J 2:56

Greenberg J (1949) The potentiation of the antimalarial activity of chlorguanide by *p*-aminobenzoic acid competitors. J Pharmacol Exp Ther 97:238–242

Greenberg J (1954) The effect of analogues of folic acid on the activity of sulfadiazine against *Plasmodium gallinaceum*. Exp Parasitol 3:351–357

Greenberg J, Richeson EM (1950) Potentiation of the antimalarial activity of sulfadiazine by 2,4-diamino-5-aryloxypyrimidines. J Pharmacol Exp Ther 99:444:449

Greenberg J, Boyd BL, Josephson ES (1948) Synergistic effect of chlorguanide and sulfadiazine against *Plasmodium gallinaceum* in the chick. J Pharmacol Exp Ther 94:60–64

Gregory KG, Peters W (1970) The chemotherapy of rodent malaria, IX. Causal prophylaxis, part I: A method for demonstrating drug action on exoerythrocytic stages. Ann Trop Med Parasitol 64:15–24

Griciute L, Tomatis L (1980) Carcinogenicity of dapsone in mice and rats. Int J Cancer 25:123–129

Gupta SK, Chakravarti RN, Mathur IS (1955) The therapeutic activity of some sulphones and sulphoxides in experimental tuberculosis of guinea-pigs. Br J Pharmacol Chemother 10:113–115

Hall WEB (1938) The sulphanilamides in tertian malaria. J Pharmacol 63:353–356

Halmekoski J, Mattila MJ, Mustakallio KK (1976) Metabolism and hemolytic effects of dapsone in man. Br J Clin Pharmacol 3:961P

Harinasuta R, Viravan C, Reid HA (1967) Sulphormethoxine in chloroquine-resistant falciparum malaria in Thailand. Lancet 1:1117–1119

Hawking F (1953) Milk diet, *p*-aminobenzoic acid, and malaria (*P. berghei*). Preliminary communication. Br Med J 1:1201–1202

Hawking F (1966) Chloroquine resistance in *Plasmodium berghei*. Am J Trop Med Hyg 15:287–293

Hawking F, Gammage K (1962) Chloroquine resistance produced in *Plasmodium berghei*. Trans R Soc Trop Med Hyg 56:263

Hawking F, Thurston JP (1951) A strain of monkey malaria (*Plasmodium cynomolgi*) made resistant to proguanil (paludrine). Trans R Soc Trop Med Hyg 44:695–701

Hawking F, Thurston JP (1952) Chemotherapeutic and other studies on the preerythrocytic forms of simian malaria (*Plasmodium cynomolgi*). Trans R Soc Trop Med Hyg 46:293–300

Helander I, Partanen J (1978) Dapsone-induced distal axonal degeneration of the motor neurons. Dermatologia 156:321–324

Herrero J (1967) The use of long-acting sulfonamides, alone or with pyrimethamine, in malaria (with special reference to sulformethoxine). Rev Soc Brasil Med Trop 1:103–136

Herting RL, Lopez F, Scherfling E, Sylvester JC, Wiegand R (1965) Clinical pharmacology of 2-sulfanilamido-3-methoxypyrazine. Antimicrob agents chemother 1964, pp 554–561. Am Soc Microbiol

Hill J (1950) The schizonticidal effect of some antimalarials against *Plasmodium berghei*. Ann Trop Med Parasitol 44:291–297

Hill J (1963) Chemotherapy of malaria. Part 2. The antimalarial drugs. In: Schnitzer RJ, Hawking F (eds). Experimental chemotherapy, vol 1, Academic, New York, pp 513–601

Hill J (1966) Chemotherapy of malaria. II. The antimalarial drugs, supplement. In: Schnitzer RJ, Hawking F (eds). Experimental chemotherapy, vol 4, Academic, New York, pp 448–462

Hill J (1975) The activity of some antibiotics and long-acting compounds against the tissue stages of *Plasmodium berghei*. Ann Trop Med Parasitol 69:421–427
Hill RA, Goodwin HM (1937) Prontosil in treatment of malaria: report of 100 cases. South Med J 30:1170
Hjelm M, DeVerdier CH (1965) Biochemical effects of aromatic amines. I. Methemoglobinemia, hemolysis and Heinz' body formation induced by 4,4'-diaminodiphenylsulfone. Biochem Pharmacol 14:1119–1128
Homeida M, Babiker A, Daneshmend TK (1980) Dapsone-induced optic atrophy and motor neuropathy. Br Med J 1:1180
Hubler WR, Solomon H (1972) Neurotoxicity of sulfones. Arch Dermatol 106:598
Huriez C, Bergoend H, Bertez ML (1972) Toxidermies bulleuses graves avec épidermolyse. Ann Dermatol Syphiligr 99:493–500
Hurly MGD (1959) Potentiation of pyrimethamine by sulphadiazine in human malaria. Trans R Soc Trop Med Hyg 53:412–415
Jacobs RL (1964) Role of *p*-aminobenzoic acid in *Plasmodium berghei* infection in the mouse. Exp Parasitol 15:213–225
Jerusalem C, Kretschmar W (1967) Untersuchungen zur Nukleinsäuresynthese der Malaria-Erreger an milchernährten Mäusen (*Plasmodium berghei*). Z Parasitenk 28:193–210
Jones TC, Cardamone JM (1968) Pseudoleukemia and dapsone. Ann Intern Med 69:639
Jopling WH, Ognibene AJ (1972) Why agranulocytosis from dapsone. Ann Intern Med 77:153
Joy RJT, Gardner WR, Tigertt WD (1969a) Malaria chemoprophylaxis with 4,4' diaminodiphenylsulfone (DDS). II. Field trial with comparison between two divisions. Milit Med 134:497–501
Joy RJT, McCarty JE, Tigertt WD (1969b) Malaria chemoprophylaxis with 4,4' diaminodiphenylsulfone (DDS). I. Field trial with comparison among companies of one division. Milit Med 134:493–496
Kabins SA (1972) Interactions among antibiotics and other drugs. J Am Med Assoc 219:206–212
Kato T, Kitagawa S (1973) Production of congenital anomalies in fetuses of rats and mice with various sulfonamides. Congenital Anomalies 13:7–15
Kazim M, Dutta GP (1980) Selection of a sulphanilamide-resistant strain of *Plasmodium berghei*. Indian J Med Res 72:632–636
Kingham JGC, Swain P, Swarbrick ET, Walker JG, Dawson AM (1979) Dapsone and severe hypoalbuminemia. A report of two cases. Lancet 2:662–664
Koller WC, Gehlmann LK, Malkinson FD, Davis FA (1977) Dapsone-induced peripheral neuropathy. Arch Neurol 34:644–646
Korolkovas A, Ferreira E, Divino Lima JD, Krettli AU (1978) Antimalarial activity of saccharidic polymers of dapsone and sulfadimethoxine. Chemotherapy 24:231–235
Krauer B, Spring P, Dettli L (1968) Zur Pharmakokinetik der Sulfonamide im ersten Lebensjahr. Pharmacol Clin 1:47–53
Krebs HA, Speakman JC (1945) Dissociation constant, solubility, and the pH value of the solvent. J Chem Soc 2:593–595
Kretschmar W (1965) The effect of stress and diet on resistance to *Plasmodium berghei* and malarial immunity in the mouse. Ann Soc Belg Med Trop 45:325–344
Kretschmar W (1966) Die Bedeutung der *p*-Aminobenzoesäure für den Krankheitsverlauf und die Immunität bei der Malaria im Tier (*Plasmodium berghei*) und im Menschen (*Pl. falciparum*). Z Tropenmed Parasitol 17:301–320, 369–390
Krettli AU, Brener Z (1968) Therapeutic activity of some sulfonamide compounds on normal and chloroquine-resistant strains of *Plasmodium berghei*. Rev Inst Med Trop São Paulo 10:389–393
Krishnaswami AK, Prakash S, Ramakrishnan SR (1954) Studies in *Plasmodium berghei*. XV. Acquired resistance to sulphadiazine. Indian J Malaria 8:9–18
Krüger-Thiemer E, Bünger P (1965) Evaluation of the risk of crystalluria with sulpha drugs. In: Proc Eur Soc Study Drug Tox, vol 6, Int Congr Series No 97, Excerpta Medica, Amsterdam, pp 185–207

Krüger-Thiemer E, Wempe E, Töpfer M (1965) Die antibakterielle Wirkung des nicht eiweißgebundenen Anteils im menschlichen Plasmawasser. Arzneimittelforsch 15:1309–1317

Krüger-Thiemer E, Berlin H, Brante G, Bünger P, Dettli L, Spring P, Wempe E (1969) Dosage regimen calculation of chemotherapeutic agents. Part 5, 2-sulfanilamido-3-methoxy-pyrazine (sulfalene). Chemotherapy 14:273–302

Laing ABG (1964) Antimalarial effect of sulphatodimethoxine (Fanasil). Br Med J 2:1439–1440

Laing ABG (1965a) Sporogony in *Plasmodium falciparum* apparently unaffected by sulphorthomidine (Fanasil). Trans R Soc Med Hyg 59:357–358

Laing ABG (1965) Treatment of acute falciparum malaria with diphenylsulphone in North-East Tanzania. J Trop Med Hyg 68:251–253

Laing ABG (1965gc) Treatment of acute falciparum malaria with sulphorthodimethoxine (Fanasil). Br Med J 1:905–907

Laing ABG (1968a) Antimalarial effects of sulphormethoxine, diaphenylsulphone and separate combinations of these with pyrimethamine: a review of preliminary investigations carried out in Tanzania. J Trop Med 71:27–35

Laing ABG (1968b) Hospital and field trials of sulphormethoxine with pyrimethamine against Malaysian strains of *Plasmodium falciparum* and *P. vivax*. Med J Malaysia 23:15–19

Laing ABG (1970) Studies on the chemotherapy of malaria. I. The treatment of overt falciparum malaria with potentiating combination of pyrimethamine and sulphormethoxine or dapsone in The Gambia. Trans R Soc Trop Med Hyg 64:562–580

Laing ABG, Pringle G, Lane FCT (1966) A study among African schoolchildren of the repository antimalarial properties of cycloguanil pamoate, 4,4′-diacetyl-diaminodiphenylsulphone, and a combination of the two drugs. Am J Trop Med Hyg 15:838–848

Laing ABG, Gooi HC, Gelber RH (1974) An acute attack of quartan malaria in a leprosy patient being treated with diaminodiphenylsulphone (DDS). Trans R Soc Trop Med Hyg 68:165

Lammintausta K, Kangas L, Lammintausta R (1979) The pharmacokinetics of dapsone in serum and saliva. Int J Clin Pharmacol Biopharm 17:159–163

Lampen JO, Jones MJ (1946) The antagonism of sulfonamide inhibition of certain lactobacilli and enterococci by pteroylglutamic acid and related compounds. J Biol Chem 166:435–448

Lampen JO, Jones MJ (1947) The growth-promoting and antisulfonamide activity of *p*-aminobenzoic acid, pteroylglutamic acid and related compounds for *Lactobacillus arabinosus* and *Streptobacterium plantarum*. J Biol Chem 170:133–146

Lehr D (1972) Sulfonamide vasculitis. J Clin Pharmacol 12:181–189

Levaditi C (1941)Phénomènes de Woods et azoïques sulfamidés, sulfoxydés et sulfonés. CR Soc Biol (Paris) 135:1109–1111

Levy L, Higgins LJ (1966) Dapsone assay based on Schiff base formation. Int J Lepr 34:411–414

Lewis AN, Ponnampalam JT (1975) Suppression of malaria with monthly administration of combined sulphadoxine and pyrimethamine. Ann Trop Med Parasitol 69:1–12

Loev B, Dowalo F, Theodorides VJ, Vogh BP (1973) A bis-*N*, O-diacetylhydroxylamine. Analog of diaminodiphenyl sulfone possessing antimalarial activity. J Med Chem 16:161–163

Maegraith BG, Deegan T, Jones ES (1952) Suppression of malaria (*P. berghei*) by milk. Br Med J 2:1382–1384

Maier J, Riley E (1942) Inhibition of antimalarial action of sulfonamides by *p*-aminobenzoic acid. Proc Soc Exp Biol Med 50:152–154

Mandell GL, Sande MA (1980) Antimicrobial agents: sulfonamides, trimethoprim, sulfamethoxazole, and urinary tract antiseptics. In: Goodman-Gilman A, Goodman LS, Gilman A (eds). The pharmacological basis of therapeutics, 6th edn, Macmillan, New York, pp 1106–1125

Manfredi G, De Panfilis G, Zampetti M, Allegra F (1979) Studies on dapsone-induced hemolytic anemia. I. Methemoglobin production and G6PD activity in correlation with dapsone dosage. Br J Dermatol 100:427–432
Manwell RD, Counts E, Coulston F (1941) Effect of sulfanilamide and sulfapyridine on the avian malarias. Proc Soc Exp Biol Med 46:523–525
Maren TH, Sonntag AC, Stenger VG (1970) The fate of the anti-malarial drug 4,4′diformamidodiphenyl sulfone (DFD) in man. Pharmacologist 12:272
Marshall PB (1945) The absorption of sulfonamides in the chick and the canary, and its relationship to antimalarial activity. J Pharmacol Exp Ther 84:1–11
Marshall EK, Litchfield JT, White HJ (1942) Sulfonamide therapy of malaria in ducks (*P. lophurae*). J Pharmacol Exp Ther 75:89–104
Martin DC, Arnold JD (1968) The drug response of a normal and a multi-resistant strain of *P. falciparum* to sulphalene. Trans R Soc Trop Med Hyg 62:810–815
Martin DC, Arnold JD (1969a) Trimethoprim and sulfalene therapy of *Plasmodium vivax*. J Clin Pharmacol 9:155–159
Martin DC, Arnold JD (1969b) Enhanced sensitivity of *Plasmodium falciparum* to sulphalene as a consequence of resistance to pyrimethamine. Trans R Soc Trop Med Hyg 63:230–235
Martindale W (1972) The Extra Pharmacopoeia, 26th edn (Wade A ed). Pharmaceutical, London
Marubini E, Soldati M, Ghione M (1968) A statistical evaluation of synergism of folic acid antagonists on experimental *Plasmodium berghei* mouse infection. Chemotherapy 13:232–241
Matveeva SA (1979) Pharmacokinetics of sulfamonomethoxine combined with ultraviolet irradiation in patients with acute pneumonia (In Russian). Ter Arkh 51:114–118
Mazzoni P (1967) Terapia della malaria acuta da *Plasmodium falciparum* con un sulfamidico ritardo. Minerva Med 58:799–802
McConnachie EW (1951) Latent infections in avian malaria in relation to the production of drug resistance. Parasitology 41:110–116
McFadzean JA (1951) Morphological changes in *Plasmodium cynomolgi* following proguanil, suphadiazine and mepacrine therapy. Trans R Soc Trop Med Hyg 44:707–716
McGuiness BW (1969) Experience with sulphormethoxine, a new long-acting sulphonamide. Br J Clin Pract 23:331–334
McKenna WB, Chalmers AC (1958) Agranulocytosis following dapsone therapy. Br Med J 1:324–325
Menk W, Mohr W (1939) Zur Frage der Wirksamkeit des Prontosils bei akuter Malaria. Archiv für Schiffs- und Tropenhygiene 43:117–125
Meyers FH, Jawetz E, Goldfien A (1980) Review of medical pharmacology, 7th edn, Lange, Los Altos, Ca.
Michel R (1968) Etude comparée de l'association sulfalène-pyriméthamine et du sulfalène seul en chimioprophylaxie palustre de masse. Méd Trop (Mars) 28:488–494
Miller AK (1944) Folic acid and biotin synthesis by sulfonamide-sensitive and sulfonamide-resistant strains of *Escherichia coli*. Proc Soc Exp Biol Med 57:151–153
Millikan LE, Harrell ER (1970) Drug reactions to the sulfones. Arch Dermatol 102:200–224
Most H, Montuori WA (1975) Rodent system (*Plasmodium berghei-Anopheles stephensi*) for screening compounds for potential causal prophylaxis. Am J Trop Med Hyg 24:179–182
Most H, Herman R, Schoenfeld C (1967) Chemotherapy of sporozoite- and blood-induced *Plasmodium berghei* infections with selected antimalarial drugs. Am J Trop Med Hyg 16:572–575
Mudrow-Reichenow L (1951) Über die chemotherapeutische Beeinflußbarkeit des *Plasmodium berghei* Vincke und Lips. Z Tropenmed Parasitol 2:471–485
Murray JF, Gordon GR, Peters JH, Levy L, Prochazka GJ (1973) Metabolic disposition of and therapeutic response to acedapsone in Filippino leprosy patients. Pharmacologist 15:207
Murray JF, Gordon GR, Gulledge CC, Peters JH (1975) Chromatographic-fluorometric analysis of antileprotic sulfones. J Chromatogr 107:67–72

Nelson T, Jacobsen J, Wennberg RP (1974) Effect of pH on the interaction of bilirubin with albumin and tissue culture cells. Pediatr Res 8:963–967

Neugodova NP, Kivman GY, Geitman IY (1977) Binding of sulfamonomethoxine and its *N*-methylglucamine salt by proteins and erythrocytes of human blood (Russian). Khim Farmatsevt Zh 11:23–36

Niven JC (1938) Sulphanilamide in the treatment of malaria. Trans R Soc Trop Med Hyg 32:413–418

Nola F Di, Soranzo ML, Cerutti L, Giuliani G (1969) Su di un caso di necrolisi epidermica tossica (sindrome di Lyell). Minerva Med 60:4176–4182

Odell GB (1959) The dissociation of bilirubin from albumin and its clinical implications. J Pediatr 55:268–274

Ognibene AJ (1970) Agranulocytosis due to dapsone. Ann Intern Med 72:521–524

Ohnhaus EE, Spring P (1975) Elimination kinetics of sulfadiazine in patients with normal and impaired renal function. J Pharmacokinet Biopharm 3:171–179

Orzech CE, Nash NG, Daley D (1976) Dapsone. In: Florey K (ed). Analytical profiles of drug substances, vol 5, Academic, New York, pp 87–114

Ott KJ (1969) The *Plasmodium chabaudi*-mouse system in chemotherapy studies. Exp Parasitol 24:194–204

Otten H, Plempel M, Siegenthaler W (1975) Antibiotica-Fibel, begründet von A. M. Walter und L. Heilmeyer, 4th edn, Thieme, Stuttgart

Padeiskaya LM, Poluchina SP, Shaevtsova SP, Perchin GN (1972) Sulfamonomethoxine: chemotherapeutic activity, tissue distribution, liquor diffusion. In: Hejzlar M, Semonsky M, Masak S (eds) Advances in antimicrobial and antineoplastic chemotherapy, vol 1. part 1. Urban and Schwarzenberg, München, pp 121–122

Paget GE, Thorpe E (1964) A teratogenic effect of a sulphonamide in experimental animals. Br J Pharmacol 23:305–312

Pakenham-Walsh R, Oxon BM (1938) Sulphonamides in malaria. Lancet 2:79

Payne HM, Hackney RL, Domon CM, Marshall EE, Harden KA, Turner OD (1953) The use of 4-amino-4′-*B* hydroxyethylaminodiphenyl sulfone (hydroxyethyl sulfone) in pulmonary tuberculosis. Am Rev Tubercul 68:103–118

Pearlman EJ, Thiemanun W, Castaneda BF (1975) Chemosuppressive field trials in Thailand. II. The suppression of *Plasmodium falciparum* and *P. vivax* parasitemias by a diformyldapsone-pyrimethamine combination. Am J Trop Med Hyg 24:901–909

Pearlman EJ, Lampe RM, Thiemanun W, Kennedy RS (1977) Chemosuppressive field trials in Thailand. III. The suppression of *Plasmodium falciparum* and *P. vivax* parasitemia by a sulfadoxine-pyrimethamine combination. Am J Trop Med Hyg 26:1108–1115

Peck CC, Lewis AN, Joyce BE (1975) Pharmacokinetic rationale for a malaria suppressant administered once monthly. Ann Trop Med Parasitol 69:141–146

Peters JH (1974) Metabolic disposition of dapsone in patients with dapsone-resistant leprosy. Am J Trop Med Hyg 23:222–230

Peters JH, Gordon GR, Colwell WT (1970a) The fluorometric measurement of 4,4′-diaminodiphenyl sulfone and its acetylated derivatives in plasma and urine. J Lab Clin Med 76:338–348

Peters JH, Gordon GR, Ghoul DC, Levy L, Tolentino JG (1970b) Acetylation of sulfamethazine and dapsone in American and Philippine subjects. Pharmacologist 12:274

Peters JH, Gordon GR, Ghoul DC, Tolentino JG, Walsh GP, Levy L (1972) The disposition of the antileprotic drug dapsone (DDS) in Philippine subjects. Am J Trop Med Hyg 21:450–457

Peters JH, Murray JF, Gordon GR, Levy L, Russell DA, Scott GC, Vincin DR, Shepard CC (1977) Acedapsone treatment of leprosy patients; response versus drug disposition. Am J Trop Med Hyg 26:127–136

Peters W (1965a) Drug resistance in *Plasmodium berghei* Vincke and Lips, 1948. I. Chloroquine resistance. Exp Parasitol 17:80–89

Peters W (1965b) Drug resistance in *Plasmodium berghei* Vincke and Lips, 1948. II. Triazine resistance. Exp Parasitol 17:90–96

Peters W (1966) Drug response of mepacrine- and primaquine-resistant strains of *Plasmodium berghei* Vincke and Lips, 1948. Ann Trop Med Parasitol 60:25–30

Peters W (1967 a) A review of recent studies on chemotherapy and drug resistance in malaria parasites of birds and mammals. Trop Dis Bull 64:1145–1175

Peters W (1967b) Chemotherapy of *Plasmodium chabaudi* infection in albino mice. Ann Trop Med Parasitol 61:52–56

Peters W (1968) The chemotherapy of rodent malaria. VII. The action of some sulphonamides alone or with folic reductase inhibitors against malaria vectors and parasites, part 2: schizontocidal action in the albino mouse. Ann Trop Med Parasitol 62:488–494

Peters W (1970) Chemotherapy and drug resistance in malaria. Academic, London

Peters W (1971 a) The chemotherapy of rodent malaria, XIV. The action of some sulphonamides alone or with folic reductase inhibitors against malaria vectors and parasites, part 4: the response of normal and drug-resistant strains of *Plasmodium berghei*. Ann Trop Med Parasitol 65:123–129

Peters W (1971 b) Potentiating action of sulfalene-pyrimethamine mixtures against drug-resistant strain of *P. berghei*. Chemotherapy 16:389–398

Peters W (1971 c) The experimental basis for the use of sulphonamides and sulphones against malaria in African communities. In: Gould GC (ed). Health and disease in Africa, East African Literature Bureau, Nairobi, pp 177–189

Peters W (1974) Prevention of drug resistance in rodent malaria by the use of drug mixtures. Bull WHO 51:379–383

Peters W (1980) Chemotherapy of malaria. In: Kreier JP (ed). Malaria, epidemiology, chemotherapy and metabolism, vol 1, Academic, New York, pp 145–283

Peters W, Ramkaran AE (1980) The chemotherapy of rodent malaria. XXXII. The influence of *p*-aminobenzoic acid on the transmission of *Plasmodium yoelii* and *P. berghei* by *Anopheles stephensi*. Ann Trop Med Parasitol 74:275–282

Peters W, Davies EE, Robinson BL (1975 a) The chemotherapy of rodent malaria. XXIII. Causal prophylaxis, part II: practical experience with *Plasmodium yoelii nigeriensis* in drug screening. Ann Trop Med Parasitol 69:311–328

Peters W, Portus JH, Robinson BL (1975 b) The chemotherapy of rodent malaria. XXII. The value of drug-resistant strains of *Plasmodium berghei* in screening for blood schizontocidal activity. Ann Trop Med Parasitol 69:155–171

Piamphongsant T (1976) Pemphigus controlled by dapsone. Br J Dermatol 94:681–686

Pinder RM (1973) Malaria. The Design, use, and mode of action of chemotherapeutic agents. Scientechnica, Bristol

Pines A (1967) Controlled trials of a sulphonamide given weekly to prevent exacerbation of chronic bronchitis. Br Med J 3:202–204

Popoff IC, Singhal GH, Engle AR (1971) Antimalarial agents. 7. Compounds related to 4,4′-bis (aminophenyl) sulfone. J Med Chem 14:550–551

Portwich F, Büttner H (1964) Zur Pharmakokinetik eines langwirkenden Sulfonamids (4-Sulfanilamido-5,6-dimethoxypyrimidin) beim gesunden Menschen. Klin Wochenschr 42:740–744

Powell RD, DeGowin RL, McNamara YV (1967) Clinical experience with sulphadiazine and pyrimethamine in the treatment of persons experimentally infected with chloroquine-resistant *Plasmodium falciparum*. Am Trop Med Parasitol 61:396–408

Ramakrishnan SP, Krishnaswami AK, Prakash S (1951) Studies on *P. berghei* n. sp. Vincke and Lips, 1948. The reaction of blood-induced *P. berghei* in albino mice to quinine and sulphadiazine. Indian J Malaria 5:455–464

Ramakrishnan SP, Basu PC, Singh H, Singh N (1962) Studies on the toxicity and action of diaminodiphenylsulphone (DDS) in avian and simian malaria. Bull WHO 27:213–221

Ramakrishnan SP, Basu PC, Singh H, Wattel BL (1963) A study of the joint action of diamino-diphenylsulphone (DDS) and pyrimethamine in the sporogony cycle of *Plasmodium gallinaceum:* potentiation of the sporontocidal activity of pyrimethamine by DDS. Indian J Malariol 14:141–148

Ramanujam K, Smith M (1951) Hemolytic anaemia during treatment of leprosy with diaminodiphenylsulphone by mouth. Lancet 1:21–22

Ramkaran AE, Peters W (1969) The chemotherapy of rodent malaria. VIII. The action of sulphormethoxine and pyrimethamine on the sporogonic stages. Ann Trop Med Parasitol 63:449–454

Ramos OL, Cabrera BD (1972) The effect of sulfamonomethoxine on both chloroquine-sensitive and -resistant *Plasmodium falciparum* and *P. vivax* infections. Southeast Asian J Trop Med Public Health, 3:562–568

Rane DS, Kinnamon KE (1979) The development of a "high volume tissue schizontocidal drug screen" based upon mortality of mice inoculated with sporozoites of *Plasmodium berghei*. Am J Trop Med Hyg 28:937–949

Rane L, Rane DS (1973) Primary screening devised for the assessment for antimalarial activity. Proc. 9th Int Congr Trop Med Malaria, Athens 1:281 (abstract no. 406)

Rapoport AM, Guss SB (1972) Dapsone-induced peripheral neuropathy. Arch Neurol 27:184–185

Ray AP, Nair CP (1955) Studies on Nuri strain of *P. knowlesi*, part IX. Susceptibility to sulphonamide substituted dihydrotriazine, sulphadiazine and mepacrine. Indian J Malariol 9:196–202

Reber H, Rutishauser G, Thölen H (1964) Clearance-Untersuchungen am Menschen mit Sulfamethoxazol und Sulforthodimethoxin. Proc 3rd int congr chemother, Stuttgart 1963, C-77 Thieme, Stuttgart, pp 1–6

Reeves DS, Bywater MJ, Holt HA (1978) Sulphonamides. In: Reeves DS, Phillipps I, Williams JD, Wise R (eds). Laboratory methods in antimicrobial chemotherapy, Churchill Livingstone, Edinburgh, pp 222–226

Reeves DS, Broughall JM, Bywater MJ, Holt HA, Vergin H (1979) Pharmacokinetics of tetroxoprim and sulfadiazine in human volunteers. J Antimicrob chemother [Suppl] 5B, 119–138

Reimerdes E, Thumin JH (1970) Das Verhalten der Sulfonamide im Organismus. Arzneimittelforsch 20:1171–1179

Rey M, Lafaix C, Diop Mar I, Sow A (1968) Le traitement du paludisme par l'association d'un sulfamide-retard et d'une pyrimidine. Bull Soc Med Afr Noire Lang Franç 13:366–376

Richards WHG (1966) Antimalarial activity of sulphonamide and a sulphone, singly and in combination with pyrimethamine against drug-resistant and normal strains of laboratory plasmodia. Nature 212:1494–1495

Richards WHG (1970) The combined action of pyrimidines and sulfonamides or sulfones in the chemotherapy of malaria and other protozoal infections. In: Garattini S, Goldin A, Hawkins F, Kopin IJ (eds). Advances in pharmacology and chemotherapy, vol 8, Academic, New York, pp 121–147

Richardson AP, Hewitt RI, Seager LD, Brooke MM, Martin F, Maddux H (1946) Chemotherapy of *Plasmodium knowlesi* infections in *Macaca mulatta* monkeys. J Pharmacol 87:203–213

Rieckmann KH (1967) A new repository antimalarial agent, CI-564, used in a field trial in New Guinea. Trans R Soc Trop Med Hyg 61:189–198

Rieckmann KH, McNamara JV, Frischer H, Stockert TA, Carson PE, Powell RD (1968) Gametocytocidal and sporontocidal effects of primaquine and of sulfadiazine with pyrimethamine in a chloroquine-resistant strain of *Plasmodium falciparum*. Bull WHO 38:625–632

Rieder J (1963) Physikalisch-chemische und biologische Untersuchungen an Sulfonamiden. Arzneimittelforsch 13:81–103

Rieder J (1972) Quantitative determination of the bacteriostatically-active fraction of sulfonamides and the sum of their inactive metabolites in the body fluids. Chemotherapy 17:1–21

Rieder J (1976) The simultaneous quantitative determination of total, "active", acetylated and conjugated sulfonamide in biological fluid. Chemotherapy 22:84–87

Riley RW, Levy L (1973) Characteristics of the binding of dapsone and monoacetyldapsone by serum albumin. Proc Soc Exp Biol Med 142:1168–1170

Rollo IM (1951) A 2,4-diamino pyrimidine in the treatment of proguanil-resistant laboratory malarial strains. Nature 168:332–333

Rollo IM (1955) The mode of action of sulphonamides, proguanil and pyrimethamine on *Plasmodium gallinaceum*. Br J Pharmacol 10:208–214
Rollo IM (1964) The chemotherapy of malaria. In: Hutner SH (ed). Biochemistry and physiology of Protozoa, vol 3, Academic, New York, pp 525–561
Rothe WE, Jacobus DP, Walter WG (1969) Treatment of trophozoite-induced *Plasmodium knowlesi* infection in the rhesus monkey with trimethoprim and sulfalene. Am J Trop Med Hyg 18:491–494
Rumler W, Woraschk J, Richter I, Gründig CA, Weigel W (1970) Über die Plazentapassage von Langzeitsulfonamiden unter besonderer Berücksichtigung von Chlorsulfisamidin. Dtsch Gesundheitswesen 25:1900–1903
Saqueton AC, Lorinez AL, Vick NA, Halmer RD (1969) Dapsone and peripheral motor neuropathy. Arch Dermatol 100:214–217
Schmidt LH (1979) Studies on the 2,4-diamino-6 substituted quinazolines. III. The capacity of sulfadiazine to enhance the activities of WR-158,122 and WR-159,412 against infections with various drug-susceptible and drug-resistant strains of *Plasmodium falciparum* and *P. vivax* in owl monkeys. Am J Trop Med Hyg 28:808–818
Schmidt LH, Harrison J, Rossan RN, Vaughan D, Crosby R (1977) Quantitative aspects of pyrimethamine-sulfonamide synergism. Am J Trop Med Hyg 26:837–849
Schneider MD (1968) Characteristics and cross-resistance patterns of chloroquine-resistant *Plasmodium berghei* infections in mice. Exp Parasitol 23:22–50
Scholtan W, Schmidt J (1962) The binding of penicillins to the proteins of blood and tissues. Arzneimittelforsch 12:741–750
Schuppli R (1968) Die Behandlung der Dermatitis herpetiformis. Dtsch Med Wochenschr 93:2343
Schvartsman S (1979) Sulfone Methemoglobinemia. Clin Toxicol 15:458
Shastri RA, Krishnaswamy K (1979) Metabolism of sulphadiazine in malnutrition. Br J Pharmacol 7:69–73
Shelly WB, Goldwein MI (1976) High dose dapsone toxicity. Br J Dermatol 95:79–82
Shepard TH (1976) Catalog of teratogenic agents, 2nd edn, Johns Hopkins University, Baltimore
Shiota T (1959) Enzymic synthesis of folic acid-like compounds by cell-free extracts of *Lactobacillus arabinosus*. Arch Biochem Biophys 80:155
Shute GT, Dowling MAC (1966) Effect of sulforthodimethoxine on parasites of *Plasmodium falciparum* and *P. malariae* on semi-immune schoolchildren in the western region of Nigeria. WHO/Mal/66.544 (cyclostyled report) WHO, Geneva
Silverman WA, Andersen DH, Blanc WA, Crozier DN (1956) A difference in mortality rate and incidence of kernicterus among premature infants allotted to two prophylactic antibacterial regimens. Pediatrics 18:614–625
Singh J, Basu PC, Ray AP (1952a) Screening of antimalarials against *Plasmodium gallinaceum* in chicks. Indian J Malaria 6:145–158
Singh J, Ray AP, Basu PC, Nair CP (1952b) Acquired resistance to proguanil in *Plasmodium knowlesi*. Trans R Soc Trop Med Hyg 46:639–649
Singh J, Nair CP, Ray AP (1956) Therapeutic effect of sulphadiazine and dihydrotriazines against blood-induced *Plasmodium cynomolgi* infection. Indian J Malaria 10:131–135
Sinton JA, Hutton EL, Shute PG (1939) Some successful trials of proseptasine as a true causal prophylactic against infection with *Plasmodium falciparum*. Ann Trop Med Parasitol 33:37–44
Smithells RW (1966) Drugs and human malformations. In: Woollam DH (ed). Advances in teratology, vol 1, Logos and Academic, New York, pp 251–278
Smithurst BA, Robertson I, Naughton MA (1971) Dapsone-induced agranulocytosis complicated by gram-negative septicemia. Med J Aust 1:537–539
Sonntag AC, Stenger VG, Maren TH (1972a) The pharmacology of the antimalarial drug 4′4-diformylamidodiphenylsulfone (DFD) in man. J Pharmacol Exp Ther 182:48–55
Sonntag AC, Stenger VG, Vogh BP, Maren TH (1972b) The pharmacology of the antimalarial drug, 4,4′-diformylamidodiphenylsulfone (DFD) in dog and monkey. J Pharmacol Exp Ther 182:34–47

Sorley ER, Currie JG (1938) Notes on the experimental use of prontosil album in the treatment of malaria. J R Nav Med Serv 24:322–325
Stauber R, Puxkandl H (1966) Die Ausscheidung des neuen Langzeitsulfonamids Fanasil in der menschlichen Galle. Wien Klin Wochenschr 78:66–70
Stickland JF, Hurdle ADF (1970) Agranulocytosis probably due to dapsone in an infantry soldier. Med J Aust 1:959–960
Stone SP, Goodwin RM (1978) Dapsone-induced jaundice. Arch Dermatol 114:947
Storey J, Rossi-Espagnet A, Mandel SPH, Matsushima T, Lietaert P, Thomas D, Brøgger S, Duby C, Gramiccia G (1973) Sulfalene with pyrimethamine and chloroquine with pyrimethamine in single dose treatment of *Plasmodium falciparum* infection. Bull WHO 49:275–282
Taylor DJ, Greenberg J (1955) Hyperactivity of metachloridine against *Plasmodium gallinaceum* in chicks maintained on a purified diet. Proc Soc Exp Biol Med 90:551–554
Taylor GML (1968) Stevens-Johnson syndrome following the use of an ultra-long acting sulphonamide. S Afr Med J 42:501–503
Terzian LA (1947) A method for screening antimalarial drugs in the mosquito host. Science 106:449–450
Terzian LA (1950) The sulfonamides as factors in increasing susceptibility to parasitic invasion. J Infect Dis 87:285–290
Terzian LA, Weathersby AB (1949) The action of antimalarial drugs in mosquitoes infected with *Plasmodium falciparum*. Am J Trop Med Hyg 29:19–22
Terzian LA, Stahler N, Weathersby AB (1949) The action of antimalarial drugs in mosquitoes infected with *Plasmodium gallinaceum*. J Infect Dis 84:47–55
Terzian LA, Stahler N, Dawkins AT (1968) The sporogonous cycle of *Plasmodium vivax* in *Anopheles* mosquitoes as a system for evaluating the prophylactic and curative capacities of potential antimalarial compounds. Exp Parasitol 23:56–66
Thompson PE (1967) Antimalarial studies on 4,4′-diaminodiphenylsulfone (DDS) and repository sulfones in experimental animals. Int J Lepr 35:605–617
Thompson PE, Werbel LM (1972) Medicinal Chemistry. A series of monographs, vol 12. Antimalarial agents: chemistry and pharmacology. Academic, New York, pp 265–300
Thompson PE, Olszewski BJ, Waitz JA (1965a) Laboratory studies of the repository antimalarial activity of 4,4′-diacetylaminodiphenylsulfone, alone and mixed with cycloguanil pamoate (CI-501). Am J Trop Med Hyg 14:343–353
Thompson PE, Olszewski B, Waitz JA (1965b) Effects of representative antimalarial drugs against three drug-resistant lines of *Plasmodium berghei* in mice. J Parasitol 51:54
Thompson PE, Waitz JA, Olszewski B (1965c) The repository antimalarial activity of 4,4′-diacetyl-aminodiphenylsulfone and cycloguanil pamoate (CI-501) in monkeys relative to release following parenteral administration. J Parasitol 51:345–349
Thompson PE, Olszewski B, Bayles A, Waitz JA (1967) Relations among antimalarial drugs. Results of studies with cycloguanil-, sulfone-, or chloroquine-resistant *Plasmodium berghei* in mice. Am J Trop Med Hyg 16:133–145
Thurston JP (1950) The action of antimalarial drugs in mice infected with *Plasmodium berghei*. Br J Pharmacol 5:409–416
Thurston JP (1951) Morphological changes in *Plasmodium berghei* following proguanil, sulphadiazine and mepacrine therapy. Trans R Soc Trop Med Hyg 44:703–706
Thurston JP (1953a) The action of dyes, antibiotics, and some miscellaneous compounds against *Plasmodium berghei*. Br J Pharmacol 8:163–165
Thurston JP (1953b) The chemotherapy of *Plasmodium berghei*. I. Resistance to drugs. Parasitology 43:246–252
Thurston JP (1954) The chemotherapy of *Plasmodium berghei*. II. Antagonism of the action of drugs. Parasitology 44:99–110
Trenholme GM, Williams RF, Fischer H, Carson PE, Rieckmann KH (1975) Host failure in treatment of malaria with sulfalene and pyrimethamine. Ann Intern Med 82:219–223
Turkel SB, Guttenberg ME, Moynes DR, Hodgman JE (1980) Lack of identifiable risk factors for kernicterus. Pediatrics 66:502–506
Van der Wielen Y (1937) Prontosil en malaria quartana. Ned Tijdschr Geneeskd 81:2905–2906

Verdraeger J (1970) Correspondence. Trans R Soc Trop Med Hyg 64:789
Vergin H, Bishop GB (1980) Bestimmung von Tetroxoprim und Sulfadiazin in Serum und Urin durch Hochdruckflüssigkeitschromatographie. Arzneimittelforsch 30:317–319
Vincke IH (1970) The effects of pyrimethamine and sulphormethoxine on the preerythrocytic and sporogonous cycle of *Plasmodium berghei berghei*. Ann Soc Belg Méd Trop 50:339–358
Vincke IH, Lips M (1948) Un nouveau *Plasmodium* d'un rongeur sauvage du Congo, *Plasmodium berghei* n. sp. Ann Soc Belg Méd Trop 48:439–454
Vivier A du, Fowler T (1974) Possible dapsone-induced peripheral neuropathy in dermatitis herpetiformis. Proc R Soc Med 67:439–440
Vogh BP, Garg LC, Sonntag AC, Maren TH (1972) 4,4'Diformylamidodiphenylsulfone (DFD): analysis of plasma and urine for unsubstituted arylamine in the presence of metabolites and acid-labile substituents on the parent compound. Clin Chim Acta 40:431–442
Vree TB, Hekster YA, Baars AM, Damsma JE, Van der Keijn E (1978) Determination of trimethoprim and sulfamethoxazole (co-trimoxazole) in body fluids of man by means of high-performance liquid chromatography. J Chromatogr 146:103–112
Wagner JG (1975) Relevant pharmacokinetics of antimicrobial drugs. Med Clin North Am 58:479–492
Waitz JA, Olszewski B, Thompson PE (1965) Antimalarial activity of sulfones in mice, rats, and monkeys. J Parasitol 51:54
Wallace S (1976) Factors affecting drug-protein binding in the plasma of newborn infants. Br J Pharmacol 3:510–512
Wallace S, Brodie MJ (1976) Decreased drug binding in serum from patients with chronic hepatic disease. Eur J Clin Pharmacol 9:429–432
Wennberg RP, Ahlfors CE, Rasmussen LF (1979) The pathochemistry of kernicterus. Early Hum Dev 3:353–372
Wiegand RG, Chun AHC, Scherfling E, Lopez F, Herting RL (1965) Chemical pharmacology of 2-sulfanilamido-3-methoxy-pyrazine. Antimicrob Agents Chemother 1964, pp 549–553 Am Soc Microb 1965
Willerson D, Rieckmann KH, Kass L, Carson PE, Frischer H, Bowman JE (1972) The chemoprophylactic use of diformyldiamino-diphenylsulfone (DFD) in falciparum malaria. Am J Trop Med Hyg 21:138–143
Willerson D, Rieckmann KH, Kass L, Carson PE, Frischer H, Richard L, Bowman JE (1974) Chemotherapeutic results in a multi-drug resistant strain of *Plasmodium falciparum* malaria from Vietnam. Milit Med 139:175–183
Williams JD (1974) The sulphonamides. Br J Hosp Med 12:722–730
Williams RL, Trenholme GM, Carson PE, Fischer H, Rieckmann KH (1975) Acetylator phenotype and response of individuals infected with a chloroquine-resistant strain of *Plasmodium falciparum* to sulfalene and pyrimethamine. Am J Trop Med Hyg 24:734–739
Williams RL, Trenholme GM, Carson PE, Fischer H, Rieckmann KH (1978) The influence of acetylator phenotype and the response to sulfalene in individuals with chloroquine-resistant falciparum malaria. Am J Trop Med Hyg 27:226–231
Wiselogle FY (1946) A survey of antimalarial drugs 1941–45. Edwards, Ann Arbor, Michigan
Woods DD (1940) The relation of *p*-aminobenzoic acid to the mechanism of the action of sulphanilamide. Br J Exp Path 21:74–90
Wyatt EH, Stevens JC (1972) Dapsone-induced peripheral neuropathy. Br J Dermatol 86:521–523
Yoshinaga T, Tsutsumi Y, Tsunoda K, Yamamura K (1970) Studies on the antimalarial property of 4-methoxy-6-sulfanilamidopyrimidine monohydrate (sulfamonomethoxine: DJ-1550) and on its effect on the chloroquine-resistant malaria. Arzneimittelforsch 20:1206–1210
Young S, Marks JM (1979) Dapsone and severe hypoalbuminemia. Lancet 2:909–909

CHAPTER 5

Dihydrofolate Reductase Inhibitors

R. FERONE

A. Introduction

While exploring structural variations of anilinopyrimidines with antimalarial activity, a group at Imperial Chemical Industries found that certain biguanides synthesised as ring-opened analogues possessed good activity against *Plasmodium gallinaceum* infections in chicks (CURD et al. 1945). Later, a group at Burroughs Wellcome who were testing various types of pyrimidines as inhibitors of nucleic acid synthesis pointed out a formal structural analogy between the most active of the biguanides, proguanil (chlorguanide), and a 2,4-diamino-5-aryloxypyrimidine which was a folic acid antagonist (FALCO et al 1949). Soon after this, it was discovered that proguanil is cyclised metabolically to a dihydrotriazine, an active metabolite which is a folic acid antagonist (CARRINGTON et al. 1951). Eventually, it was shown that the diaminopyrimidine, pyrimethamine, and the dihydrotriazine, cycloguanil, share a common locus of action – the powerful, selective inhibition of the activity of malarial dihydrofolate reductase (FERONE et al. 1969). Thus, one compound which was inadvertently synthesised as a prodrug and another which derived from a programme of synthesis of untargeted antimetabolites, together stand as prime examples of chemotherapeutic exploitation of species differences of isofunctional enzymes. These drugs have experienced 3 decades of widescale use for the prophylaxis and suppression of human malaria.

B. Proguanil (Chlorguanide)

I. Chemistry and Assay

Proguanil is N^1-*p*-chlorophenyl-N^5-isopropylbiguanide, frequently referred to as chlorguanide (Fig. 1). The hydrochloride salt is the product used commercially (Paludrine, ICI). The solubility in water is $\sim 1\%$; it is soluble in alcohol, but practically insoluble in organic solvents such as ether and chloroform.

A frequently used method of assay for proguanil in tissues and body fluids is that of SPRINKS and TOTTEY (1945), with modifications by MAEGRAITH et al. (1946), SCHMIDT et al. (1947) and SMITH et al. (1961). In this method, the sample is made alkaline and extracted into organic solvent, which is then acidified and extracted back into an aqueous phase. This is then autoclaved causing a hydrolytic cleavage to release *p*-chlorophenylanaline, which is determined by the Bratton-Marshall procedure for diazotisable amines. Recoveries of drug added to urine, blood, plas-

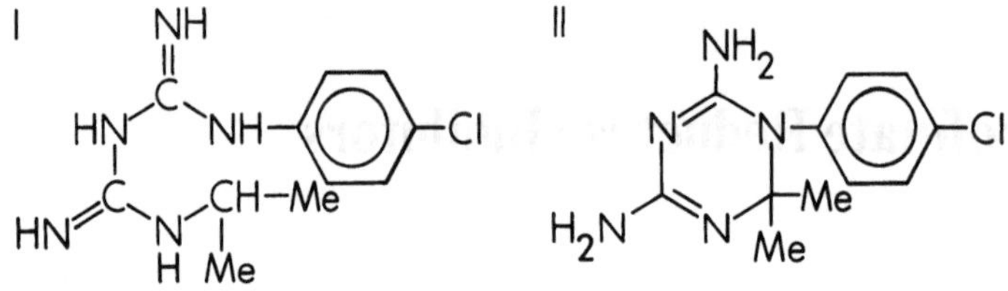

Fig 1. I. Proguanil; II. Cycloguanil

ma or faeces were 90%–100% in the 1–50μg/ml range. The method is also usable for proguanil metabolites which yield a *p*-chlorophenylaniline fragment upon hydrolytic cleavage.

A simpler method was devised for estimation of proguanil in urine (GAGE and ROSE 1946) which was adopted for use in the field (TOTTEY and MAEGRAITH 1948). The copper complex of parent compound in urine is extracted into benzene and then reacted with a solution of diethyldithiocarbamate to give a coloured product. This can be measured quantitatively in a spectrophotometer or estimated visually by comparison with serial dilutions of a standard. Since the presumed metabolites would not be determined by this method, lower values would be expected than with the hydrolytic cleavage method.

SMITH and colleagues (SMITH et al. 1961; AMSTRONG 1973) found methods to assay proguanil and the two main metabolites, *p*-chlorophenylbiguanide and cycloguanil. Cycloguanil is measured microbiologically by inhibition of growth of the folate-requiring bacterium *Streptococcus faecium* (ATCC8043), and the *p*-chlorophenylbiguanide determined by the same assay after chemical conversion to cycloguanil by condensation with acetone in hydrochloric acid.

II. Metabolism and Pharmacokinetics

Soon after proguanil was introduced, it was observed that the drug was inactive as an inhibitor of the in vitro growth of *P. gallinaceum* (TONKIN 1946) and *P. cynomolgi* (HAWKING 1947), but that sera from dosed monkeys were active against *P. cynomolgi* in vitro (HAWKING 1947). These findings suggested that proguanil was activated in vivo. In 1951, CARRINGTON et al. reported on the isolation of a proguanil metabolite from the urine of dosed rats and men, which was ten fold more potent than parent compound against *P. gallinaceum* infections in chicks. The metabolite was identified as a cyclised compound (and thus named cycloguanil); 4,6-diamino-1-*p*-chlorophenyl-2,2-dimethyl-1,3,5-dihydrotriazine (CARRINGTON et al. 1951; CROWTHER and LEVI 1953) (Fig. 1). The latter authors also identified the analogous triazine metabolite from chloroproguanil, the dichloro analogue of proguanil.

Since that time, it has been accepted by most investigators in this field that cycloguanil is the active metabolite of proguanil and that parent compound is inactive per se. Thus, in comparing sensitivities of different strains and species of plasmodia to proguanil, possible species differences of the host in activation of proguanil to cycloguanil must be taken into account. A thesis dissertation by ARMSTRONG (1973) reports on the cyclisation of proguanil to cycloguanil by the mixed function oxidase system of rabbit hepatic microsomes. The rabbit system also produced equal amounts of an *N*-dealkylated metabolite, *p*-chlorophenylbiguanide (Amstrong and Smith 1974). The rates of formation of both metabolites were induced to higher levels by pretreatment of the rabbits with phenobarbital or 3-methylcholanthrene. The authors concluded that cyclisation to cycloguanil required cytochrome P-448 whereas *N*-dealkylation probably involved P-450. Rats form low amounts of cycloguanil and rat microsomes were poor in the cyclisation reaction, although significant amounts of the *N*-dealkylated product were formed. Pretreatment of the rats with 3-methylcholanthrene greatly increased the formation of cycloguanil, supporting the conclusion that the poor ability of rats (and mice) to cyclise proguanil was due to the low levels of cytochrome P-448 normally found in these rodents compared with the levels found in rabbits. It follows from their study that conditions which effect P-448 levels in animals, including man, could effect the efficacy of proguanil as an antimalarial.

Most absorption and tissue distribution studies on proguanil have employed the *p*-chloroaniline release assay originated by Spinks and Tottey (1945). With this assay, it was found that plasma levels in man peak at 4 h after oral dosing (Maegraith et al. 1946; Chaudhuri et al. 1952) and decrease with a half-life of 15 h (Ritshel et al. 1978). Tissue analysis from human autopsies revealed higher levels of compound in kidney, liver and whole blood than in plasma. Smith et al. (1961) reported that tissue levels in the monkey and dog were much higher than in the rat. Only ≅45% of the daily dose of proguanil was recovered in the tissues and excreta of the rat, leaving 55% metabolised to materials not found by the *p*-chloroaniline release assay.

In man, half of an oral dose is excreted in the urine, mainly in the first 48 h (Maegraith et al. 1946; Chaudhuri et al. 1952; Smith et al. 1961) and only 7% -12% in the faeces (Maegraith et al. 1946). Most of the drug excreted by man is the parent compound, but 17%–43% was found as cycloguanil (Smith et al. 1961).

III. Toxicity

A table of acute toxicities of proguanil in animals was compiled by Hill (1963), the order of susceptibility appears to be mice > rat ≅ rabbit > chick > dog ≅ monkey. Oral dosing was in general three- to fivefold less toxic than intraperitoneal or intramuscular dosing. Chronic dosing to mice, rats, dogs and monkeys yielded gastrointestinal effects which were reversible when the drug was discontinued (Schmidt et al. 1947). No embryotoxic or teratogenic effects were noted in pregnant rats orally dosed with 25–50 mg/kg proguanil or cycloguanil (Chebotar 1974), although inhibition of the development of ova during cleavage was found, possibly accounting for the antifertility effect of proguanil in female mice reported by Cutting (1962).

The toxicity in man is low on the usual prophylatic doses of 100 mg daily or 300 mg weekly. Gastrointestinal symptoms with some renal complications have been observed at doses of 0.8–1 g/day but are reversed by stopping the drug (Fairley et al. 1946; Chaudhuri et al. 1952). A gross overdose of 14.5 g was followed by complete recovery (Rollo 1965).

IV. Mode of Action

The bulk of the evidence accumulated on the mode of action of proguanil points to inhibition of dihydrofolate reductase by the active metabolite, cycloguanil. Early studies with *P. berghei* in mice and *P. gallinaceum* in chicks implicated folic acid metabolism as the locus of action since *p*-aminobenzoic acid and folic acid partially reversed the growth inhibitory effect of proguanil (Thurson 1950; Greenberg 1949a, 1953) and the drug was synergistic with sulphonamides (Greenberg 1945b and many others). Falco et al. (1949) drew attention to the structural analogy of proguanil and 2,4-diamino-5-*p*-chlorophenoxypyrimidine and suggested that the former might be a folic acid antagonist and the latter might have antimalarial activity. Soon after came the evidence that proguanil is cyclised to a dihydrotriazine which is indeed a folic antagonist. The antifolate nature of cycloguanil was first shown indirectly: cycloguanil inhibition of the growth of folate-requiring lactic acid bacteria is reversed by folic acid and leucovorin (a stable cofactor form of folate); cycloguanil-resistant strains of plasmodia are usually cross-resistant to pyrimethamine; cycloguanil is synergistic with sulphonamides for inhibition of malarial growth. Later, cycloguanil was shown to be a potent inhibitor of the activity of dihydrofolate reductase from *P. berghei* (Ferone et al. 1969; Ferone 1970). The affinity of the malarial enzyme ($K_i = 0.78 \times 10^{-9} M$) is several hundred-fold stronger than the affinity of the mouse erythrocyte dihydrofolate reductase, thus documenting the selective toxicity of cycloguanil on an enzymatic basis. The parent compound, proguanil, did not inhibit the activity of dihydrofolate reductase of *P. berghei*, rat liver, or *Escherichia coli* at $2 \times 10^{-4} M$ (R. Ferone 1980, unpublished data). Since plasmodia synthesise their folate cofactors de novo and cannot utilise intact exogenous folates, then selective inhibition of the parasite dihydrofolate reductase will result in depletion of tetrahydrofolate cofactors required for cellular metabolism and thus prevent cell growth.

V. Deployment

Proguanil is used for prophylaxis and suppression of malarial infections. Most authors have stressed (a) that it not be used for treatment of acute attacks in non-immune subjects because of the slowness of action and (b) that it only be used in areas where resistance is not well established (good advice for the use of any antimicrobial agent!). The recommended dose is 100 mg daily for non-immunes and 300 mg weekly for semi-immunes (Rollo 1965). Although it is not the drug of choice for treatment of acute attacks, it can be used for non-severe attacks in semi-immunes at the dosage of 1.5–1.8 g over 5 days (Contacos 1969; Rollo 1965; Chaudhuri et al. 1952). Ritshel et al. (1978) analysed pharmacokinetic data in the literature on proguanil and recommended that a loading dose of 450 mg be given followed by 250 mg at 24-h intervals, in order to achieve steady-state plasma levels during treatment.

Proguanil is an effective agent for the prevention of drug sensitive malaria because it is a true causal prophylactic, effective in inhibition of the development of the primary erythrocytic forms, and because it inhibits schizogony of the erythrocytic form (Curd et al. 1945). It also inhibits oocyst development in the mosquito, thus preventing transmission of the disease (Omar et al. 1974). Proguanil is preferred by many for suppression and prophylaxis of malaria for these reasons, as well as the need for daily dosing which is claimed to be desirable for effective antimalarial discipline (BRUCE-CHWATT 1977).

VI. Resistance

The use of proguanil as a malaria prophylactic agent has been compromised by the appearance of resistant strains of the parasite, noted in all major geographical areas of its use (PETERS 1970; WORLD HEALTH ORGANIZATION 1965). Frequently, but not invariably, cross-resistance to pyrimethamine is also observed. In at least one case in the field, resistance to proguanil was overcome by the combination of dapsone with proguanil. BLACK (1973) reported a sharp decrease in the *P. falciparum* incidencc among Australian troops in Vietnam after dapsone (25 mg daily) was added to the daily dose of 200 mg proguanil. However, the spread in Southeast Asia of *P. falciparum* strains resistant to an antifol/sulpha combination (pyrimethamine/sulfadoxine) makes it likely that the proguanil/dapsone combination will be ineffective in that area.

C. Pyrimethamine

I. Chemistry and Assay

Pyrimethamine (Fig. 2) is an odourless, tasteless weak base (pKa 7.3) of molecular weight 248.7. It is lipophilic, with an octanol/water partition coefficient (log P) of 2.69 (CAVALLITO et al. 1978) and thus is poorly soluble in water, although moderately soluble in alcohol and in dilute acids.

A variety of methods have been used to analyse the pyrimethamine content of biological samples, including microbiological growth inhibition, UV spectroscopy,

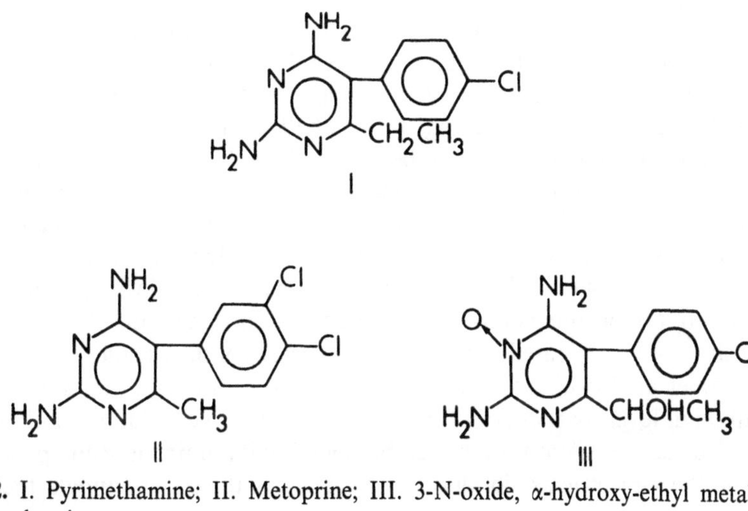

Fig. 2. I. Pyrimethamine; II. Metoprine; III. 3-N-oxide, α-hydroxy-ethyl metabolite of pyrimethamine

dye-binding, gas-liquid chromatography, thin-layer chromatography (TLC), gel filtration and high-performance liquid chromatography. In the microbiological method, sterile samples are tested for inhibition of growth of *Streptococcus faecium* ATCC 8043 (SMITH and IHRING 1957). For the dye-binding, UV, and TLC methods, the drug is first extracted from alkalinised biological samples into an organic solvent such as ethylene dichloride, before final analysis. It can be back extracted into 0.1 *N* HCl and the UV spectrum determined (SCHMIDT et al. 1953). SMITH and IHRIG (1957) found the microbiological and the UV methods to be equivalent for determination of pyrimethamine levels in the sera and urines of monkeys and men. The organic solvent extract can also be mixed with a methyl orange solution for determination of drug by the dye-binding method (SCHMIDT et al. 1953). A more sensitive and more specific technique is to separate pyrimethamine on silica gel thin-layer chromatography plates followed by quantitation of the fluorescence or UV absorbance of the drug with a scanning spectrophotometer (JONES and KING 1968; SIMMONS and DEANGELIS 1973; DEANGELIS et al. 1975). DEANGELIS et al. (1975) concentrated the drug by evaporating the organic solvent and redissolving the residue in a small volume of chloroform for application to the TLC plate, thus achieving a lower limit of detection of 5–10 ng/ml of sample. This method is also suitable for the determination of similar diaminopyrimidines and for some pyrimethamine metabolites.

Recently, high-performance liquid chromatography has been used to analyse pyrimethamine levels in biological samples (LEVIN et al. 1978; JONES and OVENELL 1979) and in feeds (COX and SUGDEN 1977). In the procedure of LEVIN et al. (1978), samples are first deproteinised in a methanol/phosphate buffer mixture and then injected directly into the high-pressure liquid chromatography column.

II. Metabolism and Pharmacokinetics

Pyrimethamine is well absorbed after oral dosing of monkeys and man. SMITH and SCHMIDT (1963) recovered 82%–84% of the radioactivity of [^{14}C]-pyrimethamine in the urine and 3.5%–5.2% in the faeces of monkeys dosed by oral, intramuscular and intravenous routes. In man, urinary excretion during the first 5 days after oral dosing accounted for 12% of the dose administered, as determined by both the UV and the microbiological assay methods (SMITH and IHRIG (1957). Drug was still being excreted 12 days after oral dosing. Plasma half-life for pyrimethamine in the mouse, rat, dog and man was found to be 6.5, 8, 23 and 85 h, respectively (CAVALLITO et al. 1978). The long half-life in man explains the prolonged suppressive antimalarial effects noted in many studies. Plasma binding of pyrimethamine in these species was 78%, 78%, 85% and 87%; for the close analogue metoprine (Fig. 2) 58% of the drug bound to plasma protein was associated with albumin and 5.6% bound to β-lipoprotein (with a binding affinity 50-fold tighter than for albumin). The drug is concentrated somewhat in the tissues of dogs (LORZ et al. 1951), rat (SCHMIDT et al. 1953; CAVALLITO et al. 1978) and monkeys (SCHMIDT et al. 1953), with high levels particularly found in lung, liver, spleen, kidney and brain. In the rat, drug concentrations in the cerebrospinal fluid, brain, lung and pancreas decreased at the same rate as did blood levels. Thus, in the larger animals, the picture of pyrimethamine pharmacokinetics is one of complete absorption, extensive plasma protein binding and moderate tissue concentration, and slow urinary excretion, with a significant amount of drug excreted for at least 11 days in man.

Only a small fraction of pyrimethamine remains as unmetabolised drug after dosing of animals and man. Most of the early reports noted the lack of total recovery of drug administered, or the presence of unidentified metabolites. Recently, a comprehensive study on the metabolism of 2-[^{14}C]-pyrimethamine (and two close analogues) in rats was reported by HUBBELL et al. (1978). At least 16 metabolites were revealed by two-dimensional TLC of rat urine. There were six glucuronide conjugates, accounting for $\cong$20% of the dose. Both *N*-1 and *N*-3 oxides were found, as well as the α-hydroxyethyl compound. The major metabolite (34% of the dose by 72 h) was the *N*-3 oxide hydroxylated on the α-position of the ethyl group (Fig. 2 III). Only a small amount of parent compound was found in the urine. The authors also reported *N*-oxides as metabolites of metoprine and trimethoprim, suggesting that *N*-oxidation of the pyrimidine ring is a major metabolic pathway for the 5-aryl-2,4-diaminopyrimidines. Interestingly, rats dosed with the *N*-1-oxide of trimethoprim reduced it to parent compound, yielding a similar pattern of excreted metabolites to trimethoprim per se. It is possible that this type of metabolic recycling may also occur with pyrimethamine.

HUBBELL et al. (1980) found sex differences in the disposition of metoprine in mice; females metabolised and eliminated the drug more rapidly than did males, resulting in higher plasma levels and a lower LD_{50} in the males. This report should alert investigators to be aware of possible sex differences in studies of similar compounds.

III. Toxicity

It was recognised in the early animal studies on pyrimethamine that two different types of toxicity were manifested by the drug; acute convulsions and delayed folate-deficiency type symptoms. The central nervous system (CNS) toxicity is usually observed at high lethal doses and is not effected by administration of folates, whereas the delayed effects, which occur at lower doses (or upon multiple dosing), can be prevented by folates. This dual mode of toxicity was reported for mice (FALCO et al. 1951), rats (SCHMIDT et al. 1953), dogs (HAMILTON et al. 1954), and rhesus monkeys (SCHMIDT et al. 1953). It also occurs in man; accidental ingestion of very high doses (>25 mg/kg) by children leading to convulsions and deaths in some cases, whereas toxicity at doses closer to therapeutic levels is usually of the folate deficiency type (HITCHINGS 1960).

COHN (1965) and DUCH et al. (1979) have identified a specific action of pyrimethamine (and close analogues) on the metabolism of the CNS. Pyrimethamine is a competitive inhibitor ($K_i = 0.5 \mu M$) of histamine *N*-methyl transferase, the enzyme primarily responsible for the metabolism of histamine in the mammalian CNS. In a detailed follow-up study of metoprine, DUCH et al. (1979) found that the drug caused prolonged elevated levels of histamine in the brains (and several other tissues) of dosed rats. A number of other compounds of interest in malaria chemotherapy also were found to be good inhibitors of histamine *N*-methyl transferase, including chloroquine, quinazolines and a dihydrotriazine.

The standard adult prophylactic dose of 25 mg pyrimethamine weekly is well tolerated (MYATT et al. 1953; DERN et al. 1955). However, this dose on a daily basis for 6 weeks caused mild to moderate megaloblastic anaemia in 6 of 12 volunteers, who returned to normal after the drug was discontinued. Other examples can be found in the literature of folate deficiency type of symptoms after daily dosing of pyrimethamine, which is not surprising in view of the long half-life (85 h) of this in man. Prolonged daily dosing is obviously not advisable. Precautions must also be taken against the concurrent administration of pyrimethamine and another dihydrofolate reductase inhibitor, such as trimethoprim or methotrexate, since the toxicity potential is the same as increasing the dosage of either alone.

Folic acid and folinic acid (leucovorin) have been used to prevent and reverse toxic folate-deficiency type symptoms of pyrimethamine. However, leucovorin is the preferred agent, since it bypasses the dihydrofolate reductase block of pyrimethamine. It can be used to prevent or reverse toxicity without compromising the antimalarial efficiency of pyrimethamine (HURLY 1959; TONG et al. 1970; CANFIELD et al. 1971). CASTLES et al. (1971) showed that simultaneous dosing with leucovorin, but not folic acid, protected beagles from the chronic toxicity of pyrimethamine. It is recommended by the manufacturer that leucovorin be administered with the large doses of pyrimethamine which are used for the treatment of toxoplasmosis in pregnant women.

High doses of pyrimethamine are teratogenic in the rat (THIERSCH 1954) and less so in hamsters (SULLIVAN and TAKACS 1971), causing resorptions and malformations. Simultaneous administrations of leucovorin, but not folic acid, prevented these effects. MORSE et al. (1976) showed that 48 mg/kg pyrimethamine p.o. on days 10, 11 and 12 of pregnancy in rats caused 85%–88% resorption or abnormalities among the pups and depressed the fetal and placental dihydrofolate reductase levels measured on day 21. Concurrent administration of 122 mg/kg leucovorin totally prevented the resorptions and abnormalities and restored the enzyme levels. It had been previously shown that folic acid did not prevent the teratogenicity of pyrimethamine in rats (ANDERSON and MORSE 1966).

MORLEY et al. (1964) used 50 mg pyrimethamine monthly to suppress malaria in pregnant women in Nigeria. The infants born had higher birth weights than an untreated control group, with no difference in the rates of stillbirths or neonatal deaths.

IV. Mode of Action

In the 1940s HITCHINGS and co-workers realised a possible structural analogy between certain 5-substituted-2,4-diaminopyrimidines which were considered folic acid antagonists on the basis of their inhibition of growth of *Lactobacillus casei* and proguanil drawn in such a way as to resemble a six-membered ring (FALCO et al. 1951). This suggestion led to the testing of many compounds of this type as antimalarials, with the eventual synthesis and choice of pyrimethamine as the most active of the series against *P. berghei* and *P. gallinaceum* (FALCO et al. 1951). Thus, in the case of pyrimethamine, the general locus of action (folate metabolism) was known before the target organism (plasmodia) was identified. Early studies in bacteria (WOOD and HITCHINGS 1959) and mammals (HITCHINGS et al. 1952) narrowed the site of action to a step in the conversion of folic to folinic acid. Finally, this site was shown to be the plasmodial dihydrofolate reductase, an enzyme with a high affinity for pyrimethamine (FERONE et al. 1969). Plasmodia, like many parasitic microorganisms, synthesise their folate cofactors de novo and cannot utilise intact exogenous folates (FERONE 1977). The folate cofactors present in the host tissues are not available for end product reversal of the inhibitory block of the drug. The effects of folic acid and leucovorin on the reversal of inhibition of plasmodial growth by dihydrofolate reductase inhibitors are most likely due to their breakdown and the subsequent utilisation of the *p*-aminobenzoate and/or pteridine moieties (ROLLO 1955).

The selective nature of the inhibition of the malarial dihydrofolate reductase compared with the host enzyme is of primary importance in determining the antimalarial effectiveness of a dihydrofolate reductase inhibitor. The affinity of the *P. berghei* enzyme for pyrimethamine is 2000-fold greater than the affinity of the mouse erythrocyte enzyme for the drug (FERONE et al. 1969). The ratio of binding affinities of host and of parasite enzyme to a compound can be useful as a fundamental determinant of potential potency and toxicity of an antiparasitic compound. Pharmacokinetic parameters determine the actual concentrations of drug at the target sites in host and parasite and thus determine the effective in vivo ratio of enzyme inhibition in the two organisms.

Inhibition of dihydrofolate reductase results in decreased pool sizes of tetrahydrofolate cofactors. In most cells, these cofactors are utilised in the de novo synthesis of purines, methionine, thymidylate and glycine/serine (HITCHINGS and BURCHALL 1965). However, plasmodia do not contain two of the folate cofactor interconverting enzymes which would be required for purine biosynthesis (PLATZER 1972). This is consistent with the observations that plasmodia do not synthesise purines de novo (SHERMAN 1979). Also, no unequivocal evidence exists for the synthesis of N^5-methyltetrahydrofolate and its utilisation for methionine synthesis by plasmodia (for discussion, see FERONE 1977; HITCHINGS 1978). However, the enzymes necessary for the synthesis of thymidylate and for the serine/glycine interconversion have been demonstrated in plasmodia. Both *P. lophurae* (PLATZER 1972) and *P. berghei* (FERONE 1980, unpublished data) contain serine hydroxymethyltransferase (serine + tetrahydrofolate $\leftrightarrow$ glycine + N^5, N^{10}-methylenetetrahydrofolate). This folate cofactor is utilised for the synthesis of thymidylate (N^5, N^{10}-methylenetetrahydrofolate + deoxyuridylate $\rightarrow$ dihydrofolate + thymidylate), catalysed by thymidylate synthase, an enzyme found in *P. lophurae* (WALSH and SHERMAN 1968), *P. chabaudi* (WALTER et al. 1970) and *P. berghei* (REID and FRIEDKIN 1973). The folate product in this reaction is dihydrofolate, which must then be reduced by dihydrofolate reductase to re-enter the tetrahydrofolate cofactor pool. It was recently reported that dihydrofolate reductase and thymidylate synthase activities from *Crithidia fasciculata* exist on a bifunctional protein. Evidence was presented which also indicates an association of these enzymes in *P. berghei* (and possibly many other protozoa) (FERONE and ROLAND 1980).

The presence of the enzymes of the thymidylate synthase cycle in plasmodia, the high affinity of the parasite dihydrofolate reductase to pyrimethamine, and the lack of utilisation of preformed pyrimidines by plasmodia (SHERMAN 1979), taken together, should result in inhibition of DNA synthesis of malaria by this drug. Although inhibition of plasmodial DNA synthesis by low concentrations of pyrimethamine has been demonstrated in long incubation-time experiments (SCHEL-

LENBERG and COATNEY 1961; MCCORMICK et al. 1971), GUTTERIDGE and TRIGG (1971) found that DNA synthesis by *P. knowlesi* was apparently inhibited by pyrimethamine only after morphological abnormalities and growth inhibition were observed. Since DNA synthesis in malaria occurs mainly during the ring and trophozoite stages, whereas pyrimethamine (and other antifolate antimalarials) cause the accumulation of abnormal schizonts, these authors suggested that inhibition of dihydrofolate reductase in malaria results in the depletion of a folate cofactor required for some function other than the synthesis of thymidylate.

V. Deployment

Pyrimethamine as an antimalarial is a potent, long-lasting, blood schizontocidal and sporontocidal agent, with pronounced activity against primary exoerythrocytic forms of plasmodia. Since it is a causal prophylatic to *P. falciparum*, it is used mainly to prevent and suppress malarial infections. Since the mid 1960s, it has also been used in combination with sulphonamides and other drugs for the treatment of chloroquine-resistant *P. falciparum* (BRUCE-CHWATT 1977).

The first report on pyrimethamine revealed it to have high activity against blood forms of *P. gallinaceum* in the chick, *P. berghei* in mice and *P. cynomolgi* in rhesus monkeys, but to be less effective against exoerythrocytic forms (FALCO et al. 1951). The *P. cynomolgi* results were confirmed and amplified by SCHMIDT and GENTHER (1953), who also noted that resistance to the drug could be rapidly developed. PETERS (1970) has summarised the studies of many laboratories on pyrimethamine against different malaria infections. Some typical values for multiple dosing of pyrimethamine for inhibition of blood-induced infections are: 0.005–0.03 mg/kg for *P. gallinaceum*; 0.05 mg/kg for *P. cynomolgi bastianellii* and *P. knowlesi*; and 0.1–0.4 mg/kg for *P. berghei*. These values illustrate the potent blood schizontocidal effects of pyrimethamine. However, in *P. cynomolgi* for instance, relapses always occurred after treatment of sporozoite-induced infections, even at doses of drug as high as 20 mg/kg (SCHMIDT and GENTHER 1953).

The drug is highly effective on the primary exoerythrocytic forms. PETERS et al. (1975) showed pyrimethamine and several other dihydrofolate reductase inhibitors to be true causal prophylactics against *P. berghei* by a technique which distinguished between activity against primary tissue schizogony and residual activity of the drugs against emerging blood forms of the parasite. Suppressive effects against sporozoite-induced infections of *P. gallinaceum* (FALCO et al. 1951), *P. cynomolgi* (SCHMIDT and GENTHER 1953) and *P. vivax* (COATNEY 1952) have been observed. Since eight or more weekly doses of 25 mg pyrimethamine starting on the day of inoculation with *P. vivax* sporozoites resulted in many suppressive cures, COATNEY et al. (1953) concluded that the drug must have some deleterious effects on the early tissue stage of the parasite. In the case of *P. falciparum*, complete protection against sporozoite-induced infections in man was achieved by the usual recommended dose of 25 mg weekly (COVELL et al. 1953).

The causal prophylactic activity of pyrimethamine against *P. falciparum*, combined with its prolonged half-life, have led to its major use as a protective and suppressive agent against malaria at a dose of 25 mg weekly. The drug can also aid in preventing transmission of malaria, since it has a pronounced inhibitory action on the development of the malaria parasite in the mosquito. FOY and KONDI (1952) first reported that sporozoites of *P. falciparum* did not develop in mosquitos which had fed on a pyrimethamine-treated patient. Since then, others have demonstrated the inhibition by pyrimethamine of oocyst development of *P. vivax* (SHUTE and MARYON 1954; TERZIAN et al. 1968), *P. cynomolgi* (OMAR et al. 1974) and *P. gallinaceum* (TERZAKIS 1971). This sporontocidal effect of the drug could be an advantage in preventing the spread of the disease in some situations.

Most investigators could recommended against the use of pyrimethamine alone for the therapy of acute attacks of *P. falciparum*, because of the slow action of the drug. Combinations of pyrimethamine and a sulphonamide with quinine (BRUCE-CHWATT 1977) are used for the treatment of chloroquine-resistant *P. falciparum*, although the recent report on the spread of resistance to the pyrimethamine-sulfadoxine combination in eastern Thailand warns of the probable loss of this vital therapeutic regimen in that area (Morbidity and Mortality Weekly Report 1980).

VI. Resistance

The ability of plasmodia to develop resistance to pyrimethamine has been well documented in the laboratory and in the field (see reviews, WORLD HEALTH ORGANIZATION 1965; PETERS 1970), and has been a major factor in limiting the use of the drug in some areas of the world. In many instances, resistance to pyrimethamine (and to chlorguanide) has been overcome by taking advantage of the synergistic effects of pyrimethamine and sulpha drug combinations (see also this part, Chap 6,16). As noted above, resistance to the combination has already occurred, as might be expected where resistance to the individual components was first established. Since most reviewers have pointed to the development of resistance as the major drawback of the drug, and it has been demonstrated that resistance is slower to develop for sulpha-dihydrofolate reductase inhibitor combinations, then it follows that such combinations should be used preferentially to pyrimethamine, particularly in areas with drug-sensitive strains of malaria.

Several pyrimethamine resistant strains of rodent malaria have been shown to contain higher levels of dihydrofolate reductase than do sensitive strains (FERONE 1977). Some of the kinetic properties of the resistant enzymes differed also, including decreased affinity for pyrimethamine. KAN and SIDDIQUI (1979) purified dihydrofolate reductase from the Uganda-Palo Alto and the Vietnam-Oak Knoll strains of *P. falciparum*. The enzyme level in the pyrimethamine-resistant Uganda-Palo Alto strain was 30- to 80-fold higher than in the drug-sensitive Vietnam-Oak Knoll strain. Increased enzyme is a mode of resistance frequently encountered for dihydrofolate reductase inhibitors of bacteria and mammalian cells (BLAKELY 1969).

References

Anderson I, Morse LM (1966) The influence of solvent on the teratogenic effect of folic acid antagonist in the rat. Exp Mol Pathol 5:134–145

Armstrong VL (1973) Metabolism of chlorguanide, a unique mixed function oxidase substrate. Diss Abstr 33:382 B

Armstrong VL, Smith CC (1974) Cyclization and *N*-dealkylation of chlorguanide by rabbit and rat hepatic microsomes. Toxicol appl Pharmacol 29:90

Black RH (1973) Malaria in the Australian army in South Vietnam. Successful use of a proguanil-dapsone combination for chemoprophylaxis of chloroquine-resistant falciparum malaria. Med J Aust 1:1265–1270

Blakley RL (1969) The biochemistry of folic acid and related pteridines. North Holland, Amsterdam

Bruce-Chwatt LJ (1977) Prevention and treatment of malaria. Trop Doct 7:17–20

Canfield CJ, Keller HI, Cirksena WJ (1971) Erythrokinetics during treatment of acute falciparum malaria. Milit Med 136:354–357

Carrington HC, Crowther AF, Davey DG, Levi AA, Rose FL (1951) A metabolite of Paludrine with high antimalarial activity. Nature 168:1080

Castles TR, Kintner LD, Lee C-C (1971) The effects of folic or folinic acid on the toxicity of pyrimenthamine in dogs. Toxicol Appl Pharmacol 20:447–459

Cavallito JC, Nichol CA, Brenckman WD Jr, DeAngelis RL, Stickney DR, Simmons WS, Sigel CW (1978) Lipid soluble inhibitors of dihydrofolate reductase. 1. Kinetics, tissue distribution, and extent of metabolism of pyrimethamine, metoprine, and etoprine in the rat, dog, and man. Drug Metab Dispos 6:329–337

Chaudhuri RN, Chakravarty NK, Chaudhuri MNR (1952) Chemotherapy and chemoprophylaxis of malaria. Br Med J 1:568–574

Chebotar NA (1974) Embryotoxic and teratogenic action of proguanil, chlorproguanil and cycloguanil in rats. Byull Eksp Biol Med 77:56–57

Coatney GR (1952) Studies on the compound 50–63. Trans R Soc Trop Med Hyg 46:496–497

Coatney GR, Myatt AV, Hernandez T, Jeffrey GM , Cooper WC (1953) Studies on human malaria XXXII. The protective and therapeutic effects of pyrimethamine (Daraprim®) against Chesson strain vivax malaria. Am J Trop Med Hyg 2:777–787

Cohn VH (1965) Inhibition of histamine methylation by antimalarial drugs. Biochem Pharmacol 14:1686–1688

Contacos PG (1969) The treatment of malaria infection. Bull NY Acad Med 45:1077–1085

Covell G, Shute PG, Maryon M (1953) Pyrimethamine (Daraprim) as a prophylactic against a West African strain of *P. falciparum*. Br Med J 1:1081–1083

Cox GB, Sugden K (1977) Determination of pyrimethamine, ethopabate and sulfaquinoxaline in poultry feeding stuffs by high-performance liquid chromatography using a weak cation-exchange column packing. Analyst 102:29–34

Crowther AF, Levi AA (1953) Proguanil: isolation of metabolite with high antimalarial activity. Br J Pharmacol Chemother 8:93–97

Curd FHS, Davey DG, Rose FL (1945) Studies on antimalarial drugs. X. Some biguanide derivatives as new types of antimalarial substances with both therapeutic and causal prophylactic activity. Ann Trop Med Parasitol 39:208–216

Cutting W (1962) Antifertility effects of biguanides. Antibiot Chemother 12:671–675

DeAngelis RL, Simmons WS, Nichol CA (1975) Quantitative thin-layer chromatography of pyrimethamine and related diaminopyrimidines in body fluids and tissues. J Chromatogr 106:41–49

Dern RJ, Beutler E, Arnold J, Lorincz A, Block M, Alving AS (1955) Toxicity studies of pyrimethamine (Daraprim). Am J Trop Med Hyg 4:217–220

Duch DS, Dowers S, Edelstein M, Nichol CA (1979) Histamine: elevation of brain levels by inhibition of *N*-methyltransferase. In Usdin E, Burchardt RT, Creveling CR (eds) Transmethylation. Elsevier North Holland, New York, pp 287–295

Fairley NH, Blackburn CRB, Mackerras MJ, Gregory TS, Tonge JI, Black RH, Lemerle TH, Ercole QN, Pope KG, Dunn SR, Swann MSA, Abhurst TAF (1946) Researches on Paludrine (M4888) in malaria: an experimental investigation undertaken by the L.H.Q. Medical Research Unit (A.I.F.), Cairns, Australia. Trans R Soc Trop Med Hyg 40:105–162

Falco, EA, Hitchings GH, Russell PB, Vanderwerff H (1949) Antimalarials as antagonists of purines and pteroylglutamic acid. Nature 164:107–108

Falco EA, Goodwin LG, Hitchings GH, Rollo IM, Russell PB (1951) 2,4-diaminopyrimidines – a new series of antimalarials. Br J Pharmacol 6:185–200

Ferone R (1970) Dihydrofolate reductase from pyrimethamine-resistant *Plasmodium berghei.* J Biol Chem 245:850–854
Ferone R (1977) Folate metabolism in malaria. Bull WHO 55:291–298
Ferone R, Roland S (1980) Dihydrofolate reductase: thymidylate synthase, a bifunctional polypeptide from *Crithidia fasciculata.* Proc Natl Acad Sci USA 77:5802–5806
Ferone R, Burchall JJ, Hitchings GH (1969) *Plasmodium berghei* dihydrofolate reductase. Isolation, properties and inhibition by antifolates. Mol Pharmacol 5:49–59
Foy H, Kondi A (1952) Effect of Daraprim on the gametocytes of *Plasmodium falciparum* Trans R Soc Trop Med Hyg 46:370
Gage JC, Rose FL (1946) The estimation of Paludrine in urine. Ann Trop Med Parasitol 40:333–336
Greenberg J (1949a) Inhibition of the antimalarial activity of chlorguanide by pteroylglutamic acid. Proc Soc Exp Biol Med 71:306–308
Greenberg J (1949b) The potentiation of the antimalarial activity of chlorguanide by *p*-aminobenzoic acid competitors. J Pharmacol Exp Ther 97:238–242
Greenberg J (1953) Reversal of the activity of chlorguanide against *Plasmodium gallinaceum* by free or conjugated *p*-aminobenzoic acid. Expt Parasitol 2:271–279
Gutteridge WE, Trigg PI (1971) Action of pyrimethamine and related drugs against *Plasmodium knowlesi in vitro.* Parasitology 62:431–444
Hamilton L, Philips FS, Sternberg SS, Clarke DC, Hitchings GH (1954) Hematological effects of certain 2,4-diaminopyrimidines, antagonists of folic acid metabolism. Blood 9:1062–1081
Hawking F (1947) Activation of Paludrine *in vitro.* Nature 159:409
Hill J (1963) Chemotherapy of malaria. Part 2. The antimalarial drugs. In: Schnitzer RJ, Hawking F (eds) Experimental chemotherapy, vol I. Academic New York, pp 513–601
Hitchings GH (1960) Pyrimethamine. The use of an antimetabolite in the chemotherapy of malaria and other infections. Clin Pharmacol Ther 1:570–589
Hitchings GH (1978) The metabolism of plasmodia and the chemotherapy of malarial infections. In: Wood C (ed) Tropical medicine from romance to reality. Academic London, pp 79–98
Hitchings GH, Burchall JJ (1965) Inhibition of folate biosyntheses and function as a basis for chemotherapy. Adv Enzymol 27:417–468
Hitchings GH, Falco EA, Vanderwerff H, Russell PB, Elion GB (1952) Antagonists of nucleic acid derivatives. VII. 2,4-diaminopyrimidines. J Biol Chem 199:43–56
Hubbell JP, Henning ML, Grace ME, Nichol CA, Sigel CW (1978) *N*-oxide metabolites of the 2,4-diaminopyrimidine inhibitors of dihydrofolate reductase, trimethoprim, pyrimethamine and metoprine. In: Garrod JW (ed) Biological oxidation of nitrogen. Elsevier-North Holland Biomedical, New York, pp 177–182
Hubbell JP, Kao JC, Sigel CW, Nichol CA (1980) Sex-dependent disposition of metoprine in mice. In: Nelson JD, Grassi C (eds) Current chemotherapy and infectious disease, vol II. pp 1620–1621 The American Society for Microbiology Washington DC
Hurly MGD (1959) Administration of pyrimethamine with folic and folinic acids in human malaria. Trans R Soc Trop Med Hyg 53:410–411
Jones CR, King LA (1968) Detection and fluorescent measurement of pyrimethamine in urine. Biochem Med 2:251–259
Jones CR, Ovenell SM (1979) Determination of plasma concentrations of dapsone, monoacetyl dapsone and pyrimethamine in human subjects dosed with Maloprim J Chromatogr 163:179–185
Kan SC, Siddiqui WA (1979) Comparative studies on dihydrofolate reductases from *Plasmodium falciparum* and *Aotus trivirgatus.* J Protozool 26:660–664
Levin EM, Meyer RB JR, Levin VA (1978) Quantitative high-pressure liquid chromatographic procedure for the determination of plasma and tissue levels of 2,4-diamino-5-(3,4-dichlorophenyl)-6-methyl-pyrimidine (metoprine) and its application to the measurement of brain capillary permeability coefficients. J Chromatogr 156:181–187
Lorz DC, Lee GP, Hitchings GH (1951) Distribution of 2,4-diamino-pyrimidine in the tissues of the dog. Fed Proc 10:320

Maegraith BG, Tottey M, Adams ARD, Andrews WHH, King JD (1946) The absorption and excretion of Paludrine in the human subject. Ann Trop Med Parasitol 40:493–506

McCormick GJ, Canfield CJ, Willet GP (1971) *Plasmodium knowlesi: In vitro* evaluation of antimalarial activity of folic acid inhibitors. Exp Parasitol 30:88–93

Morbidity and Mortality Weekly Report (1980) *Plasmodium falciparum* malaria contracted in Thailand resistant to chloroquine and sulfonamide-pyrimethamine. Morbid Mortal Weekly Rep 29:493–495

Morley D, Woodland M, Cuthbertson WFJ (1964) Controlled trial of pyrimethamine in pregnant women in an African village. Br Med J 1:667–668

Morse LM, Pinckaers M, Houg JG (1976) The effect of 5-formyltetrahydrofolic acid on pyrimethamine-induced congenital abnormalities in the rat. Nutr Rep Int 13:93–99

Myatt AV, Hernandez T, Coatney GR (1953) Studies on human malaria XXXIII. The toxicity of pyrimethamine (Daraprim) in man. Am J Trop Med Hyg 2:788–794

Omar MS, Collins WE, Contacous PG (1974) Gametocytocidal and sporontocidal effects of antimalarial drugs on malaria parasites. II. Action of the folic reductase inhibitors, chlorguanide, and pyrimethamine against *Plasmodium cynomolgi*. Exp Parasitol 36:167–177

Peters W (1970) Chemotherapy and drug resistance in malaria. Academic London

Peters W, Davies EE, Robinson BL (1975) The chemotherapy of malaria, XXIII Causal prophylaxis, part II: practical experience with *Plasmodium yoelii nigeriensis* in drug screening. Ann Trop Med Parasitol 69:311–328

Platzer EG (1972) Metabolism of tetrahydrofolate in *Plasmodium lophurae* and duckling erythrocytes. Trans NY Acad Sci 34:200–208

Reid VE, Friedkin M (1973) Thymidylate synthetase in mouse erythrocytes infected with *Plasmodium berghei*. Mol Pharmacol 9:74–80

Ritshel WA, Hammer GV, Thompson GA (1978) Pharmacokinetics of antimalarials and proposals for dosage regimens. Int J Clin Pharmacol Biopharm 16:395–401

Rollo IM (1955) The mode of action of sulfonamides, proguanil and pyrimethamine on *Plasmodium gallinaceum*. Br J Pharmacol 10:208–214

Rollo IM (1965) Drugs used in the chemotherapy of malaria. In: Goodman LS, Gilman A (eds) The pharmacological basis of therapeutics, 3rd edn. Macmillan, New York pp 1087–1127

Schellenberg KA, Coatney GR (1961) The influence of antimalarial drugs on nucleic acid synthesis of *Plasmodium gallinaceum* and *Plasmodium berghei*. Biochem Pharmacol 6:143–152

Schmidt LH, Genther CS (1953) The antimalarial properties of 2,4-diamino-5-*p*-chlorophenyl-6-ethylpyrimidine (Daraprim). J Pharmacol Exp Ther 107:61–91

Schmidt LH, Hughes HB, Smith CC (1947) On the pharmacology of *N*-para-chloro-phenyl-*N*-isopropylbiguanide (Paludrine). J Pharmacol Exp Ther 90:233–253

Schmidt LH, Hughes HB, Schmidt IG (1953) The pharmacological properties of 2,4-diamino-5-*p*-chlorophenyl-6-ethylpyrimidine (Daraprim). J Pharmacol Exp Ther 107:92–130

Sherman IW (1979) Biochemistry of *Plasmodium* (malarial parasites). Microbiol Rev 43:453–495

Shute PG, Maryon M (1954) The effect of pyrimethamine (Daraprim) on the gametocytes and oocysts of *Plasmodium falciparum* and *Plasmodium vivax*. Trans R Soc Trop Med Hyg 48:50–63

Simmons WS, DeAngelis RL (1973) Quantitation of pyrimethamine and related diaminopyrimidines *in situ* by enhancement of fluorescence after thin-layer chromatography. Anal Chem 45:1538–1540

Smith CC, Ihrig J (1957) The pharmacological basis for the prolonged antimalarial activity of pyrimethamine. Am J Trop Med Hyg 6:50–57

Smith CC, Schmidt LH (1963) Observations on the absorption of pyrimethamine from the gastrointestinal tract. Exp Parasitol 13:178–185

Smith CC, Ihrig J, Menne R (1961) Antimalarial activity and metabolism of biguanides. I. Metabolism of chlorguanide and chlorguanide triazine in rhesus monkeys and man. Am J Trop Med 10:694–703

Spinks A, Tottey M (1945) Studies of synthetic antimalarial drugs. XII. Determination of N^1-*p*-chlorophenyl-N^5-methyl-N^5-isopropylbiguanide (4430) and N^1*p*-chlorophenyl-N^5-isopropylbiguanide (Paludrine): a preliminary report. Ann Trop Med Parasitol 39:220–224
Sullivan GE, Takacs E (1971) Comparative teratogenicity of pyrimethamine in rats and hamsters. Teratology 4:205–210
Terzakis JA (1971) *Plasmodium gallinaceum*: Drug-induced ultrastructural changes in oocysts. Exp Parasitol 30:260–266
Terzian LA, Stahler N, Dawkins AT Jr (1968) The sporogonous cycle of *Plasmodium vivax* in anopheles mosquitoes as a system for evaluating the prophylactic and curative capabilities of potential antimalarial compounds. Exp Parasitol 23:56–66
Thiersch JB (1954) Effect of certain 2,4-diamino-pyrimidine antagonists of folic acid on pregnancy and rat fetus. Proc Soc Exp Biol Med 85:571–577
Thurston JP (1950) Action of Proguanil on *P. berghei*. Inhibition by *p*-aminobenzoic acid. Lancet 259–438
Tong MJ, Strickland GT, Votteri BA, Gunning J-J (1970) Supplemental folates in the therapy of *Plasmodium falciparum* malaria. JAMA 214:2330–2333
Tonkin IM (1946) The testing of drugs against erythrocytic forms of *P. gallinaceum in vitro*. Br J Pharmacol 1:163–173
Tottey M, Maegraith BG (1948) Field method of estimating Paludrine in urine. Trans R Soc Trop Med Hyg 41:438–439
Walsh CJ, Sherman IW (1968) Purine and pyrimidine synthesis by the avian malaria parasite, *Plasmodium lophurae*. J Protozool 15:763–770
Walter RD, Mühlpfordt H, Königk F (1970) Vergleichende Untersuchungen der Deoxythymidylatsynthase bei *Plasmodium chabaudi, Trypanosoma gambiense* und *Trypanosoma lewisi*. Z. Tropenmed Parasitol 21:347–357
Wood RC, Hitchings GH (1959) Effect of pyrimethamine on folic acid metabolism in *Streptococcus faecalis* and *Escherichia coli*. J Biol Chem 234:2377–2380
World Health Organization (1965) Resistance of malaria parasites to drugs. WHO Tech. Rep Ser 296

Novel Methods of Drug Development

CHAPTER 6

Drug Combinations

W. PETERS

A. Introduction

In this chapter discussion is limited to the different types of antimalarial drug combinations that have been described in experimental situations or for clinical use. The possible value of drug combinations in the prevention of drug resistance will be covered in Chap. 16. Combinations of drugs may be considered under several headings, namely those that are complementary (e.g. against different stages of a parasite), combinations that are additive but acting against the same stages and those that are synergistic. All have their place in the control of malaria. While this chapter is written within the context of "Novel Methods of Drug Development", some of the older drug combinations will be referred to for the sake of completion and as a guide to future developments.

B. Complementary Combinations

I. Drugs Affecting Different Stages of the Life Cycle

The classical example of a complementary combination is the sequential use of chloroquine followed by primaquine for the radical cure of infection due to *Plasmodium vivax*. In this case chloroquine cures the acute attack by its blood schizontocidal action but is devoid of activity against the exoerythrocytic stages. Primaquine, which has only modest action if any against the asexual erythrocytic stages, is a potent tissue schizontocide and completes a radical cure by destroying the tissue forms (probably hypnozoites) that are responsible for relapses of this infection and of *P. ovale*.

Primaquine also has a marked gametocytocidal action on all species of *Plasmodium*, and this action fortunately is retained against the gametocytes of chloroquine-resistant *P. falciparum* (RIECKMANN et al. 1968). A single dose of 45 mg primaquine base effectively sterilises the gametocytes for several days following treatment with, for example, a sulphonamide-pyrimethamine combination which, by itself, may be followed by a wave of gametocytaemia, and primaquine is therefore of considerable potential value for reducing the transmission of such strains. Moreover, chloroquine itself, which has no action on mature gametocytes of *P. falciparum*, may promote the growth of the sporogonic stages of mosquitoes that have fed on chloroquine-treated people infected with resistant strains (WILKINSON et al. 1976).

II. Drugs Affecting the Same Stages of the Life Cycle

As distinct from drugs that have an additive action on, for example, asexual erythrocytic stages, attention has been drawn in recent years to a different type of complementary effect, namely the sequential use of one drug with a rapid blood schizontocidal effect, quinine, to overcome the acute attack, followed by a second but slowly acting compound, a tetracycline or clindamycin, to destroy lingering blood stages. In areas where chloroquine-resistant *P. falciparum* is prevalent, such as Vietnam, up to 90% of patients treated with standard doses of quinine alone may have recrudescences of their infections (HUNSICKER et al. 1967). Yet quinine, even in these patients, normally provides rapid relief of symptoms and reduction of the parasitaemia. The addition of a tetracycline to the regimen (CLYDE 1974) is usually followed by radical cure. However, because of the need to avoid the use of antibiotics other than in infections with bacteria that are sensitive to them (unfortunately a Utopian ideal rarely realised), most authorities prefer to recommend that initial therapy with quinine should be followed by an appropriate sulphonamide-pyrimethamine combination such as sulphadoxine-pyrimethamine (Fansidar).

A number of clinical investigators who have studied the action of mefloquine in patients infected with chloroquine-resistant *P. falciparum* have suggested that, here too, quinine and mefloquine should be used sequentially since the response to mefloquine may be rather slower than that to quinine (HALL 1977). It should in this case be noted, however, that both compounds have precisely the same mode of action, mefloquine being both more potent and much longer acting than quinine (PETERS et al. 1977).

An interesting sidelight on the use of complementary combinations should be recalled. Following observations by ARNOLD et al. (1954) that weekly administration of 45 mg primaquine for eight consecutive weeks was as effective in producing a radical cure of vivax malaria as the usual 14-day course and less hazardous to G6PD-deficient individuals, VIVONA et al. (1961) demonstrated that eight single weekly doses of 300 mg chloroquine base with 45 mg primaquine base during the repatriation process was very effective in bringing about the radical cure of latent infections of *P. vivax* acquired in Korea. This was apparently the rationale for the famous CP tablet that came to form the foundation of antimalarial chemoprophylaxis for US military personnel in the Vietnam war. Unfortunately it was not appreciated (a) that much of the malaria in Vietnam was *P. falciparum* and (b) that the local strains of *P. falciparum* were going to prove highly resistant to chloroquine. Persistence in the deployment of the CP tablet, even allowing for failure in many cases to take the drugs, resulted by 1966 in a malaria attack rate in US troops of 1% of the command per combat day (TIGERTT 1966).

C. Additive Combinations

In this context we consider additive combinations to be combinations of drugs that have dissimilar modes of action but that affect the same stages of the parasite life cycle. One of the first such combinations to be used on a large scale was chloroquine with pyrimethamine. Two rationales were given for using this pair: (a) that

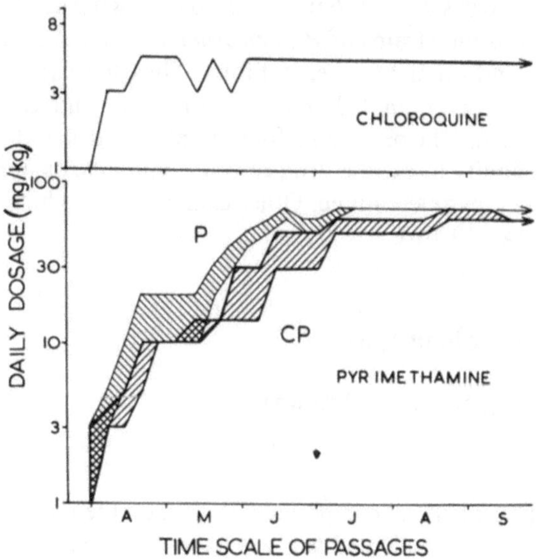

Fig. 1. The failure of a mixture of chloroquine and pyrimethamine to delay the development of resistance to either drug when administered by the serial technique to mice infected with *P. berghei* NK65. The *top line* shows the daily doses of chloroquine used in the CP line (exposed to both drugs) and the *shaded area CP* in the *lower part of the figure* shows the doses of pyrimethamine used in this line. Pyrimethamine doses could be increased as rapidly as in the *P line* exposed only to pyrimethamine (PETERS et al. 1973)

the chloroquine would protect by virtue of its potent blood schizontocidal action and that pyrimethamine would be valuable for its sporontocidal effect which would help to reduce transmission of the parasites in an endemic area; (b) that the use of two drugs with supposedly different modes of action on the blood stages would minimise the risk of resistance developing to one or both compounds.

Chloroquine-pyrimethamine mixtures in various doses were used on a large scale in malaria eradication and control programmes. With the blessing of WHO, this combination and another consisting of amodiaquine with primaquine (a complementary mixture in the sense just described) were dispensed far and wide in Africa, Asia and the New World. What was not appreciated, unfortunately, was that there was no experimental back-up to support the contentions on which these combinations were used. A retrospective study in rodent malaria indicated clearly that the combination of chloroquine with pyrimethamine did *not* prevent the development of resistance by *P. berghei* to both drugs, and, indeed, the process was barely even slowed down (RABINOVITCH 1965; PETERS et al. 1973), as shown in Fig. 1.

Moreover, it became clear from these and other experiments that, once parasites had become resistant to chloroquine and to pyrimethamine, they probably shared metabolic adaptations that enabled them to overcome nutritional deficiencies imposed on them in the presence of drug. This may indeed help to explain two interesting observations. Firstly, only by starting from parent lines already rendered resistant to pyrimethamine was it possible to develop chloroquine-resistant lines of *P. vinckei* (POWERS et al. 1969) or *P. chabaudi* (ROSARIO 1976). Secondly, most chloroquine-resistant strains of *P. falciparum* are, in addition, resistant also to pyrimethamine (and often to other antifols). Thus the use of additive combinations should not be promoted until experimental studies have produced enough evidence to justify the belief that, for example, the drugs at least do not enhance each other's ability to expose drug-resistant mutants, as appears to be the case with chloroquine-pyrimethamine. Other examples of additive combinations are discussed in PETERS (1970a).

D. Potentiating Combinations

I. Compounds Acting on Folate Pathways

1. Basic Principles

It has long been appreciated that compounds which exert their actions at sequential points on a particular metabolic pathway are likely to potentiate each other's actions. Yet almost the only examples of this promising approach to antimicrobial chemotherapy are those in which two stages of the pathway leading to tetrahydrofolate (FH_4) are blocked. Sulphonamides and sulphones block the condensation of *p*-aminobenzoic acid (PABA) with pteridine in the formation of dihydropteroate which is subsequently condensed with glutamate to form dihydrofolate (FH_2). The step from FH_2 to FH_4 is catalysed by the enzyme dihydrofolate reductase (DHF)[1], which, in turn, is blocked by a number of compounds including some of the most potent antimalarials, e.g. proguanil and its active triazine metabolite, cycloguanil, related triazines such as clociguanil and WR 99210, pyrimethamine and the quinazoline WR 158122. FH_4 is involved in the intermediate metabolism of purines and pyrimidines, e.g. pathways leading to thymidylate synthesis and orotic-acid incorporation into DNA, as well as in the utilisation of purines (SHERMAN 1979).

As long ago as 1948 GREENBERG et al. recognised that the antimalarial effect of sulphadiazine against *P. gallinaceum* was potentiated by proguanil. ROLLO (1955) showed that pyrimethamine, too, acted synergistically with sulphadiazine against this parasite. Since then potentiation with DHF inhibitors and sulphonamides or sulphones has been the accepted rule. Other points of attack have also been identified but never adequately exploited in the folate pathway. Thus, for example, AVIADO et al. (1968) found that two pteridine compounds, triamterene and WR 3090, acted synergistically with dapsone against *P. berghei*. KISLIUK et al. (1967) found that tetrahydrohomopteroic acid appeared to block the development of either drug-sensitive or pyrimethamine-resistant *P. cynomolgi*, possibly by inhibiting the activity of dihydropteroate synthase (FERONE 1977). The toxicity was, unfortunately, not sufficiently selective for this compound to be developed further, and no studies were reported on possible potentiation of this compound with pyrimethamine itself or sulphonamides.

Following the same reasoning, KINNAMON et al. (1976) described the potentiating activity of two quinazolines, WR 158122 and its tetrahydro analogue WR

1 This should now be referred to as tetrahydrofolate dehydrogenase

180872, against *P. berghei* in mice. Marked potentiation of the two compounds was observed in that model, but only a modest degree against *P. cynomolgi* in rhesus monkeys (KINNAMON and DAVIDSON 1980). The authors reasoned that, while WR 158122 acts as a DHF inhibitor, WR 180872 may block the next step beyond FH_4.

O'SULLIVAN and KETLEY (1980) indicated that enzymes involved in dihydro-orotate metabolism are susceptible to block by appropriate antimetabolic drugs. Several investigators have shown that enzymes involved in the synthesis of uridine monophosphate from dihydro-orotate are present in malaria parasites. The level of these enzymes in *P. berghei* is 100 times greater than that in mouse liver. 5-Azaorotate inhibits this pathway. GERO and O'SULLIVAN (1979) have identified in *P. berghei* dihydro-orotate dehydrogenase, the activity of which is associated with ubiquinone and mitochondrial respiration.

The key to success with drugs that block essential steps in the folate or any other metabolic pathway is (a) that certain steps should be essential for the target organisms but not for the hosts or (b) that the enzyme used by the host has a lower affinity for the drug than the enzyme of the parasite. Here, for example, lies the explanation for the highly selective antiplasmodial toxicity of pyrimethamine, the affinity of which for *P. berghei* DHF is some 10^4 greater than it is for DHF of the mouse. Here, too, lies the reason for the value of sulphonamides, since mammalian tissues can utilise preformed FH_2 while plasmodia have to form their own. At this point consideration should be given to *P. cynomolgi* and *P. vivax* against which, in contrast, for example, to *P. knowlesi, P. berghei,* and *P. falciparum,* sulphonamides are of little value. While it seems probable that *P. cynomolgi* and *P. vivax* can utilise preformed FH_2 at least to some degree, no data appear to have been published on this point which is of considerable practical value. The marked potentiating action of sulphadoxine-pyrimethamine against *P. falciparum,* for example, is in most cases sufficient to control the infection even of parasites which are resistant to pyrimethamine used on its own, as indeed do similar combinations used in pyrimethamine-resistant *P. berghei* infections. Nevertheless, in areas such as Thailand where both *P. vivax* and *P. falciparum* are present, many *P. vivax* infections break through regular prophylactic administration of sulphadoxine-pyrimethamine (PEARLMAN et al. 1977). It is very likely that these parasites are resistant to pyrimethamine alone, to which they were exposed for a number of years in the past, and that the sulphonamide component of the mixture is incapable of controlling the growth of *P. vivax,* which is basically insusceptible to PABA antagonists, an observation made long ago by FAIRLEY (1945) and COATNEY et al. (1947). In *Aotus* monkeys SCHMIDT et al. (1977) found that a sulphadiazine-pyrimethamine mixture failed to cure a few infections with strains of *P. falciparum* that were highly resistant to pyrimethamine. In a meticulous quantitative study they commented on the remarkably high levels of potentiation between these drugs in human and simian malaria, but also cautioned against expecting such combinations to be 100% successful in treating patients with multiple drug-resistant falciparum malaria.

2. Some Novel Inhibitors Possibly Acting on Folate Synthesis and Folate-Linked Synthetic Processes

a) Cycloguanil Potentiation with Menoctone

There is ample evidence to show that cycloguanil and related triazines, e.g. clociguanil, are DHF inhibitors. FERONE et al. (1969), for example, showed that these compounds bind more tightly to plasmodial DHF than to that of host tissue. In *P. berghei* PETERS (1970b) demonstrated a strong synergistic action between cycloguanil and the naphthoquinone menoctone, which is now believed to act as an analogue of ubiquinone. This phenomenon was difficult to explain but was sufficiently marked to suggest that the two compounds were acting at two different points on a single biosynthetic pathway. Since cycloguanil inhibits DHF it seemed possible that menoctone was blocking some step beyond FH_4. Recently JAFFE (1980) in certain filarial infections has found that these organisms are susceptible to a deficiency of folate and that the inhibitory effect of this deficiency is potentiated by menoctone, which, he suggests, acts as a competitive inhibitor of ubiquinone 7; this, in turn, is a cofactor in the oxidation of methyl FH_4. It has now been shown that menoctone is also a potent inhibitor of the dihydro-orotate dehydrogenase of *P. berghei*, with a K_i value of 1.8×10^{-8} *M* (GERO and O'SULLIVAN 1979). Thus the potentiating action of cycloguanil and menoctone may well be due, ultimately, to a block of uridine monophosphate synthesis from dihydro-orotate, a hypothesis that has not, however, yet been tested. If this is the case potentiation should also be observed between cycloguanil and 5-azaorotate and other synthetic pyrimidine analogues which are also potent inhibitors of dihydro-orotate dehydrogenase.

Such a combination appears particularly promising since, in contrast to malaria parasites, mammalian tissues can utilise preformed folates and preformed pyrimidines such as uridine. Thymidine analogues should also be of interest in this context since the parasites may also synthesize this pyrimidine with the aid of thymidylate synthase from uridine monophosphate (GUTTERIDGE and COOMBS 1977).

Since the sporogonic stages of *Plasmodium* depend more on mitochondrial enzymes (for aerobic glycolysis) than the erythrocytic asexual stages (HOWELLS et al. 1972) and are sensitive to DHF inhibitors, it would be anticipated that cycloguanil-menoctone should possess an exceptionally powerful gametocytocidal or sporontocidal effect, and this possibility should be investigated.

b) Sulphadiazine and Chlorcycloguanil with a Quinolone

RYLEY and PETERS (1970) reported that a quinolone ester (ICI 56780) (Fig. 2, II) which was a potent blood schizontocide against *P. berghei* displayed a marked and unanticipated synergism with sulphonamides. The mode of action of similar quinolones has been investigated in relation to coccidiosis, since several related compounds have proved effective in this indication (RYLEY and BETTS 1973).

It has been suggested that the coccidiostatic activity of quinolones may be due to an inhibitory action on coccidial thymidine synthetase, which, in turn, interferes

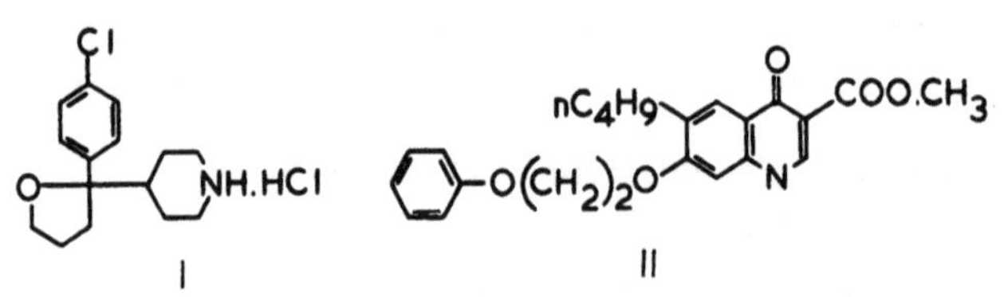

Fig. 2. Structures of experimental antimalarial drugs. *I*, BA 41799; *II*, ICI 56780

with DNA synthesis. It has also been shown that anticoccidial quinolones inhibit respiration of mitochondria isolated from oocysts, suggesting that their primary mode of action may be inhibition of electron transport (GUTTERIDGE and COOMBS 1977), perhaps in this manner resembling menoctone in its proposed mode of antimalarial action. Either mode of action of the quinolones might explain their synergistic action with sulphonamides or with chlorcycloguanil (an antifol) against *P. berghei* as shown by RYLEY and PETERS (1970) in vivo. It would be interesting to see if quinolones also potentiate with inhibitors of dihydro-orotate dehydrogenase.

As there are many similarities between the life cycles, structure and physiology of the coccidia and *Plasmodium,* it is to be anticipated that their response to various drugs would also bear certain similarities. Thus, for example, both are susceptible to sulphonamides and to DHF inhibitors, although not necessarily to the same compounds since major differences in the location of the various species affect their accessibility to drugs, and the tissue distribution and pharmacokinetics will differ accordingly. Nevertheless much could be learned about potentially valuable compounds and drug combinations for use in malaria from a careful study of anticoccidial agents (see, e.g. CHAPMAN 1978), e.g. clopidol (Fig. 3,III) with methyl benzoquate (Fig. 3,II), which have a potentiating effect. While it is true that those engaged in drug screening in the pharmaceutical industry are sometimes involved in both antiplasmodial and anticoccidial models, these almost invariably focus on single substances, and studies on drug combinations are rarely undertaken. Moreover, there is often little affinity of thought, much less collaboration between workers in the two fields.

c) Sulphadiazine with a Tetrahydrofuran

Significant potentiation against asexual erythrocytic stages of *P. berghei* was reported between a novel tetrahydrofuran derivative (BA 41799) (Fig. 2,I) and sulphadiazine and PETERS (1970c) suggested that the furan acted as a DHF inhibitor. However, no kinetic studies were made on isolated DHF and, in retrospect, it seems quite possible that the site of action of BA 41799 was other than on DHF itself. Certainly the compound bears no structural similarity to the familiar diamino-substituted ring systems seen in most DHF inhibitors. In a Dreiding molecular model analysis of BA 41799 CHENG (1971) drew a parallel to other apparently unrelated compounds which certainly are not DHF inhibitors such as the aminoalcohols. Since, being too toxic, this compound never reached clinical trial, no further attempt was made to clarify its mode of action even though this might have revealed a novel approach for further and rational chemical synthesis. Like other DHF inhibitors, BA 41799 was also active as a causal prophylactic (PETERS et al. 1975).

d) 2,4-Diamino-6-Substituted Quinazolines with Sulphonamides

A number of compounds in this series have been reported to be potent antimalarials and one in particular, WR 158122, has proved especially active against rodent and simian malarial strains that are sensitive to DHF inhibitors. These compounds are themselves DHF inhibitors and WR 158122, for example, shows marked potentiation with sulphadiazine against drug-sensitive and pyrimethamine-resistant strains of *P. falciparum* and *P. vivax* in *Aotus* monkeys (SCHMIDT 1979 a). Following the suggestion of FRIEDKIN et al. (1971), the tetrahydro derivative of WR 158122 was synthesised to see whether it would act perhaps at the step in folate metabolism beyond FH_4, namely the conversion of FH_4 to N^5,N^{10} derivatives. KINNAMON et al. (1976) found that the activity of the tetrahydro derivative named WR 180872 was strongly potentiated by sulphadiazine against *P. berghei* as was that of WR 158122. Moreover, the two quinazolines potentiated each other's action, although to a lesser degree than that observed by each with sulphadiazine. In a subsequent study KINNAMON and DAVIDSON (1980) found that the evidence of synergism between the two quinazolines was far less convincing against *P. cynomolgi bastianellii* in rhesus monkeys than against *P. berghei* in mice. However, this is perhaps simply another reflection of fundamental differences in the enzymes of the folate pathways of different *Plasmodium* species (such as we noted earlier between *P. falciparum* and *P. vivax* in their response to sulphonamides).

II. Other Compounds

1. Diamidines and Inhibitors of DNA Synthesis

Diamidines possess a modest level of activity against asexual erythrocytic stages of *P. berghei*. Diminazene aceturate (Berenil), for example, has an ED_{90} of 30 mg/kg (daily × 4) against the drug-sensitive N strain and only a little more than this against the highly chloroquine-resistant RC strain (PETERS et al. 1975). Interestingly it is more than three times less active against the cycloguanil-resistant B strain. The same compound is also active as a causal prophylactic against *P. yoelii nigeriensis* (PETERS et al. 1975 d) and is well known as an anti-babesial, anti-trypanosomal and anti-leishmanial agent. The toxicity of diamidines against haemoflagellates has been reported to depend upon their interference with kinetoplast-DNA replication, but nothing is known of their mode of action against *Plasmodium* or *Babesia,* which in any case do not have a kinetoplast and have not yet been shown conclusively to possess extracellular (mitochondrial) DNA. Nevertheless it would be interesting to explore whether diamidines exhibit any synergism with other compounds that intervene at a very early stage of DNA synthesis of malaria parasites such as the DHF inhibitors.

2. A Novel Dihydroacridinedione

RAETHER and FINK (1979) described the blood schizontocidal activity of floxacrine (HOE 991) (Chap. 15) against *P. berghei* (drug-sensitive and drug-resistant) and *P. vinckei* in mice, and against *P. cynomolgi bastianellii* in rhesus monkeys. Resistance to floxacrine (Fig. 3,I) developed rapidly in *P. berghei* and *P. cynomolgi*. The drug was found also to have a causal prophylactic effect against *P. cynomolgi,* but at a dose level that caused a serious haemorrhagic syndrome in some monkeys (SCHMIDT 1979 b). The compound was less effective against *P. fal-*

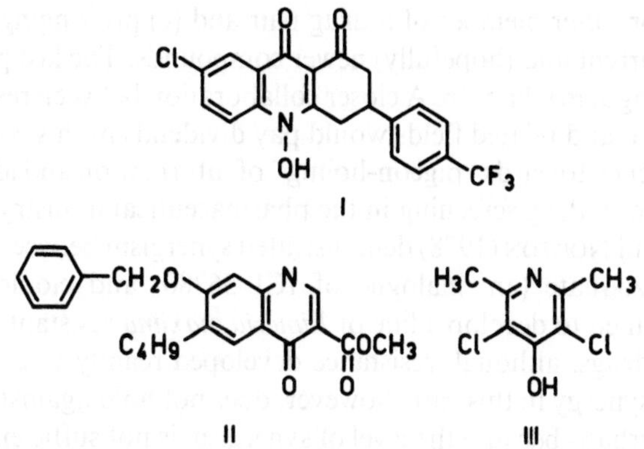

Fig. 3. Structures of antimalarial and anticoccidial drugs. *I*, floxacrine; *II*, methyl benzoquate; *III*, clopidol

ciparum or *P. vivax* in *Aotus* monkeys and resistant strains readily developed in these species and *P. cynomolgi*. Moreover floxacrine showed no secondary tissue schizontocidal activity against the latter parasite. Neither PABA nor folic acid reversed the action of floxacrine on the asexual blood stages of *P. berghei*. Further studies are in progress to find a "partner" compound that will slow down the rate at which resistance develops to floxacrine.

3. Erythromycin and Chloroquine

An unexpected type of potentiation was described by WARHURST et al. (1976), who found that the greatly reduced activity of chloroquine against the slightly chloroquine-resistant NS line and the highly resistant RC line of *P. berghei* was considerably enhanced when this drug was administered to mice together with erythromycin. This antibiotic, by itself, has little activity against any line of *P. berghei* and the combined activity of the two drugs was no more than additive against the drug-sensitive N strain of *P. berghei*. Potentiation appeared in direct proportion to the increase in chloroquine resistance. The action was not antagonised by supplementary PABA so that an indirect effect of the antibiotic by reducing biosynthesis of PABA by a suppressed intestinal flora does not appear to explain these observations. On the contrary, minocycline, which has a marked effect on the intestinal flora and a direct antimalarial action, does not show potentiation with chloroquine against any strain of *P. berghei* (KADDU et al. 1974). WARHURST (1977) suggested that the activity of erythromycin on chloroquine-resistant *P. berghei* might be due to an abnormal permeability of the parasite mitochondria under the influence of chloroquine, the antibiotic being little or unable to enter the mitochondria (its site of action in other eukaryotes such as yeasts) of *P. berghei* that are not in contact with chloroquine.

E. Conclusion

The use of antimalarials in combination offers many opportunities for (a) the exploration of novel, rational ways of producing drug synergism, (b) overcoming resistance to one or other member of a drug pair and (c) prolonging the useful life of some of the current and (hopefully) newer compounds. The last point is considered at greater length in Chap. 16. A closer collaboration between research workers in the antimalarial and related fields would pay dividends in this context. There is at present a tendency towards "pigeon-holing" of information and ideas, especially by those occupied in drug screening in the pharmaceutical industry. Thus, for example, JOYNER and NORTON (1978) demonstrated synergism between the coccidiostats methyl benzoquate (an analogue of ICI 56780) and clopidol (Fig. 3,III) (Chap. 15) and failed to develop a line of *Eimeria maxima* resistant to a 1:12 mixture of the two drugs, although resistance developed readily to each component used alone. The synergy in this case, however, does not hold against the individual resistant lines, perhaps because the level of synergism is not sufficiently great. Clopidol, the mode of action of which is still unknown, also has a moderately good action against asexual stages of *P. berghei* (GENTHER and SMITH 1977). Perhaps this action would be potentiated by other antimalarials?

References

Arnold J, Alving AS, Hockwald RS, Clayman CB, Dern RJ, Beutler E, Jeffery GM (1954) The effect of continuous and intermittent primaquine therapy on the relapse rate of Chesson strain vivax malaria. J Lab Clin Med 44:429–438

Aviado DM, Brugler B, Bellet J (1968) Pathologic physiology and chemotherapy of *Plasmodium berghei* V. Suppression of parasitaemia, diuresis and cardiac depression by pteridines. Exp Parasitol 23:294–302

Chapman HD (1978) Drug resistance in Coccidia. In: Long PL, Boorman KN, Freeman BM (eds) Avian coccidiosis. British Poultry Science, Edinburgh

Cheng CC (1971) Structure and antimalarial activity of aminoalcohols and 2-(*p*-chlorophenyl)-2-(4-piperidyl) tetrahydrofuran. J Pharm Sci 60:1596–1598

Clyde DF (1974) Treatment of drug-resistant malaria in man. Bull WHO 50:243–249

Coatney GR, Cooper WC, Young MD, Burgess RW, Smarr RG (1947) Studies in human malaria II. The suppressive action of sulfadiazine and sulfapyrazine against sporozoite-induced vivax malaria (St. Elizabeth strain). Am J Hyg 46:105–118

Fairley NH (1945) Chemotherapeutic suppression and prophylaxis in malaria. An experimental investigation undertaken by medical research teams in Australia. Trans R Soc Trop Med Hyg 38:311–355

Ferone R (1977) Folate metabolism in malaria. Bull WHO 55:291–298

Ferone R, Burchall JJ, Hitchings GH (1969) *P. berghei* dihydrofolate reductase. Isolation, properties and inhibition by antifolates. Mol. Pharmacol 5:49–59

Friedkin M, Crawford EJ, Plante LT (1971) Empirical vs rational approaches in chemotherapy. Ann NY Acad Sci 186:209–213

Genther CS, Smith CC (1977) Antifolate studies. Activities of 40 potential antimalarial compounds against sensitive and chlorguanide triazine resistant strains of folate-requiring bacteria and *Escherichia coli*. J Med Chem 20:237–243

Gero AM, O'Sullivan WJ (1979) Studies on dihydroorotate dehydrogenase from human spleen and the malarial parasite, *Plasmodium berghei*. Proc Aust Biochem Soc 12:9

Greenberg J, Boyd BL, Josephson ES (1948) Synergistic effect of chlorguanide and sulfadiazine against *Plasmodium gallinaceum* in the chick. J Pharmacol Exp Ther 94:60–64

Gutteridge WE, Coombs GH (1977) Biochemistry of parasitic protozoa. Macmillan, London

Hall AP (1977) Sequential treatment with quinine and mefloquine or quinine and pyrimethamine-sulfadoxine for falciparum malaria. Br Med J I:1626–1628

Howells RE, Peters W, Homewood CA (1972) Physiological adaptability of malaria parasites. In: Van den Bossche H (ed) Comparative biochemistry of parasites. Academic, New York, pp 235–258

Hunsicker LG, Schwarz RA, Barnwell FM (1967) Malaria from Vietnam. Ann Intern Med 66:1046

Jaffe J (1980) Filarial folate-related metabolism as a potential target for selective inhibitors. In: Van den Bossche J (ed) The host-invader interplay. Elsevier-North Holland, Amsterdam, pp 219–234

Joyner LP, Norton CC (1978) The activity of methyl benzoquate and clopidol against *Eimeria maxima:* synergy and drug resistance. Parasitology 76:369–377

Kaddu JB, Warhurst DC, Peters W (1974) The chemotherapy of rodent malaria, XIX. The action of a tetracycline derivative, minocycline, on drug-resistant *Plasmodium berghei.* Ann Trop Med Parasitol 68:41–46

Kinnamon KE, Davidson DE (1980) *Plasmodium cynomolgi:* folic acid antagonist combinations for treatment of malaria in rhesus monkeys. Exp Parasitol 49:277–280

Kinnamon KE, Ager AL, Orchard RW (1976) *Plasmodium berghei:* combining folic acid antagonists for potentiation against malaria infections in mice. Exp Parasitol 40:95–102

Kisliuk RL, Friedkin M, Schmidt LH, Rossan RN (1967) Antimalarial activity of tetrahydrohomopteroic acid. Science 156:1616–1617

O'Sullivan WJ, Ketley K (1980) Biosynthesis of uridine monophosphate in *Plasmodium berghei.* Ann Trop Med Parasitol 74:109–114

Pearlman EJ, Lampe RM, Thiemanun W, Kennedy RS (1977) Chemosuppressive field trials in Thailand. III. The suppression of *Plasmodium falciparum* and *Plasmodium vivax* parasitaemias by a sulfadoxine-pyrimethamine combination. Am J Trop Hyg 26:1108–1115

Peters W (1970 a) Chemotherapy and drug resistance in malaria. Academic, London

Peters W (1970 b) A new type of antimalarial drug potentiation. Trans R Soc Trop Med Hyg 64:462–464

Peters W (1970 c) The chemotherapy of rodent malaria, XII. Substituted tetrahydrofurans, a new chemical family of antimalarials. The action of 2-(*p*-chlorophenyl)-2-(4-piperidyl)-tetrahydrofuran against *Plasmodium berghei* and *Plasmodium chabaudi.* Ann Trop Med Parasitol 64:189–202

Peters W, Portus JH, Robinson BL (1973) The chemotherapy of rodent malaria, XVII. Dynamics of drug resistance, part 3: influence of drug combinations on the development of resistance to chloroquine in *P. berghei.* Ann Trop Med Parasitol 67:143–154

Peters W, Davies EE, Robinson BL (1975) The chemotherapy of rodent malaria, XXIII. Causal prophylaxis, part II: practical experience with *Plasmodium yoelii nigeriensis* in drug screening. Ann Trop Med Parasitol 69:311–328

Peters W, Howells RE, Portus J, Robinson BL, Thomas S, Warhurst DC (1977) The chemotherapy of rodent malaria, XXVII. Studies on mefloquine (WR 142,490). Ann Trop Med Parasitol 71:407–418

Powers KG, Jacobs RL, Good WC, Koontz LC (1969) *Plasmodium vinckei:* Production of chloroquine-resistant strain. Exp Parasitol 26:193–202

Rabinovich SA (1965) Experimental investigations of antimalarial drug Haloquine. III. Investigation of the possibility to restrain the development of chemoresistance to chloridine (Daraprim) by combined administration of chloridine with Haloquine. Med Parazitol (Mosk) 34:434–439

Raether W, Fink E (1979) Antimalarial activity of floxacrine (HOE 991). I. Studies on blood schizontocidal action of floxacrine against *Plasmodium berghei, P. vinckei* and *P. cynomolgi.* Ann Trop Med Parasitol 73:505–526

Rieckmann KH, McNamara JV, Frischer H, Stockert TA, Carson PE, Powell RD (1968) Gametocytocidal and sporontocidal effects of primaquine and sulfadiazine with pyrimethamine in a chloroquine-resistant strain of *P. falciparum.* Bull WHO 38:625–632

Rollo IM (1955) The mode of action of sulphonamides, proguanil and pyrimethamine on *Plasmodium gallinaceum.* Br J Pharmacol Chemother 10:208–224

Rosario VE (1976) Genetics of chloroquine-resistance in malaria parasites. Nature 261:585–586

Ryley JF, Betts MJ (1973) Chemotherapy of chicken coccidiosis. Adv Pharmacol Chemother 11:221–293

Ryley JF, Peters W (1970) The antimalarial activity of some quinolone esters. Ann Trop Med Parasitol 64:209–222

Schmidt LD (1979a) Studies on the 2,4-diamino-6-substituted quinazolines. III. The capacity of sulfadiazine to enhance the activities of WR-158,122 and WR-159,412 against infections with various drug-susceptible and drug-resistant strains of *Plasmodium falciparum* and *Plasmodium vivax* in owl monkeys. Am J Trop Med Hyg 28:808–818

Schmidt LD (1979b) Antimalarial properties of floxacrine, a dihydroacridinedione derivative. Antimicrob Agents Chemother 16:475–485

Schmidt LH, Harrison J, Rossan RN, Vaughan D, Crosby R (1977) Quantitative aspects of pyrimethamine-sulfonamide synergism. Am J Trop Med Hyg 26:837–848

Sherman IW (1979) Biochemistry of *Plasmodium* (malarial parasites). Microbiol Rev 43:453–495

Tigertt WD (1966) Present and potential malaria problem. Milit Med [Suppl] 131:853–856

Vivona S, Brewer GJ, Conrad M, Alving AS (1961) The concurrent weekly administration of chloroquine and primaquine for the prevention of Korean vivax malaria. Bull WHO 25:267–269

Warhurst DC (1977) Chloroquine-erythromycin potentiation of *P. berghei*. Ann Trop Med Parasitol 71:383

Warhurst DC, Robinson BL, Peters W (1976) The chemotherapy of rodent malaria, XXIV. The blood schizontocidal action of erythromycin upon *Plasmodium berghei*. Ann Trop Med Parasitol 70:253–258

Wilkinson RN, Noeypatimanondh S, Gould DJ (1976) Infectivity of falciparum patients for anopheline mosquitoes before and after chloroquine treatment. Trans R Soc Trop Med Hyg 70:306–307

CHAPTER 7

Repository Preparations

D. F. Worth and L. M. Werbel

A. Introduction

I. The Need

The nature and extent of the malaria problem and the details surrounding those agents both available and under development for treatment of active disease have been addressed in various sections of this volume. We propose to discuss here a specific need which exists in malaria chemotherapy, that is for agents with prolonged activity – the so-called repository drugs. This therapeutic requirement has only in recent years received attention, and it is certainly not yet attracting substantial research. Early efforts in this field were reviewed in 1969 (Elslager 1969) and again in 1974 (Elslager 1974). It is our intention to place in perspective both past and recent research in this brief survey.

The obvious question which deserves response, of course, is "why?" Why are long-acting or repository antimalarial drugs needed? Justification of the need is reasonably simple. First from an overall point of view, there are of course a variety of drugs available today for the treatment of malaria. However, reduction of parasite levels in vectors to a point where transmission stops, with the ultimate aim of eliminating the disease within an endemic region, requires that nearly all people within that region be protected from infection for the duration of at least one transmission season. This requires a continuous maintenance of an effective schizontocidal level of a drug in the blood of most individuals. Currently available drugs are effective for only short periods of time, and would require frequent dosing to accomplish this goal. This would present insurmountable problems both in the logistics of drug distribution to the population and the ensuing costs. In Africa, for example, perhaps only 20% of the population is within ready access of the appropriate health care facilities. Thus the need is great for an agent which could lead to the ultimate elimination of the disease problem.

More specifically, long-acting agents are needed for the protection of those "at risk" individuals entering an infected area. An interesting example is the recent discussion (Bruce-Chwatt 1977) concerning the question of how best to protect airline pilots flying regularly into malarious areas. The problems besetting currently available agents are perhaps best placed in perspective in this context. Chloroquine, for example, is recommended at 300 mg base once a week in areas not containing the drug-resistant parasite. Concern is voiced, however, over the potential for neuroretinal changes with long-term drug therapy. Proguanil at 100–200 mg daily or pyrimethamine at 25 mg once a week are suggested as causing fewer side effects, but they are also less certain to afford protection because of resistance to the antifol types. Maloprim, a mixture of 12.5 mg pyrimethamine and 100 mg dapsone, given weekly is also recommended, with the caveat that care be taken not to exceed the prescribed dose because of the possibility of haemolytic side effects. Finally Fansidar, a mixture of 25 mg pyrimethamine and 500 mg sulfadoxine, is recommended as effective for chloroquine-resistant *P. falciparum* given weekly, biweekly or even monthly. This would seem a not too comforting situation were one about to enter a malarious area of the world.

Finally we must consider the properties of available antimalarial drugs. Mefloquine, for example, a relatively recent entry into the field, possesses a variety of very attractive properties. It has been noted, however (DOBERSTYN et al. 1979), that the rapid absorption of the drug may be the cause of the gastrointestinal intolerance sometimes noted with its use. Therefore a slower released form of the drug would be desirable. Moreover it appears from recent pharmacokinetic studies (RITSCHEL et al. 1978) that most antimalarial drugs are overdosed utilising the prescribed dosage regimens. Thus the maximum drug levels achieved were from 6 to 8.5 times larger than the minimum levels and regimens were recommended to achieve less fluctuation. The concept of a long-acting or repository agent also attempts to provide a minimum constant effective blood level of drug over a longer period of time, thus leading to decreased potential for toxic side reactions.

How then to approach solutions to these obvious needs? It is possible that the tremendous advances recently towards in vitro cultivation of the plasmodia (Part I, Chaps. 3, 6) will aid greatly in the eventual development of an effective vaccine for malaria. However, successful achievement of such a prophylactic approach at the present time must still be regarded realistically, no matter what one's personal prejudices, as a distant prospect. Today the need exists, as PETERS has pointed out (PETERS 1978), for a new technology which would allow the administration of a drug at intervals of no less than 3 months. Such a goal is, in fact, one of the priority targets of the Malaria Chemotherapy Scientific Working Group of the WHO Special Programme for Research and Training in Tropical Diseases (TDR).

II. Attributes of a Repository Preparation

Our primary purpose in this review is to treat that aspect of repository antimalarial drugs which might lead to eradication of the disease in specific endemic regions. Thus we will be concerned with those approaches that have the potential to provide a preparation which will protect against infection for at least 3 months after a single dose. A longer period of protection, preferably encompassing at least one complete transmission season, would be even more desirable. This implies, of course, that sufficient drug can be administered, and that absorption into the blood can be sufficiently slow to last for 3 months, and yet be fast enough to afford continuous schizontocidal concentrations. The preparation must also be relatively innocuous, since once administered it is usually impossible, or at best extremely difficult, to remove it from the patient. Inferred, therefore, are safeguards against the sudden release of relatively large amounts, i.e. systemically toxic levels, of drug from the injection site. The drug or a metabolite must not, moreover, be transported preferentially and stored in any organ to the extent of causing toxic manifestations. Finally, there should be little or no local irritation after intramuscular dosing. While ideally the drug should be effective after oral administration, for the present at least this seems a rather unlikely prospect. Such a preparation must, of course, in addition share those other properties common to all antimalarial agents such as: broad activity against the various life cycle forms as well as sensitive and drug-resistant strains, limited potential for development of resistance, fast-acting, cheap, long shelf-life.

B. Approaches to Repository Antimalarial Drugs

Two basic approaches to the development of long-acting antimalarial agents are apparent. The first is concerned with the search for substances which, after oral administration, are bound by host tissues from which they are slowly released. The second relies on prolonging the effects of compounds with known antimalarial activity. The duration of action of a drug is, of course, dependent on the rate at which it is absorbed, metabolically altered or destroyed, and excreted. Thus the persistence of a drug can be prolonged by delaying its degradation and excretion, or by slowing its rate of absorption. Such effects may be feasible either through structural modification, physical change, use of an external device or even simply by a change of route of administration.

I. Tissue-Held Drugs

This approach utilises oral drug administration and relies on subsequent binding to, and slow release from, deep tissue sites. Several classes of antimalarial substances in addition to the 4-aminoquinolines, quinolinemethanols and diaminoquinazolines detailed below persist in tissues for relatively long periods following oral administration. None, however, has been demonstrated to have appreciable repository activity in man. The weakly antimalarial compound RC-12, 4-(2-bromo-4,5-dimethoxyphenyl)-1,1,7,7-tetraethyldiethylenetriamine, showed encouraging prophylactic activity against *P. cynomolgi* infections in the monkey (SODEMAN et al. 1972). The antiamoebic and weakly antimalarial agent, bialamicol, is retained for long periods in the tissues of both dog and man after oral dosing. Its lack of repository action against *P. berghei* in mice may be a result of its relatively low potency (ELSLAGER 1969).

II. Drugs Incorporated in Polymers and in Physical Devices

This approach (ROBINSON 1978) employs drugs known to be highly active clinically placed within a polymer matrix or some form of device, such as the Alza Minipump, which is implanted or injected intramuscularly and from which the drug is released at a slow, controlled rate. Such a polymer approach was used in the early testing of the quinazoline WR 158122 (to be described in detail below) and sulphadiazine by WISE et al. (1979). Quinine has also been placed in a polymerised polymethacrylate carrier (PINAZZI et al. 1978), but antimalarial properties of the preparation were not described. Dapsone and sulphadimethoxine were incorporated into saccharidic polymers, but only a slight increase in activity against *P. berghei* infections in mice was achieved (KOROLKOVAS et al. 1978).

Chloroquine incorporated into silicone discs was shown in vitro to release drug in microgram quantities for over 4 months, but no results against the infection are included (FU et al. 1973). The recent Alza Minipump delivery technology in its various forms has been applied to several disease areas (CHANDRASEKARAN et al. 1978). The only application to malaria is a somewhat unusual example wherein the antimalarial effect of primaquine given once daily to mice with *P. berghei* was compared with the drug given continuously by constant release from an implanted "osmotic mini pump" (JUDGE and HOWELLS 1979 a). It was concluded that no reduction in total dose of primaquine required was achieved by the use of such a slow release preparation.

JUDGE and HOWELLS (1979 b) used similar drug/polymer mixtures and evaluated their chemotherapeutic effects with *P. berghei*. Primaquine, cycloguanil and menoctone implants resulted in local tissue necrosis. Chloroquine implants were ineffective in contrast to those containing pyrimethamine, sulphadiazine, and sulfadoxine. At a drug concentration of 0.5%, pyrimethamine protected from infection for between 5 and 6 months.

A somewhat different approach involved the preparation of a slow-release form of quinine from slowly eroding, timed-release tablets prepared with variable amounts of a swellable gum, carbomer, and cellulose acetate hydrogen phthalate at different compaction pressures. Once again this was an in vitro feasibility study with no chemotherapy attempted (CHOULIS and PAPADOPOULOS 1975).

III. Poorly Soluble Salts and Derivatives

This approach, which has been perhaps the most successful to date, is akin to the aforementioned utilisation of a polymer matrix for slow release, in that the preparation is injected intramuscularly or subcutaneously. Now, however, the drug is presented as a poorly soluble salt or biodegradable derivative suspended in an aqueous or lipid vehicle. Upon injection the insoluble material is deposited in the tissues, forming a depot from which the active drug is very slowly released into the circulation. Previous examples of this approach were developed in the work of ELSLAGER et al. (1969 a, b, c, d) and WORTH et al. (1969). Detailed accomplishments of this approach with cycloguanil pamoate are outline below.

C. Laboratory Test Methods

I. Biological Response

1. Screening in Mice

THOMPSON et al. (1963) devised a simple, yet elegant, method for screening potentially repository antimalarial compounds utilising single *P. berghei* challenges in mice. Groups of 25 mice were treated subcutaneously with a suspension of the candidate drug. One, 3, 5, and 7 weeks post-treatment, subgroups of five mice each in parallel with vehicle controls were challenged intraperitoneally with 15 million parasites in blood obtained from donor mice during the ascending phase of parasitaemia. Protection from infection was then determined by examination of Giemsa-stained smears of peripheral blood 7 and 14 days postchallenge. Results were expressed as the number of weeks that 50% of the mice were protected (PMW) by the standard 400-mg/kg dose (ELSLAGER 1969). Utilisation of this method allowed both comparisons of the PMW with other potential agents and an assessment of the dose/response relationship. An initial rough estimate of local irritation at the injection site was also made. The use of this screen pointed the way towards the development of cycloguanil pamoate (PMW > 8) (THOMPSON et al. 1963) and Dapolar, a combination of cycloguanil pamoate and acedapsone (DADDS) (THOMPSON et al. 1965 a–c).

More recently a screening strategy designed to detect both causal prophylactic or blood schizontocidal activities after simultaneous oral and subcutaneous dosing was described by SCHOFIELD et al. (1981). In contrast to the method of THOMPSON et al. (1963), mice are challenged intravenously with 40,000 *P. yoelli yoelii* sporozoites. The screening plan is divided into two stages. The first stage is designed to expose those compounds which possess no appreciable prolonged activity and thus require no further testing. Groups of five mice are challenged 3 days post-treatment, protection is assessed 7 days postchallenge from Giemsa-stained blood smears and host deaths are recorded 14 days postchallenge. Only compounds demonstrating antimalarial activity are then passed on to the second stage. For this, subgroups of five mice each are challenged 1, 2 or 3 weeks after oral and subcutaneous dosing. Results are then compared with those from the control drug, diformyldiaminodiphenyl sulphone (DFD), and a DFD index (DFDI) ranging from 0.0 to 4.0 is assigned to each test drug. A DFDI of 0.0 indicates no observed antimalarial activity, while a DFDI of 4.0 indicates complete protection from the 3-week challenge.

A third variant of the mouse test was described by WISE et al. (1976). This test uses multiple intraperitoneal challenges with *P. berghei*-infected blood after a single subcutaneous dose of drug/polymer preparations in an aqueous suspension. A group of five mice is used for each dose level. The mice are challenged immediately after drug administration. At 7-day intervals thereafter, blood smears are examined for parasites and all negative mice are rechallenged. The test is terminated when all mice have died or at 15 weeks post-treatment. This method makes very efficient use of the test animals, in that only five mice are needed for each dose level. However, when animals die without a confirmed infection, the results are difficult to interpret.

Testing for repository activity frequently requires careful control. When poorly soluble salts or derivatives are used, the crystal size, shape and compatibility with the vehicle needs examination. If polymeric carriers are used, the polymer characteristics must be controlled. In addition to the sham-dosed animal control groups, it is sometimes necessary to include also groups treated with drug-free polymer or derivatising agents. Further control groups can be treated with a soluble form of the drug under study, both orally and parenterally, to confirm parasite susceptibility and prolongation of activity.

2. Tests in Monkeys

Normally mouse testing is followed by testing in monkeys, where more versatility is available. Several of the best compounds identified by the mouse tests have received further evaluation in monkeys. THOMPSON et al. (1963, 1965 a, b, c) used rhesus monkeys and challenged intravenously with 15 million *P. cynomolgi* trophozoites obtained from donor monkeys in the ascending phase of parasitaemia. Thus the animals were treated intramuscularly with an oleaginous or aqueous suspension of a potential repository agent and challenged with malaria at various intervals up to 1 year later. Until there was evidence to the contrary, the tendency was to challenge each monkey only once to preclude concerns that active immunisation might contribute to resistance to patent infections from later challenges (Thompson et al. 1963). These concerns were later somewhat alleviated by observing breakthroughs in animals that were given as many as six previous challenges (Schmidt et al. 1963). A much greater concern is the development of resistant parasites during the period when drug-restrained, subpatent infections are present. By subinoculating blood from rhesus monkeys previously treated with cycloguanil pamoate and challenged with *P. cynomolgi* sporozoites into normal animals, Schmidt et al. (1963) found that three of seven subjects had low level parasitaemias well before the infections were detected on thick films, in one monkey for 67 days.

Monkeys may also be used to determine if a repository drug has radically eliminated challenge parasites, or is acting as a long-term suppressant. To accomplish this, Schmidt et al. (1963) treated rhesus monkeys with cycloguanil pamoate, then challenged 1 week later with *P. cynomolgi* sporozoites. The animals were then held nearly 300 days and splenectomised. When none developed observable parasitaemia, they were rechallenged with sporozoites. When six of the eight animals were found susceptible to infection, it was concluded that the drug had functioned essentially as a prophylactic.

The tests for repository action described above were all performed with *P. cynomolgi*. However, it has been noted by Schofield et al. (1981) that *Aotus trivirgatus griseimembra* infected with *P. falciparum* or *P. vivax* can now be considered in tertiary preclinical testing.

II. Rate of Release Studies

In contrast to the examination of the duration of a biological response, a direct measurement of the rate of release of active drug component may be made. This method is particularly useful for comparing different formulations designed to release slowly the same chemotherapeutic agent. The ultimate aim is the development of a system of constant, controlled rate of release. The two basic needs are a method of obtaining samples at appropriate time intervals and a sufficiently sensitive assay procedure.

The simplest methods utilise in vitro techniques. As examples, Wise et al. (1978) measured the release of ^{35}S from various polymeric devices containing sulphadiazine placed in an extraction thimble over several months. Fu et al. (1973) placed silicone discs incorporating chloroquine phosphate in an aqueous buffer placed in a shaker bath and measured drug release by ultraviolet spectroscopy for up to 126 days. In contrast, Chien et al. (1974), Chien (1978), and Flynn and Smith (1971) have described more sophisticated mechanical devices which may be used for in vitro diffusion studies.

Release rate studies have also of course been carried out in vivo. A major added difficulty is that of drug metabolism. There must therefore be some assurance that the assay system employed actually measures only the antimalarial component or components released. A second practical difficulty is that only a limited amount of biological fluid containing a very low drug concentration is normally available. Since the most significant measurements are often those at the time when the drug concentrations released are near the minimum required for the desired biological effect, very sensitive assay methods are highly desirable. For this reason, radio-labelled drugs are most commonly used. A decided advantage of in vivo release studies is that they may be combined with measurements of antimalarial protection. With cumulative excretion curves, it is also possible to estimate when essentially all of a drug has been released from a repository depot. Using the polymeric preparations referred to above incorporating [^{35}S] sulphadiazine, WISE et al. (1978) compared release rates from mice with the drug preparations implanted subcutaneously with those obtained in vitro. In addition, WISE et al. (1979a, b) later used tritium-labelled sulphadiazine mixed with 2,4-diamino-6-(2-naphthylsulphonyl)-quinazoline-2-[^{14}C] (WR 158122) to measure simultaneously the release of both drugs after subcutaneous injection in mice and intramuscular injection in rhesus monkeys. After it was found that mefloquine (WR 142490) possessed prophylactic activity in humans (RIECKMANN et al. 1974), a kinetic study was completed in human volunteers. Estimates of blood concentrations as long as 83 days after oral administration (DESJARDINS et al. 1979b) were possible using high-pressure liquid chromatography (GRINDEL et al. 1977).

A rather different assay method was employed by WERBEL et al. (1984) in studies conducted with pyrimethamine pamoate in *Macaca fascicularis*. A series of dilutions of serum samples taken periodically from the monkeys after intramuscular drug injection were assayed in vitro for *P. falciparum* growth suppression, utilising the semiautomated methodology developed by DESJARDINS et al. (1979a). Direct comparison with a series of known pyrimethamine concentrations then allowed an estimation of the effective pyrimethamine serum concentrations. In addition, these monkeys were periodically challenged with *P. cynomolgi* utilising the method of THOMPSON et al. (1963).

D. Major Types of Drugs Investigated

I. 4-Aminoquinolines

Perhaps the structural class which has shown the greatest potential for the approach involving a drug bound to the tissues is the 4-aminoquinolines related to chloroquine. Several compounds related to 12,278 RP (I) (SCHNEIDER et al. 1965) showed definite repository activity in experimental systems including mice and monkeys, and even in clinical trials (WORLD HEALTH ORGANIZATION 1967). None, however, displayed properties adequate for their selection as a repository drug. More recent effort has centred on tripiperaquine (II) (M1020) (LABORATORY OF MALARIA RESEARCH, SHANGHAI 1975).

In mice this material, given in a single dose of 500 mg/kg, protected against *P. berghei* infections for as long as 50 days. In monkeys infected with trophozoite-induced *P. cynomolgi*, a single oral dose of 100 mg/kg of the phosphate salt "afforded a significant suppressive effect for 30 days". In man M1020 phosphate (0.6 g) was

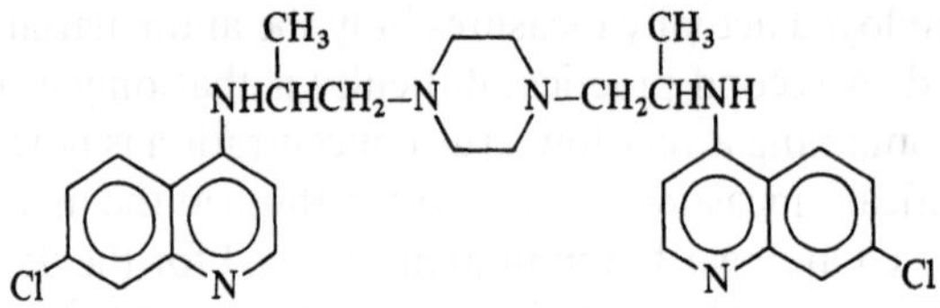

I

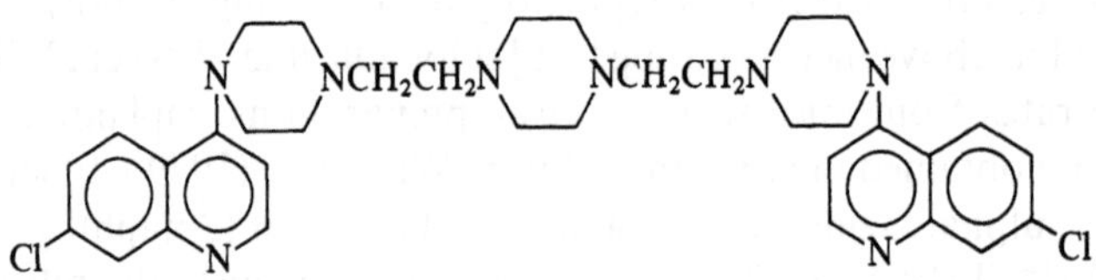

II

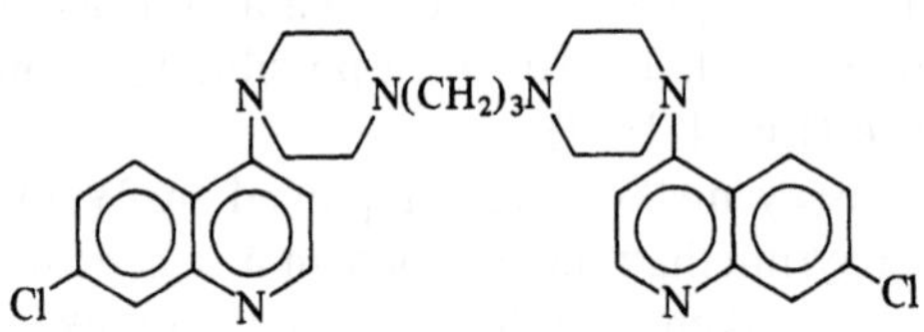

III

Fig. 1. 4-Aminoquinoline structures I–III

given with 0.25 g sulfadoxine and 0.025 g pyrimethamine as a single oral dose monthly. The incidence of malaria was reduced 65.1% compared with that prior to treatment. *P. vivax,* however, is suppressed for only 2 weeks. The data do not indicate a significant superiority to 13,228 RP (III). Significantly also, nearly 20% of the subjects treated with M1020 complained of mild abdominal discomfort or diarrhoea.

II. Quinolinemethanols

An early quinolinemethanol (IV) synthesised during World War II appeared to persist in the tissues for relatively long periods following oral administration (WISELOGLE 1946). Although the drug was effectively absorbed from the gastrointestinal tract, the plasma level fell very slowly after drug administration was discontinued. Four weeks after the last dose, only 50% of the drug had disappeared from the plasma, and from 1% to 5% of the drug was still present as long as 3 months after the last dose. Most subjects, unfortunately, developed a marked skin sensitivity to sunlight (phototoxicity) which persisted for long periods after discontinuance of drug administration.

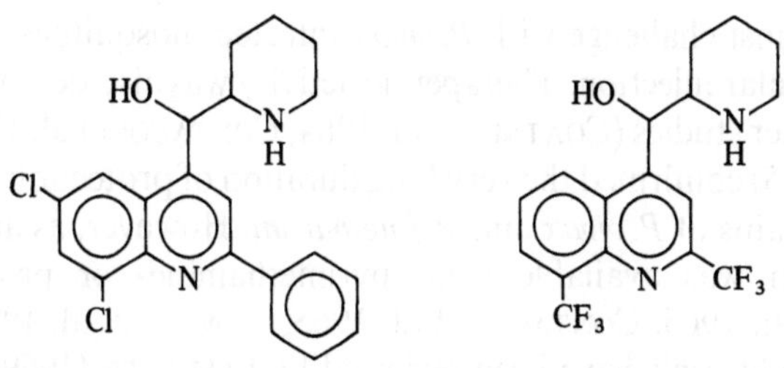

IV V

Fig. 2. Quinolinemethanol structures IV and V

The recently developed quinolinemethanol (V) (mefloquine) has also shown single-dose therapeutic efficacy and prolonged effectiveness as a prophylactic drug (see also Chap. 9). In preliminary studies even against a drug-resistant strain of *P. falciparum*, the development of patent parasitaemia was prevented when non-immune persons were exposed to infected mosquitoes 2 weeks after medication, and it was delayed when exposure occurred 3 weeks after drug administration (RIECKMANN et al. 1974). This efficacy has been explained by the findings of a very large apparent volume of distribution and a long half-life.

III. Cycloguanil Pamoate

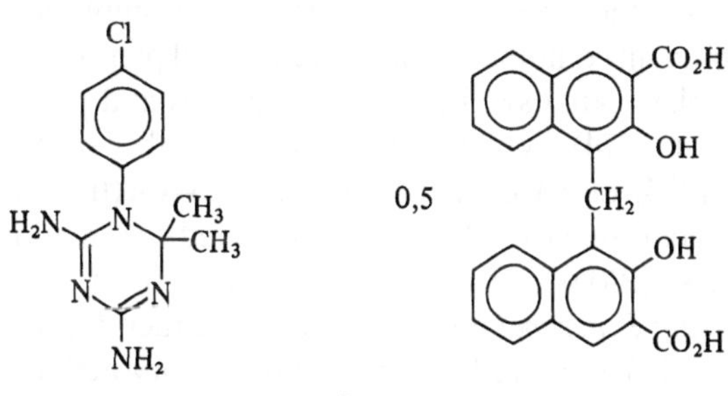

VI

Fig. 3. Cycloguanil pamoate (VI)

This agent (VI) has received far more study than any other repository antimalarial. The compound contains the active metabolite of proguanil (HAWKING and PERRY 1948) as the antimalarial component and is an example of a poorly soluble salt given by injection and released slowly from the injection site. It was the outstanding member of a large group of salts reported by ELSLAGER (1969) and tested initially by THOMPSON et al. (1963). In mice, a single subcutaneous injection of 360 mg/kg protected against infection from *P. berghei* for 8 weeks. Rhesus monkeys given single intramuscular doses were protected from challenge with *P. cynomolgi* trophozoites or sporozoites for 7–40 weeks (THOMPSON et al. 1963; SCHMIDT et al. 1963). Furthermore, when infections did finally break through in the treated monkeys SCHMIDT et al. (1963) found no evidence of drug-resistant parasites. Initial trials in humans (COATNEY et al. 1963) showed that protection was conferred for

9–12 months against challenge with *P. vivax*-infected mosquitoes, after a single 5-mg/kg intramuscular injection. Therapeutic activity was also demonstrated in four volunteers. Further studies (Coatney et al. 1964; Contacos et al. 1964, 1965, 1966; Powell et al. 1965) confirmed the very long duration of protection against normal, drug-sensitive strains of *P. vivax* and *P. falciparum*. However, as anticipated, little or no protection was available from pyrimethamine- or proguanil-resistant strains (Chin et al. 1965; Contacos et al. 1965; Powell et al. 1964). The results from extensive field trials have been reviewed by Elslager (1969) and minimum protection periods summarised as follows: for *P. vivax*, 6 months for normal strains, none for proguanil-resistant strains; for *P. malariae*, 5 months; for *P. falciparum*, 4 months for normal strains, 2 months for strains partially resistant to proguanil and pyrimethamine, and none for strains resistant to both proguanil and pyrimethamine.

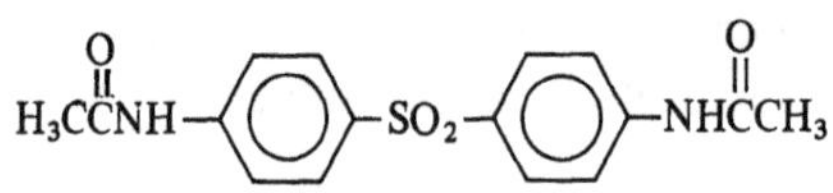

VII

Fig. 4. Acedapsone (VII)

In an effort to overcome the lack of activity against the resistant strains, efforts were directed towards the development of a repository sulphone or sulphonamide derivative that would, in combination with cycloguanil pamoate, provide a sequential block for the plasmodial synthesis of pyrimidines and purines (Thompson et al. 1965 b; Elslager 1974). While testing a large number of dapsone derivatives (Elslager 1969, 1974; Elslager et al. 1969 a, b, c; Worth et al. 1969) in mice it was found that acedapsone (VII, DADDS) protected the majority of animals for longer than 10 weeks (PMW > 10) (Thompson et al. 1965 a), and it was chosen for further testing. Using *P. berghei* highly resistant to either dapsone or cycloguanil, it was found that a 1 : 1 mixture had broader repository action against the drug-resistant lines than did either drug alone (Thompson et al. 1965 a). In monkeys, a single intramuscular dose of 25 mg/kg each of acedapsone and medium particle size cycloguanil pamoate in lipid suspension protected for 112–228 days against *P. cynomolgi* trophozoite challenges (Thompson et al. 1965 a). Following clinical studies (Chin et al. 1967 a, b; Black et al. 1966) this mixture was subjected to extensive field trials. The results from these trials have been reviewed by Elslager (1969, 1974) and minimum protection periods summarised as follows: for *P. vivax*, 5 months for normal strains, none for proguanil-resistant strains; for *P. falciparum*, 4 months for proguanil- and pyrimethamine-resistant strains, approximately 2 months for Southeast Asian strains resistant to proguanil, pyrimethamine, and 4-aminoquinolines, and 3–4 months for certain Brazilian strains possibly resistant to chloroquine.

Despite the early promise and a great deal of clinical work, neither cycloguanil pamoate nor the acedapsone-cycloguanil pamoate mixture are currently in use. Prominent among the reasons for this are the variable durations of protection afforded from resistant or partially resistant parasites and the prevalence of local intolerance at the injection site encountered in some of the field trials. Interestingly, the use of intramuscular acedapsone for control of leprosy emerged from this work (RUSSELL et al. 1979) continues.

IV. Pyrimethamine Pamoate

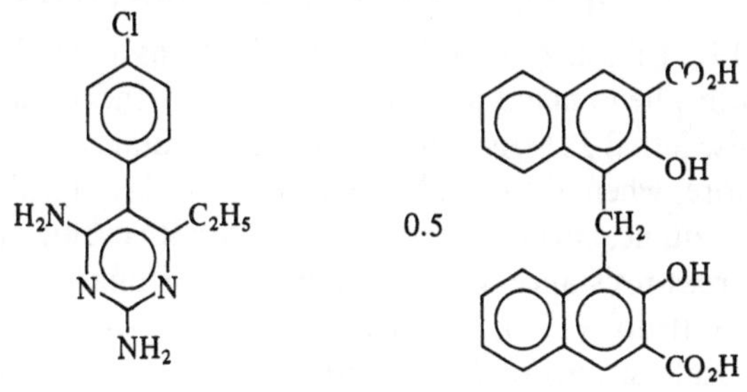

VIII

Fig. 5. Pyrimethamine pamoate (VIII)

This preparation (VIII) (ELSLAGER and WORTH 1966), along with a host of other pyrimethamine salts (ELSLAGER 1969), was tested utilising the method of THOMPSON et al. (1963). A single 400-mg/ml subcutaneous injection was found to protect mice for >8 weeks (PMW>8). More recently (WERBEL et al. 1984), pyrimethamine pamoate was compared with a pyrimethamine-impregnated lactic/glycolic acid copolymer. Results from preliminary mouse tests are shown in Table 1.

Subgroups of mice were challenged 1, 3, 5, 7, and 9 weeks post-treatment, and protection was assessed 1 week postchallenge. Although no striking differences were seen in the duration of protection between the salt and polymer forms in this test, the pamoate did protect more mice from the 5-week challenge than did the polymer composite. Initial tests with the pamoate in cynomolgus monkeys

Table 1. Duration of protection from *P. berghei* infections for mice given a subcutaneous injection of pyrimethamine pamoate or a pyrimethamine/polymer composite

	Post-treatment *P. berghei* challenge Mice protected/mice in subgroup				
	1 week	3 week	5 week	7 week	9 week
400 mg/kg					
Pamoate	5/5	4/5	3/5	1/5	0/5
Polymer	5/5	4/5	0/5	0/5	0/5
Base	0/5	0/5	0/5	Test Terminated	Test Terminated
200 mg/kg					
Pamoate	5/5	3/5	2/5	0/5	0/5
Polymer	5/5	4/5	0/5	0/5	0/5
Vehicle	0/5	0/5	0/5	0/5	0/5

indicated that single intramuscular injections of 50 or 200 mg/kg conferred protection from *P. cynomolgi* challenge for 3–4 months (WERBEL et al. 1984). At this time, serum levels were generally below 100 ng/ml when assayed in vitro for inhibition of *P. falciparum* (see Sect. C.II).

V. 2,4-Diamino-6-(2-Naphthylsulphonyl)Quinazoline (WR 158122)

ELSLAGER et al. (1979) characterised this material (IX) as a member of a new class of compounds with phenomenal antimalarial activity. Indeed it was curative in mice with otherwise lethal *P. berghei* infections at subcutaneous doses as low as 5 mg/kg. Furthermore, when given orally to mice, it displayed little or no cross-resistance with chloroquine, negligible cross-resistance with cycloguanil and less than two- to sixfold cross-resistance with dapsone. Unfortunately this rosy picture faded a bit when SCHMIDT (1973) found a high level of cross-resistance with pyrimethamine for certain strains of *P. falciparum* and *P. vivax* in owl monkeys, and a facile development of drug-resistance with subcurative treatment. However, since related diaminoquinazolines were known to act synergistically with dapsone (THOMPSON et al. 1970), testing with drug combinations was pursued. Indeed SCHMIDT (1973) found a 16- to 64-fold enhancement of potency when combinations of IX and sulphadiazine were given to monkeys infected with various pyrimethamine and chloroquine-resistant *P. falciparum* and *P. vivax* strains. More importantly, there was no development of parasite drug-resistance. Increased effectiveness of combination therapy was also seen in initial clinical studies (ROZMAN and CANFIELD 1979).

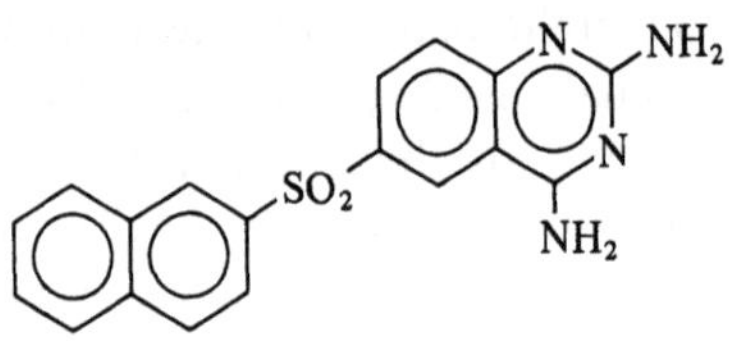

Fig. 6. WR 158122 (IX) IX

Repository testing has been done with WR 158122 alone (WISE et al. 1976; WERBEL et al. 1981), sulphadiazine alone (WISE et al. 1978) and the combination (WISE et al. 1979 a). WISE et al. (1976) prepared a powder containing a glycolic/lactic acid polymer incorporating the diaminoquinazoline containing tracer amounts of ^{14}C. This was then injected subcutaneously into mice at various dose levels. After the inital 3 weeks, during which there were relatively high values, the weekly release was nearly constant as measured by the radioactivity in the urine and faeces. The mice were also challenged weekly with *P. berghei*, utilising the third variant of the mouse test described above. At doses of 80–640 mg/kg complete protection was obtained for 3–5 weeks. Unfortunately, controls dosed with unformulated drug or drug-free polymer were not reported. WERBEL et al. (1981) tested the unformulated diaminoquinazoline base using the method of THOMPSON et al. (1963). After a 400-mg/kg dose, protection was complete through the challenge 5 weeks post-treatment. Thus the use of the polymer formulation to decrease significantly the rate of release of this drug in mice must be questioned. WERBEL et al. (1981)

also found from challenges 7–19 weeks post-treatment that 20%–80% of the mice were protected and that, in contrast to the controls and mice treated with pyrimethamine pamoate, most of the susceptible animals lived at least 2 weeks postchallenge.

WISE et al. (1979 a) then compared mixtures of the diamino-quinazoline-2-[^{14}C] and [^{3}H] sulphadiazine as a pure drug mix, and incorporated into a glycolic/lactic acid polymer, in mice and rhesus monkeys. In mice, the release rates for the sulphadiazine component were very similar, with 20%–39% released the 1st week and only 40%–42% recovered throughout the 13-week test period. Little or no drug was found in either the urine or feaces after 60 days. The urinary excretion of the diaminoquinazoline was also similar, with 26% recovery from both the pure drug mixture and the polymer formulation. The faecal excretion did vary, however. Over 13 weeks, 54% and 24% of drug from the pure drug mixture and polymer formulation respectively were eliminated by this route. In monkeys, excretion of sulphadiazine was virtually complete after 3 weeks, and 74%–93% recovery was obtained from the urine and faeces. Thus the polymer did not significantly retard the release of tritiated materials from the sulphadiazine injected. Without explanation, however, higher plasma levels were reported for the polymer-formulated drug 1–6 weeks postinjection. The recovery of radioactive materials over the 13-week experiment from the diaminoquinazoline was greater, 47% vs 30%, from the monkey given the pure drug mixture, than those treated with the polymer.

Overall, these experiments indicate that the diaminoquinazoline possesses repository activity which may be enhanced by formulation with a polymer. However, more work is needed to evaluate the possible advantages of a polymer formulation. In addition, the drug needs to be used with a sulphonamide or sulphone, and much more work is required to find a system which will provide an acceptable, simultaneous release of the two agents.

E. Closing Comments

The advantages of an agent that would protect from infection over an entire transmission season seem obvious. However, the inherent problems involved have, so far, prevented the successful development and implementation of such an agent. Perhaps one of the greatest needs is the intimate cooperation of people from several diverse disciplines, such as polymer chemistry, bioengineering, parasitology, pharmacokinetics, and malariology. With the continued concern for increased exposure to malaria and the advances and heightened cooperation between these disciplines, the eventual development of repository agents for chemoprophylaxis seems likely.

References

Black RH, Hennessy WB, McMillian B (1966) Studies on depot antimalarials: 2. The effect of a single injection of the depot antimalarial CI-564 on relapsing vivax malaria acquired in New Guinea. Med J Austr 2:808–811

Bruce-Chwatt LJ (1977) Prolonged malaria prophylaxis. Br Med J 2:1287

Chandrasekaran SK, Benson H, Urquhart J (1978) Methods to achieve controlled drug delivery, the biomedical approach. In: Robinson JR (ed) Sustained and controlled release drug delivery systems. Dekker, New York, pp 557–593

Chien YW (1978) Methods to achieve sustained drug delivery. The physical approach: implants. In: Robinson JR (ed) Sustained and controlled release drug delivery systems. Dekker, New York, pp 211–349
Chien YW, Lambert HJ, Grant DE (1974) Controlled release from polymeric devices I: Technique for rapid *in vitro* release studies. J Pharm Sci 63:365–369
Chin W, Lunn JS, Buxbaum J, Contacos PG (1965) The effect of cycloguanil pamoate (CI-501) against a chlorguanide-resistant Chesson strain of *Plasmodium vivax*. Am J Trop Med Hyg 14:922–924
Chin W, Contacos PG, Coatney GR, Jeter MH, Alpert E (1967a) Evaluation of CI-564, a 1:1 mixture of cycloguanil pamoate (CI-501) and 4,4′-diacetylaminodiphenylsulfone (CI-556), against multiresistant falciparum malarias. Am J Trop Med Hyg 16:580–584
Chin W, Coatney GR, King HK (1967b) An evaluation of CI-564 against blood-induced chlorguanide-sensitive and chlorguanide-resistant strains of vivax malaria. Am J Trop Med Hyg 16:13–14
Choulis NH, Papadopoulos H (1975) Timed-release tablets containing quinine sulfate. J Pharm Sci 64:1033–1035
Coatney GR, Contacos PG, Lunn JS, Kilpatrick JW, Elder HA (1963) The effect of a repository preparation of the dihydrotriazine metabolite of chlorguanide, CI-501, against the Chesson strain of *Plasmodium vivax* in man. Am J Trop Med Hyg 12:504–508
Coatney GR, Contacos PG, Lunn JS (1964) Further observations on the antimalarial activity of CI-501 (Camolar®) against the Chesson strain of vivax malaria. Am J Trop Med Hyg 13:383–385
Contacos PG, Coatney GR, Lunn JS, Kilpatrick JW (1964) The antimalarial activity of CI-501 (Camolar®) against falciparum malaria. Am J Trop Med Hyg 13:386–390
Contacos PG, Coatney GR, Lunn JS, Chin J (1965) Resistance to cycloguanil pamoate (CI-501) by falciparum malaria in West Pakistan. Am J Trop Med Hyg 14:925–926
Contacos PG, Coatney GR, Lunn JS, Chin W (1966) The urinary excretion and the antimalarial activity of CI-501 (Cycloguanil-pamoate, Camolar®) against vivax and falciparum malaria. Am J Trop Med Hyg 15:281–286
Desjardins RE, Canfield CJ, Haynes JD, Chulay JD (1979a) Quantitative assessment of antimalarial activity *in vitro* by a semiautomated microdilution technique. Antimicrob Agents Chemother 16:710–718
Desjardins RE, Pamplin CL, von Bredlow J, Berry KG, Canfield CJ (1979b) Kinetics of a new antimalarial, mefloquine. Clin Pharmacol Ther 26:372–379
Doberstyn EB, Phintuyothin P, Noeypatimanondh S, Teerakiartkamjorn (1979) Single-dose therapy of falciparum malaria with mefloquine or pyrimethamine-sulfadoxine. Bull WHO 57:275–279
Elslager EF (1969) Progress in malaria chemotherapy Part 1. Repository antimalarial drugs. Prog Drug Res 13:171–212
Elslager EF (1974) New perspectives on the chemotherapy of malaria, filariasis, and leprosy. Prog Drug Res 18:99–172
Elslager EF, Worth DF (1966) Pyrimidine compounds. U.S. Patent 3,236,849
Elslager EF, Gavrilis ZB, Phillips AA, Worth DF (1969a) Repository drugs. IV. 4′,4‴-Sulfonylbisacetanilide (acedapsone, DADDS) and related sulfanilylanilides with prolonged antimalarial and antileprotic action. J Med Chem 12:357–363
Elslager EF, Phillips AA, Worth DF (1969b) Repository drugs. V. 4′,4‴-[*p*-Phenylenebis(methylidyneimino-*p*-phenylenesulfonyl)]bisacetanilide (PSBA) and related 4′,4‴-[bis(imino-*p*-phenylenesulfonyl)]bisanilides, a novel class of long-acting antimalarial and antileprotic agents. J Med Chem 12:363–367
Elslager EF, Capps DB, Worth DF (1969c) Repository drugs. VII. *N*-Allylidene-4,4′-sulfonyldianiline and *N*-(benzylidene and -1-naphthylmethylene)-*N*′-methylene-4,4′-sulfonyldianiline polymers with prolonged antimalarial and antileprotic action. J Med Chem 12:597–599
Elslager EF, Tendick FH, Werbel LM (1969d) Repository drugs. VIII. Ester and amide congeners of amodiaquine, hydroxychloroquine, oxychloroquine, primaquine, quinacrine, and related substances as potential long-acting antimalarial agents. J Med Chem 12:600–607

Elslager EF, Hutt MP, Jacob P, Johnson J, Temporelli B, Werbel LM, Worth DF (1979) Folate antagonists. 15. 2,4-Diamino-6-(2-naphthylsulfonyl)quinazolines and related 2,4-diamino-6-[(phenyl and naphthyl)-sulfinyl and sulfonyl]quinazolines, a potent new class of antimetabolites with phenomenal antimalarial activity. J Med Chem 22:1247–1257

Flynn GL, Smith EW (1971) Membrane diffusion I: design and testing of a new multi-featured diffusion cell. J Pharm Sci 60:1713–1717

Fu JC, Kale AK, Moyer DL (1973) Drug-incorporated silicone discs as sustained release capsules. I. Chloroquine diphosphate. J Biomed Mater Res 7:71–78

Grindel JM, Tilton PF, Shaffer RD (1977) Quantitation of the antimalarial agent, mefloquine, in blood, plasma, and urine using high-pressure liquid chromatography. J Pharm Sci 66:834–837

Hawking F, Perry WLM (1948) Activation of paludrine. Br J Pharm 3:320–325

Judge BM, Howells RE (1979a) A comparison of the response of *Plasmodium berghei* to primaquine diphosphate following drug administration by repeated daily injections and by a constant release system. Trans R Soc Trop Med Hyg 73:327–328

Judge BM, Howells RE (1979b) The use of drug polymer mixture implants for sustained antimalarial effects in mice. Br Soc Parasitol Proc 79:ii–iii

Korolkovas A, Ferreira EI, Lima JD, Krettli AU (1978) Antimalarial activity of saccharidic polymers of dapsone and sulfadimethoxine. Chemotherapy 24:231–235

Laboratory of Malaria Research, Shanghai Institute of Parasitic Diseases (1975) Preliminary studies on tripiperaquine (M1020). Chin Med J (Engl) 1:419–424

Peters W (1978) Medical aspects – comments and discussion II. Symp Br Soc Parasitol 16:25–40

Pinazzi C, Rabadeux JC, Pleurdeau A, Niviere P, Paubel JP, Benoit JP (1978) Synthesis and polymerization of polymethacrylates containing the quinine residue. Comparative study of the toxicity and immunogenicity of the free and polymeric form. Makromol Chem 179:1699–1706

Powell RD, Brewer GJ, DeGowin RL, Alving AS (1964) Studies on a strain of chloroquine-resistant *Plasmodium falciparum* from Vietnam. Bull WHO 31:379–392

Powell RD, DeGowin RL, Eppes RB (1965) Studies on the antimalarial effects of cycloguanil pamoate (CI-501) in man. Am J Trop Med Hyg 14:913–921

Rieckmann KH, Trenholme GM, Williams RL, Carson PE, Frischer H, Desjardins RE (1974) Prophylactic activity of mefloquine hydrochloride (WR 142490) in drug-resistant malaria. Bull WHO 51:375–377

Ritschel WA, Hammer GV, Thompson GA (1978) Pharmacokinetics of antimalarials and proposals for dosage regimens. Int J Clin Pharmacol 16:395–401

Robinson JR (1978) Sustained and controlled release drug delivery systems. Dekker, New York

Rozman RS, Canfield CJ (1979) New experimental antimalarial drugs. In: Garattini S, Goldin A, Hawking F, Kopkin IJ (eds) Advances in pharmacology and chemotherapy, vol 16. Academic, New York, pp 31–32

Russell DA, Worth RM, Jano B, Fasal P, Shepard C (1979) Acedapsone in the prevention of leprosy: field trial in three high prevalence villages in Micronesia. Am J Trop Hyg 28:559–563

Schmidt LH (1973) Infections with *Plasmodium falciparum* and *Plasmodium vivax* in the owl monkey – model systems for basic biological and chemotherapeutic studies. Trans R Soc Trop Med Hyg 67:446–470

Schmidt LH, Rossan RN, Fisher KF (1963) The activity of a repository form of 4,6-diamino-1-(*p*-chlorophenyl)-1,2-dihydro-2,2-dimethyl-*s*-triazine against infections with *Plasmodium cynomolgi*. Am J Trop Med Hyg 12:494–503

Schneider J, Bonury M, Le Quellac J (1965) *Plasmodium berghei* et chimiotherapie. Ann Soc Belg Med Trop 45:435–439

Schofield P, Howells RE, Peters W (1981) A technique for the selection of long-acting antimalarial compounds using a rodent malarial model. Ann Trop Med Parasitol 74:521–531

Sodeman TM, Contacos PG, Collins WE, Smith CS, Jumper JR (1972) Studies on the prophylactic and radical curative activity of RC-12 against *Plasmodium cynomolgi* in *Macaca mulatta*. Bull WHO 47:425–428

Thompson PE, Olszewski BJ, Elslager EF, Worth DF (1963) Laboratory studies on 4,6-diamino-*l*-(*p*-chlorophenyl)-1,2-dihydro-2,2-dimethyl-*s*-triazine pamoate (CI-501) as a repository antimalarial drug. Am J Trop Med Hyg 12:481–493

Thompson PE, Olszewski B, Waitz JA (1965a) Laboratory studies on the repository antimalarial activity of 4,4′-diacetylaminodiphenylsulfone, alone and mixed with cycloguanil pamoate (CI-501). Am J Trop Med Hyg 14:343–353

Thompson PE, Bayles A, Olszewski B, Waitz JA (1965b) Studies on a dihydrotriazine and sulfone, alone and in combination, against *Plasmodium berghei* in mice. Am J Trop Med Hyg 14:198–206

Thompson PE, Waitz JA, Olszewski B (1965c) The repository antimalarial activities of 4,4′-diacetylaminodiphenylsulfone and cycloguanil pamoate (CI-501) in monkeys relative to local release following parenteral administration. J Parasitol 51:343–349

Thompson PE, Bayles A, Olszewski B (1970) Antimalarial activity of 2,4-diamino-6-[(3,4-dichlorobenzyl)nitros-amino]quinazoline (CI-679 base) and CI-679 acetate, laboratory studies in mice and rhesus monkeys. Am J Trop Med Hyg 19:12–26

Werbel LM, Jacobs RL, Steinkampf RW, Worth DF (1981) Repository effects of 2,4-diamino-6-(2-naphthylsulfonyl)quinazoline in mice. Personal observations

Werbel LM, Jacobs RL, Steinkampf RW, Worth DF (1981b) Repository antimalarial activity of pyrimethamine pamoate. Am J Trop Med Hyg, Submitted for publication

Wise DL, McCormick GJ, Willet GP, Anderson LC (1976) Sustained release of an antimalarial drug using a copolymer of glycolic/lactic acid. Life Sci 19:867–874

Wise DL, McCormick GJ, Willet GP, Anderson LC, Howes JF (1978) Sustained release of sulfadiazine. J Pharm Pharmac 30:686–689

Wise DL, Gresser JD, McCormick GJ (1979a) Sustained release of a dual antimalarial system. J Pharm Pharmacol 31:201–204

Wise DL, Fellman TD, Sanderson JE, Wentworth RL (1979b) Lactic/glycolic acid polymers. In: Gregoriades G (ed) Drug carriers in biology and medicine. Academic, London, pp 237–270

Wiselogle FY (1946) A survey of antimalarial drugs, 1941–1945, 2 Vols. Ann Arbor, Michigan

World Health Organization (1967) Chemotherapy of malaria, Report of a WHO scientific group. WHO Tech Rept Ser No 375

Worth DF, Elslager EF, Phillips AA (1969) Repository drugs. VI. 4′-[*N*-(aralkylidene-, -benzylidene-, and -naphthylidene)sulfanilyl]anilides, 4′-[*N*-[(dimethylamino)methylene]sulfanilyl]anilides, and related sulfanilylanilides with prolonged antimalarial and leprotic action. J Med Chem 12:591–596

CHAPTER 8

Cell Targeting of Primaquine

A. TROUET, P. PIRSON, R. BAURAIN, and M. MASQUELIER

A. Introduction

Primaquine, 6-methoxy-8-(4′-amino-1′-methylbutyl-amino)quinoline (PQ), is still the drug of choice for the complete eradication of the exoerythrocytic liver forms of *Plasmodium vivax* and *Plasmodium ovale* (BRUCE-CHWATT 1980). The clinical use of PQ as a causal prophylactic and therapeutic agent is, however, curtailed by its toxic side effects, especially for those patients having glucose-6-phosphate dehydrogenase-deficient erythrocytes (TARLOV et al. 1962). Much research has, therefore, been pursued in the hope of developing new 8-aminoquinoline derivatives possessing a higher therapeutic index.

TROUET (1978) proposed that the selectivy and the therapeutic activity of antiprotozoal drugs such as PQ would be improved significantly by associating them with lysosomotropic carrier molecules. This concept of targeting drugs with the help of selective carriers relies on the observation that cells possess at their surface receptors which interact selectively with ligands present in the extracellular medium. After binding to the receptor these ligands are taken up by endocytosis and transferred into or through the lysosomes (SCHNEIDER et al. 1981). If a drug is adequately linked to such a ligand, it will inherit its selectivity. Several criteria must, however, be fulfilled by the ligand and the drug-carrier conjugate before such a drug targeting effect can be achieved. The ligand or carrier should recognise as selectively as possible a given cell type, be endocytosed after interaction with the cell surface and be transferred into the lysosomes. The association between the drug and the carrier should remain stable in the bloodstream and the extracellular fluids, and the drug has to remain inactive while it is carried from its site of administration to its site of action. This linkage between the drug and the carrier should, on the other hand, be reversible in the presence of lysosomal hydrolases and, if this condition is fulfilled, the drug will be released in an active form inside the lysosomes of the target cells after endocytosis of the drug-carrier conjugate. The drug itself should be resistant to the lysosomal enzymes and be able to exert its pharmacological effect inside the lysosomes or be able to diffuse in the other cell compartments. The drug carrier conjugate should finally be non-immunogenic and gain access to the target cells by its ability to cross the anatomical barriers which it will encounter after its administration. This latter condition implies that the lysosomotropic drug carriers will require parenteral routes of administration since they are very unlikely to be taken up by the gastrointestinal tract. Infections of the central nervous system will not benefit either from this type of targeted therapy since the blood-brain bar-

Table 1. Criteria to be fulfilled by a lysosomotropic drug-carrier conjugate

The carrier should be:
1. Selective for the target cell surface
2. Endocytosed by the target cell and be transferred into the lysosomal compartment
3. Degradable
4. Non-immunogenic
5. Able to permeate through the anatomical barriers separating the administration site and the target

The drug should be resistant to lysosomal enzymes and pH.
The drug-carrier conjugate should be:
1. Stable in the bloodstream and extracellular spaces
2. Pharmacologically inactive
3. Sensitive to the lysosomal enzymes or pH such as to release the drug in an active form
4. Non-Immunogenic

rier will not allow the passage of the drug-carrier conjugate unless its permeability is altered by the infectious process. All these criteria are summarised in Table 1.

We have tried to apply this drug-carrier concept to the treatment of the intrahepatic stage of malarial infection since two carrier types seemed to be good candidates for targeting PQ to the liver. First, liposomes seem to have a tropism towards cells of the liver and spleen (SEGAL et al. 1974; KIMELBERG 1976). Moreover, sodium stibogluconate (Pentostam) included in liposomes has a greatly increased chemotherapeutic effect in experimental leishmaniasis (BLACK et al. 1977; ALVING et al. 1978; NEW et al. 1878). Glycoproteins characterised by terminal galactose sugar residues have, on the other hand, been shown by ASHWELL and MORELL (1974) to be taken up selectively by the hepatocytes through receptor-mediated endocytosis (MOREL et al. 1971; TOLLESHAUG et al. 1977). These asialoproteins can easily be prepared by removing enzymatically the terminal sialic acid residues from fetoprotein.

We have tested the lysosomotropic drug-carrier concept by analysing the chemotherapeutic properties of PQ included in liposomes on one hand, and linked to asialofetuin, on the other. As a test system we have used the mouse model with sporozoite-induced infection of *Plasmodium berghei*. The usefulness of this model for assessing the activity of PQ has been documented by PETERS (1970), GREGORY and PETERS (1970), and FINK (1974). The chemotherapeutic objective of this work on PQ-carrier conjugates was to develop a derivative of PQ which would be curative in a single-dose treatment of *P. berghei*-infected mice. Since this cannot be reached with PQ due to its toxicity, this goal could be achieved either by decreasing the toxicity of PQ or by increasing its chemotherapeutic activity, and both effects can be expected if a true lysosomotropic PQ-carrier conjugate is developed.

B. Chemotherapy Methods

I. Experimental Malaria Infection

P. berghei sporozoites (Anka strain) were isolated from *Anopheles stephensi* as described by PIRSON et al. (1980), 18 days after a blood meal on parasitised mice.

Within 35 min of the dissection of the mosquitoes, 10,000–30,000 sporozoites were injected intravenously into male TB_{ESP} mice weighing between 18 and 22 g.

II. Chemotherapeutic and Toxicity Parameters

After inoculation of the sporozoites and drug administration the mice were kept for a maximum of 50 days. The infection rate (number of infected mice/total number of mice) was assessed daily by checking Giemsa-stained blood smears. The number of days that the mice survived was used to calculate the median survival time (MST), and the percentage of increase in life span (ILS) was calculated as follows: (MST treated/MST control $-1) \times 100$. The percentage of long-term survivors (LTS) was established at the end of the 50-days observation period. Dose-dependent drug efficacy, expressed as CPD_{50} (causal prophylactic activity), was calculated from the relationship between cure rate and the dose administered.

The overall toxicity of PQ and its derivatives was estimated by determining the dose that kills 50% of non-infected mice (LD_{50}). The data were calculated by logit weighted transformation. The maximal tolerated dose (MTD) was defined as the highest dose that induces a weight loss of less than 5% in non-infected animals.

III. Primaquine

Stock solutions of primaquine diphosphate at 5 and 10 mg/ml were prepared in sterile phosphate buffered saline, the pH being finally adjusted to 7.2 with 0.1 *M* KOH.

C. Primaquine Entrapped in Liposomes

Liposomes have already been widely studied as drug carriers and have the great advantage that a large variety of drugs can be entrapped in them without major technical or chemical problems (Gregoriadis 1979).

I. Preparation of Primaquine Liposomes

Small multilamellar liposomes were prepared according to the method of Bangham et al. (1974) and PQ was entrapped in their aqueous phase as described by Pirson et al. (1980). The liposomes consisted of phosphatidyl choline, phosphatidyl serine and cholesterol in a molar ratio of 4 : 1 : 5 and incorporated 97 ± 11 g PQ/mol total lipids. Radioactively labelled PQ liposomes were prepared by using ^{3}H-labelled primaquine diphosphate, with a specific radioactivity 0f 4 mCi/mmol, obtained by catalytic exchange of tritium.

II. Toxicity and Therapeutic Activity

When injected intravenously into TB_{ESP} mice PQ liposomes were about 3.6 times less toxic than PQ with regard to the LD_{50} and about 4.3 times less in terms of MTD (Table 2). Empty liposomes are not toxic and do not modify the toxicity of PQ when given together with the drug.

Table 2. Toxicity of primaquine and its derivatives

Drug[a]	MTD[b]	LD_{50}[c]
Primaquine	24.6	38.6
PQ-liposomes	105.4	138.8
Leu-PQ	38.6	50.9
Ala-Leu-PQ	50.9	72.0
Ala-Leu-Ala-Leu-PQ	≧ 50.9	≧ 72.0

[a] All doses are expressed in milligrams PQ diphosphate equivalents/kg body wt
[b] Maximal tolerated dose
[c] Dose killing 50% of the TB_{ESP} mice

Table 3. Antimalarial activity of primaquine free and entrapped in liposomes

Drug[a]	Dose[b] (mg/kg)	ILS (%)	LTS/N[c]	CPD_{50}[d]	TI[e]
Controls	–	0	0/178	–	–
Primaquine	6.25	46	0/6	22.5	1.7
	12.5	58	11/33		
	15.0	166	10/23		
	20.0	110	25/55		
	25.0	> 320	50/94		
	30.0	91[f]	2/9		
PQ-liposomes	20	109	4/14	26.7	5.2
	25	255	9/18		
	30	273	10/20		
	40	> 355	21/24		
	60	> 355	8/8		
	70	> 355	12/12		
Liposomes[g]	–	0	0/12	–	–

[a] Drugs were given intravenously 3 h after inoculation of the *P. berghei* sporozoites to TB_{ESP} mice
[b] Dose expressed in milligrams PQ diphosphate/kg body wt
[c] Long-term survivors over the number of mice treated
[d] Causal prophylactic dose for 50% of the mice
[e] Therapeutic index: ratio of LD_{50} over CPD_{50}
[f] Toxic dose
[g] At the concentration of 0.7 mmol total lipids/kg corresponding to the lipid amount of the 100% curative dose of PQ liposomes

The best therapeutic effect with PQ and PQ liposomes was obtained when mice were treated 3 h after the sporozoites inoculation. As shown by the results summarised in Table 3 the optimal dose of free PQ was 25 mg/kg, which induced an ILS in excess of 320% and about 50% long-term survivors. At 30 mg/kg PQ was toxic and it was therefore impossible to obtain a 100% cure rate with PQ given as a single i.v. injection. At doses up to 25 mg/kg PQ liposomes had an activity equal to that of PQ but their lower toxicity allowed the administration of single curative doses of about 60 mg/kg.

No significant residual therapeutic activity could be demonstrated on the erythrocytic stage of the infection, and the curative effect of PQ liposomes was thus a true prophylactic activity against the exoerythrocytic stage of *P. berghei.*

III. Pharmacokinetics and Tissue Distribution

As described previously by TROUET et al. (1981), when PQ was injected i.v. as PQ liposomes, 45% of it was eliminated in a first rapid phase with a half-life of 48 s, while the remaining PQ disappeared more slowly from the plasma with a half-life of 7.9 min. PQ entrapped in liposomes was eliminated more slowly from the plasma than free PQ, the concentration of which fell to 15% of its initial value within 1 min, with an estimated half-life of 17 s. During the first 20 min after the administration of PQ liposomes there was a discrepancy between the levels of PQ and the associated lipid constituents of the liposomes, indicating that ±10% of the primaquine entrapped inside the liposomes became rapidly dissociated upon intravenous injection. When PQ was mixed with empty liposomes it disappeared from the plasma exactly as the free drug.

Distribution of PQ in various tissues was determined 20 and 120 min after one i.v. administration of [^{3}H]-PQ and [^{3}H]-PQ liposomes as described by TROUET et

Table 4. Concentration of [^{3}H] primaquine in selected tissues after i.v. administration of free and entrapped drug

Tissues	Time [a]	Free primaquine [b]	Primaquine-liposomes [b]
Liver	20	589± 113	907± 53
	120	530± 62	882± 56
Spleen	20	616± 65	1,960±430
	120	364± 26	1,400±120
Heart	20	257± 64	52± 29
	120	286± 62	42± 19
Kidney	20	382± 58	103± 21
	120	523± 57	114± 9
Lungs	20	3,706±1,250	267± 36
	120	3,538±1,560	118± 24
Stomach	20	63± 16	62± 16
	120	37± 5	84± 31
Duodenum	20	38± 9	38± 10
	120	15± 3	54± 30
Rectum	20	131± 79	22± 8
	120	35± 24	45± 21
Brain	20	23± 2	6
	120	4± 1	4
Muscles	20	28± 2	0
	120	5± 1	0

[a] Sampling time in minutes after i.v. administration of the drug
[b] Results are expressed in pmoles primaquine equivalents/mg proteins. Means ±SE of six experiments

al. (1981). The amount of [^{3}H]-PQ found in the tissues was corrected for the [^{3}H]-PQ still present in the contaminating blood, and the amount of PQ-associated radioactivity found in the tissues was expressed as picomoles of primaquine/per milligram of tissue protein. The results given in Table 4 indicate that the concentration of PQ was about doubled in the liver and increased more significantly in the spleen when it was administered as PQ liposomes. These results are in accordance with several reports from the literature indicating that intravenously injected liposomes are mainly concentrated by spleen and liver both of which are rich in phagocytic cells (KIMELBERG 1976; RAHMAN et al. 1974; STEGER and DESNICK 1977). Moreover, more than 50% of the liposomes trapped by the liver are taken up by the Kupffer cells (FREISE et al. 1980). When injected entrapped in liposomes PQ is, on the other hand, less concentrated in heart, kidneys, lungs, muscles, and brain, the most striking decrease being observed in the lungs, heart, and muscles.

IV. Discussion

Trapping of PQ in liposomes results in important changes in the pharmacokinetics and tissue distribution parameters of PQ. The reduced toxicity of PQ liposomes can be related to the lower uptake of PQ by tissues such as lung, brain, heart, and muscle. This decreased uptake is probably related to the poor phagocytic activity of tissues such as the heart and muscles and to the existence of anatomical barriers impermeable to the liposomes, such as in the case of the brain and, perhaps, the lungs.

The chemotherapeutic activity of PQ is not increased by trapping it in liposomes even if the concentration in the liver is slightly increased. However, liposomes and their PQ content are more precisely targeted towards the Kupffer cells and the concentration of PQ will probably not be increased in the hepatocytes themselves.

The main therapeutic advantage of PQ liposomes is thus the result of a reduced overall toxicity. The therapeutic index of PQ liposomes is, as a consequence, about three times higher than that of PQ, allowing the injection of a higher, single dose of PQ which is able to cure 100% of the infected mice.

D. Primaquine Linked to Asialofetuin

The linkage of PQ to proteins by a covalent bond is much more difficult to achieve in view of the various criteria to be met by a lysosomotropic drug-carrier conjugate (Table 1). Primaquine can be linked via its free NH_2 group to a carboxylic side chain of the carrier protein by formation of an amide bond. This is, however, not an ideal substrate for peptidases and the carrier molecule may well cause steric hindrance. A similar problem was encountered when the antitumour drug daunorubicin was linked to protein carriers. The major problem was indeed to obtain an amide bond between the NH_2 group of daunorubicin and the protein which would be hydrolysed by lysosomal enzymes and restore active daunorubicin with a free NH_2 group (TROUET et al. 1982). This problem was successfully solved by intercalating between the NH_2 group of daunorubicin and the protein carrier the tetrapeptidic spacer arm, alanyl-leucyl-alanyl-leucyl. To obtain a good hydrolysis rate it is very important that the first amino acid linked to the drug is a leucine (MASQUELIER et al. 1980). Without repeating with PQ all the preliminary experiments performed with daunorubicin we synthesised as a first step the tetrapeptide derivative of PQ, using leucyl-PQ (leu-PQ) and alanyl-leucyl-PQ (ala-leu-PQ) as intermediates. As a second step we linked alanyl-leucyl-alanyl-leucyl-PQ (ala-leu-ala-leu-PQ) to asialofetuin but we also tested the toxic and chemotherapeutic properties of the amino acid and peptide derivatives of PQ.

I. Amino Acid and Peptide Derivatives of Primaquine

1. Methods of Synthesis

N-L-leucyl-primaquine was synthesised from primaquine base and *N*-carboxyanhydride of L-leucine as described for the synthesis of *N*-L-leucyl-daunorubicin by MASQUELIER et al. (1980). *N*-L-alanyl-L-leucyl-primaquine was obtained by reacting leu-PQ with the *N*-trityl-L-alaninate of *N*-hydroxysuccinimide (STELAKATOS et al. 1959; ANDERSON et al. 1964). *N*-L-alanyl-L-leucyl-L-alanyl-L-leucyl-primaquine was synthesised, like ala-leu-PQ, by using ala-leu-PQ and leu-ala-leu-PQ successively as starting material.

2. Toxicity and Therapeutic Activity

Leu-PQ was slightly less toxic than PQ (1.3–1.5 times) both in terms of MTD and LD_{50} values, while ala-leu-PQ and ala-leu-ala-leu-PQ were two times less toxic than PQ (Table 2).

The therapeutic activity of leu-PQ was very close to that of PQ, with a slightly higher CPD_{50} value (Table 5). The lower toxicity of leu-PQ permitted, however, the injection of 35 mg/kg of PQ equivalents, which cured about 75% of the infected animals as compared with the 50% after administration of PQ.

Ala-leu-PQ and ala-leu-ala-leu-PQ were more active than PQ since their CPD_{50} values were respectively 1.4 and 1.8 times lower than those of PQ. This higher activity combined with a lower toxicity resulted in a 100% cure rate being achieved with 35 mg/kg of PQ equivalents. This was half the dose of PQ required when administered inside liposomes (Table 3).

3. Hydrolysis in the Presence of Serum and Lysosomal Hydrolases

In an attempt to understand the interesting chemotherapeutic properties of ala-leu-PQ and ala-leu-ala-leu-PQ and to check to what extent they can be considered as prodrugs of PQ, we examined their hydrolysis into PQ in the presence of serum and of lysosomal hydrolases since serum and lysosomes are the most likely sites where they are susceptible to transformation enzymatically into their parent drug.

The drugs were incubated in the presence of 10% calf serum at pH 7.5 and in the presence of a purified lysosomal fraction at pHs 4.5 and 6. The appearance of digestion products and of the parent compound was monitored by high-pressure liquid chromatography according to the method described by TROUET et al. (1981).

While in the presence of serum leu-PQ was stable, while ala-leu-PQ was slowly transformed into leu-PQ, 50% being transformed after 15 min and 80% after 60

Table 5. Antimalarial activity of aminoacid and peptide derivatives of primaquine

Drug [a]	Dose [b] (mg/kg)	ILS (%)	LTS/N [c]	CPD_{50} [d]	TI [e]
Controls	–	0	0/184	–	–
Leu-PQ	7	0	0/9	25.9	1.9
	20	32	2/15		
	25	100	7/14		
	30	58	7/20		
	35	> 163	15/20		
	40	106 [f]	7/14		
Ala-leu-PQ	10.9	33	3/27	16.4	4.5
	12.5	> 194	5/9		
	17.5	> 194	16/27		
	25.0	> 194	9/9		
	31.5	> 194	22/27		
	35.0	> 194	18/18		
Ala-leu-Ala-Leu-PQ	6.25	20	0/7	12.3	> 5.9
	12.5	> 194	8/14		
	25.0	> 194	12/14		
	31.5	> 194	8/8		

[a] Drugs were given intravenously 3 h after inoculation of the *P. berghei* sporozoites to male TB_{ESP} mice
[b] Doses are expressed in milligrams PQ diphosphate equivalents/kg body wt
[c] Long-term survivors over the number of mice treated
[d] Dose curing 50% of the treated mice (causal prophylactic dose 50%)
[e] Therapeutic index: ratio of LD_{50} over CPD_{50}
[f] Toxic dose

min. In the presence of lysosomal enzymes, however, leu-PQ, ala-leu-PQ and ala-leu-ala-leu-PQ were rapidly hydrolysed into PQ; 85%–100% were converted into PQ within 4–12 min (TROUET et al. 1981).

4. Discussion

Quite unexpectedly the amino acid or peptide derivatives of PQ display interesting chemotherapeutic properties. The elucidation of the cellular mechanisms and pharmacokinetic properties which could explain these results requires more detailed in vivo tissue distribution studies. We suggest, however, that since the activity of leu-PQ is very similar to that of PQ, it is either active by itself or has to be hydrolysed into PQ within the cells, most probably within the lysosomes, and it could in this latter case be acting as a prodrug of PQ. In any case, its lower toxicity could result from an altered uptake by different tissues and cells resulting from the additional leucyl group.

Ala-leu-PQ and ala-leu-ala-leu-PQ are even more probably prodrugs which have to be hydrolysed into PQ or leu-PQ before becoming active. This activation could occur either in the serum, inside the cells or in both on the basis of the in vitro hydrolysis experiments. Here again, and more than for leu-PQ, the differential cellular uptake and tissue distribution of these derivatives could explain their interesting chemotherapeutic properties.

II. Asialofetuin-Primaquine Conjugates

Primaquine was subsequently linked to asialofetuin (ASF) with the intercalation of the tetrapeptide ala-leu-ala-leu between the drug and the carrier protein. As described above, ASF is a glycoprotein with terminal galactose sugar residues which is selectively recognised and taken up by hepatocytes (ASHWELL and MORELL 1974; MORELL et al. 1971; TOLLESHAUG et al. 1977).

1. Methods of Synthesis

Asialofetuin was prepared by the action of *Clostridium perfringens* neuraminidase on a calf fetuin (Sigma Chemicals, St. Louis, Mo) as described by CORFIELD et al. (1978). The ASF thus obtained retained less than 10% of its original sialic acid residues. A first conjugate (succ-ASF-ala-leu-ala-leu-PQ) was prepared by succinylating at a first step 85% of the ε-amino lysine residues of the protein, and linking subsequently the tetrapeptide-PQ in the presence of carbodiimide. A binding ratio of five to six PQ molecules per molecule of ASF was consistently obtained.

A second conjugate (ASF-ala-leu-ala-leu-PQ) involving a minimal modification of the carrier protein was prepared by linking succinyl-ala-leu-ala-leu-PQ to ASF at a drug/protein molar ratio varying between 5 and 8.

2. Therapeutic Activity

ASF-ala-leu-ala-leu-PQ cured 100% of the infected mice at a dose of 25 mg PQ/kg and 50% of the animals could be cured with doses close to 10 mg/kg (Table 6). This conjugate was thus definitely more active than PQ and PQ liposomes.

Succ-ASF-ala-leu-ala-leu-PQ was, on the other hand, significantly less active and less toxic than PQ since it did not cure all the animals even at 50 mg/kg.

Table 6. Antimalarial activity of asialofetuin-primaquine conjugates

Drug[a]	Dose[b] (mg/kg)	ILS (%)	LTS/N[c]	CPD_{50}[d]
Controls	–	0	0/45	–
ASF-ala-leu-ala-leu-PQ	6.25	100	1/12	12.8
	10.0	170	5/12	
	12.5	160	7/16	
	15.0	>400	7/12	
	20	>400	5/6	
	25	>400	12/12	
Succ(ASF)-ala-leu-ala-leu-PQ	6.25	26	0/7	38.5
	12.5	68	0/7	
	25	68	1/7	
	35	>163	4/7	
	50	>163	5/8	

[a] Drugs were given intravenously 3 h after inoculation of the *P. berghei* sporozoites to male TB_{ESP} mice
[b] Doses are expressed in milligrams PQ diphosphate equivalents/kg body wt
[c] Long-term survivors over the number of treated mice
[d] Dose curing 50% of the treated mice (causal prophylactic dose 50%)

3. Discussion

The therapeutic results obtained with ASF-ala-leu-ala-leu-PQ are in accordance with the drug-carrier concept since the therapeutic effectiveness of PQ was increased and this resulted most probably from a higher concentration of the drug inside the hepatocytes. In contrast to PQ liposomes, the beneficial effect is not simply the result of a decrease in toxicity. The targeting effect of ASF-ala-leu-ala-leu-PQ was indirectly confirmed by the results obtained with succ-ASF-ala-leu-ala-leu-PQ, which was less active than PQ and than ASF-ala-leu-ala-leu-PQ. The major difference between these two conjugates was the extensive succinylation of the carrier protein in the case of succ-ASF-ala-leu-ala-leu-PQ, which most probably decreases or even destroys the specificity of ASF for the hepatocyte receptors, and thus transforms succ-ASF to a non-specific carrier. Like PQ liposomes thus later conjugate was less toxic than PQ, but it seemed to be less active than PQ liposomes, with a CPD_{50} value about 1.4 times less. This suggests that it is taken up by various tissues, with a lower specificity for the liver and spleen as compared with liposomes.

Although further studies are needed to complete the results presented here, the higher activity of ASF-ala-leu-ala-leu-PQ is most probably due to the targeting of PQ to the hepatocytes resulting from specific binding by these cells of the ASF carrier, followed by its endocytosis and the intralysosomal activation of the conjugated PQ.

E. Conclusions

Using sporozoite-induced *P. berghei* malaria in mice we have shown that it is possible to improve the chemotherapeutic index of PQ against the exoerythrocytic stage of infection, by associating or linking the drug to carriers such as liposomes or asialoglycoproteins. In both cases a 100% curative single dose of PQ could be given as the result of either a decreased toxicity when PQ was entrapped in liposomes, or of an increased therapeutic activity when the drug was linked to ASF.

When considering the various criteria listed in Table 1, we can discuss briefly how the two conjugate types comply with the conditions to be fulfilled by lysosomotropic drug-carrier conjugates. The selectivity of liposomes seems to be restricted since, if they are more selectively taken up by spleen and liver, their liver target cells are the Kupffer cells rather than the hepatocytes. Asialofetuin is more selective since it is taken up by the hepatocytes, and ASF-ala-leu-ala-leu-PQ seems to have inherited at least part of this selectivity in contrast to succ-ASF-ala-leu-ala-leu-PQ. Both carrier types, liposomes and ASF, are endocytosable and can be transferred to the lysosomes to be degraded. They will be poorly immunogenic if homologous ASF is used or if homologous proteins such as serum albumin are transformed into glycoproteins selective for hepatocytes by the addition of galactosyl residues (GLYNN 1978). ASF has access to the hepatocytes as demonstrated by the in vivo studies of ASHWELL and MORELL (1974) and MORELL et al. (1971). For liposomes, however, the ability to permeate through the capillary structures of the liver will depend very much on their size, and the small multilamellar vesicles are better suited for this purpose than the large multilamellar ones, and perhaps less than the small unilamellar vesicles (GREGORIADIS 1979; FREISE et al. 1980).

PQ liposomes are relatively stable in the bloodstream, only ±10% of PQ being released from the vesicles within the first minutes after i.v. administration. We have not yet checked the stability of ASF-ala-leu-ala-leu-PQ but, by analogy with the results obtained with daunorubicin-protein conjugates, its stability will probably be found satisfactory. As a corollary to the stability criteria, the drug conjugates are pharmacologically inactive and can be activated intracellulary after endocytosis and intralysosomal processing.

The resistance of PQ to lysosomal enzymes was not studied in vitro but can be deduced from the retained and enhanced activity of PQ associated with the carriers. The immunogenicity of the PQ-carrier conjugates remains to be checked and one should look more specifically for the occurrence of immunological, including allergic, reactions, against PQ linked to carrier proteins.

As a side product of this research, the amino acid and peptide derivatives of PQ were shown to have very interesting inherent chemotherapeutic properties.

For the future it will be very important to determine whether variations and modifications in the peptide spacer arm can modulate the speed of intralysosomal hydrolysis and thus provide us with conjugates and peptide derivatives characterised by a much slower rate of activation which could be used for prophylaxis.

Acknowledgements. This investigation received financial support from the UNDP/World Bank/WHO Special Programme for Research and Training in Tropical Diseases.

References

Alving CR, Steck E, Chapman WL, Waits VB, Hendricks LD, Schwartz GM, Hanson WL (1978) Therapy of leishmaniasis: superior efficacies of liposome encapsulated drugs. Proc Natl Acad Sci USA 75:2959–2963

Anderson GW, Zimmerman JE, Callahan FM (1964) The use of esters of *n*-hydroxysuccinimide in peptide synthesis. J Am Chem Soc 86:1839–1842

Ashwell G, Morell AG (1974) The role of surface carbohydrates in the hepatic recognition and transport of circulating glycoproteins. Adv Enzymol 41:99–128

Bangham AD, Hill MW, Miller NGA (1974) Preparation and use of liposomes as models of biological membranes. In: Korn S (ed) Methods in membrane biology, vol I. Plenum, New York, pp 1–68

Black CDV, Watson GJ, Ward RJ (1977) The use of Pentostam liposomes in the chemotherapy of experimental leishmaniasis. Trans R Soc Trop Med Hyg 71:550–552

Bruce-Chwatt LJ (1980) Essential malariology; chapter 8 Chemotherapy and chemoprophylaxis, William Heinemann Medical Books, London, pp 169–208

Corfield AP, Beau JM, Schauer R (1978) Desialylation of glycoconjugates using immobilized *Vibrio cholerae* neuraminidase preparation, properties and use of the bound enzyme. Hoppe Seylers Z Physiol Chem 359:1335–1342

Fink E (1974) Assessment of causal prophylactic activity in *Plasmodium berghei yoelii* and its value for the development of new antimalarial drugs. Bull WHO 50:213–222

Freise J, Muller WH, Brolsch C, Schmidt FN (1980) In vivo distribution of liposomes between parenchymal and non-parenchymal cells in rat liver. Biomed J 32:118–123

Glynn W (1978) Effect of reductive lactosamination on the hepatic uptake of bovine pancreatic ribonuclease A dimer. J Biol Chem 253:2070–2072

Gregoriadis G (1979) Liposomes. In: Gregoriadis G (ed) Drug carriers and medicine. Academic, London, pp 287–341

Gregory KG, Peters W (1970) The chemotherapy of rodent malaria. IX. Causal prophylaxis. Part I: a method for demonstrating drug action on exo-erythrocytic stages. Ann Trop Med Parasitol 64:15–24

Kimelberg HK (1976) Differential distribution of liposome-entrapped [^{3}H]-methotrexate and labelled lipids after intravenous injection in a primate. Biochim Biophys Acta 448:531–550

Masquelier M, Baurain R, Trouet A (1980) Amino acid and dipeptide derivatives of daunorubicin. I. Synthesis, physicochemical properties and lysosomal digestion. J Med Chem 24:1166–1170

Morell AG, Gregoriadis G, Scheinberg IH, Hickman J, Ashwell G (1971) The role of sialic acid in determining the survival of glycoproteins in the circulation. J Biol Chem 246:1461–1467

New RRC, Chance ML, Thomas SC, Peters W (1978) Antileishmanial activity of antimonial entrapped in liposomes. Nature 272:55–56

Peters W (1970) Chemotherapy and drug resistance in malaria. Academic, New York

Pirson P, Steiger RF, Trouet A, Gillet J, Herman F (1980) Primaquine liposomes in the chemotherapy of experimental murine malaria. Ann Trop Med Parasitol 74:384–391

Rahman YE, Rosenthal MW, Cerny EA, Moretti ES (1974) Preparation and prolonged tissue retention of liposome encapsulated chelating agents. J Lab Clin Med 83:640–646

Schneider YJ, Octave JN, Limet JN, Trouet A (1981) Functional relationship between cell surface and lysosomes during pinocytosis. In: Schweiger HG (ed) International Cell Biology 1980–1981. Springer, Berlin Heidelberg New York, pp 590–600

Segal AW, Wills EJ, Richmond JE, Slavin G, Black CDV, Gregoriadis G (1974) Morphological observation on the cellular and subcellular destination of intravenously administered liposomes. Br J Exp Pathol 55:320–327

Steger LD, Desnick RJ (1977) Enzyme therapy. VI. Comparative in vivo fates and effects on lysosomal integrity of enzyme entrapped in negatively and positively charged liposomes. Biochim Biophys Acta 464:530–546

Stelakatos GC, Theodoropoulos DM, Zervas L (1959) On the trityl method for peptide synthesis. J Am Chem Soc 81:2884–2887

Tarlov AR, Brewer GJ, Carson PE, Alving AG (1962) Primaquine sensitivity. Arch Intern Med 109:209–234

Tolleshaug H, Berg T, Nilsson M, Norum KR (1977) Uptake and degradation of ^{125}I-labelled asialofetuin by isolated rat hepatocytes. Biochim Biophys Acta 499:73–84

Trouet A (1978) Increased selectivity of drugs by linking to carriers. Eur J Cancer 14:105–111

Trouet A, Pirson P, Steiger R, Masquelier M, Baurain R, Gillet J (1981) Development of new derivatives of primaquine by association with lysosomotropic carriers. Bull WHO 59:449–458

Trouet A, Masquelier M, Baurain R, Deprez-De Campeneere D (1982) A covalent linkage between daunorubicin and proteins that is both stable in serum and reversible by lysosomal hydrolases, as required for a lysosomotropic drug-carrier conjugate: *in vitro* and *in vivo* study. Proc Natl Acad Sci USA 79:626–629

Recent Developments in Antimalarials

CHAPTER 9

Drugs with Quinine-like Action

T. R. SWEENEY

A. Introduction

The drugs to be discussed in this chapter all belong to the general chemical class arylaminoalcohols, and are related structurally to quinine. It is customary to refer to them as derivatives of methanol and they are further classified according to their particular aromatic ring system, e.g. quinolinemethanols, phenanthrenemethanols, pyridinemethanols, etc. Since all of the arylaminoalcohols discussed in this chapter were developed in the US Army programme at the Walter Reed Army Institute of Research and since only two have been officially named, they are referred to by their Walter Reed (WR) numbers. The antimalarial arylaminoalcohols have been reviewed previously (ROZMAN and CANFIELD 1979; CANFIELD 1980; SWEENEY 1981).

The arylaminoalcohol-type antimalarials are fast-acting blood schizontocides. They have no activity against the tissue stages of the parasite and hence are not used as causal prophylactic agents or radical curative agents against relapsing malarias. Because of their potent action against the blood forms of the parasites they are useful as "suppressive prophylactics" against both relapsing and non-relapsing malarias and as radical curative agent against non-relapsing malarias.

Several hundred arylaminoalcohols were screened for antimalarial activity in the *P. berghei*-mouse model during the course of the US Army programme; many reached the stage of advanced testing and a number were investigated clinically.

The compounds synthesized may be represented by the general formula $ArCHOH(CH_2)_nCH_2NR_1R_2$, in which R_1 and R_2 are H or alkyl or in which the moiety $CH_2NR_1R_2$ is in a cyclic form such as piperidyl or quinuclidinyl. Ar represents an aromatic nucleus, monocyclic or polyclic, benzenoid or heterocyclic, substituted or unsubstituted. While a detailed discussion of structure/activity relationships is beyond the scope of this chapter, it is of immediate interest to note that a specific aromatic ring is not required for activity. All of the ring systems tested showed activity provided they contained an appropriate side chain and appropriate ring substituents. Activities among the aryl types varied, of course, but gross overlaps were common depending upon the nature of the substituents. It is of interest that, in the Army programme, a number of highly active arylaminoalcohols were identified in aryl series other than the ones discussed in this chapter but, because of the adequacy and number of the ones in hand, there was no incentive to develop additional analogues that would, in all likelihood, have the same profile of activity. The arylaminoalcohol-type drugs that will be discussed in this chapter are in the class of 4-quinolinemethanols, 9-phenanthrenemethanols or 4-pyridinemethanols. Representatives of these classes that will be discussed are those that have progressed to the point where they can be considered as alternatives to mefloquine (CANFIELD 1980). This restriction precludes a discussion of some highly active trifluoromethyl-substituted dihydroquine derivatives (BROSSI 1976) (see also Chap. 2).

Because these alternative drugs are all of the same chemical class, i.e. arylaminoalcohols, there is the danger that the emergence of a strain of plasmodia resistant to one would be cross-resistant to all. Using a laboratory strain of *P. berghei* in which mefloquine resistance had been induced, studies with infections in mice showed that the strain was resistant to all six of the drugs considered to be alternatives to mefloquine (CANFIELD 1980). Whether or not such cross-resistance shown by an unnatural strain of *P. berghei* in the mouse is indicative of what might be expected with a naturally resistant strain of *P. falciparum* in man, the probability of the emergence of such cross-resistance, should one of the drugs become widely used, is not ureasonable. On the other hand, when tested against natural drug-resistant malaria in the owl monkey (SCHMIDT et al. 1978a), mefloquine was just as effective against both the multidrug-resistant (including quinine) Smith strain and the chloroquine- and quinine-resistant, pyrimethamine-susceptible Oak Knoll strain of *P. falciparum* as it was against the quinine-susceptible Malayan Camp-CH/Q strain of *P. falciparum*. Natural resistance to mefloquine has recently been reported. While the possibility of the development of widespread resistance to mefloquine, or one of the other alternative arylaminoalcohols, cannot be ignored, the event does not seem imminent.

B. Quinolinemethanols

Interest in the quinolinemethanols evolved from the antimalarial action of the cinchona alkaloids and quinine. The identification of the carbostyril, 2-hydroxycinchonine, as the major urinary metabolite of cinchonine (WISELOGLE 1946) and 2-hydroxyquinine as a product of the in vitro action of rabbit liver on quinine (MEAD and KOEPFLI 1944) led to the deduction (RAPPORT et al. 1946) that the blocking of the 2-position through the introduction of a substituent at this position should hinder the oxidation of the alkaloids to the carbostyrils and thus increase their effectiveness as antimalarials. This line of reasoning proved to be fruitful when it was found that the 2-phenyl derivative of cinchonidine was more active against avian malaria than cinchonidine (WISELOGLE 1946). When similar reasoning was applied to the α-(2-piperidyl)-4-quinolinemethanol-type compounds, which may be regarded as quinine derivatives with a simplified side chain, the introduction of a 2-phenyl substituent was found to increase activity against avian malaria (RAPPORT et al. 1946). During the malaria investigations of World War II, 120 compounds of the 2-phenyl-4-quinolinemethanol class were synthesised and screened in birds. Ten of these eventually were studied in man although only six were actually tested for antimalarial activity (WISELOGLE 1946). The most promising drug to emerge was 6,8-dichloro-2-phenyl-α-(2-piperidyl)-4-quinolinemethanol (SN 10275). When this drug was tested in volunteers, all patients treated with it exhibited a long-lasting phototoxic reaction varying from mild to severe (PULLMAN et al. 1948), and it is possibly for this reason that the potential of this class of compounds was never developed. Since the time that SN 10275 was tested, the *P. berghei*-mouse model has become established as the model of choice for screening large numbers of compounds. Using this model, the 2-phenyl-4-quinolinemethanols were reinvestigated in the US Army programme and the potent activity of SN 10275 in the avian model was confirmed in the mouse model. The phototoxicity of the compound that was noted in patients was confirmed in mice (ROTHE and JACOBUS 1968). In general it was found that, in this class, all of the more active antimalarials showed considerable phototoxicity in mice. The effectiveness of quinine against some chloroquine-resistant strains of *P. falciparum* indicated that the elimination of phototoxicity with retention of high antimalarial activity in the 4-quinolinemethanol type compounds was a reasonable and highly desirable objective. This objective was achieved with the development of WR 30090 in the 2-phenyl-4-quinolinemethanol class and with the development of mefloquine in a third generation class of 4-quinolinemethanols, the 2-trifluoromethyl-substituted analogues.

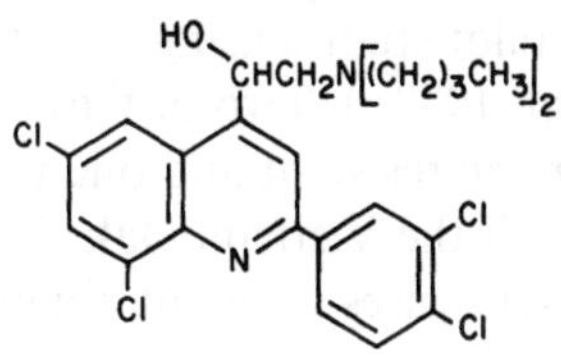

Fig. 1. WR 30090 α-[(Dibutylamino) methyl]-6,8-dichloro-2-(3,4-dichlorophenyl)-4-quinolinemethanol

I. WR 30090

The drug WR 30090 (Fig. 1) was originally synthesised by LUTZ et al. (1946) as part of the World War II antimalarial programme. It was included in the Survey of Antimalarial Drugs (WISELOGLE 1946) but was not evaluated in man until this was done in the current antimalarial programme of the US Army. The decision to proceed to human studies was based upon the high activity of the compound against avian and murine malarias, its lack of appreciable phototoxicity and encouraging pharmacological findings. The following discussion pertains to the hydrochloride salt unless otherwise stated.

1. Activity in Animal Models

The drug WR 30090 has been tested in a number of animal models. Against *P. gallinaceum* in chicks, a therapeutic index of 186.5 was obtained; the corresponding therapeutic index for quinine was 28 (COATNEY et al. 1953). Against *P. lophurae* in the duck, it had a quinine equivalent of 20. In the *P. berghei*-mouse model (OSDENE et al. 1967), against a blood-induced infection, the compound was 100% curative when a single dose of 160 mg/kg was administered subcutaneously and, in addition, it produced a significant increase in survival time, compared with controls, at a dose as low as 10 mg/kg (STRUBE 1975). In another study (AVIADO and BELEJ 1970) using *P. berghei* infections in mice, a dose of 10 mg/kg administered subcutaneously or 25 mg/kg administered orally brought about a 97%–100% suppression of parasitaemia. When orally administered and tested in mice against a susceptible strain of *P. berghei*, it was found to be approximately 60 times as active as quinine (THOMPSON 1972). In another study with a susceptible strain of *P. berghei* an SD_{90} of 2.7 mg/kg per day in the "4-day test" was obtained when WR 30090 was administered orally (PETERS et al. 1975a). Against strains of *P. berghei* rendered moderately resistant to chloroquine, WR 30090 showed no appreciable loss in activity compared with the susceptible strain, but against *P. berghei* rendered highly resistant to chloroquine a high degree of cross-resistance with chloroquine was found (THOMPSON 1972; PETERS et al. 1975a).

The drug WR 30090 has been tested against trophozoite-induced infections of *P. cynomolgi* in rhesus monkeys (DAVIDSON et al. 1976). When administered orally it was curative at a dose of 100 mg/kg. It is interesting and surprising that, under the same conditions, the curative dose of quinine was only 31.6 mg/kg. This relative activity stands in contrast to the relative activity of the two drugs against avian and murine malaria. The good activity of WR 30090 against *P. berghei* in the mouse did not carry over in pilot studies using five strains of *P. falciparum* in the *Aotus* monkey (SCHMIDT et al. 1978a). Two of these strains were chloroquine resistant, two were pyrimethamine resistant and one was multidrug resistant. With the exception of infections with the Vietnam Oak Knoll (VnOK) strain, which is chloroquine resistant, consistent cures were not obtained at total doses as high as 280 mg/kg; an SD_{90} of 195 mg/kg, total dose, was obtained with the VnOK strain. It would appear from these studies that chloroquine resistance was not a factor in the relative response of these strains to WR 30090.

2. Biochemistry

It has been found (FITCH 1969) that *P. berghei*-infected erythrocytes have three classes of binding sites for chloroquine, viz. low, intermediate and high affinity. The important difference between chloroquine-susceptible and chloroquine-resistant infections was that there was a deficiency of high-affinity binding sites in erythrocytes with the latter infections, i.e. they did not concentrate chloroquine as did those erythrocytes with susceptible infections. This fact provides a reasonable explanation for chloroquine resistance. It follows, then, that chloroquine-resistant parasites may exhibit cross-resistance to other drugs if binding to the same receptors is essential for activity. The question arises, therefore, whether such binding could be used to predict cross-resistance. A number of drugs were studied and found to inhibit competitively chloroquine binding to high-affinity receptors (FITCH 1972). The apparent inhibition constant, K_i, for the high-affinity receptor of chloroquine-susceptible *P. berghei* was 5×10^{-7} *M* for chloroquine and 2×10^{-6} *M* for WR 30090, indicating that the binding site will interact with WR 30090. If the therapeutic dose of the drug is appropriately related to the dissociation constant (the K_i may be used as an estimate of the dissociation constant) such correlations may be used to predict cross-resistance. However, the cross-resistance pattern of *P. falciparum* in the owl monkeys is different from that of *P. berghei* in the mouse and predictions based upon the latter would not be valid for the former (FITCH 1972).

The possibility of predicting cross-resistance would also seem to be inherent in the haemozoin-clumping phenomenon. Exposure to chloroquine brings about a clumping of haemozoin in intraerythrocytic malaria parasites, in vitro or in vivo (WARHURST et al. 1971; WARHURST and BAGGALEY 1972). This clumping can be competitively inhibited by quinine and other quinine-like drugs. Studies have suggested that the inhibitors act by competing with chloroquine for a common binding site. Various quinolinemethanols, including WR 30090, inhibit chloroquine-induced clumping. Although there are overall similarities in the clumping site of WARHURST and the high-affinity binding site of FITCH, the two sites are distinct (WARHURST and THOMAS 1975). Data from a series of compounds indicated that the clumping site is more structure-specific than is the high-affinity site. The results of the study of the quinine-like drugs also indicated that WR 30090 acts in vivo by means of a metabolite (WARHURST et al. 1972).

Phase contrast and electron microscopic studies of the chloroquine-induced pigment clumping in intraerytheorytic parasites showed that WR 30090 as well as other arylaminoalcohols not only could inhibit chloroquine-induced pigment clumping when given before chloroquine, but could also reverse the process when given afterwards (EINHEBER et al. 1976). It was suggested that such an inhibition-reversal phenomenon could serve as an indicator of the bioavailability of various formulations of candidate antimalarial drugs possessing the ability to produce the inhibition-reversal effect.

Although WR 30090 was not studied, the closely related compound SN 10275 was studied for its interaction with DNA (HAHN and FEAN 1969). It was found that the affinities of SN 10275 for DNA resembled those of quinine but, on the average, ten times more SN 10275 was bound than quinine. It was proposed that the binding of synthetic quinolinemethanols resembles that of quinine and that the greater antimalarial potency of SN 10275 compared with quinine is a direct result of the greater number of SN 10275 molecules being bound.

3. Toxicology

When tested in the standard *P. berghei*-mouse model for antimalarial activity, WR 30090 produced no acute toxicity when administered at 640 mg/kg either subcutaneously in a peanut oil vehicle or orally in a methylcellulose/Tween 80 vehicle. The drug caused a phototoxic reaction in mice when they were exposed to ultraviolet irradiation. The minimum effective phototoxic dose upon intraperitoneal administration was 50 mg/kg. This dose was ten times the amount required to bring about the same response with SN 10275, the antimalarial 2-phenyl-4-quinolinemethanol that was abandoned earlier because of its phototoxicity. Hence WR 30090 can only be classified as moderately phototoxic. In swine (BAY et al. 1970), the drug had only minimal phototoxicity. In volunteers, phototoxicity was observed in only four out of 39 subjects; the reaction was ephemeral and absent 24 h after cessation of drug administration (MARTIN et al. 1973). During the treatment of 26 patients with acute *P. falciparum* malaria in Vietnam no photosensitivity was observed (CANFIELD et al. 1973).

A subacute oral toxicity study in albino rats was conducted by POWERS (1968 a). Dosage levels of 500, 1,000, and 2,000 mg/kg per day were investigated, the drug being administered daily for 20 days. There were no drug-related changes in appearance or behaviour of the rats nor were there pharmacotoxic signs. In the groups of rats receiving the two higher doses body weight gains and food consumption were significantly lower. In another study (LEE et al. 1971 a) groups of rats were administered 250, 500 or 1,000 mg/kg per day orally for 84 days. No signs of toxicity were noted at the lowest dose but, at the two higher doses, there was a slight depression in growth rate and food consumption. A mild reticulocytopaenia in the rats receiving the two highest doses was also noted.

Single oral doses of 80, 270 or 940 mg/kg of WR 30090 to beagles caused no ill effects (LEE et al. 1967). However, a dose of 500 mg/kg per day for 14 days brought about weight loss, occasional emesis, diarrhoea, anorexia, and ataxia. An elevated myeloid/erythroid ratio in the rib marrow was noted in all of the dogs after the 14-day regimen because of depression of the erythrocytic elements. The appearance of large portions of the drug in the faeces suggested poor gastrointestinal absorption. Similar toxic effects were noted when beagles were administered 25, 50, 125 or 250 mg/kg per day of WR 30090 orally for 14 days (LEE et al. 1968 a, b) although effects were less severe at the lowest dose. Administration of 12.5 mg/kg per day for 14 days produced no adverse symptoms (LEE et al. 1968 c).

Beagles receiving 10, 20 or 40 mg/kg per day of WR 30090 for 91 days showed depressed weight gains. Also observed were persistent inflammatory lesions and vacuolar degeneration in the liver, effects which were dose related. The increase in the incidence and severity of inflammatory lesions in the lung and other tissues with increase in dosage may have been the result of an increased susceptibility of natural infections (LEE et al. 1971 b).

4. Pharmacology

In two bile-duct-cannulated dogs receiving respectively 10 mg (2 μCi) and 4.3 mg (4.3 μCi) WR 30090-[^{14}C] intravenously, 3% and 13% of the dose was excreted in the urine and bile respectively in one dog in 6 h and 1.7% and 15% respectively in the other dog in 4 h (MU et al. 1975). The disappearance of the drug from the plasma appeared to be multiphasic. The highest concentration of the ^{14}C was found in the liver, lung, spleen, heart, and kidney. Four rats were given WR 30090-[^{14}C] intraperitoneally, two receiving the drug in an ethanol vehicle, and two in an olive oil vehicle. Only 0.1%–0.5% of the drug-derived radioactivity was excreted in the urine. About 85% was excreted in the faeces when the drug was administered in ethanol but only 4.9%–6.0% when it was administered in olive oil. Apparently absorption was influenced by the vehicle (MU et al. 1975).

The acceleration of heart rate normally associated with the inhalation of chloroform by mice was reduced by pretreatment of the mice with WR 30090. Such pretreatment also decreased the incidence of ventricular fibrillation, which is also normally associated with chloroform inhalation (AVIADO and BELEJ 1970). The mice receiving the WR 30090 showed no change in the noradrenaline content of the heart. In dogs the intravenous infusion of the drug at the rate of 1 mg/kg per min brought about a fall in cardiac output with doses up to 80 mg/kg, but at a dose of 100 mg/kg the rate remained unchanged. The lethal dose was in excess in 100 mg/kg but was not determined (AVIADO and BELEJ 1970). The absence of a depletion of noradrenaline in the mouse heart and an increase in cardiac output in the dog was in contrast to the effect of the drug SN 10275 (AVIADO and BELEJ 1970).

5. Determination in Biological Fluids

In a study (MENDENHALL et al. 1979) of the determination of mefloquine in plasma and whole blood using a plastic ion-selective electrode, it was shown that solutions of WR 30090 in dilute aqueous acid could be quantified. The response potential was linearly related to the drug concentration. Measurements could be made with ±4% accuracy and ±2% precision with a sensitivity approaching $10^{-9}M$. The studies reported were primarily for the determination of mefloquine, and the actual determination of WR 30090 in blood was not reported. The implication, however, is that the method could be applied to WR 30090. The method will be described in more detail under the discussion of mefloquine.

In a study of the bioavailability of WR 30090, blood concentrations were determined using high-performance liquid chromatography (HPLC) (STELLA et al. 1978). In the procedure used, 5 ml whole blood were mixed with two drops of 15% ethylenediaminetetra-acetic acid solution. The resulting solution was extracted three times with 5-ml portions of ether, the extracts combined, evaporated and dried in vacuo overnight over $CaCl_2$ in the dark. The residue was taken up in 100 ml 20% chloroform-80% heptane (standard reagent grades) and 5–10 ml of the solution injected onto the HPLC column. The column was 1.8-mm id stainless steel, 50 cm long, had a silica stationary phase and was equipped with a 280-mm UV detector. With a fresh column the mobile phase was 10% (V/V) methanol in the stock solvent, 20% (V/V) dioxane-heptane. With time, as the column was used, the separation of WR 30090 from the blood components became less efficient and it was necessary to decrease the amount of methanol in the mobile phase to obtain good separation; the sensitivity also decreased. A standard solution of WR 30090 was injected before and after each blood sample as an external standard. The average area of the standard peaks was used to define the column sensitivity. Recovery was 80% for samples containing 20 ng or more of WR 30090 in 5 ml whole blood.

6. Storage and Formulation

While the compound WR 30090 (free base) in solution is rapidly degraded in the presence of ultraviolet light, in the presence of normal laboratory fluorescent lighting the degradation is very much slower (OKADA et al. 1975). In addition to irradiation, the rate of breakdown is affected by the nature of the solvent and the concentration of the solution. The degradation is both UV-irradiation-initiated and catalysed; removal of the irradiation source quenches the degradation. The hydrochloride salt of WR 30090 was degraded also but only after exposure to UV light for more than 24 h. The degradation products were numerous and different from those obtained from the free base. The major degradation product of the free base was 2-(3′,4′-dichlorophenyl)-6,8-dichloro-4-quinolinecarboxaldehyde; it was isolated by column chromatography. Because of this sensitivity to ultraviolet light, solutions of the compound, including extracts of blood, should be appropriately protected.

Solutions of the drug WR 30090 HCl are subject to a loss of the base because of adsorption on the walls of the container (THAKKER et al. 1979). Adsorption, which involves only the free base, appears to be a multilayer-forming process. Adsorption is minimised under conditions that increase solubility of the compound, e.g. decreasing the pH of the solution. Loss from solution was also minimised when the hydrophobicity of glass surfaces was reduced by coating them with silicone or methacrylate polymer.

The effect of formulation on the delivery of WR 30090 has been studied (STELLA et al. 1978). When the bioavailability in dogs was compared, a solution of WR 30090 base in oleic acid contained in a soft gelatin capsule proved to be a significantly more efficient formulation than WR 30090 HCl in a hard gelatin capsule.

7. Clinical Studies

The fate of WR 30090-[^{14}C] when administered orally was studied in one volunteer (MU et al. 1975). About 95% of the ingested drug-derived ^{14}C was excreted in the faeces. Almost all of the urinary ^{14}C consisted of metabolites. There was evidence of a number of metabolites in the faeces and less than 10% of the ^{14}C was excreted as unchanged drug. The decline of the level of ^{14}C in the plasma was slow and multiphasic, the apparent half-lives of disappearance from the two phases being 4 and 26 h respectively. The drug was found to be highly bound (99.1%) to human plasma albumin as determined by the molecular sieve technique.

In a study utilising volunteers infected with several strains of *P. falciparum* and the Chesson strain of *P. vivax*, WR 30090 was found to be an effective blood schizontocide against both types of infection (MARTIN et al. 1973). The best cure rate was obtained with a dose of 230 mg every 8 h for 6 days. With this regimen 100% cure rates were obtained against *P. falciparum* infections with the chloroquine-susceptible Uganda I strain and the moderately chloroquine-resistant Malayan Camp, Malayan (Tay) and Philippine (Per) strains. Nineteen out of 23 volunteers were cured of infections with the highly chloroquine-resistant Vietnam Smith and Vietnam Crocker strains. Three days of therapy were sufficient to achieve 100% cures against the chloroquine-resistant Marks strain. Against a blood-induced infection of Chesson *vivax*, six of seven volunteers were cured. The drug failed to cure sporozoite-induced infections. For all strains except the Vietnam Smith, parasitaemia was cleared by the 4th day of therapy, but the Smith strain required 5–9 days. Lysis of fever was completed in not more than 72 h. The drug was well tolerated and no significant adverse effects were noted.

CLYDE et al. (1973) studied the suppressive prophylactic activity of WR 30090 against the chloroquine- and pyrimethamine-resistant Philippine (Per), Malaya (Tay), and Vietnam Smith strains of *P. falciparum* and the Chesson and Vietnam strains of *P. vivax* in non-immune volunteers. The drug, 690 mg, was administered at weekly intervals commencing on the day of mosquito-induced infection for the falciparum suppression studies. Of a total of 11 subjects receiving eight weekly doses, ten were cured; of those receiving seven weekly doses, four of four were cured; with subjects receiving one, two or three weekly doses (one subject at each level) cures were not achieved. At a dose of 460 mg, six of six subjects were cured with eight weekly doses; treatment for 3 or 4 weeks (one subject each) was not curative. When tested against *P. vivax* infections, with the subjects receiving weekly doses of 690 mg for 8 weeks, beginning either 1 week before infection or on the day of infection, two of nine subjects developed parasitaemia during the course of treatment; two of six subjects receiving weekly doses of 460 mg on the same regimen also developed parasitaemia during treatment. Most of the subjects in whom *P. vivax* was successfully suppressed subsequently developed malaria after completion of the prophylactic course. The drug, therefore, was less effective as a suppressive prophylactic and ineffective as a radical curative agent against *P. vivax*. No side effects were noted during treatment.

In a field study in Vietnam (CANFIELD et al. 1973), of 26 patients acutely ill with multidrug-resistant *P. falciparum* malaria who were placed on a regimen of 230 mg WR 30090 every 8 h for 6 days, 23 were cured. The average time of response to the therapy as measured by fever clearance was 88 h and detectable parasitaemia was eliminated in 4 days. It was concluded that treatment with WR 30090 was a major advance against drug-resistant *P. falciparum*. The drug produced higher cure rates than any other single drug that had been used up to that time (the phenanthrenemethanol, WR 33063, which produced a comparable cure rate, will be discussed in another section). No adverse effects from the drug including photosensitisation were noted.

In a study in southeast Thailand using selected volunteers from patients with chloroquine-resistant falciparum malaria who required hospitalisation for treatment, 68 volunteers were treated with WR 30090, 250 mg every 8 h for 6 days (HALL et al. 1975). A cure rate of 86% was obtained, with a mean parasite clearance time of 72 h and a mean fever clearance time of 58 h. In contrast to the absence of side effects reported by MARTIN et al. (1973) and CANFIELD et al. (1973), headache, backache, and urticaria appeared to be associated with the drug in this study.

In summary, WR 30090 was an effective drug against multidrug-resistant *P. falciparum*. It was well tolerated in therapeutic doses. The chief drawback to its use was inconvenience. It had to be administered in a large dose which necessitated divided doses over a considerable period of time; under certain field conditions such a regimen can be a liability.

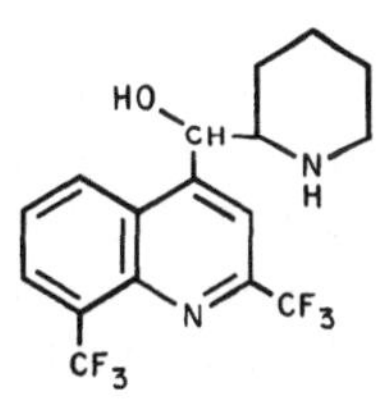

Fig. 2. Mefloquine (WR 142490). *dl-Erythro*-α-(2-piperidyl)-2,8-bis(trifluoromethyl)-4-quinolinemethanol

II. Mefloquine

Mefloquine, WR 142490 (Fig. 2), is a representative of what may be considered the third generation of quinolinemethanols. The first generation is represented by quinine and other cinchona alkaloids, the second by compounds such as WR 30090 and SN 10275 in which the cinchona side chain is modified and a 2-phenyl substituent is introduced, and the third by mefloquine, in which the 2-phenyl moiety is replaced by a trifluoromethyl group. Each step in this evolution has brought about an improvement in the therapeutic index of the repesentative drugs.

Mefloquine, along with the 2,6- and 2,7-bistrifluoromethyl isomers, was originally synthesised by OHNMACHT et al. (1971) but an improved synthesis has been patented by GRETHE and MITT (1978). The synthesis of radiolabelled mefloquine, *dl*-erythro-α-(2-piperidyl)-2,8-bis(trifluoromethyl)-4-quinolinemethanol-α-[^{14}C]-hydrochloride, has also been reported (YANKO and DEEBEL 1980).

The following discussion pertains to the hydrochloride salt unless otherwise stated.

1. Activity in Animal Models

When administered subcutaneously to mice in a single dose in peanut oil on the 3rd day after a blood-induced infection with *P. berghei* (OSDENE et al. 1967), the minimum "active" dose (the dose that doubles the mean survival time of the treated mice compared with controls) of mefloquine was 10 mg/kg; the drug was 100% curative at 40 mg/kg. It was twice as effective as the 2,7-bis(trifluoromethyl)-isomer and four times as effective as the 2,6-bis(trifluoromethyl)-isomer (OHNMACHT et al. 1971). The minimum active dose of 10 mg/kg in this model is at least eight times smaller than that of chloroquine (CARROLL and BLACKWELL 1974) and 64 times smaller than that of quinine (STRUBE 1975). In the "4-day test" for blood schizontocidal activity (PETERS 1965) against a drug-sensitive strain of *P. berghei* in the mouse, PETERS et al. (1977a) found the 50% and 90% effective dose levels of mefloquine to be 1.5 and 3.8 mg/kg respectively.

In a detailed study of the effect of mefloquine hydrochloride on *P. berghei* infections in mice, RICHLE (1980), using the "4-day test", obtained ED_{50} and ED_{90} values of 1.8 mg/kg and 4.0 mg/kg respectively, which are close to the values obtained by PETERS et al. (1977a). In other trials RICHLE (1980) studied the suppressive prophylactic activity when single doses of 2.5–200 mg/kg of mefloquine were administered orally at 6, 24, 48, 72 or 96 h before infection. The extent of the reduction in parasitaemia and mean survival time depended upon the dose and time lapse but, even after 96 h, parasitaemia was much reduced compared with controls, and mean survival time was increased. Both chloroquine and quinine were much less effective in this type of experiment. In experiments designed to study the effect of mefloquine against established infections (RICHLE 1980), it was found that, after a single oral dose of 400 mg/kg on day 4 following a blood infection, parasitaemia continued to rise and did not start to decline until 24 h after drug administration. It then declined steadily to 1% by 124 h. By 1 week 80% of the mice were clear of infection and by 2 weeks all were clear. Similar results were obtained when the drug was administered on day 2 or 3. Thus, under these conditions, mefloquine was rather slow acting. Morphological changes in parasites were not microscopically detectable until 48 h after treatment; in comparison changes were detectable 24 h and 72 h following similar treatment with chloroquine and quinine respectively. Despite these changes, blood taken from infected mice 48 or 72 h after mefloquine treatment was capable of infecting clean mice. Mefloquine was clearly superior to chloroquine and quinine when survival times were measured following a single oral dose of 400 mg/kg to mice with established infections. None of the quinine-treated mice survived for 3 weeks and none of the chloroquine-treated mice survived for 5 weeks, but 39 out of 49 of the mefloquine-treated animals were alive at 6 weeks.

Against lines of *P. berghei* especially developed to have high resistance against the drugs cycloguanil, pyrimethamine, and the sulphonamides respectively, mefloquine was as active as it was against the parent drug-susceptible line (PETERS et al. 1977b). Against a strain of *P. berghei* moderately resistant to chloroquine (NS strain) some cross-resistance was evident while against a strain highly resistant to chloroquine (RC strain) significant cross-resistance was present. It must be emphasised, however, that the RC strain is an "unnatural" one and has far greater resistance to chloroquine than the most chloroquine-resistant natural strains. PETERS et al. (1975a) have suggested that the value of such tests lies in predicting the ability of parasites, already able to tolerate chloroquine, to develop tolerance to new compounds.

The possibility of the emergence of a mefloquine-resistant strain of plasmodia, should the use of the drug become widespread, has been considered. PETERS et al. (1977a) have shown that *P. berghei* in rodents can readily develop resistance to mefloquine through successive passages in mice when exposed to drug selection pressure. This resistance was induced more easily in parasites that are already resistant to chloroquine. However, the rate at which resistance was acquired was slower when mefloquine was administered in a mixture with pyrimethamine, sulphaphenazole or primaquine than it was when administered alone. This effect was not apparent when mefloquine was mixed with a drug devoid of inherent antimalarial activity. The acquired resistance to mefloquine was unstable in the absence of drug pressure. This inhibitory effect was confirmed and extended to a combination of mefloquine with a 2:1 mixture of sulfadoxine and pyrimethamine (MERKLI et al. 1980). The development of resistance to this combination was greatly inhibited (MERKLI and RICHLE 1980).

The exceptional promise of mefloquine was highlighted by results obtained when it was tested against acute *P. falciparum* infections in the owl monkey (SCHMIDT et al. 1978a). The compound was equally effective against the chloroquine-resistant, pyrimethamine-sensitive Vietnam Oak Knoll strain and the chloroquine-sensitive, pyrimethamine-resistant Malayan Camp-CH/Q strain and only slightly less effective against the multidrug-resistant Smith strain. The activity was a function of the total dose of drug delivered, single doses being as effective as three or seven fractional doses delivered over as many days. It was also shown that the doses that were effective against various strains of *P. falciparum* were at least as effective against the blood schizonts of the Vietnam Palo Alto and New Guinea Chesson strains of *P. vivax* (SCHMIDT et al. 1978a). Against the above strains of *P. falciparum* mefloquine was at least ten times more active than WR 30090 and had a much larger therapeutic index. Against the chloroquine-susceptible Malayan Camp-CH/Q strain of *P. falciparum*, mefloquine was five times as active as chloroquine and had a significantly better therapeutic index.

In the study of the activity of mefloquine against the various drug-resistant and drug-susceptible strains of *P. falciparum* and *P. vivax* in the owl monkey, SCHMIDT et al. (1978a) found that in no case was the dose required to cure a previously treated infection greater than that required to cure previously untreated infections. This fact indicated that, at least in this model, the development of resistance to mefloquine does not occur rapidly.

When tested against sporozoite-induced infections of *P. cynomolgi* (a relapsing malaria) in the rhesus monkey, mefloquine was ineffective against early and persistent tissue schizonts. Thus, like WR 30090 and other quinolinemethanols, it has neither causal prophylactic nor radical curative activity against relapsing malarias (SCHMIDT et al. 1978 a). However, data obtained by SCHMIDT et al. (1978 a) indicated that, like chloroquine, mefloquine could serve as an effective companion drug to primaquine in a radical curative regimen.

2. In Vitro Activity

A rapid, semiautomated, microdilution technique for measuring the activity of potential antimalarial drugs against cultured intraerythrocytic asexual forms of *P. falciparum* was developed by DESJARDINS et al. (1979 a). Antimalarial activity of a drug is indicated by its ability to inhibit the uptake of a radiolabelled nucleic acid precursor by the parasites. The method is able to quantitate the extent of resistance among different strains of parasites to antimalarial drugs.

When the inhibitory effect of mefloquine was compared with that of quinine and chloroquine against both the drug-susceptible Uganda I strain and the multidrug-resistant Smith strain of *P. falciparum*, the ID_{50} (the 50% inhibitory dose) of chloroquine was almost 20 times as great for the resistant strain as for the susceptible strain, and the ID_{50} of quinine about four times as great. In contrast, the ID_{50} of mefloquine was essentially the same for both strains. The absence of cross-resistance in vitro is thus consistent with the lack of cross-resistance in the rodent and owl monkey models.

A study to determine the susceptibility of chloroquine-resistant *P. falciparum* malaria to mefloquine in vitro was carried out by ANTUÑANO and WERNSDORFER (1979). Using isolates from Boa Vista, Brazil and Villavicencio, Colombia and employing a modified RIECKMANN et al. (1978) technique, mefloquine was found to be in the order of seven times as effective as chloroquine.

3. Biochemistry

Being a blood schizontocide and a structural analogue of quinine, it is not surprising that mefloquine behaves like quinine under certain experimental conditions. In vitro, neither compound alone causes clumping of haemozoin in *P. berghei* trophozoites but both are competitive inhibitors of the clumping caused by chloroquine (PETERS et al. 1977 a). Mefloquine, however, has a very high affinity for the "clumping site", with a Ki value of $4.1 \times 10^{-7} M$, about 100 times that of quinine. Morphological changes induced in *P. berghei* at both the light and electron microscopic levels were similar and most obvious in the pigment. SCHMIDT et al. (1978 a) noted also that morphological changes in the early ring stages of *P. falciparum* and *P. vivax* brought about by mefloquine were identical to those produced by quinine.

The findings of BROWN et al. (1979) on the effects of mefloquine on *E. coli* would seem to be pertinent. Mefloquine caused an immediate loss of bacterial viability, rapidly suppressed the uptake and/or incorporation of precursors of protein,

DNA and RNA, inhibited nucleic acid and protein synthesis, lysed spheroplasts and inhibited NADH oxidase, an enzyme located in the cytoplasmic membranes of *E. coli*. The accumulated evidence indicates that a drug-membrane interaction is responsible for the antibacterial effects of mefloquine. The morphological changes in the malaria parasite brought about by mefloquine (PETERS et al. 1977a; SCHMIDT et al. 1978a) may be similarly related to membrane impairment. It is known that mefloquine has a high affinity for red-cell membranes (MU et al. 1975; CHEVLI and FITCH 1981).

JEARNPIPATKUL et al. (1980) have shown that *P. berghei* haemozoin binds mefloquine and have suggested haemozoin as a drug-binding and concentrating site in the parasite cytoplasm.

An extensive body of experimental evidence indicates that chloroquine complexes with DNA, both plasmodial and bacterial, and that the binding involves intercalation between the base pairs of the DNA as well as electrostatic forces (HAHN 1974). The increase in the length and rigidity of DNA as the result of intercalation interferes with template function and inhibits DNA-dependent nucleic acid polymerase reactions. The blood schizontocidal agents mepacrine and quinine behave similarly and it has been proposed that the chemotherapeutic action of the chloroquine-related compounds (8-aminoquinolines are excluded) rests upon this molecular mechanism (HAHN 1974). Arylaminoalcohols with antimalarial activity, in addition to quinine, have also been reported to complex with DNA (HAHN and FEAN 1969; PANTER et al. 1973; OLMSTEAD et al. 1975). This possible mode of antimalarial action for the 4-aminoquinolines and 4-quinolinemethanols gained general acceptance; mefloquine was postulated to intercalate with DNA, this being related to its antimalarial action. It was suprising, therefore, when DAVIDSON et al. (1975, 1977) reported that mefloquine *a* (Fig. 3) does not intercalate with calf thymus DNA and binds only weakly by electrostatic attraction at low ionic strength. In addition, mefloquine had no inhibitory effect on RNA transcription by *E. coli* RNA polymerase in a standard assay system. Both the carboxamide analogue *b* and analogue *c* had very weak antimalarial activity. However, analogue *b* could intercalate whereas analogue *c* could not. DAVIDSON et al. (1975, 1977) concluded from their studies that the ability of quinolinemethanols to intercalate with DNA is dependent upon the nature and position of the substituents on the quinoline ring. While all of the analogues (*a, b, c*) have a bulky (extending beyond the thickness of the aromatic ring system) substituent at the 4-position *a* and *c* have an additional bulky group at the 2-position. The carboxamido group of *b* is not considered bulky because it can be rotated to a planer position. Molecular models indicated that the proximity of bulky groups in the 2- and 8-positions prevents stacking because the two subsituents cannot lie cleanly in opposite grooves of the double helix. The trifluoromethyl group of *b*, however, can project into one groove of the DNA double helix while the side chain can be in the opposite groove; hence this complexation allows stacking. It would appear, therefore, that the antimalarial activity of mefloquine is not primarily associated with intercalative complexing with DNA. It will be recalled that mefloquine did inhibit macromolecular synthesis in *E. coli* (BROWN et al. 1979) but because mefloquine does not bind to DNA this inhibition was considered a secondary effect. Thus while specific effects of mefloquine are known, the primary mode of action remains unexplained.

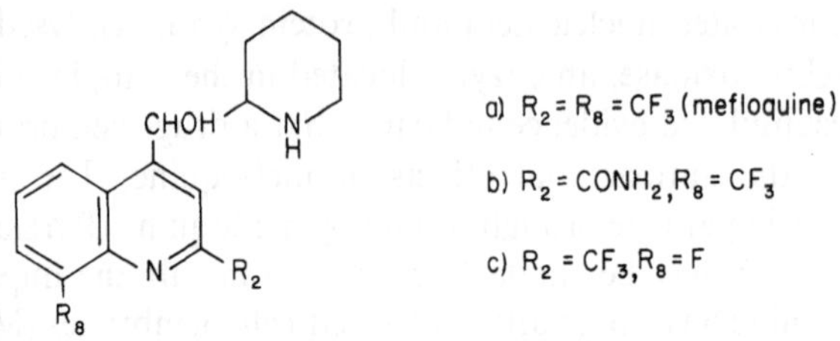

Fig. 3. Mefloquine analogues. *a*, mefloquine; *b*, 2-carboxamido; *c*, 8-F

Another interesting facet of the subject of the mode of action of mefloquine is the question of why mefloquine is active against naturally chloroquine- or multi-drug-resistant plasmodia. Although *P. berghei* CS (chloroquine sensitive) and *P. berghei* CR (chloroquine resistant) lines are equally susceptible to chloroquine upon equal exposure in vitro (FITCH 1977), under in vivo conditions erythrocytes parasitised with *P. berghei* CS accumulated chloroquine to a much greater extent than did *P. berghei* CR-infected erythrocytes. Hence chloroquine resistance in this model can be attributed to the parasite being exposed to an ineffective concentration of the drug (MACOMBER et al. 1966; FITCH 1969). Under in vitro conditions the pattern of mefloquine accumulation in parasitised erythrocytes differed considerably from that of chloroquine. While the accumulation of chloroquine by *P. berghei* CS-infected erythrocytes was greater than the accumulation by *P. berghei* CR-infected eryhtrocytes, there was, in contrast, no difference in the accumulation of mefloquine (FITCH et al. 1979). Uninfected erythrocytes accumulated more than half as much mefloquine as infected erythrocytes; in contrast, uninfected erythrocytes accumulated only trace amounts of chloroquine. While there are large differences between the drugs with respect to accessibility to drug receptors and strength of binding, chloroquine competitively inhibits mefloquine accumulation and vice versa. Based upon their accumulated data FITCH et al. (1979) have suggested that there may be a common process of accumulation and a common group of receptors for chloroquine and mefloquine. However, in the case of chloroquine, the erythrocyte may require modification by active metabolism in the presence of the parasite, a process requiring energy, before latent high-affinity receptors become accessible to the drug, whereas these same receptors may require little or no modification to bind mefloquine. Thus the undiminished accumulation of mefloquine by *P. berghei* CR-infected erythrocytes provides a rational explanation for the effectiveness of mefloquine against chloroquine-resistant malaria.

4. Toxicology

Single doses of 120 mg/kg or 420 mg/kg of mefloquine administered orally to beagles brought about no adverse effects during a 9-week observation period (LEE et al. 1972a). Repeated doses of 5 mg/kg per day orally for 28 consecutive weeks were non-toxic and also were non-toxic to rats (LEE et al. 1972b). A dose of 30 mg/kg per day on the same schedule caused occasional diarrhoea and emesis and lesions in the lymph tissues and/or liver in dogs. In rats, this dose caused lymphocytopaenia but no other adverse effects. Doses of 150 mg/kg per day were patently toxic, with deaths occurring in both species. This dose brought about depression and atrophy of lymphoid tissue and inflammation and degeneration of cardiac and skeletal muscle in the rats; serum glutamic oxaloacetic transaminase (SGOT) and blood urea nitrogen (BUN) levels were elevated. In the dogs, 150 mg/kg per day caused extensive lesions in the lymphoid tissue. Degenerative changes occurred in the intestine, liver, kidney and testis. This dose in dogs also brought about reticulocytopaenia, lymphopaenia and elevated SGOT, serum glutamic pyruvic transaminase (SGPT), alkaline phosphatase and BUN. Mefloquine administered orally at a dose of 5 mg/kg per week for 52 weeks to rats and beagles (LEE et al. 1974a, b) was without adverse effect in either species. Doses at 25 or 125 mg/kg with the same schedule were also without effect in the dogs; reduced weight gain without other effects was noted in the rats.

In other studies KORTE et al. (1978) also found that low doses, 6 mg/kg or 13.5 mg/kg, administered daily, orally, for 28 days were not toxic to beagles. At a dose of 30 mg/kg day on the same schedule weight gain was slightly suppressed. Toxic signs were evident at 68 mg/kg day with lymphoid atrophy, hepatic degeneration and increased BUN. In studies where mefloquine was administered orally for 90 consecutive days to dogs and monkeys KORTE et al. (1979) found no observable effects in either species at 13.5 mg/kg per day. At higher doses of 30 mg/kg per day or 68 mg/kg per day, with the same schedule, changes noted in monkeys were an increase in the weight of the liver and heart. In dogs, both of the higher doses produced a dose-related depression of lymphoid tissues along with weight loss and diarrhoea. A dose of 68 mg/kg per day, fatal to one of four dogs, caused moderate hepatic vacuolar degeneration, portal inflammation and/or bile duct hyperplasia with increase in SGOT, alkaline phosphatase, SGPT, lactic dehydrogenase (LDH) and α-hydroxybutyrate dehydrogenase (HBD). No histopathological changes were noted in the testes, prostate or epididymis nor were there changes in serum testosterone levels in either species.

In a study of the effects of mefloquine hydrochloride on reproduction in mice and rats by MINOR et al. (1976), female rats that consumed 50 mg/kg per day before mating until weaning produced young with decreased body weights and survival rate, effects attributed to malnourishment. These effects were not observed at a dose of 5 mg/kg per day. Male rats that consumed 50 mg/kg per day for 13 weeks showed a reduced growth, reduced fertility index, elevated SGOT and epididymal lesions; again, these effects were not observed at the 5 mg/kg per day level. When administered to rats and mice from day 6 through day 15 of gestation some anomalies were noted at a dose of 100 mg/kg but not at 10 mg/kg. A dose of 70 mg/kg per day from gestational day 16 until weaning produced toxicity in both dams and pups but toxicity was not observed when the dose was 7 mg/kg per day. Cross-fostering experiments indicated that toxicity to the pups was produced during the postnatal period.

5. Pharmacology

Pulmonary and cardiovascular effects produced by the infusion of mefloquine methanesulphonate in the anaesthetised dog were investigated by CALDWELL and NASH (1977). A dose rate of 1 mg/kg per min over 20 min produced little or no observable effects. However, during infusion at the rate of 2 or 3 mg/kg per min over 20 min, tidal volume was depressed but at the same time respiratory rate was increased. Measurements returned to control values after infusion. Dynamic airways resistance decreased during infusion but then rose above control values. Arterial blood pressure and cardiac contractile force decreased during drug administration but subsequently returned to control values. Central venous pressure and pulmonary artery pressure rose during drug infusion but returned to control levels subsequently. The magnitude of the observed effects appeared to be a function of the rate of drug delivery rather than the total dose of drug.

Cardiovascular and antiarrhythmic effects produced by mefloquine methanesulphonate after the intravenous administration of a dose of 5 mg/kg to cats were investigated by HEMWALL and DIPALMA (1979). The drug had an antifibrillatory potency about one-fifth of that observed with quinidine and had a slower onset of effect. Initially the drug caused a rapid drop in arterial pressure accompanied by a transient rise in mean aortic flow, changes comparable to those produced by an equivalent dose of quinidine. Mefloquine did, however, induce a greater and more sustained bradycardia than quinidine.

THONG et al. (1979), in a study of the effect of mefloquine on the immune response in mice, found that, in vitro, both human and mouse lymphocyte proliferative responses to mitogens were suppressed at a drug concentration of 1 μg/ml. The viability of mouse lymphocytes was severely affected at the higher dose of 4 μg/ml; a higher proportion of human lymphocytes, however, remained viable at this concentration. Antibody responses to sheep erythrocytes were impaired at a total dose of 60 mg/kg but not at 30 mg/kg. Delayed-type hypersensitivity responses to this antigen were not affected even at the higher dose level.

When mefloquine-α-[^{14}C] was administered intraperitoneally to rats, about 77% of the ^{14}C was excreted in the faeces and 3%–4% in the urine in 6 days (MU et al. 1975). The pattern of excretion in bile-cannulated rats suggested significant enterohepatic recirculation. It was concluded from ethyl acetate extraction data that urine and faeces contained practically no unchanged mefloquine, whereas gastric juice and bile contained significant amounts. There was evidence for at least three metabolites or decomposition products of mefloquine, all unidentified but more polar than mefloquine, in faeces and urine. Mefloquine was highly bound to plasma proteins and tissues with extensive tissue localisation. Studies with red blood cells in vitro indicated a high affinity of the drug for red-cell membranes.

After either oral or intraperitoneal administration of mefloquine-[^{14}C] to mice (ROZMAN et al. 1978) about 70% of the ^{14}C was excreted in the faeces and, in contrast to the urinary excretion in the rat (MU et al. 1975), about 20% in the urine. In addition, an appreciable portion of the administered ^{14}C was excreted as unchanged drug, again in contrast to the excretion pattern in the rat (MU et al. 1975). Elimination half-lives of mefloquine in plasma and red-blood cells were calculated to be 17.0 and 18.6 h, respectively. Tissue localisation was apparent with the major 24-h concentrations of mefloquine-derived radioactivity in the liver and lungs. Large amounts were located in the gastrointestinal tract and the residual carcass. Tissue extracts contained a high percentage of mefloquine as determined by TLC; the heart, in contrast, contained primarily metabolites. The disposition of *dl-threo*-α-(2-piperidyl)-2,8-bis(trifluoromethyl)-4-quinolinemethanol HCl (mefloquine is the *erythro* racemate) was described by CHUNG et al. (1979).

In another study, JAUCH et al. (1980) administered mefloquine-[^{14}C] hydrochloride to rats intraperitoneally and compared metabolic patterns in faeces and biological fluids. A large portion of the mefloquine-derived ^{14}C appeared in the faeces (82.2%) while 6.3% appeared in the urine. Metabolites in the faeces were separated by TLC and identified by radio-gas chromatography (GC) and GC/mass spectrometry (MS) analysis after trimethylsilylation. In the urine, blood and bile metabolites were identified by TLC. Several metabolites (*a, b, c;* Fig. 4) were identified or proposed, *d.*

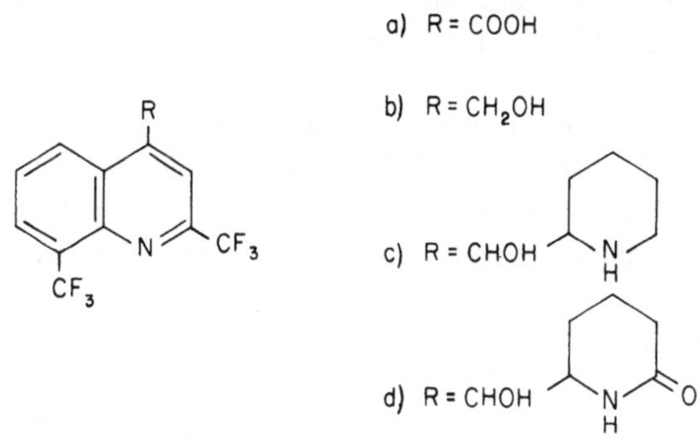

Fig. 4. Mefloquine metabolites *a–d* (see text for details)

The metabolites, as well as mefloquine, were all found in faeces, blood, urine, and bile. In contrast to earlier studies in rats (MU et al. 1975), the main component in the faeces was mefloquine. Only a small amount of mefloquine was found in the urine, the main component being the acid, *a*. The main component of the bile was the parent although appreciable amounts of metabolites *a* and *b* were present, partially as conjugates. The blood contained mefloquine and the acid *a* as the main components. Thus, with urine as the exception, the metabolic pattern of blood, bile (after conjugate hydrolysis) and faeces are rather similar.

6. Determination in Biological Fluids

High-performance liquid chromatography has been used successfully to effect separation and quantitation of mefloquine from whole blood, plasma and urine specimen extracts (GRINDEL et al. 1977). A chromatograph equipped with a 280-nm absorbance monitor was used. Extracts of whole blood or plasma were chromatographed on a column of 10-μm fully porous silica bonded with a monomolecular layer of cyanopropylsilane; the mobile phase was ether-dioxane-acetic acid (3:2 V/V+0.5%). For urine extracts, a column of 10-μm fully porous silica bonded with a monomolecular layer of octadecylsilane and a mobile phase of methanol-0.1 *M* NaH_2PO_4(3:2 V/V) was used. An analogue of mefloquine, *dl*-2,8-bis (-trifluoromethyl(-4-[1-hydroxy-3-(*N-tert*-butylamino)propyl]quinoline phosphate (WR 184806), was used as an internal standard in a dioxane-methanol (7:3 V/V) (196 μg/ml) solution. Extraction was accomplished by agitating a mixture of 9.8 μg of the standard (50 μl), 5 ml whole blood, plasma, or urine and 5 ml 0.065 *M* phosphate buffer (pH 7.4) with 10 ml ethyl acetate. The extraction was repeated twice, the combined extracts taken to dryness at 40° under nitrogen and the residue reconstituted in 500 μl of the appropriate mobile phase; 50-μl aliquots were injected into the chromatograph. Quantitation was achieved by measuring peak area ratios of mefloquine to the standard and relating them to a least-squares linear regression curve of the peak area ratio of mefloquine/standard versus the amount of mefloquine injected. The lower limit of sensitivity for the assay was 0.05 μg/ml mefloquine for blood or plasma samples and 0.25 μg/ml for urine samples.

Utilising optimal analytical conditions for the assay of blood, plasma, and urine samples spiked with known concentrations of mefloquine, the relative accuracy was ±3% of the amount added with relative standard deviations less then 10% over the range 0.05–5.00 μg/ml for blood and plasma and over the range 0.25–5.0 μg/ml for urine.

Mefloquine has also been determined in biological fluids using a plastic ion-selective electrode (MENDENHALL et al. 1979). The plastic electrode-calomel electrode pair was immersed in a stirred aqueous sample solution and the potential measured with a digital ion analyser. Quantitation was accomplished by comparison of the unknown solution potential with a standard curve constructed from plastic electrode analysis of samples containing known amounts of analyte prepared in the appropriate matrix, i.e. whole blood, plasma, or water. Solutions containing mefloquine in $10^{-4} N$ H_2SO_4 could be quantified by direct measurement. The potential response was linearly related to concentration over three orders of magnitude, while measurement could be made with ±4% accuracy and ±2% precision over the linear concentration range. Sensitivity to $10^{-7} M$ could be obtained. The direct determination of mefloquine in buffered plasma resulted in the loss of two orders of magnitude in sensitivity compared with aqueous solutions. This loss in sensitivity was attributed to the extensive protein binding of mefloquine. The determination of mefloquine in blood required an extraction of the drug. Direct extraction from neutral or basic solution was unsatisfactory. An effective separation of the drug involved an initial ether extraction to remove extraneous interfering materials, followed by ether extraction of the aqueous phase to which had been added trichloroacetic acid to pH 3. The extracted drug was reconstituted in aqueous buffer, pH 6, and the concentration determined using the plastic electrode. The procedure using spiked blood samples indicated a linear potential-concentration response to $10^{-6} M$ drug. Measurements could be made with ±8% accuracy and ±6% precision. Derivatisation of the isolated drug by alkylation with benzyl bromide in the presence of an HBr acceptor increased detector sensitivity an order of magnitude.

Gas-liquid chromatography (GLC) has also been used successfully to determine mefloquine in whole blood (NAKAGAWA et al. 1979). The procedure involved solvent or ion pair extraction of the drug, trimethylsilylation and GLC determination using electron-capture or flame-ionisation detection. Quantitation was achieved by using a related antimalarial drug, a pyridinemethanol, as an internal standard in a peak height ratio method. Ion pair extraction involving ether extraction in the presence of trichloroacetic acid gave higher recovery and better reproducibility than did solvent extraction using ethyl acetate. The detection limit for mefloquine was 1 ng/ml and the limit of accurate determination 10 ng/ml using electron-capture detection; the detection limit using flame-ionisation detection was 100 ng/ml. The latter mode of detection was therefore limited to drug levels greater than 100 ng/ml and the electron-capture mode was used for levels of 10–1,000 ng/ml.

Another method for the quantitative determination of mefloquine in plasma or whole blood by direct densiometric measurement after thin-layer chromatography has been developed by SCHWARTZ (1980). The method also allowed the determination of the main mefloquine metabolite, 2,8-bis(trifluoromethyl)-4-quinoline carboxylic acid, using a single extraction. The method involved the isopropyl acetate extraction of a sample of whole blood or plasma that had been mixed with a sodium chloride saturated Tris-HCl buffer of pH 8. The solvent was removed in a stream of nitrogen and the residue reconstituted in a small volume of the same solvent and quantitatively spotted on a TLC plate. Plasma (or blood) standards containing known amounts of mefloquine and its metabolite were also carried through the procedure and the reconstituted standard solution spotted side by side with the sample. The plates were developed with the mixed solvent system dichloromethane-methanol-acetic acid (80:10:10, V/V). The plate was scanned at 30 nm and reflectance measured using a chromatogram spectral photometer. Peak surfaces were then measured. Peak surfaces determined for plasma standards were found to fit a linear regression line up to a concentration of about 600 ng/ml for mefloquine and up to 1,800 ng/ml for the metabolite. Slopes determined for the respective compounds with the standards were used to calculate the concentrations of the respective compounds in the samples. Recoveries of mefloquine were 91%–99% and of the metabolite 62%–69%. The overall standard deviation of the method measured for mefloquine concentrations in the range 200–600 ng/ml and for the metabolite in the range 600–1,800 ng/ml was less than ±5%. Operating under optimal conditions of sensitivity, a 100-ng standard of mefloquine in plasma gave a mean peak height of approximately 10 mm and a mean peak surface of 45 mm^2.

7. Clinical Studies

In the clinical studies described, mefloquine was used as the hydrochloride salt.

The tolerance for mefloquine was appraised by TRENHOLME et al. (1975) in volunteers by a single-dose, double-blind study with 19 dose levels rising from 5 to 2,000 mg. A gamut of blood and enzyme determinations, physical examinations and electrocardiograms revealed no drug-related abnormalities to the 1,500-mg dose level. In the 1,750- to 2,000-mg range, transient dizziness and nausea were noted in four out of eight of the volunteers. Phototoxicity was not observed in any of the 42 participants of the study. In another study of mefloquine (CLYDE et al. 1976) ten volunteers were administered 250 mg and four administered 500 mg at weekly intervals for 7 weeks; no adverse effects were noted. A biweekly dose of 500 mg for 6–8 weeks also produced no side effects in four volunteers. One volunteer receiving two 1,000-mg doses of mefloquine 4 weeks apart and two volunteers receiving three 1,000-mg doses 4 weeks apart experienced mild epigastric discomfort without vomiting or diarrhoea shortly following each administration of drug. In a 1-year tolerance study, no clinical or laboratory evidence of intolerance was obtained when 500 mg mefloquine was administered weekly (ROZMAN and CANFIELD 1979).

In a kinetic study involving one human subject given 1 g mefloquine orally, SCHWARTZ et al. (1980) found maximum plasma levels of 0.9–1.0 μg/ml of the drug within 2–12 h of administration. The metabolite, 2,8-bis(trifluoromethyl)-quinoline-4-carboxylic acid, appeared in the blood 2–4 h after drug administration and rose to a maximum concentration of 1.1–1.4 μg/ml within 1 or 2 weeks. The average terminal half-lives of elimination of unchanged mefloquine from plasma, after the oral administration of 1 g of the drug to each member of three groups of human subjects, three members to a group, ranged from 12.3 ± 2.2 to 27.5 ± 5.4 days. The groups were of different racial, geographical, and dietetic backgrounds and sampling was non-uniform. DESJARDINS et al. (1979b) studied the kinetics of mefloquine in 20 adult male volunteers, divided into groups of four, at dose levels of 250 mg, 500 mg, 1,000 mg, and 1,500 mg; the drug was administered orally in a single dose as 250-mg tablets. One group received an aqueous suspension of 500 mg. The drug was eliminated slowly with a mean whole blood $t_{1/2}$ of 13.89 ± 5.31 days and a range of 6.48–22.65 days. No significant differences in elimination could be attributed to the dose or formulation administered. However, the rate of absorption of the drug was much faster when it was administered as an aqueous suspension rather than as a tablet. It was pointed out by DESJARDINS et al. (1979b) that, because of the wide individual kinetic variation, it is anticipated that occasional treatment failures may occur when the drug is used for single-dose therapy on a large scale.

In a delayed infection study of the suppressive activity of mefloquine (RIECKMANN et al. 1974), adult male volunteers were given a single oral dose of 1 g mefloquine and, at fixed intervals thereafter, were infected with Vietnam (Marks) strain of *P. falciparum* by mosquito bite. Subjects infected 14–16 days after medication were protected. A 21-day interval between medication and infection delayed but did not prevent patency. The mean prepatent period for treated subjects was 29 days as opposed to 10 days for the controls. Suppressive prophylactic studies with mefloquine were reported by CLYDE et al. (1976). Volunteers administered 250 mg or 500 mg of the drug weekly for 7 weeks were protected from a mosquito-induced infection of the multidrug-resistant Smith strain of *P. falciparum* when challenged on the 1st day of medication. Volunteers on a biweekly 500-mg schedule for 6–8 weeks were also protected. A regimen of 1,000 mg every 4 weeks for 8 weeks was likewise protective. Mefloquine was less effective against Chesson and El Salvador (Gue.) strains of *P. vivax*. Doses of 50 mg or 100 mg weekly failed to extend appreciably the prepatent period following mosquito-induced infection. Parasitaemia did not appear while weekly doses of 250 mg or 500 mg were being administered, but did appear 7 or more weeks after the termination of medication.

PEARLMAN et al. (1980), in a double-blind study, evaluated the efficacy of mefloquine in suppressing naturally acquired malaria in an area of northeastern Thailand highly endemic for *P. vivax* and chloroquine-resistant *P. falciparum*. Mefloquine was shown to be more effective than a sulfadoxine-pyrimethamine combination in suppressing both falciparum and vivax infections. Three regimens for mefloquine administration were tested, viz. a single dose of 180 mg weekly, 360 mg weekly or 360 mg biweekly. No apparent difference was noted in the efficacy of the three schedules.

TRENHOLME et al. (1975) reported on the therapeutic efficacy of mefloquine against two multidrug-resistant strains of *P. falciparum* (Vietnam Marks and Cambodian Buchanan) and one drug-sensitive strain (Ethiopian Taemenie). A single dose of 400 mg given to ten volunteers with patent parasitaemia following mosquito-induced infections with the drug-resistant strains cleared all subjects of fever and parasitaemia but only two were cured. This same dose cleared fever and parasitaemia in two subjects infected with the Ethiopian strain, but only one was cured. A dose of 1,000 mg cured 10 out of 12 subjects with resistant-strain infections and a dose of 1,500 mg was 100% curative. When tested in a limited number of partially immune subjects the drug was 100% curative with a single dose of 500 mg. Against blood-induced infections of Chesson *vivax* in a limited number of partially immune volunteers, single doses of 400 mg or 1,000 mg were curative. Against mosquito-induced infections parasitaemia was cleared but all subjects relapsed. This result, showing a lack of tissue schizontocidal activity, was consistent with the findings in animal studies.

During a field study in Thailand involving patients with naturally acquired, chloroquine-resistant, *P. falciparum* malaria, a sequential treatment consisting of a short course of quinine (average of four doses, equivalent to 2 g base) followed by a single 1.5-g dose of mefloquine was 100% curative in 35 patients (HALL 1976; HALL et al. 1977). With mefloquine alone, a cure rate of 94% was obtained with 31 patients. In the combination sequential treatment, a regimen of fewer than four doses of quinine was less effective. The results of a comparison of the therapeutic effectiveness of mefloquine and a pyrimethamine-sulfadoxine combination (Fansidar) were reported by DOBERSTYN et al. (1979). The study was conducted in central Thailand, an area endemic for chloroquine-resistant falciparum malaria, on patients with naturally acquired malaria. A single oral dose of 1.5 g mefloquine cured all of 37 patients with falciparum malaria, whereas a single dose of a combination of 75 mg pyrimethamine plus 1.5 g sulfadoxine cured 34 of 38 patients. The rates of decrease of parasitaemia and fever with the two treatments were similar, but gastrointestinal side effects were more common in the mefloquine-treated group. The undesirable side effects with mefloquine may have been associated with the particular formulation that was used.

8. Summary

Mefloquine is an orally well-tolerated drug with a biological half-life of about 2 weeks. It is therapeutically effective in single doses against both chloroquine-resistant and chloroquine-sensitive *P. falciparum*, with a cure rate approaching 100%. It is a suppressive prophylactic against both falciparum and vivax malaria. It does not have tissue schizontocidal activity and hence does not produce radical cures with relapsing malarias.

III. WR 184806

The compound WR 184806 (Fig. 5) is a structural analogue of mefloquine. While the substituted quinoline nucleus of mefloquine has been retained, the side chain of WR 184806 is a 3-*tert*-butylaminopropanol moiety. The compound was first

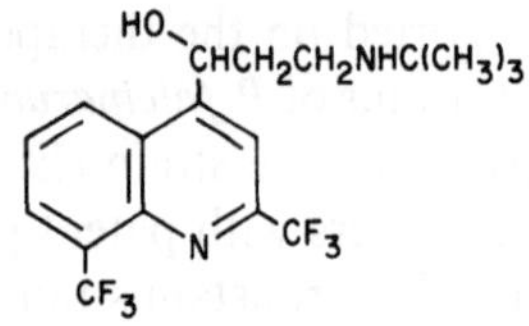

Fig. 5. WR 184806. *dl*-3-*t*-Butylamino-1-[2,8-bis(trifluoromethyl)-4-quinolyl]propanol

synthesised by BLUMBERGS et al. (1975) to determine the antimalarial effect of the attachment of an aminopropanol side chain to the mefloquine nucleus. This longer side chain was known to confer high antimalarial activity (COLWELL et al. 1972) in other arylaminoalcohol-type antimalarial compounds. The following discussion of this drug will pertain to the phosphate salt unless another salt is specifically mentioned.

1. Activity in Animal Models

When WR 184806 hydrochloride was suspended in peanut oil and administered subcutaneously to mice infected with *P. berghei* (OSDENE et al. 1967), cures were obtained at a dose of 160 mg/kg but toxicity was observed at 320 mg/kg. The compound was "active", i.e. the mean survival time of the treated mice compared with untreated controls was at least doubled, at a dose as low as 10 mg/kg (BLUMBERGS et al. 1975). The phosphate salt, when tested in this same model, also produced cures at a dose of 160 mg/kg and was 100% curative at 640 mg/kg without toxicity. When WR 184806 phosphate was administered orally to mice infected with *P. berghei*, it was 29 times as effective as quinine in reducing parasitaemia. A highly chloroquine-resistant strain of *P. berghei* (THOMPSON 1972) was also very resistant to WR 184806. However, cross-resistance with the antifolate-type antimalarials pyrimethamine, cycloguanil and dapsone was negligible.

Against blood-induced infections of *P. cynomolgi* in the rhesus monkey (DAVIDSON et al. 1976), WR 184806 was curative when administered orally at 10 mg/kg per day for seven consecutive days but ineffective at a dose of 3.16 mg/kg per day.

Both pilot and in-depth evaluations of the activity of WR 184806 against various human drug-susceptible and drug-resistant strains of *P. falciparum* and *P. vivax* in owl monkeys have been carried out by SCHMIDT et al. (1978a, b). Against both the chloroquine-quinine-resistant Vietnam Oak Knoll and the multidrug-resistant Vietnam Smith strains of *P. falciparum* the drug was as effective orally when administered in a single dose as it was when the same dose was administered in three or seven fractions on consecutive days. Doses required for the regular cure of the Smith strain (CD_{90} = 60–80 mg/kg) were much larger than those required for the Oak Knoll strain (CD_{90} = 25–27 mg/kg). The Palo Alto strain of *P. vivax* was more susceptible to the drug (CD_{90} = 14–18 mg/kg) than was the Oak Knoll strain of *P. falciparum* and markedly more susceptible than the Smith strain of *P. falciparum*. When administered intravenously, there was no significant difference between the CD_{90}s obtained with the single dose or fractional three daily dose regimens against the Oak Knoll strain of *P. falciparum* or the Palo Alto strain of *P. vivax*. In addition, the CD_{90}s obtained by intravenous administration approached the values obtained for the respective infections when the drug was administered orally, a fact suggesting good oral absorption.

2. In Vitro Activity

The in vitro antimalarial activity of WR 184806 was determined according to the method of DESJARDINS et al. (1979a). The method is based upon the inhibition of the uptake of [G-^{3}H]hypoxanthine by intraerythrocytic parasites which serves as an indicator of antimalarial activity. Comparison of the 50% inhibitory concentrations (ID_{50}), calculated from concentration-response curves of drug-susceptible and drug-resistant strains, indicated an activity of WR 184806 comparable to chloroquine against a drug-susceptible strain but, unlike chloroquine, an equal activity against a drug-resistant strain.

3. Toxicology

Acute oral LD_{50}s observed by LEE et al. (1974c) in several animal species were as follows: rats 2.09 g/kg, mice 1.9 g/kg, guinea pigs 110 mg/kg. The LD_{50} values obtained with intraperitoneal administration were: rats 384 mg/kg, mice 317 mg/kg, and guinea pigs 180 mg/kg.

Daily oral doses of 25 or 100 mg/kg up to 28 days produced no adverse effects in rats. Repeated doses of 250, 500 or 1,000 mg/kg per day were lethal, the deaths occurring between the 3rd and 13th day, the greater the dose the earlier the death. Toxic signs prior to death included hyperactivity, anorexia, weight loss, soft faeces or diarrhoea, bloody nasal discharge and convulsions. Peripheral blood changes included a decrease in lymphocytes with a corresponding increase in neutrophils, an increase in monocytes and elevations of SGOT, SGPT, and BUN levels. Lesions included severe gastroenteritis, pneumonia, atrophy and/or necrosis of the reproductive organs, depletion or necrosis of lymphoid tissues, thymic involution and vacuolar degeneration of the hepatic cord cells. Target organs were the lungs, gastrointestinal tract, reproductive organs, lymphoid tissue and liver; bone marrow was not affected.

A single oral dose of 420 mg/kg to beagles caused no toxic signs. Other than weight loss during the 1st week, there were no effects from a single dose of 940 mg/kg over a 4-week observation period (LEE et al. 1974d). Daily oral doses of 1 or 5 mg/kg for 28 days caused no adverse effects. Other than occasional emesis in some dogs during the 1st week, 20 mg/kg per day for 28 days caused no toxic signs while no changes in peripheral blood elements or blood chemistry and no lesions were observed at necropsy. Repeated doses of 80 mg/kg per day were lethal in 6 to 19 days. Toxicity was evidenced by emesis, anorexia, weight loss, ataxia, and tremors. Haematological changes included erythrocytopaenia, reticulocytopaenia, and lymphopaenia. Also observed were elevations of SGOT, SGPT, and alkaline phosphatase. Histopathological examination revealed degenerative and/or inflammatory lesions of the gastrointestinal tract, liver, and kidney as well as involution of the thymus, lymphoid depletion and bone marrow depression, especially the erythroid elements. Hence target organs were the gastrointestinal tract, liver, kidney, lymphoid tissues, and bone marrow.

Infusion of WR 184806, prepared in a dextrose-water or 0.1% H_3PO_4 vehicle, into the marginal ear veins of rabbits at a dose of 4 mg/kg caused inflammation, oedema and venous occlusion (HACKER et al. 1978). Microscopic lesions included vascular necrosis, thrombosis, haemorrhage, oedema, and epidermal vesicle formation. The incidence and severity of the lesions were dose related.

The mutagenic potential of WR 184806 evaluated using the *Salmonella*/microsome plate test (HODGSON et al. 1977 a) indicated that the drug was not mutagenic.

In tolerance studies preliminary to studying the effectiveness of WR 184806 against *P. falciparum* and *P. vivax* in the owl monkey, SCHMIDT et al. (1978 b) found that the drug was fully tolerated in oral doses of 10, 20, or 30 mg/kg base administered either as a single dose or as three fractional doses on consecutive days. Single doses of 40 mg/kg were lethal to two of four monkeys and a single dose of 60 mg/kg was lethal to two treated monkeys. Three consecutive daily doses of 30 mg/kg were lethal to two of four monkeys. Severe chronic convulsions were observed prior to death.

4. Pharmacology

When WR 184806-[^{14}C] phosphate, labelled on the hydroxyl-bearing carbon, was administered orally to female albino mice at a dose of 10 mg/kg, the drug-derived ^{14}C was primarily excreted in the faeces (71%) and 26% was excreted in the urine. Plasma levels of WR 184806 peaked at 0.4–0.5 µg/ml, total ^{14}C, expressed as drug equivalents, peaking at 1.65–2.00 µg/ml. The concentration of WR 184806 in erythrocytes reached peak levels of 1.5–1.8 µg/ml, total ^{14}C peaking at 2.5–2.9 µg/ml. The drug was well absorbed (77%–85% by 2–8 h) and was deposited mainly in the lungs, liver, skeletal muscle, kidneys, small intestine, and residual carcass. The drug-derived ^{14}C within these deposition sites was predominantly as WR 184806. In vitro equilibrium dialysis studies indicated extensive binding of the drug to plasma. Evidence for the presence of urinary metabolites was obtained by TLC (GRINDEL et al. 1976).

5. Determination in Biological Fluids

WR 184806 has been used as an internal standard in the quantitative determination of mefloquine in blood, plasma, and urine by HPLC (GRINDEL et al. 1977). High and consistent recoveries of WR 184806 from spiked whole blood were accomplished. While the method has not, apparently, been applied to the determination of WR 184806, it would appear to be adaptable with another compound, for example mefloquine, selected as the internal standard. The drug WR 184806 has also been used as an internal standard in the chromatographic determination of WR 180409 in blood (STAMPFLI et al. 1979).

6. Clinical Studies

A single-dose safety and tolerance study of WR 184806 in healthy male volunteers was performed by REBA and BARRY (1976 a). The rising dose, double-blind method was used with oral doses ranging from 5 mg to 1,400 mg. Below a dose of 1,000 mg there were no symptoms or findings that indicated intolerance. Two of the four subjects receiving 1,000 mg had transient light-headedness. At the 1,200-mg and 1,400-mg levels all subjects showed symptoms of intolerance: light-headedness, headache, nausea, difficulty in focusing and concentrating, insomnia and unusual dreams. These symptoms disappeared in 24 h. No significant haematological, biochemical, urinary or electrocardiographic alterations were attributed to drug ingestion. In a study of the tolerance for multiple doses, total doses of 900, 1,350, 1,800, 2,250, 2,700, and 3,600 mg were administered in nine equal fractional doses, one every 8 h, to six groups of volunteers (REBA and BARRY, 1976b). No drug-related symptoms were observed at doses as high as 1,800 mg. At the 2,250 mg level and above, symptoms similar to those observed with the high single dose were noted in some of the subjects. All symptoms were mild and temporary. No drug-related effects were noted in clinical laboratory examination, haematology or electrocardiograms. No phototoxic effect from the drug was noted.

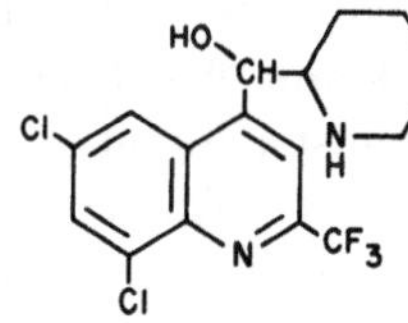

Fig. 6. WR 226253. *dl*-2-Trifluoromethyl-6,8-dichloro-α-(2-piperidyl)-4-quinolinemethanol

IV. WR 226253

The compound, WR 226253 (Fig. 6), is a variation of mefloquine in which the 8-trifluoromethyl group of the latter is replaced by chlorine atoms at the 6- and 8-positions. Its synthesis (PINDER and BURGER 1968) was prompted by the idea that the replacement of the 2-phenyl substituent in the very active but phototoxic compound SN 10275 by a trifluoromethyl group may block the metabolic oxidation of the 2-position and may also reduce or eliminate phototoxicity. It was more recently realised (R. E. Strube, personal communication) that WR 226253 might enjoy an economic advantage over mefloquine if it were developed in that the intermediate 2-trifluoromethyl-6,8-dichloro-cinchoninic acid could be made in one step from the reaction of commercially available dichloroisatin with 1,1,1-trifluoroacetone rather than by the multistep process originally used. The practicality of the isatin synthesis was confirmed (NOVOTNY and STARKS 1977). An improved method of preparing 2-trifluoromethyl cinchoninic acids has been patented (QUIMBY 1981). The ease of synthesis coupled with the biological activity of the compound, as will be discussed below, makes it a possibly attractive alternative to develop should mefloquine falter.

1. Activity in Animal Models

The compound WR 226253 hydrochloride was highly active in the *P. berghei*-mouse model (OSDENE et al. 1967). When suspended in peanut oil and administered subcutaneously, cures were obtained at a dose as low as 40 mg/kg and "activity" (by definition, a doubling of survival time compared with untreated controls) was observed at 20 mg/kg.

The effectiveness of WR 226253 · HCl against trophozoite-induced infections with the chloroquine-quinine-pyrimethamine-resistant Vietman Smith strain of *P.*

falciparum and the pyrimethamine-resistant Vietnam Palo Alto strain of *P. vivax* in the owl monkey was studied by SCHMIDT et al. (1978b). Against the Smith strain of *P. falciparum*, CD_{90}s of 8–12 mg/kg were obtained when the drug was administered either as a single dose or as the same total dose in three or seven fractions on consecutive days. The data also indicated that, in the *Aotus* model, WR 226253 was five to ten times as active as WR 184806 and twice as active as mefloquine against infections with the multidrug-resistant Smith strain of *P. falciparum*. The drug WR 226253 was also highly active against infections of the Palo Alto strain of *P. vivax* with CD_{90}s of 5.5–7.0 mg/kg. Again, the activity was a function of the total dose, a single dose being as effective as the same total amount administered in three or seven equal fractions on as many days. The CD_{90} values indicated that WR 226253 was appreciably more active against infections with the blood schizonts of *P. vivax* than infections with the blood schizonts of *P. falciparum*. Against a multidrug-resistant strain of *P. falciparum*, the drug was seven times as active as was chloroquine against a 4-aminoquinoline-susceptible strain. As was the case with mefloquine and WR 184806, recurring infections in owl monkeys resulting from initial therapeutic failures with subcurative doses of WR 226253 were invariably eradicated by doses of WR 226253 that cured previously untreated infections, this finding suggesting that WR 226253-resistant parasites had not emerged as the result of treatment with the subcurative doses.

2. In Vitro Activity

WR 226253 was highly active in vitro as an inhibitor of the uptake of radiolabelled hypoxanthine by intraerythrocytic *P. falciparum* (DESJARDINS et al. 1979a; CANFIELD 1980). It had an ID_{50} (the 50% inhibitory dose) of 1.0 ng/ml compared with an ID_{50} of 7.8 ng/ml for mefloquine.

3. Toxicology

The acute oral and intraperitoneal toxicity of WR 226253, as the methanesulphonate salt, in rats, mice, and guinea pigs is shown in Table 1 (LEE et al. 1979a, b).

By the oral route of administration the drug was most toxic to the guinea pig and least toxic to the mouse. When the drug was administered intraperitoneally no significant difference in toxicity was noted. Toxic signs were similar in all species; these were principally lethargy after oral administration, whereas intraperitoneal administration produced convulsions, loss of muscular coordination and cyanosis.

Table 1. Acute toxicity of WR 226253 · CH_3SO_3H in rodents

Species	Sex	LD_{50} (mg/kg)	
		Oral	Intraperitoneal
Rat	Male	1,134	57.4
	Female	1,450	47.0
Mouse	Male	1,798	44.3
Guinea pig	Male	745	41.8

In rats and mice, deaths occurred during the 1st and 2nd week following drug administration by either route of administration; guinea pigs died primarily during the 1st week.

In a study by LEE et al. (1979b), male rats were administered 6.5, 10, 30, or 50 mg/kg per day of WR 226253 methanesulphonate in the diet for 90 days. No toxic signs were noted in any rat at any drug dose level nor were there statistically significant differences in body weight or food consumption. However, rats treated with 50 mg/kg per day had a significant increase in the relative number of neutrophils compared with both baseline and control values. Assays performed on aortic blood taken just prior to necropsy from rats that were fed 10, 30, or 50 mg/kg per day revealed significantly lower serum levels of LDH, α-HBDH and creatine phosphokinase (CPK) compared with controls. Only in rats fed 50 mg/kg per day were statistically significant differences in organ weight noted. Significant epididymal lesions were noted microscopically in rats fed 50 mg/kg per day; these included epithelial vacuolar degeneration, swollen nuclei, nuclear necrosis and a decreased number of spermatids and necrotic spermatids. These results suggested that WR 226253 and mefloquine are of approximately equal toxicity with respect to reproductive tissue.

The drug WR 226253 · H_3PO_4 was not mutagenic when subjected to the *Salmonella*/microsome plate test (HODGSON et al. 1977b).

C. Phenanthrenemethanols

The phenanthrenemethanols are a class of compounds whose antimalarial properties have long been recognised. These aminoalcohols were studied in the World War II antimalarial investigations and about 200 of them were listed in the WISELOGLE (1946) compendium. The largest number in this listing were 9-phenanthrenemethanols but there were also an appreciable number of the 3-isomers as well as a smaller number of the 2-isomers. Of the 2-isomers that were listed, almost all had a partially saturated phenanthryl nucleus and about one-half of the 9-isomers were also of this type. Thus about 50 9-phenanthrenemethanols were tested for antimalarial activity in avian models. This isomeric class proved to be the most promising and four were selected for trials in man (WISELOGLE 1946). Two of the four selected were of the 1, 2, 3, 4-tetrahydrophenanthrene class (SN 1796, SN 5241) and two were fully aromatic (SN 8867, SN 9160). All four of the compounds were active against blood-induced vivax malaria but had only about one-half of the potency of quinine. Absorption of the compounds from the gastrointestinal tract was erratic and incomplete. Thus, at the time, the phenanthrenemethanols did not evoke the interest that the more active quinolinemethanols did. In retrospect, the poor showing made by the class is understandable because the compounds examined were, almost exclusively, either unsubstituted in the nucleus or had only one halogen substituent. More recent investigations have shown the superior worth of polyhalo substitution in the nucleus.

Early in the current antimalarial drug development programme of the US Army, the decision was made to reinvestigate the phenanthrenemethanols. The tetrahydrophenanthrenemethanols were considered too toxic to pursue (WISELOGLE 1946; COATNEY et al. 1947, 1953; RUIZ et al. 1970).

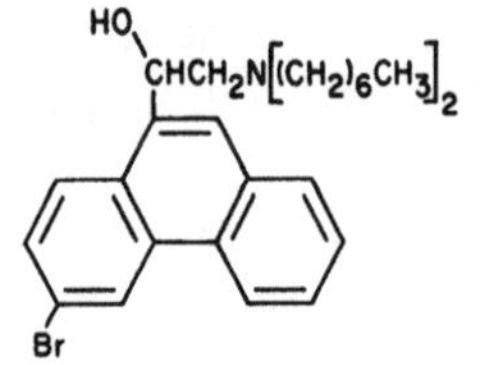

Fig. 7. WR 33063. 6-Bromo-α-[(di-*n*-heptylamino)methyl]-9-phenanthrenemethanol

I. WR 33063

Probably the best phenanthrenemethanol to emerge from the World War II antimalarial programme was SN 13465 (WR 33063) (Fig. 7). It was originally synthesised by MAY and MOSETTIG (1946). Because of its late appearance, it was not tested in man in that programme although the 6-chloro analogue, SN 9160, was so tested. Because of its relatively high antimalarial activity in avian and mouse models and its lack of phototoxicity, it received continued attention during the current programme of synthesis and testing of new phenanthrenemethanols and served as a standard for comparison.

Resolution of WR 33063 has been accomplished by crystallisation of its *d*-tartrate salt from 40% *d*-tartaric acid solution in aqueous methanol (PEARSON and ROSENBERG 1975). A series of various salts and esters of WR 33063 were prepared and found to be less water soluble than the hydrochloride. None of these derivatives were superior to the hydrochloride salt in antimalarial activity when tested in the *P. berghei*-mouse model (HARMON et al. 1973). All of the subsequent discussion pertains to the hydrochloride salt.

1. Activity in Animal Models

The drug WR 33063 was as effective as quinine against a blood-induced infection of *P. gallinaceum* in the chick when administered orally (WISELOGLE 1946) and, in this same model, it had the highest therapeutic index of any of the phenanthrenemethanols listed in the compendium of COATNEY et al. (1953). In the *P. berghei*-mouse model (OSDENE et al. 1967), WR 33063 effected cures at 80 mg/kg and above, with activity at 40 mg/kg and no apparent toxicity at the highest dose tested, 640 mg/kg (HARMON et al. 1973).

In another *P. berghei*-mouse model in which antimalarial activity was assessed by the degree to which a drug suppressed parasitaemia, WR 33063 was found to be five times as potent as quinine when administered in the diet or by gavage (THOMPSON 1972). Against strains of *P. berghei* especially developed to have high resistance to cycloguanil, pyrimethamine, or dapsone, WR 33063 was fully active; however, against chloroquine-resistant lines it exhibited a diminished activity proportional to the degree of chloroquine resistance (THOMPSON 1972). PETERS et al. (1975a) also found a high degree of cross-resistance to WR 33063 by a highly chloroquine-resistant strain of *P. berghei* when evaluated in the "4-day test". Since the degree of resistance in the laboratory-developed chloroquine-resistant strains of *P. berghei* is much greater than that present in naturally occurring strains of *P.*

falciparum, it was suggested that, regardless of the low activity against the chloroquine-resistant *P. berghei,* WR 33063 may, in fact, be useful against chloroquine-resistant *P. falciparum* (THOMPSON 1972).

While WR 33063 demonstrated appreciable potency in avian and murine models, the response to WR 33063 of blood-induced infections with *P. cynomolgi* in the rhesus monkey was minimal. With a dose of 100 mg/kg per day administered orally for seven consecutive days, one of two monkeys showed a slight suppression in parasitaemia but the drug was ineffective at levels of 31.6 or 10 mg/kg per day. In contrast, quinine was curative at 31.6 mg/kg per day and markedly suppressive at 10 mg/kg per day (DAVIDSON et al. 1976). In addition, it was less potent than any of a group of 16 new phenanthrenemethanols subsequently developed in the US Army programme when tested against infections with various strains of *P. falciparum* in the owl monkey model (SCHMIDT et al. 1978c). Against infections with various strains of *P. falciparum*, viz. the chloroquine-resistant Vietnam Oak Knoll and Vietnam Monterey strains and the pyrimethamine-resistant Malayan Camp-CH/Q and Uganda Palo Alto strains, it had a CD_{90} (milligrams per kilogram total dose of base required for cure of 90% of infections) of 1,400 mg/kg, whereas the CD_{90}s of the new compounds ranged from the most potent of the group with a CD_{90} of 23–27 mg/kg to the least potent with a CD_{90} of 350–700 mg/kg.

2. Biochemistry

The exposure of intraerythrocytic *P. berghei* to chloroquine and antimalarials of related structure, in vitro or in vivo, brings about a clumping of parasite haemozoin (WARHURST et al. 1971; WARHURST and BAGGALEY 1972). While the aminoalcohol type antimalarials (e.g. quinine) do not induce clumping as does chloroquine, they are able to inhibit chloroquine-induced pigment clumping (CIPC) (WARHURST et al. 1972) if introduced beforehand, or reverse the process if introduced after the fact (EINHEBER et al. 1976). The drug WR 33063 inhibited CIPC, but it was less active than mefloquine in vitro; in vivo, a dose of 30 mg/kg given 1 or 2 h before chloroquine inhibited clumping up to 100% (WARHURST et al. 1972).

FITCH (1972) has shown that WR 33063 competitively inhibited the binding of chloroquine to the high-affinity drug receptor of *P. berghei*, a fact indicating that both drugs interact reversibly with the same binding site. The magnitude of the apparent K_i of Fitch correlates with the therapeutic activity of a number of antimalarials (FITCH 1972) against *P. berghei* as does the clumping K_i of WARHURST and THOMAS (1975). However, the K_i of WR 33063 measured for the clumping site had a value of 29 nmol/litre compared with a value of 1,000 nmol/litre for the high-affinity site. WARHURST and THOMAS (1975) have concluded that, while the clumping and high-affinity sites have similarities, they are distinct.

3. Toxicology

In a study of the short-term effects of WR 33063, albino rats were administered daily oral doses of the drug of 62.5, 250 and 1,000 mg/kg per day for 14 consecutive days (POWERS 1968b). No compound-related effects were observed in physical appearance, behaviour, growth, food consumption, clinical laboratory results, survival, or gross and microscopic pathology. A marginal increase in thyroid activity was noted in the highest dose level animals on histopathological evaluation. In a companion study (POWERS 1968c), three groups of male rhesus monkeys were administered, respectively, 62.5, 250 and 1,000 mg/kg of WR 33063 for 14 consecutive days. No drug-related effects were observed in physical appearance, appetite, body weight or clinical laboratory findings. No histological changes were noted at the 62.5-mg/kg level but there were drug-related alterations of the spleen and kidney at the 1,000-mg/kg level.

The drug was not phototoxic (STRUBE 1975) when evaluated according to ROTHE and JACOBUS (1968).

The drug was not mutagenic when evaluated by the *Salmonella*/microsome plate test (HODGSON et al. 1977c).

4. Pharmacology

Following a single oral 30-mg/kg dose of tritium-labelled WR 33063 hydrochloride to rhesus monkeys, the biliary excretion of the label was highest during the 1st day and was complete by the end of the 2nd week. The amount excreted was 10% of the dose administered (SMITH et al. 1972).

When a single 30-mg/kg dose of tritiated WR 33063 was orally administered to owl monkeys, the urinary excretion of ^{3}H varied from 0.6% to 4.4%. The tritiated water content of the urine increased from 5% of the total ^{3}H on day 1 to 70% on day 4. After an oral dose of WR 33063-[^{3}H] to humans, tritiated water accounted for 70% of total urinary ^{3}H on day 7 and 85% on day 14 (SMITH and WEIGEL 1971a).

After a single oral dose of WR 33063-[^{14}C] to rhesus monkeys (HIREMATH 1975a), blood and plasma levels of the drug peaked 4 h after administration at 1.07 and 2.87 μg/ml respectively; the estimated average plasma half-life was 7 h. Approximately 77.55% of the administered label was recovered in 15 days, 2.70% in the urine and 74.85% in the faeces. High concentrations of ^{14}C were found in the liver, lung, cerebrum, kidney, and heart.

In a study of the cardiopulmonary effects of WR 33063 (RUIZ et al. 1970) it was found that the drug did not influence cardiac output, blood pressure, heart rate or pulmonary resistance in anaesthetised dogs with a dose of 15 mg/kg administered by intravenous infusion. Doses of 100 to 200 mg/kg administered subcutaneously did not affect the serotonin content of the brain or heart of mice, nor of the lungs of rabbits. Such a dose increased the serotonin content of lung tissue in mice (SADAVONGVIVAD and AVIADO 1969) but doses smaller than 100 mg/kg were without effect.

5. Clinical Studies

Tolerance studies of WR 33063 in 52 normal, male volunteers were carried out by ARNOLD et al. (1973). Increasing dosages from 50 mg/day for three consecutive days to 4.6 g/day for ten consecutive days were studied. Both single- and divided-dose regimens were used. The drug was well tolerated. There were no significant changes in haematocrit, nor in total white blood cell (WBC), differential WBC or platelet counts. No drug-related changes were noted in serum chemistry nor upon physical examination. There was no evidence of cardiac toxicity, adverse renal effect or phototoxicity. In the therapeutic phase of the same study, 59 volunteers received blood-induced infections with one of seven different strains of *P. falciparum* that varied in drug response from the susceptible Uganda I strain to the multidrug-resistant Smith strain. In addition, some volunteers received inoculations of the Chesson strain of *P. vivax*. A total dose of 1.6 g/day administered in four divided doses for 6 days produced a 100% cure rate of infections of the drug-susceptible African Uganda I and Caribbean Haitian strains of *P. falciparum*. In addition, this regimen produced a 100% cure rate with the chloroquine- and pyrimethamine-resistant Malayan Camp strain and the multidrug-resistant Marks strain of *P. falciparum*. With this same regimen two of three subjects were cured of infections with the Braithwaite strain and 18 of 23 subjects infected with the highly drug-resistant Smith strain were cured. This regimen alco cured four of five subjects with Chesson vivax infections.

In another study by CANFIELD et al. (1973), thirteen patients from Vietnam with falciparum malaria were hospitalised in the United States after treatment with established drug combinations had resulted in multiple recrudescences. Two of these patients received WR 33063 in combination with sulphalene and 11 received WR 33063 alone, 400 mg every 6 h for 6 days. All patients responded promptly and none had a subsequent recrudescence. Other than one complaint of transient tinnitus there were no side effects or laboratory evidence of intolerance. Another group of patients acutely ill with falciparum malaria and hospitalised in Vietnam were administered 400 mg WR 33063 every 6 h for 10 days. Of the 25 patients treated, 23 were cured while one patient suffered a recrudescence and one did not respond to the therapy. The clinical response was prompt. The average time for patients' fevers to decrease to 37.2 °C was 48 h. There were no abnormal haematological effects and no drug-related abnormalities in the clinical chemistry findings.

CLYDE et al. (1973) tested the suppressive prophylactic activity of WR 33063 in two volunteers who received a mosquito-induced infection of the multidrug-resistant Smith strain of *P. falciparum*. Weekly doses of 800 mg of the drug, commencing on the day of exposure to infected mosquitos, failed to delay significantly the development of infection. No side effects from the drug were observed. The quinolinemethanol, WR 30090, which was also tested in this same study, was more effective than WR 33063. With a weekly dose of 690 mg WR 30090, suppression and suppressive cures were achieved in 14 of 18 subjects; with a weekly dose of 460 mg, six of eight subjects were cured.

The results of a preliminary clinical trial in Thailand comparing the efficacy and toxicity of WR 33063 and quinine sulphate have been reported by SEGAL et al. (1974). Patients were Thai males with symptomatic falciparum malaria from areas of Northeast Thailand known to be endemic for chloroquine-resistant malaria. Subjects were randomly assigned to a group receiving 600 mg WR 33063 every 8 h for 6 days or to a group receiving quinine sulphate, 540 mg base, every 8 h for 6 days. The two drugs as administered were equally effective with cure rates of over 90%. The mean times for parasite and fever clearance were essentially identical. Treatment with quinine sulphate produced a greater number of reported symptomatic complaints than did treatment with WR 33063. No drug-related haematologi-

Table 2. Comparison of WR 33063, WR 30090, and quinine (Hall et al. 1975)

	Mean clearance time (h)		Failure rate	Symptomatic complaints[a]
	Parasitaemia	Fever		
WR 33063	77	54	8	91/69
WR 30090	72	58	14	119/68
Quinine	70	64	15	164/70

[a] Number of symptomatic complaints/number of patients treated

cal or biochemical abnormalities were detected during or following treatment with either drug.

In an extension of the study by Segal et al. (1974), Hall et al. (1975) compared the effectiveness and toxicity of WR 33063 with that of WR 30090 and quinine in patients from southeast Thailand, another area of multidrug-resistant falciparum malaria. A dose of an assigned drug was administered to a patient every 8 h for 6 days (18 doses). Doses of the drugs used were 600 mg WR 33063, 250 mg WR 30090, and 540 mg quinine. In this study, WR 33063 was highly effective. In comparison with WR 30090 and quinine (Table 2) it had the highest cure rate, cleared fever most rapidly and had the lowest toxicity. It was concluded that WR 33063 appeared to be a more promising drug than WR 30090.

II. WR 122455

The drug WR 122455 (Fig. 8) was one of a series of 9-phenanthrenemethanols containing fluorine atoms or fluorine-containing groups in the 3- and/or 6-positions of the phenanthrene ring that were synthesised by Nodiff et al. (1971) to explore the effect of such substituents on antimalarial activity. It consists of one of the two possible racemates and has been assigned the ±erythro configuration; the other racemate was isolated by Olsen (1972). All four of the theoretically possible enantiomers have been prepared and characterised (Carrol and Blackwell 1974). Both racemates and all of the optical isomers show potent antimalarial activity in the *P. berghei*-mouse model.

Various salts of WR 122455 have been prepared and their solubility determined. The lactate was 200 times as soluble as the hydrochloride (Agharkar et al. 1976). The following discussion pertains to the hydrochloride salt.

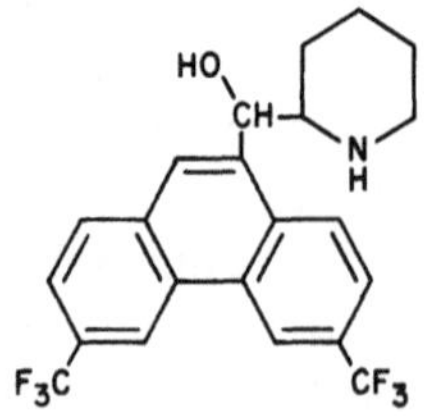

Fig. 8. WR 122455. *dl-erythro*-3,6-bis(trifluoromethyl)-α-(2-piperidyl)-9-phenanthrenemethanol

1. Activity in Animal Models

In the *P. berghei*-mouse model of RANE (OSDENE et al. 1967) WR 122455 administered subcutaneously in peanut oil was 100% curative against a blood-induced infection at a dose of 80 mg/kg and above, effected a partial cure rate at a dose of 40 mg/kg and was "active" at a dose of 10 mg/kg (NODIFF et al. 1971). When evaluated for blood schizontocidal activity in the "4-day test" against the drug-sensitive *N* strain of *P. berghei* the drug produced 90% suppression of parasitaemia (ED_{90}, mg/kg) in duplicate experiments, with donor passage material obtained at different times, as follows: subcutaneous administration, $ED_{90}=18.0$, 18.5; intraperitoneal administration, $ED_{90}=12.0$, 18.0; oral administration, $ED_{90}=8.0$, 12.5 (PORTER and PETERS 1976). The oral route was the most effective. In a direct comparison of dose-activity response in the "4-day test", WR 122455 had about one-third of the activity of chloroquine but 12–15 times the activity of quinine (PORTER and PETERS 1976).

In a study of the blood schizontocidal activity of WR 122455 against strains of *P. berghei* specially developed for resistance to established antimalarials, PETERS and PORTER (1976) found that strains highly resistant respectively to cycloguanil, pyrimethamine, sulphaphenazole or primaquine and a strain moderately resistant to chloroquine were all essentially normally responsive to WR 122455. However, a strain highly resistant to chloroquine was also highly resistant to WR 122455. It was also found (PETERS and PORTER 1976) that a strain of *P. berghei* moderately resistant to WE 122455 could be readily developed; this resistant strain showed a distinct cross-resistance to quinine. It was also found that resistance to WR 122455 could be developed much more easily in a strain of *P. berghei* moderately resistant to chloroquine than it could in a normal strain. In view of the spread of chloroquine-resistant falciparum malaria, the latter finding elicited a warning against the widescale use of WR 122455 or similar drugs other than in suitable combinations, in order to minimise the danger of the development of resistance (PETERS and PORTER 1976). The relevance of this finding involving chloroquine-resistant *P. berghei* in relation to chloroquine-resistant *P. falciparum* was questioned by SCHMIDT et al. (1978c). In delayed infection-type experiments, PORTER and PETERS (1976) showed that a dose of 200 or 400 mg/kg WR 122455 administered subcutaneously to mice completely suppressed parasitaemia when the mice were challenged with blood-induced infections of drug-sensitive *P. berghei* 1 week later; when challenged 3 weeks after drug administration the larger dose still was 90% effective.

It has been shown by PORTER and PETERS 1976) that there was no potentiation of blood schizontocidal action when WR 122455 was given with either chloroquine or primaquine.

SCHMIDT et al. (1978c) studied the antimalarial activity of WR 122455 against acute infection with various strains of *P. falciparum* in owl monkeys. When administered orally for seven consecutive days WR 122455 was fully active against strains of *P. falciparum* susceptible to chloroquine as well as those resistant to chloroquine, pyrimethamine, quinine or to all three of these drugs, with a CD_{90} of approximately 25 mg/kg. The drug was four times as active as chloroquine against chloroquine-sensitive strains. However, the time to effect parasite clearance was considerably longer than that required by chloroquine or quinine for susceptible strains or that required by mefloquine for drug-resistant strains. It was also shown by SCHMIDT et al. (1978c) that the activity of WR 122455 was a function of the total dose administered, a single dose being essentially as effective as the same amount administered in three or seven fractional doses in as many days.

In a duration of action study (SCHMIDT et al. 1978c) a dose of 35 mg/kg of WR 122455 provided 100% protection to monkeys challenged with blood schizonts 24 h after dosage, but protected only 50% of the monkeys when there were challenged 1 week after dosage. All monkeys were susceptible to challenge 3 weeks after drug dosage although there were delays in the onset of patency in many of the challenged monkeys.

The prophylactic activity of WR 122455 was assessed in the *P. cynomolgi*-rhesus monkey model (SCHMIDT et al. 1963). Doses of the drug as large as 20 mg/kg delivered on day minus 1 and minus 2 h before sporozoite inoculation, and daily thereafter for 7 days, were without effect on the development of the pre-erythrocytic forms of *P. cynomolgi,* thus demonstrating the absence of prophylactic activity. Treatment of established parasitaemias from sporozoite-induced infections with 5 or 20 mg/kg WR 122455 for 7 days cleared parasitaemia but infections relapsed following cessation of drug delivery. Retreatment of the relapses with chloroquine promptly cleared parasitaemias but relapses again recurred. This pattern of response indicated that WR 122455 has no radical curative activity against a relapsing malaria. The drug WR 122455 was also shown to have no causal prophylactic activity when tested in the *P. berghei*-mouse model (PORTER and PETERS 1976; PETERS et al. 1975b).

2. Biochemistry

DAVIES et al. (1975) and PORTER and PETERS (1976) observed the morphological changes in the trophozoites of drug-susceptible *P. berghei* at regular intervals after the intraperitoneal administration of a single 100-mg/kg dose of WR 122455 to infected mice. Most impressive was the rapidity of morphological changes and the apparent disappearance of haemozoin within 6–12 h following drug administration. The changes were similar to those produced in parasites by the treatment of infected mice with quinine but quite different from the changes produced by chloroquine. SCHMIDT et al. (1978c) observed changes in parasite morphology after treatment of *P. falciparum*-infected owl monkeys with WR 122455. Alterations were not noted until the day of the initial decrease in parasitaemia, a lag time of 48–72 h after drug administration.

The drug WR 122455, like other aminoalcohol-type antimalarials, did not cause in vitro clumping of the haemozoin of drug-sensitive *P. berghei.* However, it competitively inhibited clumping induced by chloroquine. Using the graphical analysis of WARHURST and THOMAS (1975), the dissociation constant (Ki) of WR 122455 at the clumping site was calculated as $2.26 \times 10^{-8} M$ (PORTER and PETERS 1976), which may be compared with the apparent Ki of $7\text{–}10^{-7} M$ calculated for the high-affinity receptor of chloroquine-sensitive *P. berghei* (FITCH 1972). The antagonism of WR 122455 by chloroquine may be related to the competitive binding between the compounds (PORTER and PETERS 1976).

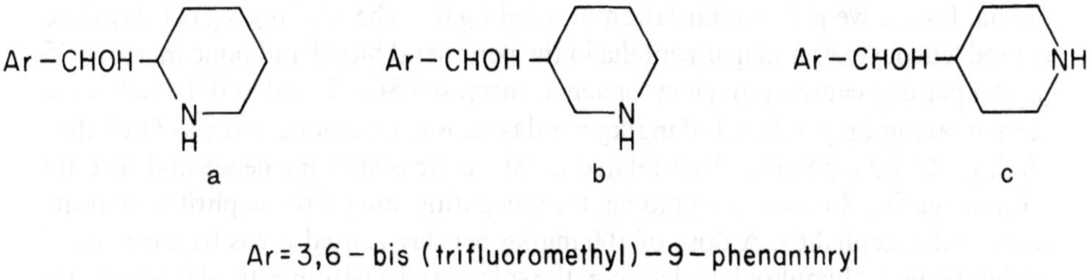

Fig. 9. Isomeric 3,6-bis(trifluoromethyl)-α-piperidyl-9-phenanthrenemetanols *a–c*

Ultraviolet absorption data have shown a strong, but undefined, interaction of WR 122455 with calf thymus DNA (PORTER and PETERS 1976). A connection between such interaction and antimalarial activity has not been established.

An interesting correlation of structure with antimalarial activity was made by CHIEN and CHENG (1973). The 3,6-bis(trifluoromethyl)-α-piperidyl-9-phenanthrene methanols *a* and *b* (Fig. 9) exist in two racemic conformations, *threo* and *erythro*, whereas *c* (Fig. 9) exists only in one. Both of the racemates of *a* have high antimalarial activity whereas only one of the racemates of *b* is active; *c* is inactive. Based upon molecular models (CHIEN and CHENG 1976) the minimum distance possible between the oxygen and nitrogen atoms of *a* is 2.5 Å and the maximum distance is 3.5 Å. With the 3 piperidyl racemates, *b*, the minimum *N–O* distances is 2.6Å but the maximum distance can be as much as 5Å. It was postulated that conformers favouring the former *N–O* distance can fit the "active site" and are biologically active; those conformations favouring the latter *N–O* distance cannot fit and are, therefore, inactive. The active conformations allow hydrogen bonding between the carbinol and amino functions (CHIEN and CHENG 1973; CHENG 1971).

3. Toxicology

During testing in the *P. berghei*-mouse model of RANE (OSDENE et al. 1967), no early deaths attributed to toxicity of WR 122455 occurred in doses as high as 640 mg/kg. In this test the drug is dissolved or suspended in peanut oil and administered subcutaneously in a single dose (NODIFF et al. 1971). In contrast, PORTER and PETERS (1976) found that a single dose of 450 mg/kg administered to mice as a saline suspension, killed four of five mice when administered subcutaneously, intraperitoneally or orally. On daily administration for 7 days, a dose of 10 mg/kg was found to be tolerated when administered by any route. The maximum fully tolerated dose was 30 mg/kg on oral administration and 60 mg/kg on intraperitoneal or subcutaneous administration (PORTER and PETERS 1976). (The unexpectedly high oral toxicity may have been compounded by mechanical damage caused during repeated gavage.)

The acute and subacute oral toxicity of WR 122455 in rodents was studied by LEE et al. (1970 a). In mice the acute LD_{50} was found to be 780 mg/kg by oral administration and 192 mg/kg by intraperitoneal administration. This result is in contrast to the 7-day regimen (PORTER and PETERS 1976) where the drug was better tolerated by the intraperitoneal route. Doses of 12.5 mg/kg per day or higher administered for 28 days to rats caused various dose-related adverse effects, viz. anorexia, loss of weight or retardation of weight gain. The 12.5-mg/kg per day dose caused leucocytosis and neutrophilia in the peripheral blood and bone marrow; 25 mg/kg per day caused reticulocytopaenia. Increased SGOT and SGPT levels were seen at 50 mg/kg per day, 100 mg/kg per day caused diarrhoea and was fatal after 10 days. In rats, possible drug-related lesions increased in incidence and severity with increasing dose viz. pneumonia, focal hepatitis, interstitial nephritis, myocarditis, and encephalitis. A dose of 100 mg/kg per day caused myositis, necrosis of skeletal muscle, lymphoid depletion in the spleen and gastrointestinal tract inflammation.

In a study of the oral toxicity in dogs (LEE et al. 1970b) single doses of 80 or 280 mg/kg administered to mongrels caused weight loss,, and single doses of 420 mg/kg or 940 mg/kg caused emesis. Single doses of 50, 100 or 200 mg/kg administered to young beagles caused vomiting within 2–5 h; a second dose of 50 mg/kg, administered 1 week later to the dogs that had received the two higher doses, caused vomiting in four of the eight dogs again (LEE et al. 1970 c). Except for the vomiting no definitely drug-related symptoms or changes were noted (LEE et al. 1970b, c). Administered daily to beagles for 28 days (LEE et al. 1970b), a dose of 20 mg/kg per day caused lesions in lymphoid tissues and the fundic part of the stomach. Damage was more severe at the higher doses of 40 mg/kg per day and 80 mg/kg per day. There were changes in peripheral blood elements, lymphoid tissue damage with destruction of small lymphocytes, lesions of the digestive tract and elevation of the marrow myeloid/erythroic ratio due mainly to an increase in maturing neutrophils. Target organs were lymphoid tissues and bone marrow. All drug-related toxicities that were produced by the 80-mg/kg per day dose in beagles gradually disappeared when the drug was discontinued and it was concluded that the toxicities were reversible (LEE et al. 1970d).

The toxicity of WR 122455 to rhesus monkeys, when administered orally and daily for 4 weeks, was studied by POWERS (1970). No toxic signs were seen at a dose of 5 mg/kg per day. Vomiting, diarrhoea and anorexia were observed with a dose of 20 mg/kg per day. At a dose of 80 mg/kg per day, drug-related effects included increases in BUN, SGPT, SGOT, and bilirubin levels and decreases in fasting blood sugar and total protein values. Total lymphocyte counts were also decreased in some animals. Histopathological changes associated with the 80-mg/kg per day dose included adrenal cortical hypertrophy, hepatocytic necrosis, dilated gastric glands, reduction of haematogenic activity in bone marrow, and occasional lymphoid depletion in the mesenteric lymph nodes.

The drug WR 122455 was not mutagenic when evaluated by the *Salmonella*/microsome plate test (HODGSON et al. 1977d).

4. Pharmacology

After the administration of tritiated WR 122455 to female mice, orally, intraperitoneally or subcutaneously, 14-day urinary excretion accounted for less than 5% of the radiolabel regardless of the route of drug administration (ROZMAN et al. 1971). Methanol extracts of faeces showed only one major peak by TLC corresponding to the parent drug. Good oral absorption of the drug was indicated. After oral administration of tritiated WR 122455 to rats, rhesus monkeys and owl monkeys (SMITH and WEIGEL 1971 b) blood radioactivity peaked at 2 days in the rats and at 4–5 days in the monkeys. Excretion of radioactivity occurred primarily in the faeces in all species with less than 10% of the dose appearing in the urine. Enterohepatic circulation in the rat may have accounted, in part, for prolonged excretion of radioactivity (21 days) in this species. Localisation of radioactivity in the rat occurred in the lungs, liver, adrenals, spleen, pancreas, and gonads. The fate of WR 122455 in owl monkeys was investigated by WEIGEL and SMITH (1973) using one ^{14}C-labelled compound (methanol group) and one tritium-labelled compound (piperidyl ring). Blood levels of ^{14}C drug equivalents ranged from 0.45 to 2.7 µg/ml, and plasma levels from 0.2 to 1.9 µg/ml. Recovery of ^{14}C was 1.3%–3.5% in the urine, 24%–84% in the faeces and 10%–44% in tissue. Highest concentrations of ^{14}C were in the lungs, liver, spleen, bone marrow, and adrenals. Recoveries of ^{3}H and blood level data were similar to those of ^{14}C. A study of biliary excretion of ^{3}H-labelled WR 122455 in rhesus monkeys (SMITH et al. 1972) showed a peak excretion of radioactivity of 0.4%–1.1% of the dose/h, 36–120 h after a single oral dose of 5 mg/kg; excretion continued for 15–20 days and accounted for 27%–100% of the administered dose. In owl monkeys given a single oral dose of WR 122455, tritium labelled on the carbinol carbon, 65% of the urinary ^{3}H had been excreted as tritiated water by the 28th day (SMITH and WEIGEL 1971 a).

5. Clinical Studies

RINEHART et al. (1976) have reported the results of a double-blind, two by two, rising oral dose study of WR 122455 in healthy volunteers. Drug regimens involved single doses of 320 mg–1,520 mg and multiple daily doses of 480 mg administered in two portions for 3 days to a daily 960 mg administered in four portions for 3 days. With the single-dose regimens in the 880- to 1,520-mg range, four or five subjects experienced nausea, diarrhoea and/or abdominal cramps while there were no untoward symptoms at 800 mg or less. A total daily dose of 480 mg administered in two divided doses for 3, 4 or 5 days was tolerated. Six-day administration of 480 or 720 mg daily in divided doses or 3-day administration of 960 mg daily in divided doses resulted in abdominal cramps, diarrhoea and/or nausea. No clinical or laboratory abnormalities were observed in any of the subjects and no phototoxicity was evident. In efficacy studies 13 volunteers received blood-induced infections with the multidrug-resistant Smith strain of *P. falciparum* and five volunteers were similarly infected with the chloroquine-sensitive African Uganda strain of *P. falciparum*. Single doses of WR 122455 ranging from 720 to 880 mg cleared fever, symptoms, and parasites in three subjects infected with the Smith strain and one infected with the African Uganda strain; however, all recrudesced in 21–34 days. A total daily dose of 480 mg administered in two divided doses for 1, 3, 4 or 6 days cured all infections with the Smith strain; the 6-day regimen cured four of four African Uganda strain infections. Clinical response was rapid. Mean fever and parasite clearance times were 72 and 66 h respectively for the Smith strain infections, and 77 and 67 h respectively for the African Uganda strain infections. Thus WR 122455 was an effective antimalarial and with respect to cure rates, and compared favourably with WR 33063.

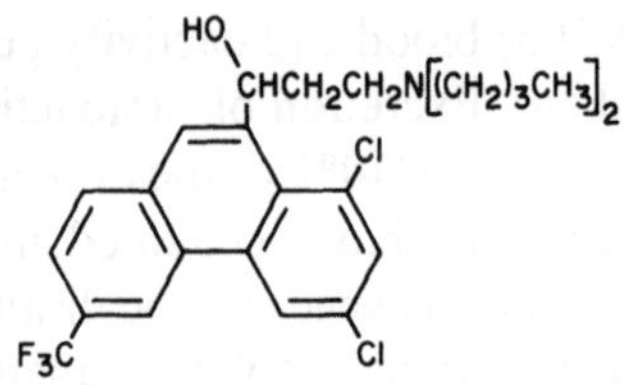

Fig. 10. Halofantrine (WR 171669). 1,3-Dichloro-6-trifluoromethyl-α-[2-dibutylamino)-ethyl]-9-phenanthrenemethanol

III. Halofantrine

Halofantrine, WR 171669 (Fig. 10), a 9-phenanthrenemethanol containing a dialkylaminopropanol side chain, was originally synthesised by COLWELL et al. (1972) as one of a series of arylaminopropanols. It was desired to compare antimalarial activity of the arylaminopropanols with that of previously tested arylaminoethanols. Earlier comparisons had indicated an activity of the 3-carbon chain at least comparable with that of the 2-carbon chain. A comparison of molecular models indicated that an aminopropanol side chain may facilitate binding to DNA more than an aminoethanol side chain.

The following discussion pertains to the hydrochloride salt unless otherwise stated.

1. Activity in Animal Models

Halofantrine showed high blood schizontocidal activity in the RANE *P. berghei*-mouse model (OSDENE et al. 1967). Administered subcutaneously in peanut oil, a single dose of 5 mg/kg was "active" (by definition, at least a doubling of survival time compared with untreated controls). At 10 mg/kg one of five mice was cured while five of five were cured with doses ranging from 20 mg/kg through 640 mg/kg with no acute toxicity (COLWELL et al. 1972). With oral administration, the drug was 59 times as effective as quinine in suppressing *P. berghei* infections in mice. There was no evidence of cross-resistance with laboratory-developed strains of *P. berghei* resistant to pyrimethamine, cycloguanil or dapsone; there was, however, appreciable (31-fold) cross-resistance with a highly chloroquine-resistant strain (THOMPSON 1972).

When evaluated for blood schizontocidal activity in the *P. cynomolgi*-rhesus monkey model (DAVIDSON et al. 1976), oral administration of the drug for 7 days beginning on day 4 after infection produced suppressive cures in all animals at doses of 10 mg/kg per day or higher. One of two monkeys was cured at a dose of 3.16 mg/kg per day but the drug was ineffective at lower tested doses. The drug was well tolerated at therapeutic doses.

Although halofantrine was of equal, or possibly slightly greater, effectiveness than WR 122455 in the *P. cynomolgi*-rhesus monkey model, it was only between one-third and one-fourth as active as WR 122455 against trophozoite-induced infections with the chloroquine-susceptible Malayan Camp-CH/Q and chloroquine-resistant Vietnam Oak Knoll strains of *P. falciparum* in the owl monkey (SCHMIDT et al. 1978c). It was, however, equally active against infections with these two strains, indicating an absence of cross-resistance with chloroquine. It was 12 times as active as WR 33063 against infections with the above strains and had an activity equal to that of chloroquine against infections with the chloroquine-susceptible Malayan Camp-CH/Q strain. A single dose of halofantrine was less active against infections with the Vietnam Oak Knoll strain than the same total dose administered in seven equal fractions over as many days (SCHMIDT et al. 1978c).

2. In Vitro Activity

In the microdilution in vitro technique of DESJARDINS et al. (1979a) where the extent of the inhibition of the uptake of tritiated hypoxanthine by parasitised erythrocytes in the presence of a drug serves as a measure of the drug's animalarial activity, the ID_{50} (the 50% inhibitory dose) of halofantrine was 2.5 ng/ml against the multidrug-susceptible African Uganda I strain of *P. falciparum* and 3.9 ng/ml against the multidrug-resistant Smith strain of *P. falciparum*. These values indicate a very high activity with essentially no cross-resistance. The comparable values for mefloquine against these strains of parasites were, respectively, 6.7 ng/ml and 7.8 ng/ml, indicating a somewhat lower activity. The respective values for quinine were 26.1 ng/ml and 109 ng/ml.

3. Biochemistry

The sequence of morphological changes brought about by halofantrine were identical to those described for the 9-phenanthrenemethanol WR 122455 (SCHMIDT et al. 1978c). However, the structural alterations appeared earlier; they were often noted 24–48 h following the first drug dose and were completed 72–96 h later.

EINHEBER et al. (1976) have studied the inhibition of chloroquine-induced clumping of haemozoin in *P. berghei* (WARHURST and BAGGALEY 1972; WARHURST et al. 1971) by halofantrine. The drug did not induce pigment clumping when used alone. However, when administered by gavage to mice infected with *P. berghei*, the drug inhibited chloroquine-induced pigment clumping if administered before chloroquine and reversed the clumping if administered after clumping had occurred.

4. Toxicology

The acute oral LD_{50} of halofantrine in male rats was determined by LEE et al. (1972c) to be 3,400 mg/kg and the acute intraperitoneal LD_{50} to be 2,050 mg/kg. Toxic symptoms included occasional diarrhoea, nasal and ocular discharge (often bloody), anorexia, weight loss, and inactiveness. The acute LD_{50} for male mice was 2,800 mg/kg. Other than nasal and ocular discharge, which were less apparent in mice, toxic signs were the same as those for rats. In 28-day toxicity studies (LEE et al. 1972c) rats were administered 25, 100 or 400 mg/kg per day by gastric intubation. At the lowest level no ill effects were observed. The incidence and severity of adverse effects at the two higher dose levels seemed to be dose related. At the 100-mg/kg level the neutrophil/lymphocyte ratio increased and there were mild thrombocytosis and elevated SGOT and BUN levels. In addition to an increased severity of these effects, a dose of 400 mg/kg per day caused reticulocytopaenia, leucocytosis and an elevation of SGPT levels. Dose-related morphological effects at the 100 mg/kg per day and 400 mg/kg per day included changes in peripheral blood elements and clinical blood chemistry and lesions of lymphoid tissues, striated muscle and bone marrow. The 400-mg/kg dose was lethal.

The acute and subacute oral toxicity of halofantrine was also studied in beagles by LEE et al. (1972d). Other than a slight weight loss in all dogs, a single dose of 180, 420, 630 or 940 mg/kg had no adverse effects. In the subacute studies, groups of dogs received 5, 15, 60 or 240 mg/kg per day for 28 consecutive days. The group receiving 5 mg/kg per day showed no adverse effects. At doses higher than 5 mg/kg per day, dose-related toxic signs were seen. These included loss of appetite, decreased growth or loss of weight, diarrhoea, emesis and ataxia. There were changes in peripheral blood elements and both SGPT and BUN levels were elevated. There were lesions of the lymphoid tissues, kidney, gastrointestinal tract, skeletal muscle and the bone marrow; the severity of these effects was dose dependent. The repeated doses of 60 mg/kg per day were lethal to some dogs during the 4th week; a dose of 240 mg/kg per day was lethal after 8 days.

Halofantrine was not mutagenic when evaluated using the *Salmonella*/microsome plate test (HODGSON et al. 1977e).

When tested in mice for phototoxicity by the method of ROTHE and JACOBUS (1968), intraperitoneal doses of 160–640 mg/kg generally elicited an erythematous response without scarring or necrosis. With oral administration there was a more severe, dose-related response. With an oral dose of 40 mg/kg there was a slight erythematous response; with doses above 80 mg/kg scarring and necrosis were commonly observed. The response was often of equal or greater severity when the mice were irradiated 5 to 10 days after drug administration.

5. Pharmacology

Other than a slowing of the heart rate, a single oral dose of 1,000 mg/kg halofantrine to mice was without cardiopneumatic effect (TEAGUE and MUNDY 1972a). Systolic, diastolic, pulse, and mean blood pressure were unaltered and no abnormalities were seen in the electrocardiogram. There was no effect on the rate or depth of respiration. Results were essentially the same when a dose of 1,000 mg/kg per day was administered for 3 days (TEAGUE and MUNDY 1972b). With the repeated doses there was a 9% loss in body weight and a depression in the usual pressor and chronotropic effect of adrenaline.

A bioavailability study was made by WINDHEUSER and HASLAM (1976) of several formulations of halofantrine, viz. a 250-mg suspension of the methanesulphonate salt in 50 ml water; 250 mg of the hydrochloride salt in a hard gelatin capsule; 250 mg of the free base, 20% by weight in oleic acid contained in a soft-gelatin capsule; and 250 mg of the methanesulphonate salt in a tablet. The formulations were administered orally to beagles after a 24-h fast. Blood levels of drug were determined by ether extraction from whole blood and subsequent quantitation using HPLC. No significant difference in bioavailability was noted for the various formulations at the 95% confidence level.

HIREMATH (1974) found that ^{14}C-labelled halofantrine was rapidly absorbed when administered orally to rats and rhesus monkeys as a single 20-mg/kg dose. Plasma levels peaked at 4–8 h in the rat and at 4–6 h in the monkey. The main route of execretion was through the faeces in both species. A high concentration of drug-derived ^{14}C was found in the lung, adrenals, spleen, liver, kidneys, and heart of the rat. In the monkey radioactivity was concentrated in the liver, lungs, cerebellum, cerebrum, lymph nodes, and testes.

6. Clinical Studies

Halofantrine has been tested in man for oral tolerance, toxicity, and effectiveness against *P. falciparum* malaria (RINEHART et al. 1976). A double-blind, two-by-two rising dose design with 40 healthy volunteers was used in the phase I study. One-day administrations were increased from a single 5-mg dose to a dose of 480 mg administered four times. Doses delivered over more than 1 day ranged from 420 mg administered three times a day for 2 days to 250 mg administered four times a day for 6 days. Single oral doses as high as 750 mg were tolerated. With multiple doses, a regimen of 420 mg three times daily for 1 day produced no symptoms, but the same daily dose given for 2 or 3 days produced mild abdominal cramps or nausea in half of the subjects. A regimen of 250 mg every 6 h for 24 doses produced epigastric pain. The severity and frequency of symptoms appeared to be dose related and disappeared 2–24 h after the last dose. No abnormalities in clinical or laboratory findings were noted.

In phase II studies, a drug regimen of 250 mg every 6 h for 12 doses (3 days) cured six of six subjects of blood-induced infections of the multidrug-resistant Smith strain of *P. falciparum* and three of three subjects with infections of the drug-susceptible African Uganda strain of *P. falciparum*. Parasitaemia was cleared in 84 h and fever in 42 h.

D. Pyridinemethanols

Thc 4-pyridinemethanols were also one of several classes of arylaminoalcohols that were investigated by the US Army in its ongoing search for new antimalarial drugs. Three compounds of this class had been tested against avian malarias in the World War II antimalarial programme (WISELOGLE 1946) but only one of these, 2,6-diphenyl-α-(dibutylaminomethyl)-4-pyridinemethanol, SN 10760, showed appreciable activity. This compound was not tested in monkeys or in man and the lead remained unexploited until it was picked up in the current US Army programme. A number of highly active 4-pyridinemethanols resulted from the investigations.

I. WR 180409

The drug WR 180409 (Fig. 11) was first synthesised by LAMONTAGNE et al. (1974). It evolved in a programme of research by these workers to increase the potency of SN 10770 after the latter compound (as WR 135642) was found to increase survival

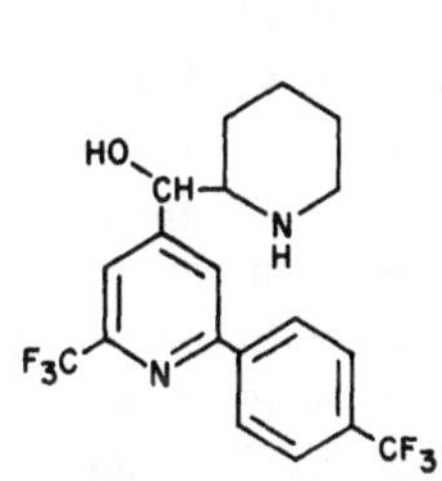

Fig. 11. WR 180409. *dl-Threo*-α-(2-piperidyl)-2-trifluoromethyl-6-(4-trifluoromethylphenyl)-4-pyridinemethanol

time but not effect cures in the *P. berghei*-mouse model (OSDENE et al. 1967). Both of the possible racemates with the WR 180409 structure were prepared and their configurations established (LAMONTAGNE et al. 1974).

Although WR 180409 was originally synthesised as the free base and hydrochloride salt, an examination of several salt forms indicated that the phosphate was more soluble than the hydrochloride and would be the preferred form for oral administration (HIGUCHI and HASLAM 1974a). All studies discussed below, therefore, were carried out using the phosphate unless otherwise indicated.

1. Activity in Animal Models

When administered subcutaneously in peanut oil to mice with blood-induced infections of *P. berghei* (OSDENE et al. 1967), the hydrochloride salt was reported to be curative at a dose of 20–640 mg/kg without toxicity and "active" at a dose of 10 mg/kg. In subsequent testing in the same model, the phosphate salt was found to be curative at 80–640 mg/kg without toxicity with "activity" at 20 mg/kg. Orally, with a 3-day regimen, a 90% suppression of parasitaemia (ED_{90}) was obtained with a dose of 3.4–4.1 mg/kg per day (quinine index 20–24) against blood-induced *P. berghei* infections in mice. In this model (THOMPSON 1972) there was evidence of cross-resistance by a strain of *P. berghei* rendered highly resistant to chloroquine; however, there was no evidence of cross-resistance by pyrimethamine or dapsone-resistant *P. berghei*.

In a *P. berghei*-rat model (MOST and MONTOURI 1975), WR 180409 showed no causal prophylactic activity against sporozoite-induced infections although suppressive activity was noted.

When tested for blood schizontocidal activity against *P. cynomolgi* in the rhesus monkey (DAVIDSON et al. 1976), an oral dose of 10 mg/kg of WR 180409 administered daily for 7 days cured four of four monkeys; a dose of 3.16 mg/kg, similarly administered suppressed parasitaemia but did not effect cures.

A study of the blood schizontocidal activity of WR 180409 against two strains of *P. falciparum* and one of *P. vivax* in owl monkeys has been made by SCHMIDT et al. (1978d). Against infections with the highly chloroquine-resistant but pyrimethamine-susceptible Vietnam Oak Knoll strain of *P. falciparum*, WR 180409 had an approximate CD_{90} of 14 mg/kg total dose when the drug was administered orally in divided doses over seven consecutive days. Against infections with the multidrug-resistant Smith strain of *P. falciparum*, it made little or no difference whether the total dose of drug was administered in a three- or seven consecutive-day schedule (CD_{90} of 24–30 mg/kg total dose). A divided-dose regimen was, however, probably superior to a single-dose schedule. Against infections with the pyrimethamine-resistant Vietnam Palo Alto strain of *P. vivax*, single, three-dose, or seven-dose regimens were essentially identical, the approximate CD_{90}s ranging from 14 to 18 mg/kg. The drug was, therefore, more effective against infections with *P. vivax* than against infections with the Smith strain of *P. falciparum*. The *P. falciparum* data also indicated that WR 180409 had therapeutic indexes at least four to eight times those of chloroquine against infections with chloroquine-susceptible strains. These superior indexes were retained against various drug-resistant strains.

In a limited study it was also shown that WR 180409 was highly effective in curing established infections with the Vietnam Palo Alto strain of *P. vivax* in the owl monkey when administered intravenously in single or three-consecutive-daily-dose regimens, CD_{90}s of 14 and 8 mg/kg respectively being obtained. There were no immediate or delayed reactions from these doses (SCHMIDT et al. 1978 d).

2. In Vitro Activity

When tested in the in vitro system of DESJARDINS et al. (1979 a), where antimalarial activity is assessed by the ability of the drug to inhibit the uptake of tritiated hypoxanthine by parasitised erythrocytes, the ID_{50}s for the drug-susceptible African Uganda I and multidrug-resistant Smith strains of *P. falciparum* were 35.4 and 48.5 ng/ml respectively. These data show that there is relatively little cross-resistance to WR 180409 in vitro, a finding consistent with in vivo testing. However, these ID_{50}s are surprisingly high compared with the ID_{50} values for other aminoalcohol antimalarials (DESJARDINS et al. 1979 a), a fact which suggests metabolite antimalarial activity.

3. Toxicology

The acute and subacute toxicity of WR 180409 in rodents was studied by LEE et al. (1976 a). The acute oral LD_{50} for male mice was 889 mg/kg. There was no difference in the acute toxicity of the drug to rats attributable to sex: the acute oral LD_{50} for male and female rats was 518 mg/kg and 508 mg/kg respectively. The acute oral LD_{50} for male guinea pigs was 285 mg/kg.

In studies of the acute oral toxicity (LEE et al. 1976 a, b) groups of rats were given single doses of 100, 300 or 900 mg/kg WR 180409 and observed for 72 h; other groups were given 316, 398, 501, 631 or 794 mg/kg and observed for 14 days. A single oral dose of 100 or 300 mg/kg caused no adverse effects except a failure to gain weight by the 300-mg/kg group. A dose of 900 mg/kg produced a number of adverse effects: weight loss, bleeding from eyes and nose, depression of lymphoid tissue, degenerative changes in the myocardium and liver, and increases in haematocrit, haemoglobin, BUN, SGOT, and SGPT. Effects were dose related, the 794-mg/kg-dose group being affected much like the 900-mg/kg-dose group. The dose of 794 mg/kg was fatal to nine of ten rats during the observation period, whereas no rats died from the 631-mg/kg dose.

In subacute toxicity studies (LEE et al. 1976 a, c) groups of rats were given 10, 30 or 90 mg/kg WR 180409 orally for 28 consecutive days. No adverse effects were noted in the group receiving 10 mg/kg. A repeated dose of 30 mg/kg was fatal to two of ten rats; there were dose-related toxic signs in all of the rats and blood changes in some. A repeated dose of 90 mg/kg was fatal to three of ten rats and caused toxic signs and blood changes in all. Toxic signs included weight loss, anorexia, haemorrhaging of the eyes and nose, diarrhoea and weakness. There were increases in erythrocyte count, haematocrit, platelet count and haemoglobin concentration, and decrease in reticulocyte count and the neutrophil to lymphocyte ratio. There were elevations of SGOT, SGPT, alkaline phosphatase and/or BUN. At the highest dose administered, 90 mg/kg, the drug caused necrosis of skeletal muscle and lymphoid depletion of the thymus and spleen. This dose also caused an increase in the incidence and severity of naturally occurring lesions in the lung.

The acute oral toxicity of WR 180409 in beagles was also studied by LEE et al. (1976 b, d). Single doses of 16 mg/kg or 37 mg/kg caused no adverse effects. Doses of 55, 80 or 420 mg/kg caused vomiting. Other than a transient increase in the neutrophil/lymphocyte ratio, with leucocytosis in one dog receiving a dose of 55 mg/kg, there were no drug-related haematological or clinical effects. In a subsequent study (LEE et al. 1976 b), a single oral dose of 55 mg/kg brought about mild elevations of SGPT, mild myocarditis, and/or myocardial degeneration in three of three dogs.

In subacute oral toxicity studies in beagles (LEE et al. 1976 d, e), groups of dogs were administered 5, 15, 30 or 45 mg/kg of WR 180409 for 28 consecutive days. At doses of 30 mg/kg or less there were no adverse signs and no lesions or changes in blood chemistry. At the 45-mg/kg level, reduced food consumption, reduced weight gain, occasional emesis and mild necrosis of the lymphoid tissue in the tonsils were found in all dogs. In one dog this dose caused severe involution of the thymus, atrophy of the germinal centres, lymphoid depletion and cellular infiltration of the lymph nodes.

The drug WR 180409 evaluated for mutagenic potential using the *Salmonella*/microsome plate test (HODGSON et al. 1977 f) was found not to be mutagenic.

4. Pharmacology

The disposition of WR 180409-[^{14}C] (label on the carbinol carbon) after oral administration to male mice was studied by CHUNG et al. (1976, 1978). Over a 240-h period about 84% and 5% of drug-derived radioactivity was excreted in the faeces and urine respectively. Plasma level radioactivity peaked at 4 h and red-cell radioactivity at 12 h. Elimination half-lives of the parent drug in plasma and in RBC were estimated to be 26.4 and 27.4 h respectively. The drug was readily absorbed and rapidly distributed throughout the body. It was strongly bound to plasma proteins. Two hours after oral administration, the major concentration of radioactivity was found in the lungs, liver, kidneys, small intestine and contents, and residual carcass; a high percentage of the radioactivity was represented by parent drug.

Findings in a companion study using rats (GALBRAITH et al. 1976) were similar. Radioactivity was largely excreted in the faeces and very little was excreted in the urine. There was chromatographic evidence for the formation of several metabolites. The drug was widely distributed, highest concentrations being found in the lungs, liver, adrenals and bone marrow.

In a study of the disposition of WR 180409-[^{14}C] in rhesus monkeys, MCCONNELL and FURNER (1977) found that ^{14}C drug-equivalents in the blood peaked between 12 and 24 h after oral dosing, the parent compound accounting for 45% of the total. Drug-equivalent elimination in faeces and urine was 59% and 24% respectively with half-lives of 1.9 and 1.7 days. No more than 50% of the drug equivalents in the faeces and 9% in the urine were parent drug; six other products were detected. High concentrations of drug equivalents were present in the liver, kidneys, lungs, and eyes. After intravenous administration, a triphasic elimination of drug equivalents from the blood was observed with half-lives of 1.2 h,, 2.9 days and 14.9 days.

5. Determination in Biological Fluids

A method for the determination of WR 180409 in whole blood has been described by NAKAGAWA et al. (1979). The method has been used for the determination of mefloquine and a brief description has been given in the section on mefloquine.

A study of the effect of changes in the composition of a multicomponent solvent system used in the chromatographic determination of WR 180409 after ethyl acetate extraction of the drug and an internal standard, WR 184806, from blood has been reported by STAMPFLI et al. (1979).

The determination of a related pyridinemethanol, WR 148946 [α-di-*n*-butylaminomethyl-2,6-bis(trifluoromethylphenyl)-4-pyridinemethanol HCl] in biological fluids has also been reported (BOUWSMA and STEWART 1976).

6. Clinical Studies

A phase I study of WR 180409 using the rising dose, double-blind method was conducted by REBA and BARRY (1977). Forty-three subjects were used in the study; 21 received placebo and the remainder received a single dose varying from 5 to 1,500 mg. There were no significant adverse effects from the drug at doses lower than 1,000 mg. At doses of 1,000 mg and greater drug-related nausea, vomiting, dizziness and subjective mental alterations were recorded. Symptoms were mild and of less than 48 h in duration. No physical or laboratory abnormalities were attributed to the drug.

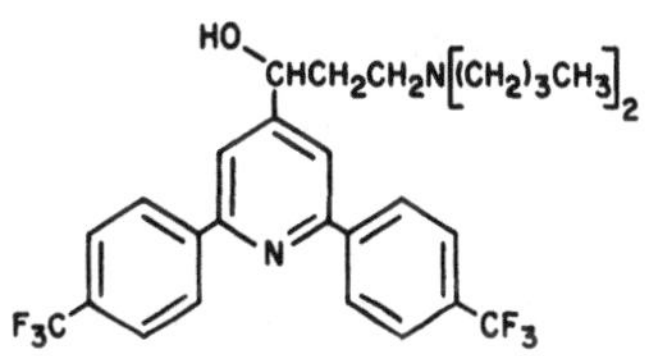

Fig. 12. WR 172435. 3-Di-*n*-butylamino-1-[2,6-bis(4-trifluoromethylphenyl)-4-pyridyl]-propanol

II. WR 172435

The pyridinemethanol WR 172435 (Fig. 12) has the same side chain as the phenanthrenemethanol, halofantrine. It was first synthesised by COLWELL et al. (1972) and submitted as the hydrochloride salt. This salt form was very sparingly soluble. In a study of several salts (HIGUCHI and HASLAM 1974b), the methanesulphonate was found to be 11 times (1.1 mg/ml) as soluble as the hydrochloride and was chosen as the salt form of the drug for all advanced studies. The following discussion pertains to the methanesulphonate unless otherwise indicated.

1. Activity in Animal Models

Against a blood-induced *P. berghei* infection in the mouse (OSDENE et al. 1967), a single subcutaneous administration of WR 172435·HCl in peanut oil produced cures with doses of 20–640 mg/kg. The compound was "active" at a level of 10 mg/kg. No acute toxicity was observed at the highest dose, 640 mg/kg.

The ability of WR 172435 · HCl to suppress parasitaemia in *P. berghei*-infected mice was evaluated by the method of THOMPSON (1972). When administered orally twice a day for 3 days, beginning 3 days after infection, the ED_{90} (dose required to suppress parasitaemia by 90%) against a drug-sensitive strain was 2.9 mg/kg per day, a value indicating the drug was 27 times more potent than quinine. Against a quinine- or mefloquine-resistant strain of *P. berghei* there was a 160-fold cross-resistance.

Pilot studies with the hydrochloride salt and expanded studies with the methanesulphonate salt of WR 172435 on the effectiveness of the drug against *P. falciparum* infections in owl monkeys were conducted by SCHMIDT et al. (1978d). The very high activity of this drug seen in the *P. berghei*-mouse model was also seen in the *P. falciparum*-owl monkey model. In pilot appraisals of the hydrochloride, approximate CD_{90}s of 28 and 32 mg/kg were obtained against infections with the chloroquine-resistant Vietnam Oak Knoll and the pyrimethamine-resistant Malayan Camp-CH/Q strains of *P. falciparum* respectively. In expanded evaluations using the methanesulphonate and the multidrug-resistant Smith strain of *P. falciparum*, it was found that a dose of the drug delivered orally in divided doses over three consecutive days or over seven consecutive days was more effective than the same total quantity of drug given in a single dose. The CD_{90} was 15–16 mg/kg in the multidose regimens. In this model, WR 172435 was at least as active, and perhaps somewhat more active, than the pyridinemethanol WR 180409. The CD_{90}s for either of these compounds against the multidrug-resistant Smith strain were between one-half and one-third the CD_{90}s of chloroquine for chloroquine-susceptible strains of *P. falciparum*. The fact that the largest dose of WR 172435 administered, 560 mg/kg, was well tolerated while the CD_{90} against the Smith strain of *P. falciparum* was 16 mg/kg indicates a therapeutic index in excess of 36.

WR 172435 was distinctly more active against blood-induced infections with the Vietnam Palo Alto strain of *P. vivax* in the owl monkey, $CD_{90} = 5–7$ mg/kg, than against infections with the Smith strain of *P. falciparum*. It was also more active than the pyridinemethanol WR 180409 against infections with *P. vivax*. In addition, the efficacies of the single-dose, three-dose or seven-dose regimens were essentially identical. The drug showed prompt control and clearance of parasitaemia.

Thus, in comparison, WR 172435 (as well as the pyridinemethanol WR 180409) was substantially more active than the phenanthrenemethanol halofantrine, slightly more active than the phenanthrenemethanol WR 122455 and similar in activity to mefloquine. In addition, parasite clearance was effected much more rapidly with either of the two pyridinemethanols than it was with either of the phenanthrenemethanols and slightly more rapidly than it was with mefloquine (SCHMIDT et al. 1978d).

2. In Vitro Activity

The in vitro activity of WR 172435, as indicated by its ability to inhibit the uptake of tritiated hypoxanthine by cultured intraerythrocytic forms of drug-sensitive and drug-resistant *P. falciparum*, was consistent with its high in vivo activity against both drug-susceptible and drug-resistant strains of *P. falciparum*. The ID_{50}s for the drug-susceptible African Uganda I and multidrug-resistant Smith strains of *P. fal-*

Table 3. Acute LD_{50} of WR 172435 in male rodents (mg/kg)

	Mice	Rats	Guinea pigs
PO	3,683	2,754	> 5,012
IP	121	254	374

ciparum were 3.2 and 7.9 ng/ml respectively. These values stand in contrast to the corresponding ID_{50}s of 35.4 and 48.5 ng/ml obtained for the pyridinemethanol WR 180409 (DESJARDINS et al. 1979 a).

3. Toxicology

Acute and subacute studies of the toxicity of WR 172435 in rodents were performed by LEE et al. (1976 f). The acute LD_{50}s in male rodents are summarised in Table 3.

Toxic signs from oral administration included anorexia, depression, rough hair coat, and weight loss; rats also had ataxia of the hind legs. Single oral doses of 30, 90 or 270 mg/kg caused no adverse signs, lesions, changes in peripheral blood elements or clinical blood chemistry over a 72-h period.

In subacute studies, groups of rats were given oral doses of 10, 20, 30, 90 or 270 mg/kg of the drug, daily for 28 days. With this regimen, doses of 10 or 20 mg/kg caused no adverse effects. Doses of 30 mg/kg caused mild lesions in lymphoid tissue. Doses of 90 mg/kg per day caused toxic signs, severe lesions and changes in peripheral blood; doses of 270 mg/kg were lethal in 7–12 days. At the 90-mg/kg level, there were severe neutrophilia and relative lymphopaenia and an increase in fasting blood glucose, SGOT and BUN. Repeated doses of 90 or 270 mg/kg caused severe lesions in the lymphoid tissues, spleen, small intestine, and skeletal muscle with mild elevation of the M/E ratio in bone marrow.

WR 172435 was not mutagenic when evaluated in the *Salmonella*/microsome plate test using five strains of bacteria (HODGSON et al. 1977 g).

4. Pharmacology

CHUNG et al. (1981) studied the disposition of WR 172435-^{14}C in mice after a single oral dose of 20 mg/kg. After 192 h 76% of the drug-derived radioactivity had been excreted in the faeces and 1% in the urine; approximately 19% was recovered in the carcass. The excretion of radioactivity in the faeces appeared to be biphasic, with a terminal phase half-life of 81.0 h. Elimination of parent drug via the faeces was monophasic with a half-life of 24 h. The concentration of radioactivity and parent drug in the plasma and red blood cells peaked 2 h after drug administration; the elimination $t_{1/2}$ of the parent drug from the plasma and red blood cells was estimated to be 63 and 67 h respectively. The major sites of radioactivity, 2 h after dosing, were the gastrointestinal tract and contents, gall bladder and bile, adrenals, spleen, lungs, kidneys, and heart. At 120 h after drug administration, the eyes and submaxillary salivary glands had acquired relatively high concentrations of radioactivity. Greater than 70% of the radioactivity in all tissues was identified as parent drug.

The disposition of WR 172435-[^{14}C] HCl in the rat after a single oral dose of 10 mg/kg was studied by HIREMATH (1975b). The drug was rapidly absorbed, with a peak plasma level of 0.71 ng/ml being reached in 2 h. Plasma drug levels were consistently higher than red blood cell levels at all times, the peak level of the latter being 0.45 ng/ml at 5 h. Estimated half-lives in plasma and red cells were 11.5 and 16 h respectively. The drug-derived radioactivity was primarily excreted in the faeces (89.50%) with only 0.10% excreted in the urine. Analysis by TLC indicated the presence of two metabolites in the faeces in addition to unchanged drug. Radioactivity was concentrated in the adrenals, liver, lungs, spleen, fat, kidneys, and skin.

The disposition of WR 172435-[^{14}C] in male rhesus monkeys was studied by HODGSON et al. (1979). A single oral dose of 35 mg/kg to male monkeys was followed over a 24-day period. At the end of this period 82% of the drug-derived radioactivity had been excreted in the faeces and 2% in the urine. Elimination of radioactivity via the faeces was biphasic with phase half-lives of 19 and 282 h. Blood level versus time data indicated a single absorption phase with a half-life of 2.8 h and two elimination phases with half-lives of 8.5 and 525 h. Significant amounts of drug-derived radioactivity were found in the liver, lungs, bile, fat, and bone marrow 9 h after dosing while appreciable concentrations of radioactivity were still present in the tissues after 92 days. An analysis of the radioactivity of tissue and faecal extracts by TLC indicated extensive metabolism of the drug.

5. Clinical Studies

A phase I study of the safety and tolerance of WR 172435 was conducted using a single oral dose in a standard double-blind, rising-dose method with healthy male subjects (REBA and BARRY 1978). Eight dose levels were used ranging from 5 mg through 1,000 mg. In one of the subjects receiving 800 mg and two of four subjects receiving 1,000 mg there were mild and temporary drug-related gastrointestinal symptoms. Seven of eighteen subjects receiving the drug had temporary leucocytosis without change in differential count. The gastrointestinal symptoms and leucocytosis appeared to be drug and dose related. It was concluded that the drug is well tolerated symptomatically up to the 1,000-mg dose level.

In a follow-up phase I double-blind study specifically designed to detect leucocytosis and gastrointestinal symptoms, 6 of 12 volunteer subjects received a single oral 1,000-mg dose of the drug by random assignment and six received a placebo (JOHNSON and BARRY 1979). In all of the subjects receiving the drug there occurred leucocytosis marked by an absolute increase in neutrophils; gastrointestinal symptoms also developed. The symptomatology and leucocytosis lasted less than 48 h.

E. Conclusions

A number of new antimalarial drugs have been developed to the point where they can be considered as alternatives to the potent antimalarial drug, mefloquine. Since they are all chemically related (they are all arylaminoalcohols) there exists the potential danger that the emergence of a strain of plasmodia resistant to one may compromise the effectiveness of all. Such an eventuality does not seem imminent.

However, research on combinations of drugs, such as is now being carried on with mefloquine and certain antifolate-type antimalarials, could result in formulations that may impede the development of drug resistance. The pursuit of such studies would seem to be a prudent course of action. New chemical classes of antimalarials unrelated to the arylaminoalcohols, e.g. the sesquiterpene lactone Qinghaosu, are needed. The development of new drugs would be facilitated by the continued study of the biochemistry and nutritional requirements of the malaria parasite and the mechanisms whereby drugs intrude on life processes.

References

Agharkar S, Lindenbaum S, Higuchi T (1976) Enhancement of solubility of drug salts by hydrophilic counterions: properties of organic salts of an antimalarial drug. J Pharm Sci 65:747–749

Antuñano FJL, Wernsdorfer WH (1979) *In vitro* response of chloroquine-resistant *Plasmodiuom falciparum* to mefloquine. Bull WHO 57:663–665

Arnold JD, Martin DC, Carson PE, Rieckmann KH, Willerson Jr D, Clyde DF, Miller RM (1973) A phenanthrene methanol (WR 33,063) for treatment of acute malaria. Antimicrob Agents Chemother 3:207–213

Aviado DM, Belej M (1970) Pharmacology of new antimalarial drugs. Pharmacology 3:257–272

Bay WW, Gleiser CA, Dukes TW, Brown RS (1970) The experimental production and evaluation of drug-induced phototoxicity in swine. Toxicol Appl Pharmacol 17:538–547

Blumbergs P, Ao M-S, LaMontagne MP, Markovac A (1975) Antimalarials. 7. 2,8-bis(-trifluoromethyl)-4-quinolinemethanols. J Med Chem 18:1122–1126

Bouwsma OJ, Stewart JT (1976) Fluorometric determination of WR-148,946 [alpha-di-*n*-butylaminomethyl)-2,6-bis(trifluoromethylphenyl)-4-pyridine methanol hydrochloride in biological fluids. Anal Lett 9:1003–1013

Brossi A (1976) The present status of malaria chemotherapy. Heterocycles 5:631–647

Brown RE, Stancato FA, Wolfe AD (1979) The effects of mefloquine on *Escherichia coli.* Life Sci 25:1857–1864

Caldwell RW, Nash CB (1977) Pulmonary and cardiovascular effects of mefloquine methanesulfonate. Toxicol Appl Pharmacol 40:437–448

Canfield CJ (1980) Antimalarial aminoalcohol alternatives to mefloquine. Acta Tropica 37:232–237

Canfield CJ, Hall AP, MacDonald BS, Neumann DA, Shaw JA (1973) Treatment of falciparum malaria from Vietnam with a phenanthrene methanol (WR 33,063) and a quinoline methanol (WR 30,090). Antimicrob Agents Chemother 3:224–227

Carroll FI, Blackwell JT (1974) Optical isomers of aryl-2-piperidylmethanol antimalarial agents. Preparation, optical purity, and absolute stereochemistry. J Med Chem 17:210–291

Cheng CC (1971) Structure and antimalarial activity of aminoalcohols and 2-(*p*-chlorophenyl)-2-(4-piperidyl) tetrahydrofuran. J Pharm Sci 60:1596–1598

Chevli R, Fitch CD (1981) The antimalarial drug, mefloquine, binds to normal erythrocyte membranes. Fed Proc 40:776

Chien P-L, Cheng CC (1973) Further side-chain modification of antimalarial phenanthrene amino alcohols. J Med Chem 16:1093–1096

Chien P-L, Cheng CC (1976) Difference in antimalarial activity between certain amino alcohol diastereomers. J Med Chem 19:170–172

Chung H, Gillum HH, Rozman RS (1976) The absorption, distribution and elimination of *threo*-α-(2-piperidyl)-2-trifluoromethyl-6-(4-trifluoromethylphenyl)-4-pyridinemethanol phosphate (WR 180,409 H_3PO_4) in mice. Fed Proc Fed Am Soc Exp Biol 35:328

Chung H, Gillum HH, Rozman RS (1978) The disposition of *threo*-α-(2-piperidyl)-2-trifluoromethyl-6-(4-trifluoromethylphenyl)-4-pyridinemethanol phosphate in mice. Drug Metab Dispos 6:82–86

Chung H, Jimmerson V, Bounds D, Keller R, Rozman R (1979) The disposition of *threo*-α-(2-piperidyl)-2,8-bis(trifluoromethyl)-4-quinolinemethanol hydrochloride (WR 177,602 HCl) in mice. Toxicol Appl Pharmacol 48:1, part 2, A10

Chung H, Jimmerson VR, Sanders JE, Bounds DW, Rozman RS, Thorne J (1981) The disposition of *dl*-3-*di*-*n*-butylamino-*l*-[2,6-bis(4-trifluoromethylphenyl)-4-pyridyl] propanol methanesulfonate in mice. Drug Metab Dispos 9:65–66

Clyde DF, McCarthy VC, Rebert CC, Miller RM (1973) Prophylactic activity of a phenanthrene methanol (WR33,063) and a quinoline methanol (WR30,090) in human malaria. Antimicrob Agents Chemother 3:220–223

Clyde DF, McCarthy VC, Miller RM, Hornick RB (1976) Suppressive activity of mefloquine in sporozoite-induced human malaria. Antimicrob Agents Chemother 9:384–386

Coatney GR, Cooper WC, Young MD, Burgess RW (1947) Human malaria IV. The suppressive action of a phenanthrene amino alcohol, NIH-204(SN-1796), against sporozoite-induced vivax malaria. Am J Hyg 46:132–140

Coatney GR, Cooper WC, Eddy NB, Greenburg J (1953) Survey of antimalarial agents. In: Public health monograph No 9, U.S. Government Printing Office. Washington

Colwell WT, Brown V, Christie P, Lange J, Reece C, Yamamoto K, Henry DW (1972) Antimalarial arylaminopropanols. J Med Chem 15:771–775

Davidson DE Jr, Johnson DO, Tanticharoenyos P, Hickman RL, Kinnamon KE (1976) Evaluating new antimalarial drugs against trophozoite-induced *Plasmodium cynomolgi* malaria in rhesus monkeys. Am J Trop Med Hyg 25:26–33

Davidson MW, Griggs Jr BG, Boykin DW, Wilson WD (1975) Mefloquine, a clinically useful quinolinemethanol antimalarial which does not significantly bind to DNA. Nature 254:632–634

Davidson MW, Griggs BG, Boykin DW, Wilson WD (1977) Molecular structural effects involved in the interaction of quinolinemethanolamines with DNA. Implications for antimalarial action. J Med Chem 20:1117–1122

Davies EE, Warhurst DC, Peters W (1975) The chemotherapy of rodent malaria, XXI Action of quinine and WR122,455 (a 9-phenanthrenemethanol) on the fine structure of *Plasmodium berghei* in mouse blood. Ann Trop Med Parasitol 69:147–153

Desjardins RE, Canfield CJ, Haynes JD (1979a) Quantitative assessment of antimalarial activity *in vitro* by a semiautomated microdilution technique. Antimicrob Agents Chemother 16:710–718

Desjardins RE, Pamplin CL III, von Bredow J, Barry KG, Canfield CJ (1979b) Kinetics of a new antimalarial, mefloquine. Clin Pharmacol Ther 26:372–379

Doberstyn EB, Phintuyothin P, Noeypatimanondh S, Teerakiartkomjorn C (1979) Single dose therapy of falciparum malaria with mefloquine or pyrimethamine sulfadoxine. Bull WHO 57:275–279

Einheber A, Palmer DM, Aikawa M (1976) *Plasmodium berghei:* Phase contrast and electron microscopical evidence that certain antimalarials can both inhibit and reverse pigment clumping caused by chloroquine. Exp Parasitol 40:52–61

Fitch CD (1969) Chloroquine resistance in malaria: a deficiency of chloroquine binding. Proc Nat Acad Sci USA 64:1181–1187

Fitch CD (1972) Chloroquine resistance in malaria: drug binding and cross resistance patterns. Proc Helminthol Soc Washington [Special Issue] 39:265–271

Fitch CD (1977) Chloroquine susceptibility in malaria: dependence on exposure of the parasites to the drug. Life Sci 21:1511–1514

Fitch CD, Chan RL, Chevli R (1979) Chloroquine resistance in malaria: accessibility of drug receptors to mefloquine. Antimicrob Agents Chemother 15:258–262

Galbraith WM, Campbell S, Tillery K, Mellett LB (1976) Disposition of WR-180,409 H_3PO_4 in the rat. Fed Proc Fed Am Soc Exp Biol 35:488

Grethe G, Mitt G (1978) Verfahren zur Herstellung von Mefloquin. Ger Offen 2.806, 909

Grindel JM, Rozman RS, Leahy DM, Molek NA, Gillum HH (1976) The absorption, distribution, and excretion in mice of a quinolinemethanol antimalarial 2,8-bis(-trifluoromethyl)-4-[1-hydroxy-3-(*N-t*-butylamino)propyl] quinoline phosphate (WR-184,806). Drug Metab Dispos 4:133–139

Grindel JM, Tilton PF, Shaffer RD (1977) Quantitation of the antimalarial agent, mefloquine in blood plasma, and urine using high-pressure liquid chromatography. J Pharm Sci 66:834–837

Hacker MP, Hong C-B, Ellis ER, Liu GK, Lee CC (1978) Local venous toxicity of α-(2-piperidyl)-2,8-bis(trifluoromethyl)-4-quinolinemethanol methanesulfonate, Mefloquine CH_3SO_3H (WR-142,490 CH_3SO_3H) and 2,8-bis(trifluoromethyl)4-[*l*-hydroxy-3-(*N-t*-bytylamino)-propyl]-quinoline phosphate (WR-184,806 · H_3PO_4) in rabbits. Interim Report No. 137, U.S. Army medical research and development command contract No. DAMD-17-74-C-4036, Jan 12

Hahn FE (1974) Chloroquine (resochin). In: Corcoran JW, Hahn FE (eds) Antibiotics, vol III. Springer, Berlin Heidelberg New York, p 58

Hahn FE, Fean CL (1969) Spectrophotometric studies of the interaction of an antimalarial quinoline methanol with deoxyribonucleic acid. Anticrob Agents Chemother 4:63–66

Hall AP (1976) The treatment of malaria. Br Med J 1:323–328

Hall AP, Segal HE, Pearlman EJ, Phintuyothin P (1975) Comparison of a 9-phenanthrene methanol (WR-33,063), a 4-quinoline methanol (WR-30,090) and quinine for falciparum malaria in Thailand. Trans R Soc Trop Med Hyg 69:342–349

Hall AP, Doberstyn EB, Karnchanachetanee C, Samransamruajkit S, Laixuthai B, Pearlman EJ, Lampe RM, Miller CF, Phintuyothin P (1977) Sequential treatment with quinine and mefloquine or quinine and pyrimethamine-sulfadoxine for falciparum malaria. Br Med J 1:1626–1628

Harmon RE, Lin TS, Gupa SK (1973) Preparation and antimalarial activity of some derivatives of 6-bromo-α-(di-*n*-heptylaminomethyl)-9-phenanthrenemethanol. J Med Chem 16:940–942

Hemwall E, DiPalma JR (1979) Cardiovascular and antiarrhythmic effects of mefloquine. Pharmacologist 21:200

Higuchi T, Haslam JL (1974a) Determination of a preferred salt form of WR-180,409 (free base). Interim Report No. 7, U.S. Army medical research and development command contract No. DADA17-73-C-3125, September

Higuchi T, Haslam JL (1974b) Determination of a preferred salt form of WR-172,435 (free base). Interim Report, U.S. Army medical research and development command contract No. DADA17-73-C-3125, February, Revised November 1975

Hiremath CB (1974) Absorption, distribution, and excretion of α-(2-di-*n*-butylaminoethyl)-1,3,dichloro-6-trifluoromethyl-9-phenanthrene methanol-C^{14}) in rats and rhesus monkeys. Fed Proc Fed Am Soc Exp Biol 33:472

Hiremath CB (1975a) Pharmacokinetics and metabolism of candidate antimalarial drugs (WR-171,669-C^{14}, WR-159,412-C^{14}, WR-33,063-C^{14}, WR-172,435-C^{14}, and WR-184,806-C^{14}) in experimental animals. Final report, U.S. Army medical research and development command contract No. DADA-17-72-C-2166, July 15

Hiremath CB (1975b) Metabolism and disposition of 3-di-*n*-butylamino-*l*-[2,6-bis(4-trifluoromethylphenyl)-4-pyridyl] propanol-1-C^{14} hydrochloride (WR-172,435-C^{14}) in the rat. Fed Proc Fed Am Soc Exp Biol 34:733

Hodgson JR, Kowalski MA, Goethem VD, Hainje M, Lee CC (1977a) Mutagenicity studies on 2,8-bis(trifluoromethyl)-4-[1-hydroxy-3-(*N-t*-butylamino) propyl] quinoline phosphate (WR-184,806 H_3PO_4). Interim report No. 125, U.S. Army medical research and development command contract No. DAMD-17-74-C-4036

Hodgson JR, Lowalski MA, Goethem VD, Hainje M, Lee CC (1977b) Mutagenicity studies on α-(2-piperidyl)-6,8-dichloro-2-trifluoromethyl-4-quinolinemethanol phosphate (WR-226,253 H_3PO_4). Interim report No. 131, U.S. Army medical research and development command contract No. DAMD-17-74-C-4036, Sept 23

Hodgson JR, Kowalski MA, Goethem DV, Hainje M, Lee CC (1977c) Mutagenicity studies on α-diheptylaminomethyl-6-bromo-9-phenanthrene methanol hydrochloride (WR-33,063 HCl). Interim report No. 132, U.S. Army medical research and development command contract No. DAMD-17-74-C-4036, September 22

Hodgson JR, Kowalski MA, Goethem DV, Hainje M, Lee CC (1977d) Mutagenicity studies on phenanthrene methanol (WR-122,455 HCl). Interim report No. 121, U.S. Army medical research and development command contract No. DAMD-17-74-C-4036, Aug 19

Hodgson JR, Kowalski MA, Goethem DV, Hainje M, Lee CC (1977e) Mutagenicity studies on 1,3,-dichloro-6-trifluoromethyl-9-[*l*hydroxy-3-(dibutylamino) propyl] phenanthrene hydrochloride (WR-171,669 HCl). Interim report No. 124, U.S. Army medical research and development command contract No. DAMD-17-74-C-4036, August 31

Hodgson JR, Kowalski MA, Goethem DV, Hainje M, Lee CC (1977f) Mutagenicity studies on DL-threo-α-(2-piperidyl)-2-trifluoromethyl-6-(4-trifluoromethylphenyl)-4-pyridinemethanol phosphate (WR-180,409 H_3PO_4). Interim report No. 129, U.S. Army medical research and development command contract No. DAMD-17-74-C-4036, September 9

Hodgson, JR, Kowalski MA, Goethem DV, Hainje M, Lee CC (1977g) Mutagenicity studies on 3-di-*n*-butylamino-*l*-[2,6-bis(4-trifluoromethylphenyl)-4-pyridyl] propanol methanesulfonate (WR-172,435 CH_2SO_3H) Interim report No. 126, U.S. Army medical research and development command contract No. DAMD-17-74-C-4036, August 32

Hodgson JR, Minor JL, Lee C-C, Chung H (1979) Pharmakokinetic studies on a new candidate antimalarial 3-di-*n*-butylamino-1-[2,6-bis(4-trifluoromethylphenyl)-4-pyridyl] propanol methanesulfonate, WR-172,435 CH_3SO_3H in rhesus monkeys. Toxicol Appl Pharmacol 48:No 1 Part 2 A8

Jauch VR, Griesser E, Osterhelt G (1980) Metabolismus von Ro 21-5998 (Mefloquine) bei der Ratte. Arzneimittelforsch 30:60–67

Jearnpipatkul A, Govitrapong P, Yuthavong Y, Wilairat P, Panijpan B (1980) Binding of antimalarial drugs to hemozoin from *Plasmodium berghei*. Experientia 36:1063–1064

Johnson JA, Barry KG (1979) WR-172,435 CH_3SO_3H: short term dosage, safety and tolerance: effect on the total and differential leukocyte counts following a single oral dose. Final report, addendum to experiment number 13, U.S. Army medical research and development command contract No. DAMD-17-75-C-5036

Korte DW Jr, Heiffer MH, Kintner LD, Lee CC (1978) Comparative acute and subacute toxicities of erythro-α-(2-piperidyl)-2,8-bis(trifluoromethyl)-4-quinolinemethanol HCl, WR-142,490 · HCl(mefloquine HCl) and its *threo* diastereomer WR-177,602 HCl, in dogs. Fed Proc Fed Am Soc Exp Biol 37:248

Korte DW Jr, Heiffer MH, Hacker MP, Kintner LD, Hong CB, Lee CC (1979) Subchronic toxicity of the antimalarial drug, mefloquine hydrochloride (WR-142,490), in monkeys and dogs. Fed Proc Fed Am Soc Exp Biol 38:680

LaMontagne MP, Markovac A, Blumbergs P (1974) Antimalarials. 6,Synthesis, anitmalarial activity, and configuration of racemic α-(2-piperidyl)-4-pyridinemethanols. J. Med Chem 17:519–523

Lee CC, Castles TR, Crawford CR, Landes AM (1967) Acute and subacute oral toxicities of 6,8-dichloro-2-(3′,4′dichlorophenyl)-α-(di-*n*-butylaminomethyl)-4-quinolinemethanol monohydrochloride (WR-30,090-E) in dogs. Interim report No. 13, U.S. Army medical research and development command contract No. DA-49-193-MD-2759, December 18

Lee CC, Castles TR, Crawford CR, Landes AM (1968a) Acute and subacute oral toxicities of 6,8-dichloro-2-(3′,4′dichlorophenyl)-α-(di-*n*-butylaminomethyl)-4-quinolinemethanol monohydrochloride (WR-30,090-E) in dogs – further study. Interim report No. 19, U.S. Army medical research and development command contract No. DA-49-193-MD-2759, April 26

Lee CC, Castles TR, Crawford CR, Landes AM (1968b) Acute and subacute oral toxicities of 6,8-dichloro-2-(3′,4′dichlorophenyl)-α-(di-*n*-butylaminomethyl)-4-quinolinemethanol monohydrochloride (WR-30,090-E) in dogs – additional study. Interim report No. 19, U.S. Army medical research and development command contract No. DA-40-193-MD-2759, February 20

Lee CC, Castles TR, Crawford CR, Landes AM (1968c) Acute and subacute oral toxicities of 6,8-dichloro-2-(3′,4′dichlorophenyl)-α-(di-*n*-butylaminomethyl)-4-quinolinemethanol monohydrochloride (WR-30,090-E) in dogs – supplement. Interim report No. 19, U.S. Army medical research and development command contract No. DA-49-193-MD-2759, July 20

Lee CC, Castles TR, Landes AM, Cronin MC, Bristow RL (1970a) Acute and sub-acute oral toxicities of phenanthrene methanol, WR-122-455 (AV-17876) in rodents. Interim report No. 35, U.S. Army medical research and development command contract No. DA-49-193-MD-2759, July 24

Lee CC, Castles TR, Landes AM, Cronin MC, Bristow RL (1970b) Acute and subacute oral toxicities of phenanthrene methanol, WR-122,455 (AV-17876), in dogs. Interim report No. 32, U.S. Army medical research and development command contract No. DA-49-193-MD-2759, Jan 21

Lee CC, Castles TR, Landes AM, Cronin MC, Bristow RL (1970c) Subacute oral toxicities of phenanthrene methanol, WR-122,455 (AV99065) in dogs. Interim report No. 38, U.S. Army medical research and development command contract No. DA-49-193-MD-2759, Oct 7

Lee CC, Castles TR, Landes AM, Cronin MC, Bristow RL (1970d) Reversal toxicity study on phenanthrene methanol WR-122,455, in dogs. Interim Report No. 36, U.S. Army medical research and development command contract No. DA-49-193-MD-2759, July 24

Lee CC, Castles TR, Landes AM, Cronin MC, Coffelt J, Hutchcraft R (1971a) Subacute oral toxicity of 6,8-dichloro-2-(3′,4′-dichlorophenyl)-alpha-(di-*n*-butylaminomethyl)-4-quinolinemethanol monohydrochloride WR-30,090 (AV-07996), in rats (84 days). Interim report No. 44, U.A. Army medical research and development command contract No. DA-49-193-MD-2759, June 21

Lee CC, Castles TR, Landes AM, Cronin MC, Coffelt J, Hutchcraft R (1971b) Subacute oral toxicity of 6,8-dichloro-2-(3′,4′-dichlorophenyl)-α-(di-*n*-butylamino-methyl)-4-quinolinemethanol monohydrochloride, WR-30,090 (AV-07996), in dogs (91 days). Interim report No. 45, U.S. Army medical research and development command contract No. DA-49-193-MD-2759, June 24

Lee CC, Kintner LD, Castles TR, Landes AM, Cronin MC, Hutchcraft R, Merle F (1972a) Acute and subacute oral toxicities of α-(2-piperidyl)-2,8-bis(trifluoromethyl)-4-quinolinemethanol hydrochloride, WR-142,490 (AY-65742), in dogs. Interim report No. 57, U.S. Army medical research and development command contract No. DA-49-193-MD-2759, Jan 21

Lee CC, Kintner LD, Castles TR, Landes AM, Cronin MC, Hutchcraft R, Merle F (1972b) Acute and subacute toxicities of α-(2-piperidyl)-2,8-bis(trifluoromethyl)-4-quinolinemethanol hydrochloride, WR-142,490(AY-65742), in rodents. Interim report No. 56, U.S. Army medical research and development command contract No. DA-49-193-MD-2759, Jan 20

Lee CC, Kintner LD, Sanyer JL, Castles TR, Landes AM, Cronin MC, Merle F (1972c) Acute and subacute toxicities of 1,3-dichloro-6-trifluoromethyl-9-[l-hydroxy-3-(dibutylamino)propyl] phenanthrene hydrochloride, WR-171,669 (BB-41223), in rodents. Interim report No. 65, U.S. Army medical research and development command contract No. DA-49-193-MD-2759, October 3

Lee CC, Kintner LD, Sanyer JL, Castles TR, Landes AM, Cronin MC, Merle F (1972d) Acute and subacute oral toxicities of 1,3-dichloro-6-trifluoromethyl-9-[l-hydroxy-3(dibutylamino)-propyl] phenanthrene hydrochloride, WR-171,669 (BB-41223) in dogs. Interim report No. 66, U.S. Army medical research and development command contract No. DA-49-193-MD-2759, October 17

Lee CC, Kintner LD, Sanyer JL, Castles TR, Reddig TW, Girvin JD, Kowalski JJ, Buchberger GL (1974a) Oral toxicity of α-(2-piperidyl)-2,8-bis(trifluoromethyl)-4-quinolinemethanol hydrochloride, WR-142,490, in rats at the completion of 52 weeks. Interim report No. 85, U.S. Army medical research and development command contract No. DAMD-17-74-C-4063

Lee CC, Kintner LD, Sanyer JL, Castles TR, Reddig TW, Girvin JD, Kowalski JJ, Buchberger GL (1974b) Oral toxicity of α-(2-piperidyl)-2,8-bis(trifluoromethyl)-4-quinolinemethanol hydrochloride, WR-142,490, in dogs at the completion of 52 weeks. Interim report No. 85, U.S. Army medical research and development command contract No. DAMD-17-74-C-4063, April 30

Lee CC, Kintner LD, Sanyer JL, Reddig TW, Girvin JD, Buchberger GL, Seifert WK (1974 c) Acute and subacute toxicity of 2,8-bis(trifluoromethyl)-4[l-hydroxy-3-(*N*-*t*-butylamino)-propyl]-quinoline phosphate, WR 184806, in rodents. Interim report No. 89, U.S. Army medical research and development command contract No. DAMD-17-74-C-4063

Lee CC, Kintner LD, Sanyer JL, Reddig TW, Girvin JD, Buchberger GL, Seifert WK (1974 d) Acute and subacute toxicity of 2,8-bis(trifluoromethyl)-4[l-hydroxy-3-(*N*-*t*-butylamino)-propyl]-quinoline phosphate, WR-184806, in dogs. Interim report No. 88, U.S. Army medical research and development command contract No. DAMD-17-74-C-4063

Lee CC, Hwang SW, Kowalski JJ, Kintner LD, Bhandari JC, Reddig TW, Girvin JD, Kroeger VE, Kemp RD (1976a) Acute and subacute toxicities of DL-*threo*-α-(2-piperidyl)-2-trifluoromethyl-6-(4-trifluoromethylphenyl)-4-pyridienemethanol phosphate, WR-180409 H_3PO_4, in rodents. Interim report No. 105, U.S. Army medical research and development command contract No. DAMD-17-74-C-4036, January 26

Lee CC, Bhandari JC, Kowalski JJ, Kemp RD (1976b) Acute toxicity studies of DL-*threo*-α-(2-piperidyl)-2-trifluoromethyl-6-(4-trifluoromethylphenyl)-4-pyridinemethanol phosphate, WR-180409 H_3PO_4 in rats and dogs. Interim report No. 108, U.S. Army medical research and development contract No. DAMD-17-74-C-4036, April 13

Lee CC, Kowalski JJ, Kintner LD, Bhandari JC, Reddig TW, Ellis ER, Kemp RD (1976c) Additional subacute oral toxicity of DL-*threo*-α-(2-piperidyl)-2-trifluoromethyl-6-(4-trifluoromethylphenyl)-4-pyridine-methanol phosphate, WR-180409 H_3PO_4 in rodents. Interim report No. 105, U.S. Army medical research and development command contract No. DAMD-17-74-C-4036, August 5

Lee CC, Hwang SW, Kowalski JJ, Kintner LD, Bhandari JC, Reddig TW, Girvin JD, Kroeger VE, Kemp RD (1976d) Acute and subacute oral toxicity of DL-*threo*-α-(2-piperidyl)-2-trifluoromethyl-6-(4-trifluoromethylphenyl)-4-pyridinemethanol phosphate, WR-180409 H_3PO_4 in dogs. Interim report No. 106, U.S. Army medical research and development command contract No. DAMD-17-74-C-4036, March 12

Lee CC, Kowalski JJ, Kintner LD, Bhandari JC, Reddig TW, Ellis ER (1976e) Additional subacute oral toxicity of DL-*threo*-α-(2-piperidyl)-2-trifluoromethyl-6-(4-trifluoromethylphenyl)-4-pyridienemethanol phosphate, WR-180409 H_3PO_4, in dogs. Interim report No. 106, U.S. Army medical research and development command contract No. DAMD-17-74-C-4036, September 29

Lee CC, Kowalski JJ, Kintner LD, Bhandari JC, Reddig TW, Girvin JD, Ellis ER, Castillo EA, Kroeger VE, Kemp RD (1976f) Acute and subacute toxicities of 3-di-*N*-butylamino-1-[2,6-bis(4-tri-fluoromethylphenyl)-4-pyridiyl]-propanol methanesulfonte, WR-172435 CH_3SO_3H, in rodents. Interim report No. 111, U.S. Army medical research and development command, contract No. DAMD-17-74-C-4036, July 30

Lee CC, Hacker MP, Elliott CL (1979a) Acute oral and intraperitoneal toxicity of α-(2-piperidyl)-6,8-dichloro-2-trifluoromethyl-4-quinolinemethanol (WR-226,253) methanesulfonate hemihydrate in rats, mice and guinea pigs. Interim report No. 144, U.S. Army medical research and development command contract No. DAMD-17-74-C-4036, March 1

Lee CC, Ellis HV III, Hacker MP, Kintner LD, Hong CB, Elliot CL, Ellis ER, Castillo EA (1979b) Toxicity of α-(2-piperidyl)-6,8-dichloro-2-trifluoro methyl-4-quinoline-methanol (WR-226253) methanesulfonate hemihydrate when fed to male rats for 90 days. Interim report No. 151, U.S. Army medical research and development command contract No. DAMD-17-74-C-4036, November 29

Lutz RE, Bailey PS, Clark MT, Codington JF, Deinet AJ, Freek JA, Harnest GH, Leake NH, Martin TA, Russell Jr, Salsbury JM, Shearer NH Jr, Smith JD, Wilson JW III (1946) Antimalarials. Alpha-alkyl and dialkyaminomethyl-2-phenyl-4-quinolinemethanols. J Am Chem Soc 68:1813–1831

Macomber PB, O'Brien RL, Hahn FE (1966) Chloroquine: physiological basis of drug resistance in *Plasmodium berghei*. Science 152:1374–1375

Martin DC, Arnold JD, Clyde DF, Al Ibrahim M, Carson PE, Rieckmann KH, Willerson D Jr (1973) A quinoline methanol (WR-30090) for treatment of acute malaria. Antimicrob Agents Chemother 3:214–219

May EL, Mosettig E (1946) Attempts to find new antimalarials. XVIII. Amino alcohols of the type-$CHOHCH_2NR_2$ derived from 3-bromo-10-acetylphenanthrene. J Org Chem 11:627–630

McConnel WR, Furner RL (1977) Studies on the absorption, distribution, metabolism, excretion, [^{14}C]WR-180,409 H_3PO_4 in rhesus monkeys. Toxicol Appl Pharmacol 41:166–167

Mead J, Koepfli JB (1944) The structure of a new metabolic derivative of quinine. J Biol Chem 154:507–515

Mendenhall DW, Higuchi T, Sternson LA (1979) Analysis of hydrophobic amine antimalarials in biological fluids with the plastic ion-selective electrode. J Pharm Sci 68:746–750

Merkli B, Richle RW (1980) Studies on the resistance to single and combined antimalarials in the *Plasmodium berghei* mouse model. Acta Tropica 37:228–231

Merkli B, Richle R, Peters W (1980) The inhibitory effect of a drug combination on the development of mefloquine resistance in *Plasmodium berghei*. Ann Trop Med Parasitol 74:1–9

Minor JL, Short RD, Heiffer MH, Lee CC (1976) Reproductive effects of mefloquine HCl(MFQ) in rats and mice. Pharmacologist 18:171

Most H, Montouri WA (1975) Rodent systems (*Plasmodium berghei – Anopheles stephensi*) for screening compounds for potential causal prophylaxis. Am J Trop Med Hyg 24:179–182

Nakagawa T, Higuchi T, Haslam JL, Shaffer RD, Mendenhall DW (1979) GLC Determination of whole blood antimalarial concentrations. J Pharm Sci 68:718–721

Nodiff EA, Tanabe K, Seyfried C, Matsuura S, Kondo Y, Chen EH, Tyagi MP (1971) Antimalarial phenanthrene amino alcohols. 1. Fluorine-containing 2- and 6-substituted 9-phenanthrenemethanols. J Med Chem 14:921–925

Novotny JF, Starks FW (1977) Synthesis of candidate antimalarials. Report No. 12, Annual summary report, U.S. Army medical research and development command contract No. DADA17-73-C-3159

Ohnmacht CJ, Patel AR, Lutz RE (1971) Antimalarials. 7. Bis(trifluoromethyl)-α-(2-piperidyl)-4 quinolinemethanols. J Med Chem 14:926–928

Okada H, Stella V, Haslam J, Yata N (1975) Photolytic degradation of α-[(dibutylamino)methyl]-6,8-dichloro-2-(3′,4′-dichlorophenyl)-4-quinoline methanol: an experimental antimalarial. J Pharm Sci 64:1665–1667

Olmstead EJ, Panter JW, Boykin DW, Wilson WD (1975) Complex formation between naphthothiopheneethanolamines and deoxyribonucleic acids. Biochemistry 14:521–516

Olsen RE (1972) Antimalarial activity and conformation of *erythro-* and *threo*-α-(2-piperidyl)-3,6-bis(trifluoromethyl)-9-phenanthrenemethanol. J Med Chem 15:207–208

Osdene TS, Russell PB, Rane L (1967) 2,4,7-triamino-6-ortho-substituted arylpteridines. A new series of potent antimalarial agents. J Med Chem 10:431–434

Panter JW, Boykin DW, Wilson WD (1973) Effect of ring and side chain substitutents on the binding of naphthothiopheneethanolamines to deoxyribonucleic acid. Spectrophotometric studies. J Med Chem 16:1366–1369

Pearlman EJ, Doberstyn EB, Sudsok S, Thiemanun W, Kennedy RS, Canfield CJ (1980) Chemosuppressive field trials in Thailand IV. The suppression of *Plasmodium falciparum* and *Plasmodium vivax* parasitemias by mefloquine (WR142,490, a 4-quinolinemethanol). Am J Trop Med Hyg 29:1131–1137

Pearson DE, Rosenberg AA (1975) Potential antimalarials. 9. Resolution of α-diheptylaminomethyl-6-bromo-9-phenanthrenemethanol by an unusual method. J Med Chem 18:523–524

Peters W (1965) Drug resistance in *Plasmodium berghei* (Vincke and Lips, 1948). I Chloroquine resistance. Exp Parasitol 17:80–89

Peters W, Porter M (1976) The chemotherapy of rodent malaria, XXVI The potential value of WR-122,455 (a 9-phenanthrenemethanol) against drug-resistant malaria parasites. Ann Trop Med Parasitol 70:271–281

Peters W, Portus JH, Robinson BL (1975a) The chemotherapy of rodent malarial, XXII The value of drug-resistant strains of *P. berghei* in screening for blood schizontocidal activity. Ann Trop Med Parasitol 69:155–171

Peters W, Davies EE, Robinson BL (1975b) The chemotherapy of rodent malaria, XXIII. Causal prophylaxis, part II: practical experience with *P. berghei nigeriensis* in drug screening. Ann Trop Med Parasitol 69:311–328

Peters W, Howells RE, Portus J, Robinson BL, Thomas S, Warhurst DC (1977a) The chemotherapy of rodent malaria, XXVII Studies on mefloquine (WR-142,490). Ann Trop Med Parasitol 71:407–418

Peters W, Portus J, Robinson BL (1977b) The chemotherapy of rodent malaria, XXVIII. The development of resistance to mefloquine (WR142,490). Ann Trop Med Parasitol 71:419–427

Pinder RM, Burger A (1968) Antimalarials. II. α-(2-piperidyl)- and -(2-pyridyl)-2-trifluoromethyl-4-quinolinemethanols. J Med Chem 11:267–269

Porter M, Peters W (1976) The chemotherapy of rodent malaria, XXV Antimalarial activity of WR-122,455 (a 9-phenanthrenemethanol) *in vivo* and *in vitro*. Ann Trop Med Parasitol 70:259–270

Powers MD (1968a) 20-day oral toxicity in rats. Final report, U.S. Army medical research and development command contract No. DADA-17-68-C-8069, February 9

Powers MB (1968b) Two-week oral toxicity-rats. Final report, U.S. Army medical research and development command contract No. DADA-17-68-C-8069, August 21

Powers MB (1968c) 14-day oral administration-monkeys. Final report, U.S. Army medical research and development command contract No. DADA-17-68-C-8069, August 15

Powers MB (1970) Four-week oral toxicity study-monkeys WR122,455 (AV 17876). Report No. 35, U.S. Army medical research and development command contract No. DADA-17-68-8069. May 22

Pullman TN, Eichelberger L, Alving AS, Jones R Jr, Craige B Jr, Whorton CM (1948) The use of SN-10,275 in the prophylaxis and treatment of sporozoite-induced *vivax* malaria (Chesson strain). J Clin Invest XXVII:12–16

Quimby DJ (1981) Preparation of 2-trifluoromethyl cinchoninic acids. US Patent 4,251,661 Feb 17

Rapport MM, Senear AE, Mead JF, Koepfli JF (1946) The synthesis of potential antimalarials. 2-phenyl-α-(2-piperidyl)-4-quinolinemethanols. J Am Chem Soc 68:2697-2703

Reba RC, Barry KG (1976a) Final report, experiment 2:WR184,806 H_3PO_4 short term safety and tolerance (single rising dose levels). U.S. Army medical research and development command contract No. DAMD-17-75-C-5036, Feb 19

Reba RC, Barry KG (1976b) Final report, experiment 2:WR184,806 H_3PO_4 short term safety and tolerance (multiple dose). U.S. Army medical research and development command contract No. DAMD-17-75-C-5036, June 2

Reba RC, Barry KG (1977) Final report experiment No. 7: WR180,409 H_3PO_4 short term dosage safety and tolerance rising single dose levels. U.S. Army medical research and development command contract No. DAMD-17-75-C-5036

Reba RC, Barry KG (1978) WR172,435 CH_2SO_3: short term dosage, safety and tolerance: single oral dose, rising dose levels. Final report, experiment Number 13, U.S. Army medical research and development command contract No. DAMD-17-75-C-5036, December

Richle RW (1980) Chemotherapeutic activity of mefloquine hydrochloride in experimental *Plasmodium berghei* malaria in mice. Current chemotherapy and infectious disease. Proceedings of the 11th ICC and the 19th ICAAC American Society of Microbiology

Rieckmann KH, Trenholme GM, Williams RL, Carson PE, Frischer H, Desjardins RE (1974) Prophylactic activity of mefloquine hydrochloride (WR142490) in drug-resistant malaria. Bull WHO 51:375–377

Rieckmann KH, Campbell GH, Sax LJ, Mrema JE (1978) Drug sensitivity of *Plasmodium falciparum*. Lancet 1:22–23

Rinehart J, Arnold J, Canfield CJ (1976) Evaluation of two phenanthrenemethanols for antimalarial activity in man: WR-122,455 and WR-171,669. Am J Trop Med Hyg 25:769–774

Rothe WE, Jacobus DP (1968) Laboratory evaluation of the phototoxic potency of quinolinemethanols. J Med Chem 11:366–368

Rozman RS, Canfield CJ (1979) New experimental antimalarial drugs. Adv Pharmacol Chemother 16:1–43

Rozman RS, Berman A, Hutchinson A, Clinton-Molero G (1971) Uptake and excretion of antimalarial phenanthrene methanols. Fed Proc Fed Am Soc Exp Biol 30:335

Rozman RS, Molek NA, Koby R (1978) The absorption, distribution, and excretion in mice of the antimalarial mefloquine, *erythro*-2,8-bis(trifluoromethyl)-α-(2-piperidyl)-4-quinolinemethanol hydrochloride. Drug Metab Dispos 6:654–658

Ruiz R, Belej M, Aviado DM (1970) Cardiopulmonary effects of antimalarial drugs II. Phenanthrenemethanols. Toxicol Appl Pharmacol 17:118–129

Sadavongvivad C, Aviado DM (1969) Influence of chloroquine and phenanthrene methanols (WR-33063) on the content of biogenic amines in the mouse lung. Milit Med [Special Issue] 134:1106–1118

Schmidt LH, Rossan RN, Fisher KF (1963) The activity of a repository form of 4,6-diamino-1-(*p*-chlorophenyl)-1,2-dihydro-2,2-dimethyl-*s*-triazine against infections with *Plasmodium cynomolgi*. Am J Trop Med Hyg 12:494–503

Schmidt LH, Crosby R, Rasco J, Vaughan D (1978a) Antimalarial activities of various 4-quinolinemethanols with special attention to WR-142,490 (mefloquine). Antimicrob Agents Chemother 13:1011–1030

Schmidt LH, Crosby R, Rasco J, Vaughan D (1978b) Antimalarial activities of the 4-quinolinemethanols WR-184,806 and WR-226,253. Antimicrob Agents Chemother 14:680–689

Schmidt LH, Crosby R, Rasco J, Vaughan D (1978c) Antimalarial activities of various 9-phenanthrenemethanols with special attention to WR-122,455 and WR-171,669. Antimicrob Agents Chemother 14:292–314

Schmidt LH, Crosby R, Rasco J, Vaughan D (1978d) Antimalarial activities of various 4-pyridinemethanols with special attention to WR-172,435 and WR-180,409. Antimicrob Agents Chemother 14:420–435

Schwartz DE (1980) Quantitative determination of thc antimalarial drug mefloquine and of its main metabolite in plasma by direct densiometric measurement on thin-layer chromatographic plates. In: Frigerio A, McCamish M (eds) Recent developments in chromatography and electrophoresis, 10. Elsevier, Amsterdam, p 69

Schwartz DE, Weber W, Richard-Lenoble D, Gentilini M (1980) Kinetic studies of mefloquine and one of its metabolites, RO 21-5104, in the dog and in man. Acta Tropica 37:238–242

Segal HE, Chinvanthananond P, Laixuthal B, Phintuyothin P, Pearlman EJ, Na-Nakorn A, Castaneda BF (1974) Preliminary study of WR-33063 in the treatment of falciparum malaria in northeast Thailand. Am J Trop Med Hyg 23:560–564

Smith CC, Weigel WW (1971a) Conversion of tritium to H_2O following oral administration of two labelled phenanthrenemethanols to primates. Pharmacologist 13:269

Smith CC, Weigel W (1971b) Metabolism of a new, tritium-labeled phenanthrene methanol with pronounced antimalarial activity. Toxicol Appl Pharmacol 19:364

Smith CC, Wolfe GF, Mattingly SF (1972) Excretion of three antimalarial drugs, WR-38,839, WR-33,063, and WR-122455, in rhesus monkeys with chronic biliary cannulae. Toxicol Appl Pharmacol 22:291

Stampfli H, von Bredow J, Osuch J, Heiffer M (1979) A multi-component solvent system for the analysis of a candidate antimalarial by normal phase HPLC. J Liq Chromatogr 2:53–65

Stella V, Haslam J, Yata N, Okada H, Lindenbaum S, Higuchi T (1978) Enhancement of bioavailability of a hydrophobic amine antimalarial by formulation with oleic acid in a soft gelatin capsule. J Pharm Sci 67:1375–1377

Strube R (1975) The search for new antimalarial drugs. J Trop Med Hyg 78:171–185
Sweeney TR (1981) The present status of malaria chemotherapy: mefloquine, a novel antimalarial. Med Res Rev 1:281–301
Teague RS, Mundy RL (1972a) Study of the effects of a large dose of WR-171,669AC (BB 41223) in the anesthetized mouse. Interim report No. 35, U.S. Army medical research and development command contract No. DADA-17-69-C-7136. June 2
Teague RS, Mundy RL (1972b) Effects of the sub-acute administration of compound WR-171,669AC (BB 41223) in large oral doses to the mouse. Interim report No. 36, U.S. Army medical research and development command contract No. DADA-17-69-C-7136, August 2
Thakker KD, Higuchi T, Sternson LA (1979) Loss of hydrophobic amine from solution by adsorption onto container surfaces. J Pharm Sci 68:93–95
Thompson PE (1972) Studies on a quinolinemethanol (WR 30,090) and on a phenanthrene-methanol (WR33,063) against drug-resistant *Plasmodium berghei* in mice. Proc Helminthol Soc Washington [Special Issue] 39:297–308
Thong YH, Ferrante A, Rowan-Kelly B, O'Keefe DE (1979) Effect of mefloquine on the immune response in mice. Trans R Soc Trop Med Hyg 73:388–390
Trenholme GM, Wiliams RL, Desjardins RE, Frischer H, Carson PE, Rieckmann KH (1975) Mefloquine (WR142,490) in the treatment of human malaria. Science 190:792–794
Warhurst DC, Baggaley (1972) Autophagic vacuole formation in *P. berghei in vitro*. Trans R Soc Trop Med Hyg 66:5
Warhurst DC, Thomas SC (1975) Pharmacology of the malaria parasite – a study of dose-response relationships in chloroquine-induced autophagic vacuole formation in *Plasmodium berghei*. Biochem Pharmacol 24:2047–2056
Warhurst DC, Robinson BL, Howells RE, Peters W (1971) The effect of cytotoxic agents on autophagic vacuole formation in chloroquine-treated malaria parasites (*Plasmodium berghei*). Life Sci 10:761–771
Warhurst DC, Homewood CA, Peters W, Baggaley VC (1972) Pigment changes in *Plasmodium berghei* as indicators of activity and mode of action of antimalarial drugs. Proc. Helminthol Soc Washington [Special Issue] 39:271–278
Weigel WW, Smith CC (1973) Fate of α-(2-piperidyl)-3,6-bis(trifluoromethyl)-9-phenanthrene methanol in owl monkeys. Proc 5th Int Congr Pharmacol 1972 Abstract No 1488
Windheuser JJ, Haslam JL (1976) Bioavailability studies of several formulations of WR171,669 in beagle dogs. Interim report No. 22, U.S. Army medical research and development command contract No. DADA17-73-C-3125, October
Wiselogle FY (1946) A survey of antimalarial drugs. Edwards, Ann Arbor
Yanko WH, Deebel GF (1980) ^{14}C-Labelled antimalarials. I. Synthesis of DL-*erythro*- and *threo*-α-(2-piperidyl)-2,8-bis(trifluoromethyl)-4-quinolinemethanol-α-^{14}C. J Label Cpds XVII:431–437

CHAPTER 10

8-Aminoquinolines

T. R. SWEENEY

A. Introduction

Over the years, the 8-aminoquinolines, as a class of antimalarial compounds, have been extensively investigated. In the compendium of WISELOGLE (1946) the activities of a large number of 8-aminoquinolines in avian models were presented along with an analysis of the toxicity of the class. COATNEY et al. (1953) compiled another body of data on the compounds and drew some conclusions with respect to structure/activity relationships. THOMPSON and WERBEL (1972) too have reviewed the class. Despite the intensive work through the World War II period, two problems associated with compounds were never really resolved; one was the inherent toxicity of the class and the other was the lack of a general correlation between the available avian models and vivax malaria. The promise of a curative drug emerging rested solely upon the known curative action of pamaquine.

The demonstration by SCHMIDT and GENTHER (1953) that a *P. cynomolgi* infection in the rhesus monkey was the counterpart, both biologically and chemotherapeutically, of a *P. vivax* infection in a human had a profound impact on the development of the 8-aminoquinolines as radical curative agents. During the post World War II period, with this knowledge in hand, older 8-aminoquinolines were reinvestigated and new ones synthesised. Four compounds emerged that were superior to pamaquine (I a), viz. pentaquine (I b), isopentaquine (I c), primaquine (I d), and SN 3883 (I e). Subsequent use in military returnees from Korea and studies with volunteers established the superiority of primaquine over the other drugs.

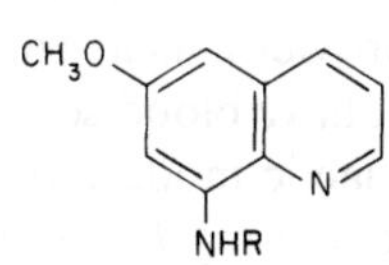

a) R = $CH(CH_3)(CH_2)_3N(C_2H_5)_2$, Pamaquine

b) R = $(CH_2)_5NHCH(CH_3)_2$, Pentaquine

c) R = $CH(CH_3)(CH_2)_3NHCH(CH_3)_2$, Isopentaquine

d) R = $CH(CH_3)(CH_2)_3NH_2$, Primaquine

e) R = $(CH_2)_4NH_2$, SN - 3883

Fig. 1. Structures of some older 8-aminoquinolines (I *a–e*)

Today, a generation later, primaquine is still the radical curative agent of choice for the treatment of relapsing malarias.

Despite the pre-eminence of primaquine, its toxicity (see Chap. 3) is a drawback and more recent investigations on the 8-aminoquinolines have had, as their goal, the development of a drug with a therapeutic index greater than that of primaquine. Classes of compounds other than the 8-aminoquinolines have, of course, been investigated. Nine classes of compounds, in addition to the 8-aminoquinolines, that have exhibited causal prophylactic activity in rodent models have been discussed by Davidson et al. (1981). Of these classes, only the 6- and 8-aminoquinolines had radical curative activity against persistent exoerythrocytic forms of *P. cynomolgi* in rhesus monkeys. The 6-aminoquinolines were substantially less active than primaquine. Two other classes of compounds, the 3- and 5-aminoquinolines, have been investigated (Khan and La Montagne 1979). With the exception of one 5-aminoquinoline which had an activity much inferior to primaquine, these classes were also inactive in the *P. cynomolgi*-rhesus model.

With the exception of 4-methyl primaquine and 8-[(s4-amino-*l*-methylbutyl) amino]-6-methoxy-4-methyl 5-(3-trifluoromethylphenoxy) quinoline succinate (WR 225448), studies on the more recently synthesised 8-aminoquinolines have not advanced beyond the stage of efficacy testing in animal models. Some toxicity studies have been carried out on the exception noted above but clinical studies are still some distance away. The discussion of recent developments in the 8-aminoquinolines (primaquine itself is discussed elsewhere in this monograph) will, therefore, be confined largely to the activity of new compounds in animal models.

B. Recent Research

Recent work in the area of 8-aminoquinolines aimed at the development of radical curative agents with therapeutic indices greater than that of primaquine has been supported by the availability of improved animal models that were not available to earlier workers. The *P. berghei*-mouse prophylactic model (Rane and Kinnamon 1979) is useful as a rapid and inexpensive means of screening a relatively large number of compounds. It does not provide a definitive test in that biologically long-lasting compounds with blood schizontocidal activity can give false-positive results. However, the model does provide a means of eliminating many compounds with short biological half-lives that have blood schizontocidal activity. Also available are secondary rodent prophylactic models, one using *P. yoelii* in the mouse (Gregory and Peters 1970) and one using *P. berghei* in the rat (Most and Montouri 1975). These models are generally used as confirmatory tests. The *P. cynomolgi*-rhesus monkey model (Schmidt et al. 1977a) provides definitive information on the radical curative activity of a potential drug in primates and is the final test of antimalarial activity prior to clinical studies. The *P. berghei*-mouse model used for the determination of blood schizontocidal activity (Osdene et al. 1967) is also useful as an aid in interpreting prophylactic activity of potential agents. Early deaths that occur in the use of this model serve as a preliminary indication of the acute toxicity of the compound being screened. A comprehensive discussion of various models has been given by Peters (1980).

I. Enantiomers of Primaquine

The drug primaquine is a racemate, the components of which have been resolved by CARROLL et al. (1975, 1978). The toxicities and curative antimalarial activities of primaquine and its *d* and *l* enantiomers were compared by SCHMIDT et al. (1977b) in order to determine if either had a sufficient advantage over primaquine to warrant evaluation for curative activity against *P. vivax* infections in volunteers. The acute oral toxicity for mice of *d*-primaquine was approximately four times that of *l*-primaquine and more than twice that of primaquine. For rhesus monkeys the relative toxicities were the reverse. The subacute oral toxicity of *l*-primaquine was found to be between three and five times that of *d*-primaquine and at least twice that of primaquine. The ability of primaquine and the two enantiomers to effect radical cure of sporozoite-induced *P. cynomolgi* infections in rhesus monkeys were essentially identical. Past experience had shown that toxicity studies with monkeys were more meaningful and more reliable than studies with rodents in the selection of candidate agents for clinical trials. Based upon this experience with monkeys, SCHMIDT et al. (1977b) concluded that the *d* enantiomer should have a twofold advantage in therapeutic index over primaquine and that the practical consequences of such an improvement would be sufficient to justify a comparison of the *d* enantiomer with primaquine in volunteers.

II. Structural Modifications of Primaquine

1. Quinoline Ring Modifications

a) 1,6-Naphthyridine Derivatives

It has been suggested from drug metabolism studies in chickens that the antimalarial action of the 8-aminoquinolines can be attributed to the metabolic formation of active 5,6-quinolinequinones (GREENBERG et al. 1961; JOSEPHSON et al. 1951a, b; DRAKE and PRATT 1951; TARLOV et al. 1962). With this in mind CARROLL et al. (1981) synthesised the 1,6-naphthyridine derivatives II and III a, b. Compound II, it was suggested, would "lock" in the 5-one structure, corresponding to the 5,6-quinolinequinone. Compound III b would be a prodrug form of the naphthyridine (III a). Both II and III b were toxic at the minimum dose tested, 40 mg/kg, when evaluated for antimalarial activity in the *P. berghei*-mouse model. When assayed for radical curative activity in the *P. cynomolgi*-rhesus monkey model III b was inactive at the maximum dose tested (10 mg/kg per day); II, however, was curative at the 3.16-mg/kg per day level but not at 1 mg/kg per day. The activity of II was, thus, much lower than that of primaquine.

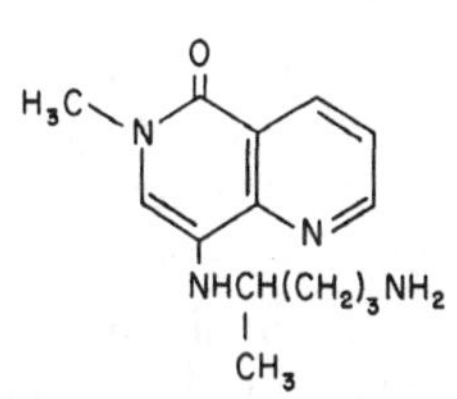

Fig. 2. 6-methyl-1,6-naphthyridine analogue of primaquine (II)

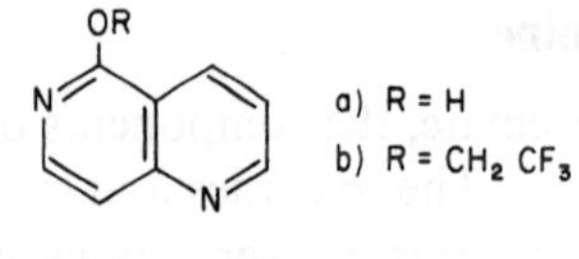

Fig. 3. 5-Substituted, 1,6-naphthyridines (III *a, b*)

b) 1,5-Naphthyridine Derivatives

PILOT and STOGRYN (1975) synthesised several 1,5-naphthyridine (IV a–c) and 1,5-naphthyridinone (V a, b) derivatives with the pentaquine- or pamaquine-type side chains. These compounds were devoid of radical curative activity in the *P. cynomolgi*-rhesus monkey model at the highest doses tested. Compound IV c, as well as its 7-chloro derivative, was prepared earlier by MCCAUSTLAND and CHENG (1970) but showed no blood schizontocidal activity in the *P. berghei*-mouse model.

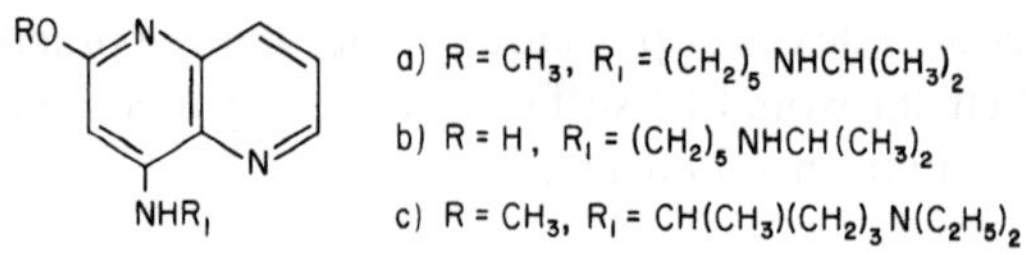

Fig. 4. 1-5,naphthyridines (IV *a–c*)

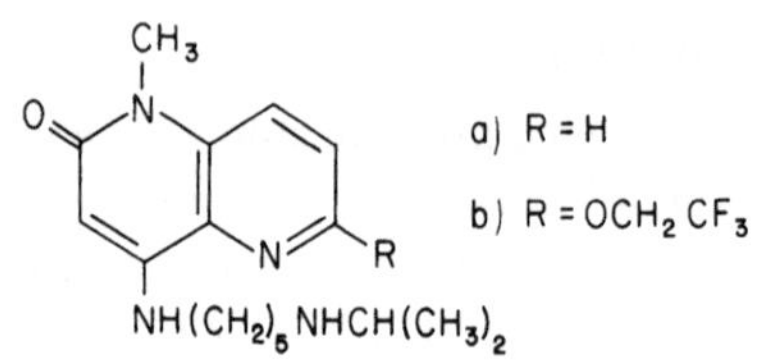

Fig. 5. 1-5,naphthyridones (V *a, b*)

c) Tetrahydroquinoline Derivatives

The compound 8-(5-diethylamino-2-pentylamino)-6-methoxy-1,2,3,4-tetrahydroquinoline (tetrahydropamaquine) exhibited high antimalarial activity against avian malarias but was ineffective, as tested, as a blood schizontocide against vivax malaria and as a prophylactic against falciparum or vivax malaria in man (WISELOGLE 1946). CARROLL et al. (1976) have extended the investigation of partially saturated pamaquine derivatives with systems of the types VI a–f and VII a, b. Compound VI e was ineffective as a radical curative agent at the highest tested dose, 10 mg/kg per day when assayed in the *P. cynomolgi*-rhesus monkey model. Compounds VII a, b were curative at this level but failed at the 1 mg/kg per day level. Thus both of these compounds were considerably less potent than primaquine as radical curative agents. The analogues VI a–f had little or no blood schizontocidal activity when assayed in the *P. berghei*-mouse model. Partial reduction of the quinoline ring would, thus seem to be disadvantageous.

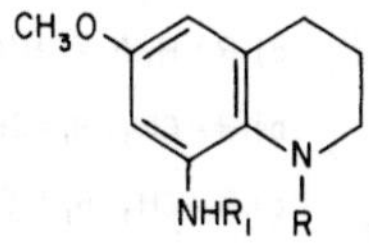

a) $R = CH_3$, $R_1 = (CH_2)_4N(C_2H_5)_2$

b) $R = n\text{-}C_4H_9$, $R_1 = (CH_2)_4N(C_2H_5)_2$

c) $R = CH_3$, $R_1 = (CH_2)_4NHCH_2C_6H_5$

d) $R = CH_3$, $R_1 = (CH_2)_4NH_2$

e) $R = CH_3$, $R_1 = CH(CH_3)(CH_2)_3NH_2$

f) $R = H$, $R_1 = CH_2CH_2N(C_2H_5)_2$

Fig. 6. Tetrahydroquinolines (VI *a–f*)

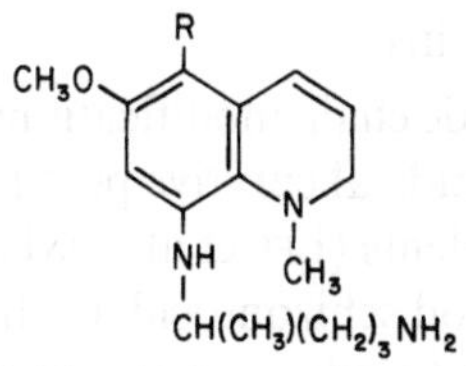

a) $R = H$

b) $R = OCH_3$

Fig. 7. Partially unsaturated primaquine analogues (VII *a, b*)

d) Naphthalene Derivatives

In consideration of the fact that the 5,6-quinolinequinone derivatives of 8-aminoquinoline-type antimalarials are not active orally but are active in vitro (see above) and the fact that the active antimalarial menoctone, 2-hydroxy-3-cyclohexyloctyl-1,4-naphthoquinone, has a resonating ion form that exists as a 1,2-naphthoquinone, ARCHER et al. (1980) synthesised several 4-[(aminoalkyl)amino]-1,2-dimethoxynaphthalenes (VII a–d) as possible prodrugs of the corresponding 1,2-naphthoquinones. These compounds had no radical curative activity when assayed in the *P. cynomolgi*-rhesus monkey model. The 1,2-naphthoquinone corresponding to the 1,2-dimethoxy "prodrug" VIII a and several related 4-[(aminoalkyl)amino]-1,2-naphthoquinones had been synthesised earlier (BULLOCK et al. 1970). These compounds had no blood schizontocidal activity in the *P. berghei*-mouse model nor prophylactic activity in the *P. gallinaceum*-bird model. They have not been tested for radical curative activity in the monkey.

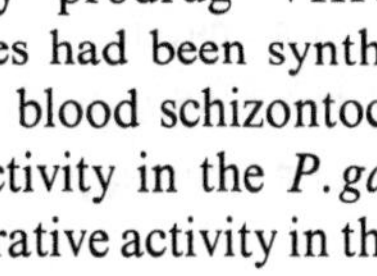

a) $R = CH(CH_3)(CH_2)_3N(C_2H_5)_2$

b) $R = CH(CH_3)(CH_2)_3NH_2$

c) $R = (CH_2)_3CH(CH_3)NH_2$

d) $R = CH(C_2H_5)(CH_2)_3NH_2$

Fig. 8. Naphthalene derivatives (VIII *a–d*)

e) Acridine Derivatives

Another modification of the primaquine ring was effected by SCOVILL et al. (1979), who synthesised the 4-amino-2-methoxyacridine derivative corresponding to primaquine (a benzoprimaquine) as well as the derivatives corresponding to 4-methylprimaquine and quinocide (IX a–c). When assayed for radical curative activity us-

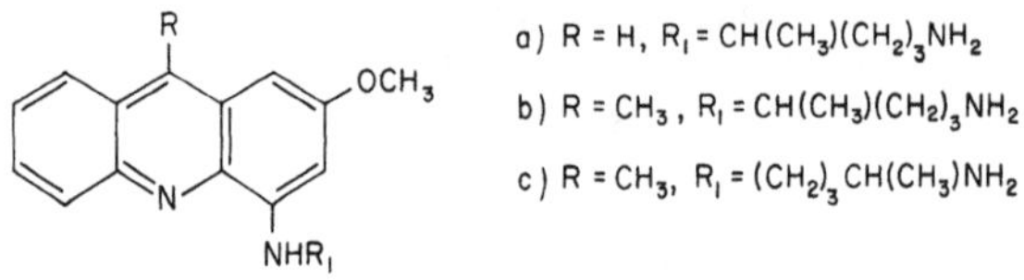

Fig. 9. Acridine derivatives (IX *a–c*)

ing the *P. cynomolgi*-rhesus monkey model, IX a cured two of three monkeys at a dose of 10 mg/kg per day but failed at a dose of 3.16 mg/kg per day.

2. Side Chain Modification

a) 4-Amino-1-Alkylbutylamino Chains

YAN et al. (1981) synthesised three side chain modifications (X a–c) of 4-methyl primaquine (XII a), a compound with radical curative potency somewhat superior to primaquine and acute toxicity in rodents (LEE et al. 1981) less than that of primaquine. Compound X a had good blood schizontocidal activity when assayed in the *P. berghei*-mouse model. It effected a 100% cure rate at a dose of 320 mg/kg and showed activity at a dose as low as 20 mg/kg. No early death toxicity was evident at the highest tested dose of 640 mg/kg. In contrast, primaquine, I d, produced no cures when administered at its minimum toxic dose (MTD) of 160 mg/kg and 4-methyl primaquine, XII a, was curative only at its MTD of 640 mg/kg. Compounds X b, c were less active than X a but were also non-toxic. The three compounds X a–c were also active in the mouse prophylactic screen. When assayed for radical curative activity in the *P. cynomolgi*-rhesus monkey model, X a was 100% curative at 0.25 mg/kg per day and cured six of seven animals at a dose of 0.125 mg/kg per day. These values indicate a radical curative potency about four times that of primaquine.

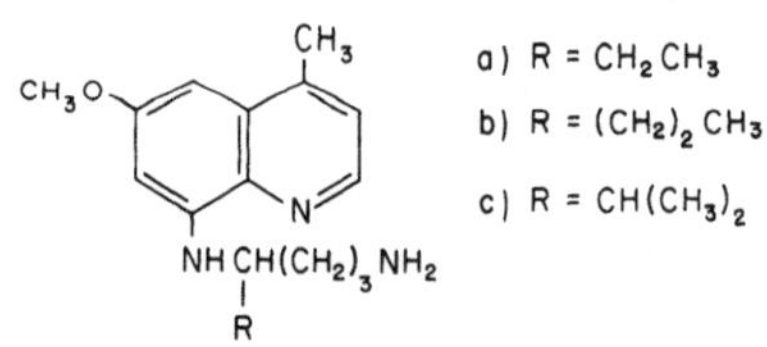

Fig. 10. Substituted 4-methyl primaquine analogues (X *a–c*)

b) Bis-piperazines

PAUL and BLANTON (1973) and SHETTY and BLANTON (1979) have synthesised a series of bis-piperazines in which two 8-aminoquinoline moieties are bridged through their side chain (XI). Groups R, R_1, R_2, and R_3 represent H or CH_3 and *n* varied from 1 to 4. The most potent blood schizontocides of the group showed only slight activity in the *P. berghei*-mouse model; none were curative. One compound ($R = R_1 = R_2 = R_3 = H$, $n = 2$) showed radical curative activity in the *P. cynomolgi*-rhesus monkey model but was somewhat less than one-tenth as active as primaquine.

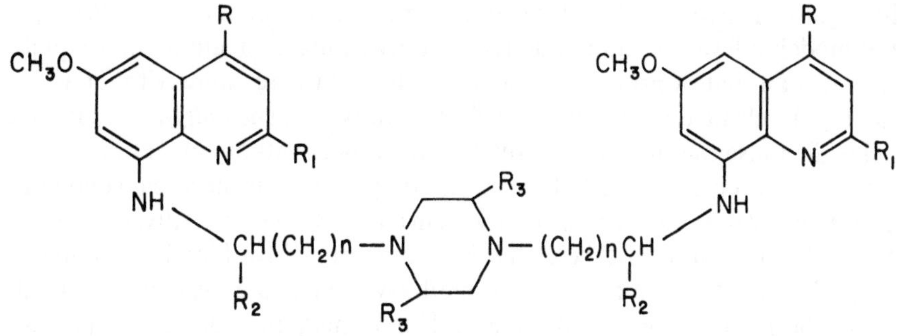

Fig. 11. Bis-piperazine derivatives of 8-aminoquinolines (XI)

c) Quinuclidine Derivatives

SINGH et al. (1969) synthesised a series of 6-methoxy-8-(quinuclidinyl-2-methyleneamino) quinolines and two derivatives of primaquine in which the primary amino group in the side chain was modified to form, respectively, a 3-quinuclidineamino and a 3-quinuclidineimino moiety. None of these analogues were active in the *P. berghei*-mouse model and were not, apparently, tested for prophylactic or radical curative activity.

3. Quinoline Ring Substituents

a) 2- and 4-Position Substituents

Data that had accrued in the World War II antimalarial drug development programme and elsewhere indicated that a 6-methoxy substituent is desirable with respect to the antimalarial activity of the 8-aminoquinolines. More recent investigations of the effect of ring substituents on antimalarial activity have, therefore, involved compounds in which the 6-methoxy substituent has usually been retained. Also, the cumulative data on the large variety of side chains investigated in the programme, the subsequent selection of primaquine as the radical curative agent of choice and additional later studies have indicated the superiority of a terminal primary amino group on the side chain. Since the primaquine side chain has a consistently high, and usually the highest, effectiveness when compared with other chains, new compounds synthesised to study the effects of various ring substituents on antimalarial activity were usually primaquine derivatives.

The synthesis of primaquine derivatives with substituents on the *N*-containing ring has been largely confined to the 2- or 4-positions. Many such derivatives have been synthesised (SHETTY and BLANTON 1978; CARROLL et al. 1979a, b, 1980; LAMONTAGNE et al. 1977).

These included derivatives containing a wide variety of functional groups as well as those containing moieties such as alkyl, alkylene, cycloalkyl, cycloalkylalkyl, and substituted-phenylthioalkyl. Several disubstituted primaquine derivatives with small alkyl or alkylene groups in the 2- and 4-positions have also been synthesised and tested. All of the above individual derivatives have not necessarily been examined in all of the animal models, but, as a group, those examined were undistinguished. Most of the derivatives were inactive in the RANE *P. berghei*-mouse model; a few had modest activity. Many exhibited acute toxicity equal to or greater than that of primaquine. Most of the derivatives were without activity at the dose levels investigated in the radical curative *P. cynomolgi*-rhesus monkey model while those that did show activity were, almost without exception, less potent than primaquine. The best of the newer compounds was the 4-ethyl derivative, (XII b), which was less toxic in the mouse than either XII a or 2-methyl primaquine, synthesised much earlier. In the *P. berghei*-mouse model for blood schizontocidal activity XII b was 100% curative at 640 mg/kg without acute toxicity and was also active in the mouse prophylactic screen. This primaquine analogue exhibited a radical curative activity in the order of that of primaquine when assayed in the *P. cynomolgi*-rhesus model. However, the absence of acute toxicity in the mouse would indicate that it may have a better therapeutic index.

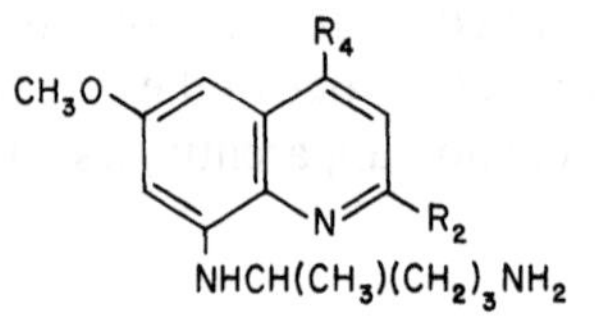

a) $R_2 = H$, $R_4 = CH_3$
b) $R_2 = H$, $R_4 = C_2H_5$
c) $R_2 = C_6H_5CH_2O$, $R_4 = H$
d) $R_2 = C_6H_5CH_2S$, $R_4 = H$
e) $R_2 = OCH_3$, $R_4 = H$
f) $R_2 = H$, $R_4 = C_6H_5O$
g) $R_2 = H$, $R_4 = C_6H_5S$

Fig. 12. 2- and 4-substituted analogues of primaquine (XII *a–g*)

The compound 4-methyl primaquine (XII a) was originally synthesised by ELDERFIELD et al. (1955). Although it was known to be a promising compound, an in-depth study of radical curative activity against infections with *P. cynomolgi* in rhesus monkeys was not carried out until much later (SCHMIDT et al. 1977 a). The compound proved to be superior to primaquine in this model with CD_{50}s (dose required to cure 50% of the mice) for a single 3-day or 7-day treatment schedule ranging from 1.7 to 2.1 mg/kg compared with a range of 2.5–3.1 mg/kg for primaquine. The CD_{90}s ranged from 3.1–4.1 mg/kg and 2.7–3.6 mg/kg for primaquine and 4-methyl primaquine respectively. In rats, mice or guinea pigs the acute toxicity of XII a (LEE et al. 1981) was less than that of primaquine (LEE et al. 1981 b). However, when the drugs were administered repeatedly the reverse was true. In dogs, a dose of 1 mg/kg per day or more for 28 consecutive days produced toxic signs, methaemoglobinaemia, thrombocytopaenia, and leucocytosis. In addition there was an elevation of SGOT and serum haptoglobin, and hypoglycaemia. At 9 mg/kg per day for 28 days hepatic degeneration and extramedullary haematopoiesis were found in some dogs. In monkeys there were toxic signs at 1 or 4 mg/kg per day as well as an increase in SGPT, BUN, and LDH with decreased haemoglobin and serum haptoglobin. The compound also caused acute erythrocytopaenia and reticulocytosis. In addition, some monkeys had degeneration of the neurones in the cerebral cortex. A dose of 6 mg/kg per day was fatal. In view of the toxicity, further development of 4-methyl primaquine seems questionable.

The 2-benzyloxy analogue of primaquine, XII c, originally synthesised by TALATI et al. (1970), and substituted-2-benzyloxy analogues (substituents 4-F, 4-CF_3, 3-CF_3, 4-Cl, 2,4-Cl_2, 4-CH_3O) as well as the 2-benzylthio analogue (XII d) and its 4-chlorobenzyl derivative were prepared by SHETTY et al. (1977) as potential antimalarials. In contrast to the parent 2-methoxy primaquine (XII e), whose MTD under *P. berghei*-mouse model conditions was 160 mg/kg, the MTD of all of the benzyloxy and benzylthio analogues was 640 mg/kg or higher. They had slight or no blood schizontocidal activity in the *P. berghei*-mouse model but some of the compounds of this series showed radical curative activity against *P. cynomolgi* infections in the rhesus monkey. The better ones, the 4-fluorobenzyloxy and 2,4-dichlorobenzyloxy derivatives, were only about one-half as potent as primaquine but, having an acute toxicity of one-fourth of that of primaquine when tested in the *P. berghei*-mouse model, a better therapeutic index was indicated. These compounds were also prophylactically active against sporozoite-induced infections in the *P. berghei*-mouse model of RANE and KINNAMON (1979).

In addition to XII c, TALATI et al. (1970) synthesised two side chain variations of XII c, viz. the aminobutylamino and aminopentylamino analogues and also synthesised the compound 2-benzyloxy-6-ethoxy-8-[3-(aminopropylamino)] quinoline. These compounds had little or no blood schizontocidal activity against *P. berghei* infections in mice. They have apparently not been tested for radical curative activity.

In another variation of the primaquine molecule, LA MONTAGNE et al. (1977) synthesised a number of substituted-phenoxy derivatives of XII f and substituted-phenylthio derivatives of XII g in which the substituents on the phenyl group were 4-Cl, 4-OCH_3, 3-CF_3, 2,4-Cl_2. All of these compounds were devoid of radical curative activity against *P. cynomolgi* infections in the rhesus monkey at the highest doses tested (10 mg/kg). Furthermore, they had no prophylactic activity in the *P. berghei*-mouse model against sporozoite-induced infections. On the other hand the 4-phenoxy primaquine derivatives exhibited fair to good blood schizontocidal activity in the *P. berghei*-mouse model with no evidence of toxicity at the highest dose level, 640 mg/kg.

b) 5- and 4,5-Position Substituents

The possibility that the in vivo activity and/or toxicity of the 8-aminoquinolines may be associated with the metabolic conversion of the quinoline moiety to a 5,6-quinolinequinone (see above) makes the 5-position of primaquine an interesting one. Partial oxidation of the 5-position in the form of a 5-OCH_3 substituent might be expected to enhace the conversion; blocking of the position, in the form of a 5-methyl substituent, for example, might be expected to have the opposite effect. A 5-phenoxy substituent would be expected to be less labile than a 5-methoxy substituent (WILLIAMS 1959) if the conversion proceeds via a 5-OH intermediate.

The compounds XIII a, b, synthesised by BURGHARD and BLANTON (1980), are of interest in this regard. In the *P. berghei*-mouse model, XIII a showed the same low blood schizontocidal activity as 4-methylprimaquine, XII a, at a dose of 160 mg/kg. However, acute toxicity was apparent at a dose of 320 mg/kg for XIII a but apparent for XII a only at a dose of 640 mg/kg. Compound XIII b showed slight blood schizontocidal activity at a dose of 10 mg/kg but was 100% lethal at a dose of 80 mg/kg. Against *P. cynomolgi* infections in rhesus monkeys, XIII a with a primaquine index (PI) of 3.5 was appreciably more potent as a radical curative agent than (XII a) (PI = 1.3); XIII b, with a PI of 1, was of lower potency than XII a.

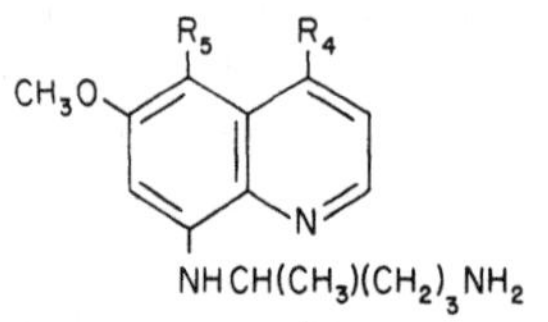

a) $R_4 = R_5 = CH_3$

b) $R_4 = CH_3$, $R_5 = F$

c) $R_4 = CH_3$, $R_5 = O(CH_2)_4CH_3$

d) $R_4 = CH_3$, $R_5 = O(CH_2)_5CH_3$

Fig. 13. 5- and 4,5-substituted analogues of primaquine (XIII *a–d*)

Results of the testing of 5,6-dimethoxy-8-aminoquinolines for antimalarial activity in avian models, reported in the compendia of WISELOGLE (1946) and COATNEY et al. (1953), indicated that many of the dimethoxy compounds where highly active. No trend in relative activity between the 5,6-dimethoxy and the 6-methoxy analogues was apparent, however.

The high therapeutic index reported in the COATNEY et al. (1953) compendium for the compound 5-(*p*-anisyloxy)-6-methoxy-8-(5-isopropylaminopentylamino) quinoline when tested against avian malaria prompted PAUL and BLANTON (1976) to re-evaluate the compound and other 5-(*p*-anisyloxy)-6-methoxy-8-aminoquinolines in animal models. The side chains evaluated were -$NH(CH_2)_5$ NHX were X = H, $CH(CH_3)_2$, 2-adamantyl, 3,4,5-trimethoxybenzyl and 2-hydroxybenzyl; also investigated was the chain $NHCH_2C_6H_4CH_2NH_2$. With the exception of the analogue with the isopropylaminopentylamino chain, which was as toxic as primaquine, all compounds were devoid of acute toxicity under the *P. berghei*-mouse model conditions at a dose of 640 mg/kg. The compounds had little or no blood schizontocidal activity when tested in this model and had no radical curative activity against *P. cynomolgi* infections in the rhesus monkey at the highest dose tested (10 mg/kg).

The parallel and high antimalarial activity of certain 6-methoxy- and 5,6-dimethoxy-8-aminoquinolines in avian models that was reported in earlier literature (WISELOGLE 1946; COATNEY et al. 1953) plus the superior activity of 4-methyl primaquine (XII a) compared with primaquine in the *P. cynomolgi*-rhesus monkey model (SCHMIDT et al. 1977 a) led LAMONTAGNE et al. (1981 a) to synthesise, for antimalarial evaluation, a number of 4-methyl-5,6-dimethoxy-8-aminoquinolines. The toxicity of these in mice and their radical curative activity against *P. cynomolgi* infections in the rhesus monkey is shown in Table 1. Primaquine (I d) and 4-methyl primaquine (XII a) are included for comparison. With the exception of XVII, which was slightly less potent than the others, the 4-methyl-5,6-dimethoxy-8-aminoquinolines with the different side chains were all in the order of 3.5–4 times more active than I d as radical curative agents and 2.5–3 times more active than XII a. The 2,4-dimethyl analogue, XXI, had the highest primaquine index. However, the greater activity of the 4-methyl-5,6-dimethoxy analogues relative to primaquine or 4-methyl primaquine was offset by their greater toxicity. With the exception of XVII, which produced some cures at 20 mg/kg, none of the compounds showed significant blood schizontocidal activity in the *P. berghei*-mouse model at non-toxic doses. Not all of the 4-methyl-5,6-dimethoxy-8-aminoquinolines of

Table 1. Radical curative activities and toxicities of 5-methoxy-8-aminoquinolines

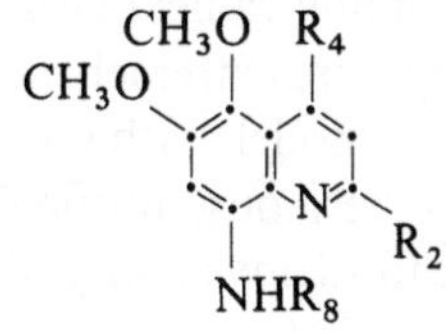

No.	R_2	R_4	R_8	PI[a]	MTD[b]
XV	H	CH_3	$CH(CH_3)(CH_2)_3NH_2$	4.0	160
XVI	H	CH_3	$CH(C_2H_5)(CH_2)_3NH_2$	3.3	80
XVII	H	CH_3	$CH(CH_3)(CH_2)_4NH_2$	1.6	40
XVIII	H	CH_3	$(CH_2)_3CH(CH_3)NH_2$	3.6	20
XIX	H	CH_3	$(CH_2)_4CH(CH_3)NH_2$	3.6	20
XX	H	H	$(CH_2)_3CH(CH_3)NH_2$	0.4	320
XXI	CH_3	CH_3	$CH(CH_3)(CH_2)_3NH_2$	4.5	40
XXII	H	H	$CH(CH_3)(CH_2)_3NH_2$	1.0	160
Id (primaquine)				1.0	160
XIIa (4-methyl primaquine)				1.3	640

[a] Primaquine index. An approximate value indicating the radical curative activity of a compound relative to primaquine in the rhesus monkey model

[b] Minimum toxic dose. The minimum dose of drug producing at least 20% drug deaths in the *P. berghei*-mouse blood schizontocidal screen

Table 1 have been examined in the prophylactic mouse screen, but those that have been examined showed activity.

Also synthesised by LaMontagne et al. (1982a) were the related 5,6-methylene- and ethylenedioxy derivatives of both 4-methyl-primaquine (XIV a, b) and 4-methyl-8-(4-amino-l-ethylbutylamino) quinoline (XIV c, d). These compounds were all devoid of radical curative activity against infections of *P. cynomolgi* in the rhesus monkey. The compounds XIV a, c were also devoid of blood schizontocidal activity against *P. berghei* infections in the mouse but were non-toxic at the highest dose tested, 640 mg/kg. Compounds XIV b, d showed slight activity without cures against the latter infection but were more toxic than primaquine.

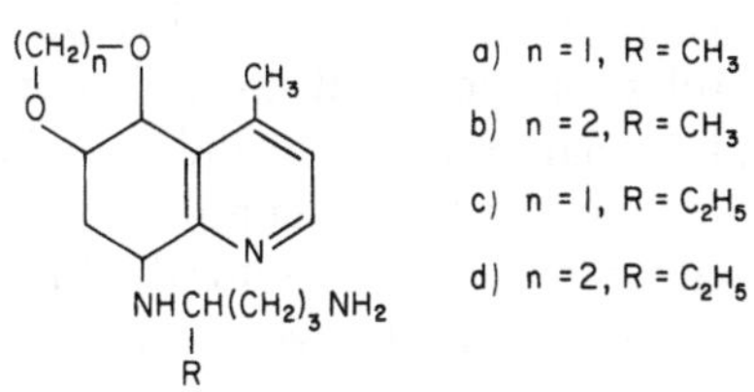

Fig. 14. 5,6-derivatives of 4-methyl primaquine and related compounds (XIV *a–d*)

Nodiff and Saggiomo (1981) extended the study of the 5-alkoxy derivatives of primaquine and 4-methyl primaquine to higher homologues. Although studies are still in progress, available data indicate that the radical curative activity of the 5-alkoxy derivatives of 4-methyl primaquine against infections of *P. cynomolgi* in rhesus monkeys peaked when the 5-alkoxy group was pentoxy or hexoxy. These two compounds (XIIIc, d) had outstanding radical curative activity with primaquine indexes of approximately 13. They were extremely potent blood schizontocides, as determined in the *P. berghei*-mouse model, with CD_{50}s of about 10 mg/kg. In addition, they were highly active in the mouse prophylactic screen. The acute early death toxicity in mice was about the same as that of primaquine, with a MTD of 160 mg/kg.

In contrast to the work of PAUL and BLANTON, Jr. (1976), in which the activities of a series of 5-(*p*-anisyloxy)-6-methoxy-8-aminoquinolines with various side chains were investigated, CHEN et al. (1977) have studied a series of 5-(substituted-phenoxy)-derivatives of primaquine and TANABE et al. (1978) a series of 5-(substituted-phenyl)thio- and 5-(substituted-anilino)derivatives of primaquine. In the 5-phenylthio series, substituents on the phenyl ring included 2-Cl; 3-Cl; 4-Cl; 3,4-$(Cl)_2$; 2,5-$(Cl)_2$; 4-CH_3, and CF_3. The 5-phenylthio derivatives of primaquine were active as radical curative agents against *P. cynomolgi* infections in rhesus monkeys. However, they were appreciably less potent than primaquine; the best one, 5-(3-trifluoromethylphenylthio) primaquine was about one-half as potent as primaquine. In addition, the 5-phenylthio derivatives showed little or no blood schizontocidal activity against *P. berghei* infections in mice. No acute early death toxicity was evident at the highest dose level, 640 mg/kg. The only anilino derivative tested, 5-(3-trifluoroanilino) primaquine, was devoid of radical curative activity.

The 5-(substituted-phenoxy) primaquine derivatives synthesised by CHEN et al. (1977) were superior to the 5-(substituted-phenyl)thio primaquine derivatives both in radical curative and blood schizontocidal activity. Further development of such derivatives was carried out by NODIFF et al. (1982) and by LAMONTAGNE et al. (1982b), who synthesised a series of 4-methyl-5-(substituted-phenoxy) primaquine derivatives. The radical curative and blood schizontocidal activity of these compounds is compared in Table 2. For this comparison the data are expressed as primaquine indexes and CD_{50}s.

The data in Table 2 show that the 5-phenoxy or 5-(substituted-phenoxy) primaquine derivatives have radical curative activities against *P. cynomolgi* infections in rhesus monkeys, varying from a fraction of the potency of primaquine to as much as 5.7 times the potency, depending upon the particular substituents on the phenyl group. Without exception, the 5-phenoxy derivatives of 4-methyl primaquine were more potent than the corresponding desmethyl analogues. The 4-methyl-5-phenoxy analogues, regardless of phenyl substituents, were generally in the order of 4.5–5.5 times more potent than primaquine and also about 3.5–4.5 times more potent than 4-methyl primaquine as radical curative agents. The PI of XXXVIII was exceptionally low. Neither the 5-phenoxy- nor the 4-methyl-5-phenoxy primaquine derivatives showed true causal prophylactic activity against sporozoite-induced *P. berghei* infections in the mouse. The anomalous high activity of the 4-methyl-5-phenoxy primaquine derivatives that was observed in the primary prophylactic *P. berghei*-mouse model was attributed to residual blood schizontocidal activity when the prophylactic activity could not be confirmed in secondary testing. The blood schizontocidal activity against *P. berghei* infections in mice was low or absent for the 5-phenoxy primaquine derivatives as seen by the high CD_{50} values. In contrast, the 4-methyl-5-phenoxy primaquine derivatives showed highly potent

Table 2. Radical curative and blood schizontocidal activities of 5-(substituted phenoxy)- and 4-methyl-5-(substituted-phenoxy) primaquine derivatives

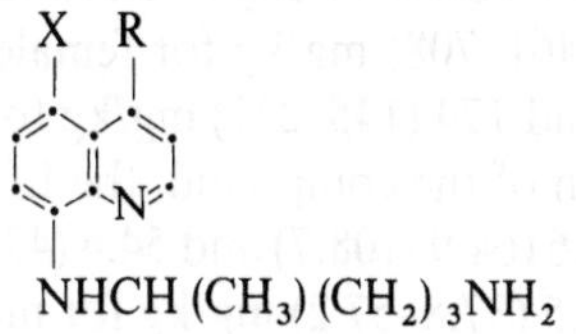

No.	R	X	PI[a]	CD_{50}[b]
XXIII	H	C_6H_5O	1.3	NC
XXIV	CH_3	C_6H_5O	4.9	28
XXV	H	$4\text{-}FC_6H_4O$	0.5	227
XXVI	CH_3	$4\text{-}FC_6H_4O$	4.4	14
XXVII	H	$4\text{-}CH_3OC_6H_4O$	0.2	666
XXVIII	CH_3	$4\text{-}CH_3OC_6H_4O$	4.3	22
XXIX	H	$3\text{-}CF_3C_6H_4O$	3.2	639
XXX	CH_3	$3\text{-}CF_3C_6H_4O$	4.8	10
XXXI	H	$2,4\text{-}Cl_2C_6H_3O$	0.5	NC
XXXII	CH_3	$2,4\text{-}Cl_2C_6H_3O$	4.7	13
XXXIII	H	$3,4\text{-}Cl_2C_6H_3O$	0.4	1,362
XXXIV	CH_3	$3,4\text{-}Cl_2C_6H_3O$	4.7	4
XXXV	H	$3\text{-}CF_3,4\text{-}FC_6H_3O$	4.0	752
XXXVI	CH_3	$3\text{-}CF_3,4\text{-}FC_6H_3O$	5.7	21
XXXVII	H	$3,5\text{-}(CF_3)_2C_6H_3O$	0.6	666
XXXVIII	CH_3	$3,5\text{-}(CF_3)_2C_6H_3O$	1.9	22
Id (primaquine)			1	NC
XIIa (4-methyl primaquine)			1.3	435

[a] See Table 1 for definition

[b] The 50% curative dose calculated from probit transformation of dose-response data obtained in the *P. berghei*-mouse model for blood schizontocidal activity.

NC, not curative

blood schizontocidal activity, a potency equalling the best of the aminoalcohol-type antimalarials. Finally, it is noteworthy that with the single exception of XXIV, none of the 5-phenoxy primaquine or 4-methyl-5-phenoxy primaquine derivatives showed any acute early death toxicity in mice at the highest of the doses tested, 640 mg/kg. The one exception, XXIV, was about as toxic as primaquine. The low toxicity and high radical curative and blood schizontocidal activity indicates a good therapeutic index for the 4-methyl-5-phenoxy primaquine class of compounds.

C. Toxicology

The compound XXX, identified in the US Army Research Programme as WR 225448, was selected for extended evaluation and toxicological and pharmacological studies. LEE et al. (1979a) have investigated the acute, single-dose, oral and intraperitoneal toxicity of WR 225448, as the succinate salt, in rodents. The LD_{50} (95% confidence limits) in rats for a 14-day observation period was 259 (128–389) mg/kg for males and 557 (461–708) mg/kg for females. For male mice the LD_{50} was 236 (191–229) mg/kg and 174 (145–237) mg/kg for male guinea pigs. With intraperitoneal administration of the compound, the LD_{50}s obtained over the same observation period were 85.6 (64.9–108.7) and 54.4 (42.2–71.4) mg/kg for male and female rats respectively, 46.5 (37.8–57.2) mg/kg for male mice and 26.7 (8.4–56.0) mg/kg for male guinea pigs. After oral administration toxic signs included lethargy, rough coat and weight loss. Immediate toxic effects following intraperitoneal administration included convulsions characterised by arching of the back, extension of the hind limbs, abdominal muscle contractions and cyanosis.

The acute oral LD_{50} for primaquine was determined by LEE et al. (1975) to be 177 (135–232) mg/kg for male rats and 224 (193–260) mg/kg for female rats. Thus WR 225448 is less acutely toxic in rats than is primaquine. The same was true with subcutaneous administration of the drugs when they were tested for blood schizontocidal activity in the *P. berghei*-mouse model. The subacute toxicity of WR 225448 succinate and primaquine diphosphate was compared by LEE et al. (1979b) following oral administration of the drugs for 28 days. Rats were administered 3, 9, 16 or 27 mg/kg of either WR 225448 or primaquine daily for 28 days. WR 225448 was lethal to eight of ten rats at a dose of 27 mg/kg per day and four of ten rats at a dose of 16 mg/kg per day. Toxic signs were also observed at the 9 mg/kg per day dose. Only mild toxic signs were observed for primaquine at 27 mg/kg per day. Several haematological alterations that were dose- and duration-of-treatment-related were noted at all dose levels of WR 225448. Similar changes, but less severe, were seen for primaquine. Tissue lesions were noted at all dose levels of WR 225448; the incidence and severity of these lesions were dose related. Lesions were observed in rats administered primaquine at the 27 mg/kg per day dose level only. Changes in clinical chemistry were also observed in rats receiving either 16 or 27 mg/kg per day WR 225448 whereas such changes were noted for primaquine only when the drug was administered at a dose of 27 mg/kg per day. Organ weight changes were observed for both drugs.

The subacute oral toxicity of WR 255448 in beagles was also studied by LEE et al. (1979c). Doses of 1, 3 or 9 mg/kg were administered daily for 28 consecutive days. General toxic signs were mild. The most consistent haematological changes noted were dose-related methaemoglobinaemia followed by compensatory reticulocytosis, elevation of haptoglobin and thrombocytopaenia. Changes in clinical chemistry were relatively mild at the 9 mg/kg per day dose level. A number of tissue lesions were observed at the high-dose level; lesions produced with the two lower dose regimens were not remarkable. In comparison with primaquine, toxic signs, changes in clinical chemistry and tissue lesions were fewer or less severe for WR 225448 succinate than for primaquine diphosphate. A dose of 9 mg/kg per day of primaquine diphosphate was lethal within 4 days. Haematological changes, however, were less severe for primaquine diphosphate.

The compound WR 225448 succinate was not mutagenic as determined in the *Salmonella*/microsome plate test (HODGSON et al. 1977).

D. Summary

There have been a number of recent efforts to uncover 8-aminoquinolines that have greater radical curative activity and a better therapeutic index than primaquine. The better therapeutic index of the *d* enantiomer of primaquine vis à vis primaquine may justify a clinical comparison. Modification of the quinoline ring of primaquine has produced compounds with little or nor activity. Such modifications included 1,5- and 1,6-naphthryidines and naphthyridinones, naphthalene analogues (deazaquinolines) partially saturated quinolines and acridines (benzquinolines). Simple modification of the side chain of 4-methyl primaquine yielded active compounds, the best one having a primaquine index of 4; bridging of two quinoline nuclei through a side chain yielded inactive compounds. Substitution of a variety of small groups on the *N*-containing ring in the quinoline moiety of primaquine resulted in compounds with little or no activity; the best of the derivatives, 4-ethyl primaquine, had activity about equivalent to primaquine as a radical curative agent. A variety of 2-(substituted-benzyloxy) primaquine analogues showed little or no blood schizontocidal activity as a class. Some of the analogues showed radical curative activity but the better ones of the group were only about one-half as potent as primaquine. A group of 4-(substituted-phenoxy) primaquine derivatives were devoid of radical curative activity in the monkey and prophylactic activity in the mouse. However, they did show fair to good blood schizontocidal activity in the mouse. The compound 5-(*p*-anisyloxy)-pentaquine and several side chain analogues were devoid of radical curative and blood schizontocidal activity. A group of 4-methyl-5,6-dimethoxy-8-aminoquinolines were characterised by high radical curative activity (several times that of primaquine), absence of blood schizontocidal activity and relatively high toxicity. Substitution of the 5-methoxy group of 4-methyl-5-methoxy primaquine by larger alkoxy groups resulted in two analogues (the 5-pentoxy and 5-hexoxy) with extremely potent radical curative and blood schizontocidal activity. The 5-(substituted phenoxy) primaquine derivatives have radical curative activity against *P. cynomolgi* infections and for some of the analogues the level of activity is very high. The 5-(substituted-phenoxy) primaquine derivatives, unlike the 4-(substituted-phenoxy) ones, had little or no blood schizontocidal activity against *P. berghei* infections. The 4-methyl-5-(substituted-phenoxy) primaquine derivatives also had potent radical curative activity and, in addition, potent blood schizontocidal activity.

E. Conclusions

To date, no new class of compounds has been uncovered that approaches the 8-aminoquinolines as a class likely to yield a drug to replace primaquine. A number of recent studies on aminoalkylamino-substituted ring systems related to the quinoline ring system have demonstrated that the retention of significant radical curative activity allows essentially no variation in the nature of the ring itself. The nature of the substituents on the quinoline ring, however, has a profound effect on activity and it is in the study of such variations that progress has been made. Investigation of variations in the side chain seem to have reached the point of diminishing returns; with very few exceptions the side chain of primaquine is better, or about as good, as any investigated. The 4-methyl-5-phenoxy- and 4-methyl-5-alkoxy primaquine derivatives seem particularly promising. The potent blood schizontocidal activity as well as the potent radical curative activity evidenced in these classes of compounds would seem to offer the possibility of a single drug that would serve as both a blood and tissue schizontocide against relapsing malarias, a goal of malaria chemotherapists that has been long contemplated. At the present time, based upon data from tests in animal models, it would appear that the combination of chloroquine and one of the newer primaquine derivatives may be better tolerated than the necessarily higher dose of a 4-methyl-5-phenoxy primaquine derivative that would be required if it were used alone. The picture will be clearer if therapeutic indices of the new primaquine derivatives are obtained and clinical trials conducted. The design of improved 8-aminoquinoline analogues would be greatly facilitated by knowledge of the nature and biological properties of the metabolites of primaquine.

References

Archer S, Osei-Gyimak P, Silbering S (1980) 4-[(Aminoalkyl)amino]-1,2-dimethoxy-naphthalenes as antimalarial agents. J Med Chem 23:516–519

Bullock FJ, Tweedie JF, McRitchie DD, Tucker MA (1970) Antiprotozoal quinones. II. Syntheses of 4-amino-1,2-napthoquinones and related compounds as potential antimalarials. J Med Chem 1:97–103

Burghard H, Blanton Jr C DeW (1980) 4,5-Disubstituted primaquine analogs as potential antiprotozoan agents. J Pharma Sci 69:933–936

Carroll FI, Berrang B, Linn CP (1975) Resolution of racemic amines with α-(2,4,5,7-tetranitro-9-fluorenylideneaminooxy) propionic acid (TAPA). Chem Ind (NY) 7:477–478

Carroll FI, Blackwell JT, Philip A, Twine CE (1976) Reduced 8-aminoquinoline analogs as potential antimalarial agents. J Med Chem 19:1111–1119

Carroll FI, Berrang B, Linn CP (1978) Resolution of antimalarial agents via complex formation with α-(2,4,5,7-tetranitro-9-fluorenylideneaminooxy) propionic acid. J Med Chem 21:326–330

Carroll FI, Berrang B, Linn CP, Twine Jr CE (1979a) Synthesis of some 4-substituted 8-amino-6-methoxyquinolines as potential antimalarials. J Med Chem 22:694–699

Carroll FI, Berrang B, Linn CP (1979b) Synthesis of 4-alkyl- and 4-alkylvinyl derivatives of primaquine as potential antimalarials. J Med Chem 22:1363–1367

Carroll FI, Berrang BD, Linn CP (1980) Synthesis of 2,4-disubstituted 6-methoxy-8-aminoquinoline analogues as potential antiparasitics. J Med Chem 23:581–584

Carroll FI, Berrang BD, Linn CP (1981) Synthesis of naphthyridinone derivatives as potential antimalarials. J Heterocycl Chem 18:941–946

Chen EH, Saggiomo AJ, Tanabe K, Verma BL, Nodiff EA (1977) Modifications of primaquine as antimalarials. 1. 5-Phenoxy derivatives of primaquine. J Med Chem 20:1107–1109

Coatney GR, Cooper WC, Eddy NB, Greenberg J (1953) Survey of antimalarial agents. Public Health Monograph No. 9, U.S. Government Printing Office, Washington

Davidson Jr DE, Ager AL, Brown JL, Chapple FE, Whitmire RE, Rossan RN (1981) New tissue schizontocidal antimalarial drugs. Bull WHO 59:463–479

Drake NL, Pratt YT (1951) Quinolinequinones. I. Quinones and hydroquinones related to pentaquine. J Am Chem Soc 73:544–550

Elderfield RC, Mertel HE, Mitch RT, Wempen IM, Werbel E (1955) Synthesis of primaquine and certain of its analogs. J Am Chem Soc 77:4816–4819

Greenberg J, Taylor DJ, Josephson ES (1961) Studies on *Plasmodium gallinaceum* in vitro. II The effects of some 8-aminoquinolines against the erythrocytic parasite. J Infect Dis 88:163–167

Gregory KG, Peters W (1970) The chemotherapy of rodent malaria, IX Causal prophylaxis, part I: A method for demonstrating drug action on exo-erythrocytic stages. Ann Trop Med Parasit 64:15–24

Hodgson JR, Kowalski MA, Goethem DV, Hainje M (1977) Mutagenicity studies on 4-methyl-5-(3-trifluoromethylphenoxy) primaquine succinate (WR-225,448 succinate). Interim report No. 136, U.S. Army medical research and development command contract No. DAMD-17-74-C-4036, Nov. 1

Josephson EJ, Greenberg J, Taylor DJ, Bami HL (1951 a) A metabolite of pamaquine from chickens. J Pharmacol Exp Ther 103:7–9

Josephson ES, Taylor DJ, Greenberg J, Ray AP (1951 b) A metabolite intermediate of pamaquine from chickens. Proc Soc Exp Biol Med 76:700–703

Khan MS, LaMontagne MP (1979) Antimalarials 11. Syntheses of 3- and 5-aminoquinolines as potential antimalarials. J Med Chem 22:1005–1008

LaMontagne MP, Markovac A, Menke JR (1977) Antimalarials 10. Synthesis of 4-substituted primaquine analogs as candidate antimalarials. J Med Chem 20:1122–1127

LaMontagne MP, Markovac A, Khan MS (1982a) Antimalarials 13. 5-Alkoxy analogues of 4-methylprimaquine. J Med Chem 25:964–968

LaMontagne MP, Blumbergs P (1982b) Antimalarials 14. 5-Aryloxy-4-methylprimaquine analogues. A highly effective series of blood and tissue schizontocidal agents. J Med Chem 25:1094–1097

Lee CC, Hwang SW, Seifert WK, Olson TW (1975) Acute oral toxicity of primaquine and 4-methyl primaquine in rats, mice, guinea pigs, and rabbits. Interim report No. 102, U.S. Army medical research and development command contract No. DAMD-17-74-C-4036 Sept 15

Lee CC, Hacker MP, Elliott CL (1979a) Acute oral and intraperitoneal toxicity of 8-[4-amino-l-methylbulyl)amino]-6-methoxy-4-methyl-5-(3-trifluoromethylphenoxy) quinoline succinate (WR-225,448 succinate) in rats, mice, and guinea pigs. Interim report No. 143, U.S. Army medical research and development command contract No. DAMD-17-74-C-4036, Feb 12

Lee CC, Hacker MP, Kintner LD, Hong CG, Elliott CL, Elwood I, Ellis, ER, Castillo EA, Ellis HV III (1979b) Toxicity of 8-[4-amino-l-methylbutyl)amino]-6-methoxy-4-methyl-5-(3-trifluoromethylphenoxy) quinoline succinate (WR-225,448 succinate) and primaquine phosphate following oral administration to rats for 28 days. Interim report No. 152, U.S. Army medical research and development command contract No. DAMD-17-74-C-4036, Dec 6

Lee CC, Hacker MP, Kintner LD, Hong CD, Elliott CL, Elwood I, Ellis, ER, Castillo EA, (1979c) Toxicity of 8-[4-amino-l-methylbutyl)amino]-6-methoxy-4-methyl-5-(3-trifluoromethylphenoxy) quinoline succinate (WR-225,448 succinate) following oral administration to dogs for 28 days. Interim report No. 146, U.S. Army medical research and development command contract No. DAMD-17-74-C-4036, May 3

Lee CC, Heiffler MH, Kintner LD (1981 a) Acute and subacute toxicities of 8-aminoquinolines. Abstracts, eighth international congress of pharmacology, IUPHAR, Tokyo, p 360

Lee CC, Kintner LD, Heiffler MH (1981 b) Subacute toxicity of primaquine in dogs, monkeys, and rats. Bull WHO

McCaustland DJ, Cheng CC (1970) 1,5-Naphthyridines. Synthesis of 7-chloro-4-(4-diethylamino-1-methyl-butylamino)-2-methoxy-1,5-naphthyridine and related compounds. J Heeterocycl Chem 7:467–473

Most H, Montouri WA (1975) Rodent systems (*Plasmodium berghei – Anopheles stephensi*) for screening compounds for potential causal prophylaxis. Am J Trop Med Hyg 24:179–182

Nodiff EA, Saggiomo AJ (1981) 5-Alkoxy-8-quinolinamines for the broad-spectrum treatment of malaria. U.S. Patent Pending, Serial No. 229487

Nodiff EA, Tanabe K, Chen EH, Saggiomo AJ (1982) Modifications of primaquine as antimalarials. 3,5-Phenoxy derivatives of primaquine. J Med Chem 25:1097–1101

Osdene TS, Russell PB, Rane L (1967) 2,4,7-Triamino-6-*ortho*-substituted arylpteridines. A new series of potent antimalarial agents. J Med Chem 10:431–434

Paul K, Blanton CDeW Jr (1973) Synthesis of 1,4-bis(6-methoxy-8-quinolylaminoalkyl) piperazines as potential prophylactic antimalarial agents. J Med Chem 16:1391–1394
Paul K, Blanton CDeW Jr (1976) 5-Aryloxy-6-methoxy-8-aminoquinolines as potential prophylactic antimalarials. J Pharm Sci 65:1527–1530
Peters W (1980) Chemotherapy of malaria. In: Krier JP (ed) Malaria, vol 1. Academic, p 145
Pilot JF, Stogryn EL (1975) Naphthyridine antimalarial agents. Final technical report for April 1, 1973–June 30, 1975, U.S. Army medical research and development command contract No. DADA17-73-C-3079
Rane DS, Kinnamon KE (1979) The development of a "high volume tissue schizonticidal drug screen" based upon mortality of mice inoculated with sporozoites of *Plasmodium berghei*. Am J Trop Med Hyg 28:937–947
Schmidt LH, Genther CS (1953) The antimalarial properties of 2,4-diamino-5-*p*-chlorophenyl-6-ethylpyrimidine (Daraprim). J Pharmacol Exp Ther 107:61–91
Schmidt LH, Fradkin R, Vaughan D, Rasco R (1977a) Radical cure of infections with *Plasmodium cynomolgi:* a function of total 8-aminoquinoline dose. Am J Trop Med Hyg 26:1116–1128
Schmidt LH, Alexander S, Allen L, Rasco J (1977b) Comparison of the curative antimalarial activities and toxicities of primaquine and its *d* and *l* isomers. Antimicrob Agents Chemother 12:51–60
Scovill JP, Klayman DL, Woods TS, Sweeney TR (1979) Primaquine analogues: derivatives of 4-amino-2-methoxyacridine. J Med Chem 22:1164–1167
Shetty RV, Blanton Jr CDeW (1978) Synthesis of 2-substituted primaquine analogues as potential antimalarials. J Med Chem 21:995–998
Shetty RV, Blanton CDeW Jr (1979) Synthesis and antiprotozoan activity of *N,N'*-disubstituted piperazines. Eur J Med Chem 14:353–356
Shetty RV, Wetter WP, Blanton CDeW Jr (1977) Synthesis of 2-benzyloxy and 2-benzylthio analogues of primaquine as potential antimalarials. J Med Chem 20:1349–1351
Singh T, Stein RG, Koelling HH, Hoops JF, Biel JH (1969) Antimalarials. Some quinuclidine derivatives of 7-chloro-4-aminoquinoline and 6-methoxy-8-aminoquinoline. J Med Chem 12:524–526
Talati SM, Lathan MR, Moore EG, Hargreaves GW, Blanton Jr CDeW (1970) Synthesis of potential antimalarials: primaquine analogs. J Pharm Sci 59:491–495
Tanabe K, Chen EH, Verma BL, Saggiomo AJ, Nodiff EA (1978) Modifications of primaquine as antimalarials. 2. 5-Phenylthio and 5-anilino derivatives of primaquine. J Med Chem 21:133–136
Tarlov AR, Brewer GJ, Carson PE, Alving AS (1962) Primaquine sensitivity. Glucose 6-phosphate dehydrogenase deficiency: an inborn error of metabolism of medical and biological significance. Arch Int Med 109:209–234
Thompson PE, Werbel LM (1972) Antimalarial agents: chemistry and pharmacology. Academic, New York
Wiliams RT (1959) Detoxication mechanisms, 2nd edn. Wiley, New York
Wiselogle FY (1946) A survey of antimalarial drugs 1941–1945. Edwards, Ann Arbor
Yan S-J, Chien P-L, Cheng CC (1981) Synthesis and antimalarial activity of 8-(l-alkyl-4-aminobutylamino)-6-methoxy-4-methylquinolines. J Med Chem 24:215–217

CHAPTER 11

Lapinone, Menoctone, Hydroxyquinolinequinones and Similar Structures

A. T. HUDSON

A. Introduction

Interest in 2-hydroxy-3-alkyl-1,4-naphthoquinones as antimalarial agents commenced in the United States in the early 1940s as a result of a massive collaborative programme between industry and academia to find a replacement for quinine (WISELOGLE 1946). Amongst the various structural types evaluated, the hydroxynaphthoquinone hydrolapachol (I) was found to be active. This prompted a joint programme of work between scientists at Harvard University, Abbott Laboratories and other research establishments. Hundreds of analogues of hydrolapachol were synthesised and their antimalarial properties comprehensively evaluated. All facets of modern drug design were employed in this work – development of structure-activity relationships, pharmacokinetic studies, receptor-binding investigations, etc. The climax of these studies occurred in 1948 when, mainly on the basis of metabolic considerations, 2-hydroxy-3-(9-hydroxy-9-pentyltetradecyl)-1,4-naphthoquinone (II) (lapinone) was synthesised (FIESER et al. 1948a) and shown to be effective in curing patients infected with *Plasmodium vivax* (FAWAZ and HADDAD 1951). However, parenteral administration of the drug at fairly high doses was required and this, coupled with the emergence of such effective agents as primaquine and chloroquine, led to a decline of interest in the hydroxynaphthoquinones.

Early in the 1960s it became apparent that drug resistance to the established antimalarials was becoming an increasing problem. Consequently, the development of a novel antiplasmodial agent once again assumed high priority. Interest in the hydroxynaphthoquinones revived and FIESER and his associates at Harvard entered into collaboration with scientists at the Sterling-Winthrop Research Institute in re-examining the potential of these compounds. Novel analogues were prepared and evaluated in the newly introduced *P. berghei* mouse screen (FIESER et al. 1967a, b). One compound, 2-hydroxy-3-(8-cyclohexyloctyl)-1,4-naphthoquinone (III) (menoctone), was selected for study in man but, disappointingly, failed to live up to its early promise (WHO 1973) and appears not to have been investigated further.

Research into the antimalarial properties of the hydroxynaphthoquinones again entered a fresh phase in the late 1960s when evidence was provided that the quinones exerted their therapeutic effect by inhibition of plasmodial electron transport at the ubiquinone (coenzyme Q) locus. This resulted in the synthesis of a wide variety of heterocyclic analogues of the 2-hydroxy-3-alkyl-1,4-naphthoquinones as

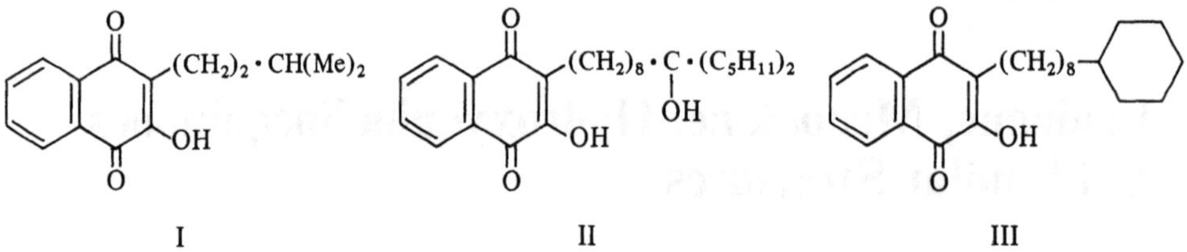

Fig. 1. Chemical structures I, hydrolapachol; II, lapinone; III, menoctone

putative ubiquinone antagonists (PORTER and FOLKERS 1974). Although several of these compounds showed considerable promise in the primary screens, as yet none appear to have been tested in man. However, the breadth of this work is such that further chemical, biochemical and biological studies will be required to evaluate comprehensively the role of ubiquinone antagonists in malaria chemotherapy.

In this review of the antimalarial properties of 2-hydroxynaphthoquinones and their hetero analogues, attention will be focused on structure-activity relationships, mode of action and pharmacokinetic behaviour. A recently published review by OLENICK (1979) has summarised work on the antibacterial, as well as antimalarial, properties of these compounds, with emphasis on their uncoupling effects on electron transport processes.

B. Chemistry

I. Structure-Activity Relationships

The discovery that the 2-hydroxy-1,4-naphthoquinone hydrolapachol (I), originally prepared by HOOKER (1936), was active against *P. lophurae* in ducks prompted the synthesis of further analogues. The activities of these compounds, numbering some 300 in all, were reported in a series of papers (FIESER et al. 1948 a) in which an in-depth structure-activity analysis was presented. The main general conclusions of this investigation were as follows:

1. The 2-hydroxyl moiety is essential for activity. Replacement of this group by OMe, H, Me, NH_2, $NHCOCH_3$, Cl or SH results in complete or extensive loss of activity.

2. Introduction of substituents into, or reduction of, the aromatic nucleus reduces activity.

3. Activity of analogues 3-substituted by an aliphatic group is maximal when nine carbon atoms are present in the side chain, e.g. IV. Introduction of cycloalkyl or aromatic groups into the chain shifts the maximum to a higher chain length.

4. The introduction of heteroatoms, halogens or double bonds into the hydrocarbon 3-substituent adversely affects activity.

5. Direct attachment of an alicyclic moiety to the 3-position is especially favourable for potent activity, e.g. V (*trans* isomer).

The above conclusions were all based on results obtained from the *P. lophurae* duck assay, compounds being administered orally. The most active compound examined in this test system was the *trans* 4′-cyclohexylcyclohexyl analogue V, with

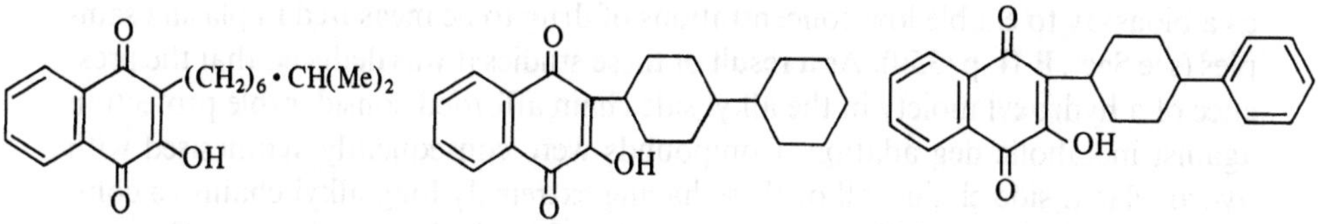

IV V VI

Fig. 2. Chemical structures IV–VI

an ED_{95} value of 0.67 mg/kg [ED_{95} is the dose (given three times daily for 4 days) required to produce a 95% reduction in parasitaemia] – compare the quinine ED_{95} of 17.35 mg/kg. The *cis* isomer of V, however, was considerably less potent – ED_{95} = 9 mg/kg. In several other pairs of *cis/trans* isomers drug efficacy was also configuration related, *trans* isomers being more active than *cis*, e.g. VI ED_{95} *trans* = 7.4 mg/kg, ED_{95} cis = 29 mg/kg.

On the basis of results obtained at an early stage of the screening programme two compounds (VII) and (VIII) were selected for study in patients infected with *P. vivax* and *P. falciparum*. Although VII was four times more potent than VIII (ED_{95} ca. 20 mg/kg) against *P. lophurae* in ducks, in man it was devoid of activity whereas VIII was seen to exert a positive, though temporary, therapeutic effect (WISELOGLE 1946; FIESER et al. 1948a).

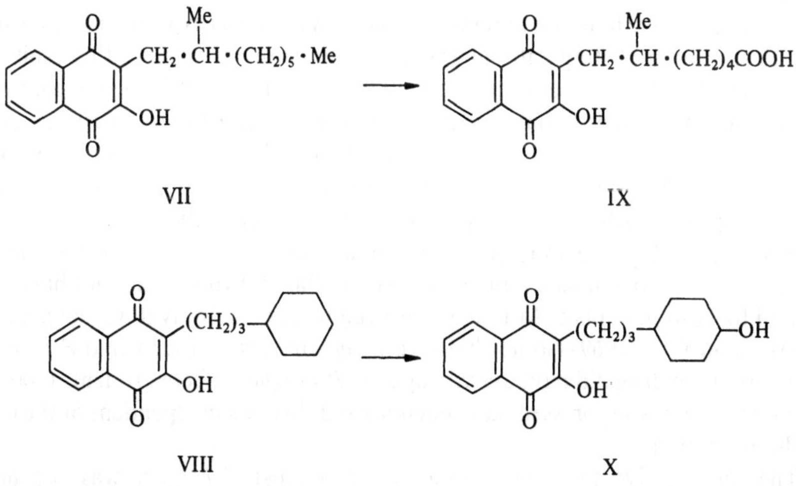

VII IX

VIII X

Fig. 3. Chemical structures VII–X

Further investigation revealed VII to be rapidly metabolised in man to the inactive acid IX whereas VIII was converted to the alcohol (X) (FIESER et al. 1948c). The latter had weak but definite antimalarial activity and persisted in blood at reasonable levels for several days. These findings rationalised the observed therapeutic effect of VIII in man and led to detailed metabolic studies on other analogues being carried out in various species, including man (see Sect. D, p. 353). A key development is this work was the introduction of an in vitro biochemical *P. lophurae* screen as a bioassay to enable low concentrations of drug to be measured in plasma samples (see Sect. B.II, p. 350). As a result of these studies it was deduced that the presence of a hydroxyl moiety in the alkyl side chain afforded considerable protection against metabolic degradation. Compounds were consequently synthesised with hydroxylated side chains, all of these having extremely long alkyl chains to compensate for the hydrophilic character introduced by the hydroxyl group (FIESER et al. 1948 a). Unfortunately, none were particularly active when given orally to *P. lophurae*-infected ducks. However, in the in vitro *P. lophurae* biochemical assay promising activity was observed. The compounds were retested in the primary duck screen and on parenteral administration several were shown to be extremely potent. The most active quinone, lapinone (II), had an ED_{95} of 4 mg/kg and was shown to have a very reasonable pharmacokinetic profile in both animals and man (FIESER et al. 1948 b). Evaluation of the drug (FAWAZ and HADDAD 1951) in patients with primary *P. vivax* infections showed it to exert a very marked therapeutic effect and 1 year after treatment six of the nine patients had not relapsed. However, fairly large quantities of drug had to be administered intravenously, 2 g/day for 4 days. This major disadvantage seems to have outweighed the initial promise shown by the drug and no further trials appear to have been carried out in man.

A resurgence of interest in the hydroxynaphthoquinones in the 1960s led to novel quinones being synthesised for evaluation in the newly established *P. berghei*-mouse assay (FIESER et al. 1967 a, b). In view of the pharmacokinetic studies of FIESER et al. (1948 b) showing the hydroxynaphthoquinones to be metabolised by similar routes in both mouse and man, this test system was expected to be particulary relevant to predicting antimalarial activity in man. Analysis of the results obtained from the *P. berghei* assay (BERBERIAN and SLIGHTER 1968) showed many hydroxynaphthoquinones to have a definite suppressive effect on the parasite. Some of these results have been tabulated in Table 1 to enable a comparison to be made between the *P. berghei* and *P. lophurae* in vivo screens. Although in general compounds appear to behave similarly in both screens, some differences in structure-activity relationships are apparent. For instance, lapinone (II) was virtually devoid of activity in the rodent assay and obviously on this showing would not have been selected for testing in man. Although this drug was given orally it was later shown (AVIADO and WILL 1969) (somewhat surprisingly in view of the in vivo *P. lophurae* results) that the drug did have activity against *P. berghei*-infected rodents (100 mg/kg daily for 3 days suppressed parasitaemia) and this was independent of the route of administration.

The most active hydroxyquinone tested against *P. berghei* was the novel analogue (III) later named menoctone – see Table 1. In addition to its suppressive effect, at high dose levels the drug was capable of effecting cures. Other novel quinones prepared by FIESER et al. (1967 b) showing good suppressive activity were the adamantyl analogues, typified by XI. These compounds were, in fact, more potent than their cyclohexyl counterparts – compare ED_{50}s of XI and VIII in Table 1. In view of this it is unfortunate that the adamantyl analogue of menoctone was not prepared.

It is apparent from the results shown in Table 1 that none of the quinones were as effective as chloroquine. However, in a later study of menoctone (PETERS et al.

Table 1. In vivo activity of 3-alkyl-2-hydroxy-1,4-naphthoquinones against *P. berghei* and *P. lophurae*

Compound	*P. lophurae*[a] ED_{95}	*P. berghei*[b] ED_{50}[c]	*P. berghei*[b] CD_{50}[d]
II	43 (5 i.m.)	>200	>200
III	Not tested	12	97
IV	9	78	>200
VIII	21	50	>100
XI	Not tested	21	> 50
Chloroquine	Not tested	5	16

[a] Data extracted from FIESER and RICHARDSON (1948)
[b] Data extracted from BERBERIAN and SLIGHTER (1968)
[c] The effective dose (mg/kg) given twice daily for 4 days intragastrically, for clearing 50% of mice of parasites
[d] The dose (mg/kg), given daily for 5 days intragastrically, required to maintain 50% of animals parasite free for 1 month

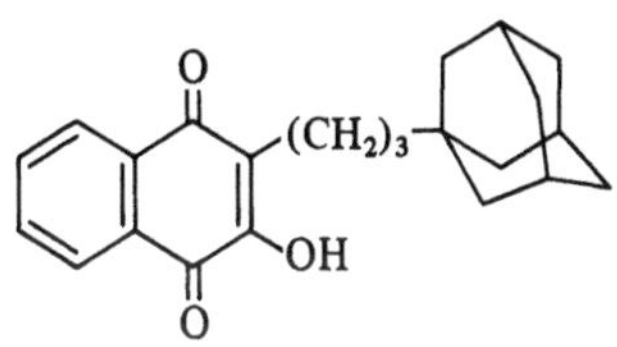

XI

Fig. 4. Chemical structure XI

1975 b) the drug was shown to be as potent as chloroquine against five species of *P. berghei* but against a cycloguanil-resistant strain it was less active.

On the basis of the results shown in Table 1 it was concluded that the activity of the quinones against the erythrocytic stages of the disease was insufficient to be of great value in treating overt malaria (BERBERIAN and SLIGHTER 1968). However, in infected rodents menoctone (III) was shown to be highly effective against pre-erythrocytic stages of the disease and to possess good causal prophylactic properties (BERBERIAN et al. 1968). The drug was considerably more active than primaquine against sporozoite-induced *P. berghei* infection in mouse, a single oral dose of 25 mg/kg of III, given 4 h prior to infection, affording complete protection. In addition, coadministration of III with either chloroquine or quinine appeared to enhance its causal prophylactic effect.

The activity of menoctone against *P. berghei* suggested that it could be valuable in chemoprophylaxis and, in combination with other drugs, in effecting radical cures. The drug was also relatively non-toxic – oral LD_{50} (mouse), $1{,}710 \pm 682$ mg/kg in contrast to primaquine – LD_{50}, 113 ± 22 mg/kg (BERBERIAN et al. 1968). However, despite these promising indications the results of clinical trials with this compound in man have been extremely disappointing. No gametocytocidal or sporontocidal effects were noted when 0.4 g or 0.5 g menoctone were administered daily by mouth for 3 days to patients infected with *P. falciparum* (Malayan Camp. strain) and only slight blood schizontocidal activity was seen (WHO 1973). Even more disappointing, the drug failed to show any causal prophylactic activity in man against two strains of *P. falciparum*. These results were explained on the basis of poor absorption of III from the gastrointestinal tract. No attempts appear to have been made to repeat this study administering the drug parenterally.

Efforts to improve the bioavailability of menoctone have been made by synthesising various prodrugs. Several interesting compounds were prepared (Razdan et al. 1971) including a water soluble derivative of menoctone (XII). Unfortunately this was unstable in aqueous solution, regenerating menoctone within minutes. This compound, along with several other prodrugs, failed to demonstrate activity greater than III in mice infected with *P. berghei* or chicks parasitised with *P. gallinaceum*. Further analogues of menoctone have been synthesised (Tullar and Lorenz 1972) containing a trimethylcylohexyl moiety (XIII). The activity of these compounds appears to be similar to menoctone with no apparent advantages.

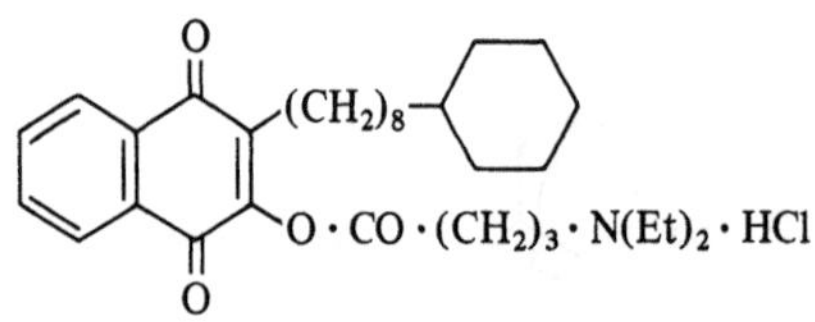

XII

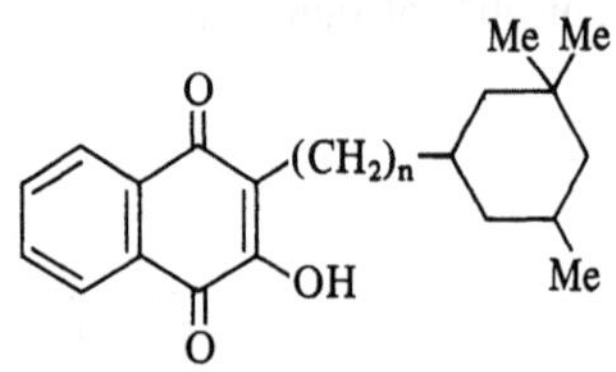

XIII n = 4–12

Fig. 5. Chemical structures XII and XIII

A fresh approach to the design of quinone antimalarials was taken when evidence was provided that the hydroxynaphthoquinones were acting as ubiquinone antagonists (see Sect. C, p. 350). A wide range of heterocyclic analogues of these compounds was prepared as putative ubiquinone antagonists. The variety of quinones synthesised and evaluated is exemplified by XIV–XXII (Porter et al. 1971, 1973; Wan et al. 1974; Bowman et al. 1973b; Friedman et al. 1973; Catlin et al. 1971; Bogentoft et al. 1972).

From the many analogues tested the 7-alkylthio-6-hydroxyquinolinequinones, typified by XVII and XVIII, emerged with greatest promise, especially as prophylactic agents. Subcutaneous administration of 10 mg/kg of XVII afforded complete protection against sporozoite-induced *P. gallinaceum* infections in chicks (Wan et al. 1974). At fairly high doses (320 mg/kg) several analogues, e.g. XVIII, were also shown to be effective in curing blood-induced *P. berghei* infections in mice (Porter et al. 1973). One compound – XVIII – was tested in *P. cynomolgi*-infected rhesus monkeys and was shown to suppress parasitaemia when given intravenously at a dosage of 3.16 mg/kg per day for 7 days (Wan et al. 1974). Attempts to achieve cures by varying the dosage and/or route of administration resulted in either severe toxicity or total loss of activity. This latter result appears to have dampened enthusiasm for the hydroxyquinolinequinones and no further investigations of their antimalarial properties appear to have been reported in detail.

It is interesting to note that, despite the synthesis and evaluation of a plethora of heterocyclic quinones, only those which can be considered close structural

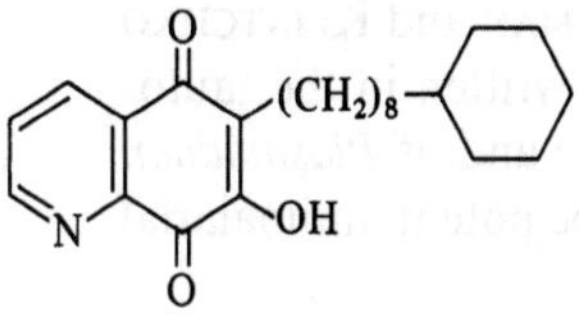

XIV

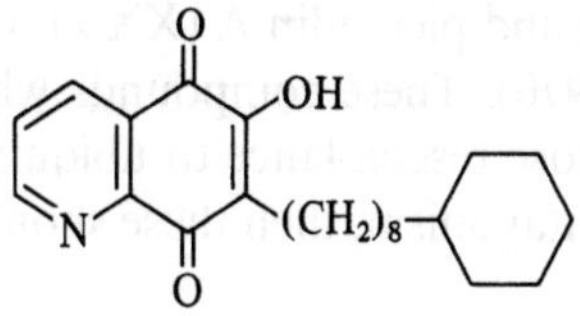

XV

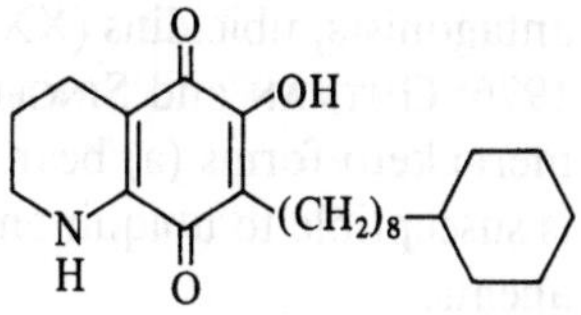

XVI

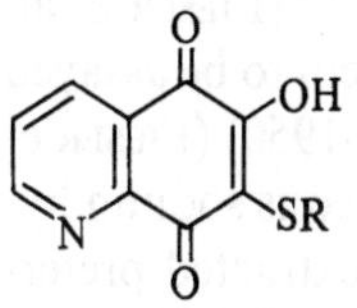

XVII $R = C_{17}H_{35}$
XVIII $R = C_{18}H_{37}$

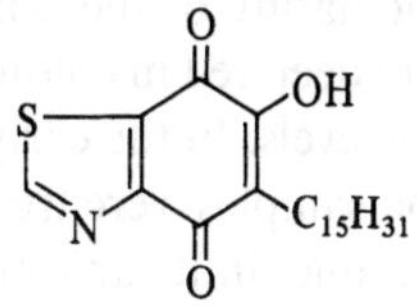

XIX

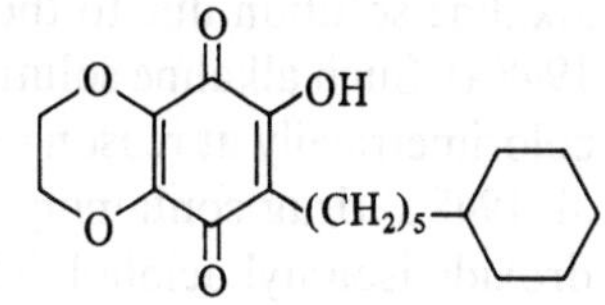

X X

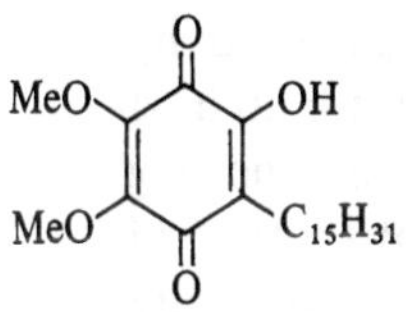

XXI

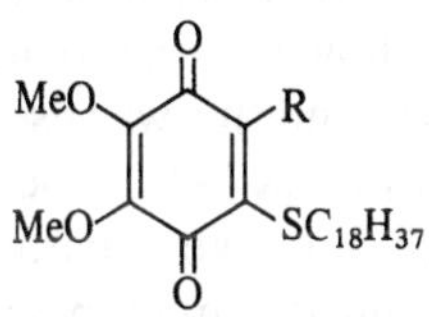

XXII R = H, Cl, NH_2, Me, $C_{18}H_{37}$

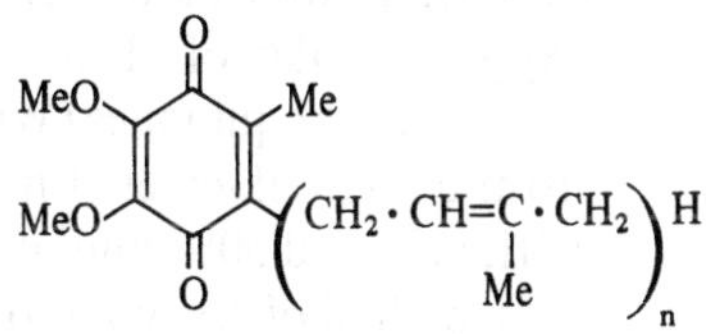

XXIII

Fig. 6. Chemical structures XIV–XXIII (XXIII, ubiquinone)

analogues of hydroxynaphthoquinones, e.g. XIV, XV, XVII, and XIX, have shown any worthwhile antimalarial activity. The benzoquinone analogues typified by XVI, XX, XXI, and XXII, despite their structural resemblance to ubiquinone XXIII, have either been inactive or their activity against *Plasmodium* has been unreported. In view of this it would be of interest to evaluate the potent ubiquinone

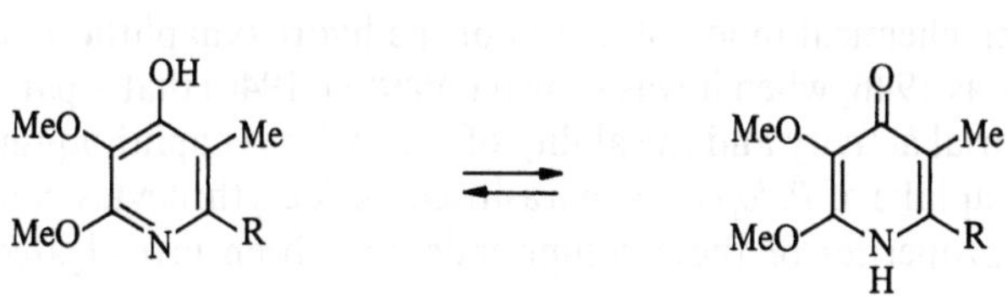

(a)

XXIV $R = (CH_2 \cdot CH{=}C(Me) \cdot CH_2)_n H$; n = 1–10

XXV $R = CH_2 \cdot CH{=}C(Me) \cdot CH{=}CH \cdot CH_2 \cdot C(Me){=}CH \cdot CH(Me) \cdot CH(OH) \cdot C(Me){=}CHMe$

Fig. 7. Chemical structures XXIV and XXV

antagonists, ubicidins (XXIV) and piericidin A (XXV) (GUTMAN and KLIATCHKO 1976; GUTMAN and SINGER 1970). These compounds when written in the tautomeric keto forms (a) bear a close resemblance to ubiquinone and, if *Plasmodium* is susceptible to ubiquinone antagonism, then these should be potent antimalarial agents.

II. Assay Methods

Hydroxyalkylnaphthoquinones are invariably yellow solids which are soluble in alkaline solution due to the acidic nature of the 2-hydroxyl moiety (FIESER et al. 1948 a). Such alkaline solutions are deep red in colour enabling them to be assayed colorimetrically at reasonably low levels. In the early studies (pre-1950) (FIESER et al. 1948 a) drug-containing plasma samples were treated with aqueous sodium hydroxide/isoamyl aclohol. The quinone, in its anionic form, was extracted preferentially into the alcohol. Measurement of the extinction coefficient of the isoamyl alcohol at 490 nm enabled the quinone concentration to be determined after correcting for the presence of carotenoid material which also absorbs in this region.

A more sensitive bioassay was introduced at a later stage in the pre-1950 work employing duck blood cells parasitised by *P. lophurae* (FIESER et al. 1948 b). The oxygen uptake of these cells was shown to be remarkably sensitive to hydroxynaphthoquinones (WENDEL 1946) and this was used as the basis for an in vitro antimalarial screen (FIESER and HEYMANN 1948). The more active quinones, e.g. VIII, achieved 50% inhibition of oxygen uptake of parasitised cells at 1×10^{-6} *M*. This method of assay was obviously limited to quinones with antirespiratory activity and metabolites such as the hydroxynaphthoquinone (IX) (see Sect. B.I, p. 344) were undetectable. However, use of this in vitro test in conjunction with the colorimetric assay did enable the blood levels of various naphthoquinones to be determined with reasonable accuracy (FIESER et al. 1948 b).

No further reports on assay procedures for antimalarial quinones have appeared since the original studies discussed above.

C. Modes of Action

Studies on the biochemical mode of action of the hydroxynaphthoquinones were initiated as early as 1946, when it was shown (WENDEL 1946) that a parallel existed betwen antimalarial activity and the ability of the hydroxynaphthoquinones to inhibit the oxygen uptake of *P. lophurae*-parasitised duck erythrocytes. Since then the antirespiratory properties of these compounds have been investigated by many

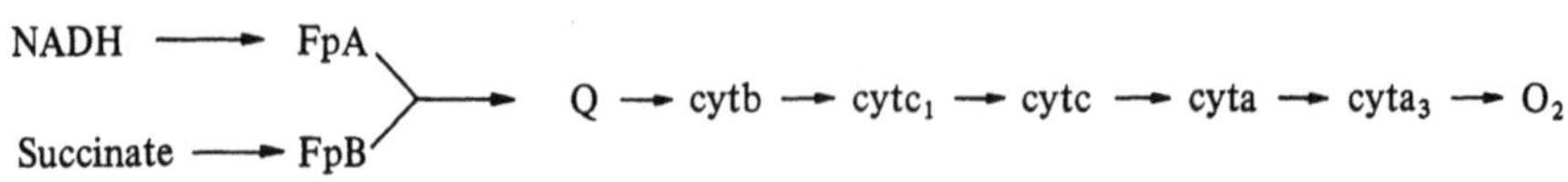

Fig. 8. Electron transport chain. *Fp*, flavoprotein; *Q*, ubiquinone; *cyt*, cytochrome. Succinate oxidase refers to the section of the chain coupling succinate to oxygen. Succinate-cytochrome c reductase refers to section of chain coupling succinate to cytochrome c

groups and attempts made to pinpoint the exact site of interaction with the electron transport chain – see OLENICK (1979) for a recent review.

For illustrative purposes a typical mammalian respiratory system can be regarded as a linear electron transport chain as shown in Fig. 8 (KLINGENBERG 1968). Studies by BALL et al. (1947) established that naphthoquinones with good activity against *P. knowlesi*, e.g. 2-hydroxy-3-(2-methyloctyl)-1,4-naphthoquinone (VII), were highly effective inhibitors of beef heart succinate oxidase and this suggested the use of this enzyme for evaluating potential antimalarial hydroxynaphthoquinones. However, in a more detailed appraisal (HEYMANN and FIESER 1948a) it was shown that, although some correlation existed between enzyme inhibition and antimalarial activity, this was not enough to be relied upon as an index of antiplasmodial potency in vivo.

Attempts to define the specific site of action in the respiratory chain acted on by the naphthoquinones were made with beef heart mitochondria and evidence was obtained that the site affected was located between cytochromes b and c (BALL et al. 1947). The similarity between the hydroxynaphthoquinones and vitamin K (XXVI) prompted experiments to reverse the electron transport blockade using the latter agent but the results obtained were inconclusive. Some years later the fundamental role of ubiquinone in electron transport processes was discovered (CRANE et al. 1957, 1959; CRANE 1960) and efforts to reverse the antirespiratory activity of the hydroxynaphthoquinones with this quinone were made by several groups, again using mammalian electron transport systems (CRANE 1960; HENDLIN and COOK 1960). The results obtained provided some evidence that the naphthoquinones did act at the ubiquinone locus in respiratory systems but were inconclusive. Reversal of inhibition required a large excess of ubiquinone and could be achieved by other compounds non-quinonoid in nature, e.g. squalene.

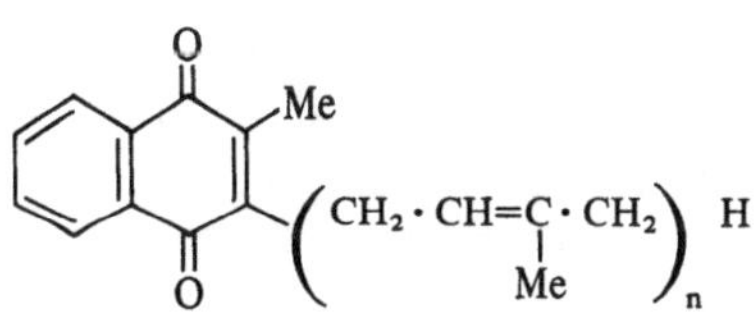

XXVI

Fig. 9. Chemical structure XXVI

Further studies on the mode of action of the hydroxynaphthoquinones were made by the group of FOLKERS [see PORTER and FOLKERS (1974) for a review on ubiquinone antagonism and malaria chemotherapy]. On the assumption that the hydroxynaphthoquinones owed their antimalarial properties to inhibition of the parasite's respiratory system, various species of *Plasmodium* were examined for the presence of the electron transporting quinones vitamin K and ubiquinone (RIETZ et al. 1967; SKELTON et al. 1969, 1970; SCHNELL et al. 1971). In all cases only the latter quinone was detected, no trace of vitamin K being observed. Furthermore the principal quinone in *Plasmodium* was shown to be ubiquinone 8 (XXIII) ($n=8$) and not ubiquinone 10 (XXIII) ($n=10$), which is the major quinone present in mammals. It was not established whether ubiquinone 8 arose by de novo synthesis or by metabolism of the host ubiquinone 10.

The above findings prompted the synthesis of putative ubiquinone antagonists for evaluation as antimalarial agents. A wide range of quinones was synthesised (see Sect. B.I, p. 344) and examined for antirespiratory properties and/or activity against *P. gallinaceum* and *P. berghei*. The most active of these compounds in the antimalarial screens, the hydroxyquinolinequinones, were also highly active against yeast and beef heart NADH and succinate oxidase preparations (BOWMAN et al. 1973 a). Furthermore it was possible to reverse the activity of menoctone (III) and the quinolinequinone analogue (XV) in the NADH-cytochrome c and succinate-cytochrome c reductase systems (see Fig. 8) by the addition of ubiquinone 6 (XXIII) ($n=6$) (SKELTON et al. 1973). Kinetic analysis indicated that both III and XV acted as competitive inhibitors of the ubiquinone enzyme systems. More detailed studies (ROBERTS et al. 1978) using yeast mitochondrial preparations provided good evidence that the quinones blocked electron transfer between cytochromes b and c_1.

Further circumstantial evidence linking the mode of action of the hydroxyquinones to inhibition of plasmodial electron transport processes was provided by BEAUDOIN et al. (1969) and HOWELLS et al. (1970). These workers showed by electron microscopy that the initial effect of menoctone against *P. fallax* or *P. berghei* was on the mitochondrion, which is where ubiquinone-mediated electron transport would be expected to occur. However, it must be emphasised that very little is known of the nature or location of the respiratory system(s) of *Plasmodium*. Cytochrome oxidase has been found in many species of *Plasmodium* but, as the majority of mammalian *Plasmodium* lack a citric acid cycle (SHERMAN 1979), the relevance of this is difficult to assess. The suggestion has been made that the oxygen utilisation of *Plasmodium* could be coupled to the pyrimidine biosynthetic pathway by the enzyme dihydroorotate dehydrogenase (GUTTERIDGE et al. 1979). Studies on this enzyme from *P. knowlesi*, *P. berghei* and *P. gallinaceum* have shown it to be similar to the mammalian enzyme and to be intimately connected to an electron transport chain. Significantly the enzyme was susceptible to inhibition by menoctone and this result was taken as evidence for a ubiquinone involvement (GUTTERIDGE et al. 1979).

At this time, dihydroorotate dehydrogenase inhibition offers the most attractive rational explanation for the antimalarial activity of the hydroxyquinones. Unlike mammals, which can both salvage preformed pyrimidines and carry out de novo biosynthesis, *Plasmodium* is totally reliant upon the latter for satisfying its pyrimidine requirements (JAFFE and GUTTERIDGE 1974). A blockade of the pyrimidine biosynthetic pathway indiscriminately on both parasite and host would hence have lethal consequences for the former but not necessarily for the latter. However, a more attractive rationalisation would be provided if the quinones could be shown to inhibit preferentially the plasmodial enzyme. Further work testing a range of hydroxynaphthoquinones against both plasmodial and mammalian dihydroorotate dehydrogenases will be required to explore this possibility. Attempts to relieve inhibition of the malaria enzyme with ubiquinone could also help to resolve the role of the latter in plasmodial biochemistry.

In addition to dihydroorotate dehydrogenase, the possibility must be considered that other malarial enzymes may have a ubiquinone cofactor requirement making them susceptible to the hydroxyquinones. In this context it is interesting to note that menoctone has recently been shown to inhibit the filarial enzyme converting 5-methyltetrahydrofolate to 5,10-methylenetetrahydrofolate when the assay was conducted in the presence of ubiquinone 7 (XXIII) ($n=7$) (JAFFE 1980). Whether this finding bears any relationship to filaria chemotherapy in vivo is not yet known.

The studies carried out to date on the mode of action of the antimalarial hydroxyquinones suggest that these compounds exert their therapeutic effects via interference with some ubiquinone-linked enzyme connected to the parasite's respiratory system. However, the evidence for this is largely circumstantial and it may well be that the antiplasmodial effects of the hydroxyquinones are not due to inhibition at any one specific site. OLENICK and HAHN (1974) have studied the effect of 2-hydroxy-3-(3-cyclohexylpropyl)-1,4-naphthoquinone (VIII) on *Bacillus megaterium* and concluded that its bactericidal action results from inhibition of ATP-linked transport of essential nutrients. The possibility of a similar effect operating in *Plasmodium* is one that should not be overlooked.

D. Pharmacokinetics and Metabolism

Extensive pharmacokinetic evaluations were carried out on the hydroxynaphthoquinones synthesised prior to 1950. Clinical trials of the cyclohexylpropylquinone (VIII) and its nonyl analogue (VII) showed both to be converted to hydroxynaphthoquinones with enhanced solubility in sodium bicarbonate solution (WISELOGLE 1946; FIESER et al. 1948a). Further studies (FIESER et al. 1948c) in non-infected patients established that VIII was rapidly degraded to the alcohol (X), which had some antimalarial activity (FIESER and HEYMANN 1948), whereas VII was converted to the inactive acid (IX) (see Sect. B.I, p. 344). The structure of X was confirmed by synthesis (DAUBEN and ADAMS 1948) and the hydroxyl moiety shown to be *trans* to the propylquinone unit. A second metabolite isolated from VIII-treated patients was shown to be isomeric with X but was not characterised further (FIESER et al. 1948c). Both isomers were considerably more resistant to metabolism than the parent compound (VIII) and persisted at reasonable levels in blood for at least 20 h.

Examination of a range of hydroxynaphthoquinones in man showed that, in each case, the alkyl side chains were oxidatively metabolised (FIESER et al. 1948c). For example, hydrolapachol (I) was metabolised to the tertiary carbinol (XXVII) while the higher homologue (XXVIII) was converted to the acid (XXIX).

In general, however, hydroxynaphthoquinones having hydrocarbon side chains terminating in methyl groups were oxidised to carboxylic acids, while quinones with a terminal cycloalkyl moiety were hydroxylated in the alkyl ring to cyclocarbinols. The acids were devoid of activity against *P. lophurae* whereas the cyclocarbinols showed some activity but were not as potent as their parent compounds, e.g. X was one-tenth as active as VIII against *P. lophurae* in vitro (FIESER and HEYMANN 1948). It was concluded that the introduction of an hydroxyl group

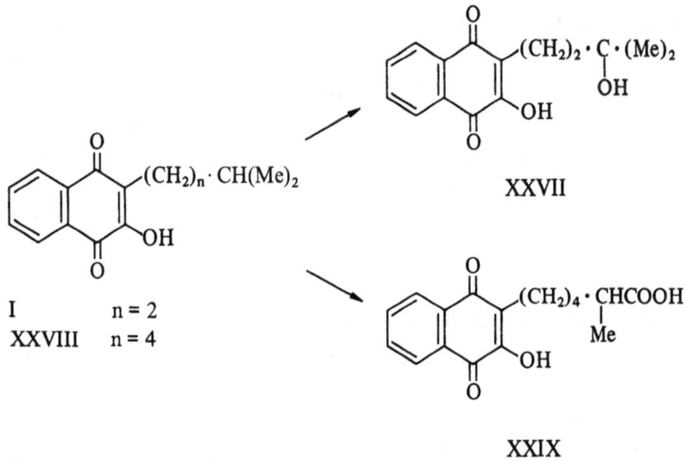

Fig. 10. Chemical structures XXVII–XXIX

into the quinone side chain was detrimental to antimalarial activity but beneficial in protecting against metabolic degradation.

The synthesis of further quinones revealed that the undesirable effects on potency resulting from the presence of an oxygen function in the side chain could be offset by increasing the carbon content of the alkyl group (FIESER et al. 1948 a). Two compounds, II (later named lapinone) and XXX, were sufficiently active against *P. lophurae* to warrant in-depth pharmacokinetic evaluation (FIESER et al. 1948 b). Significant activity in the *P. lophurae* bioassay was observed in plasma samples taken up to 20 h after intravenous administration of 0.6 g of both compounds to man. Although the observed blood levels of II were somewhat variable, on balance the compound appeared to have a longer plasma half-life than XXX. Reasonable blood concentrations of II were, however, only attained when the drug was given intravenously, low levels of drug resulting from oral or intramuscular administration. On the basis of these results II was selected for study in *P. vivax*-infected patients and shown to be effective when administered intravenously (FAWAZ and HADDAD 1951).

Other hydroxynaphthoquinones were evaluated in a similar manner to II and XXX but were all found to be very rapidly metabolised in man and consequently were judged to have little potential for malaria chemotherapy (FIESER et al. 1948 b). A particular disappointment was that the most active quinone tested against *P. lophurae*, V (*trans* isomer), seemed to be metabolised faster than any of the other analogues. Prodrugs of several of the hydroxynaphthoquinones were also examined in man, e.g. XXXI, XXXII, and XXXIII, but, although the parent drugs were readily regenerated in vivo, no pharmacokinetic advantages were apparent (FIESER et al. 1948 c).

The choice of lapinone for antimalarial testing in man and the subsequent demonstration of its efficacy against *P. vivax* (FAWAZ and HADDAD 1951) must be seen as a vindication of the assay procedures employed by FIESER et al. (1948 a). However, in the selection of this drug for clinical evaluation and the rejection of other analogues, heavy reliance was placed upon plasma drug levels (FIESER et al. 1948 b).

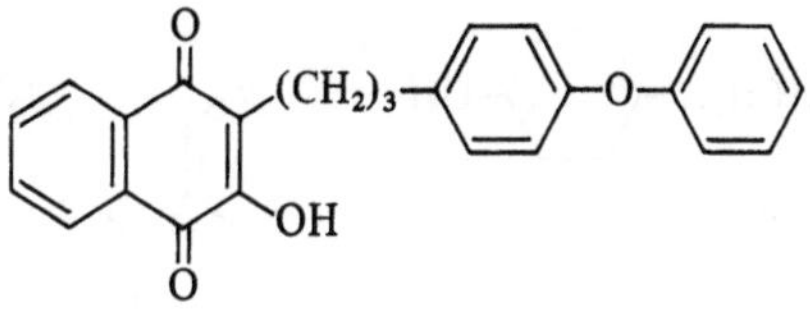

XXX ED$_{95}$ ca. 7mg/kg

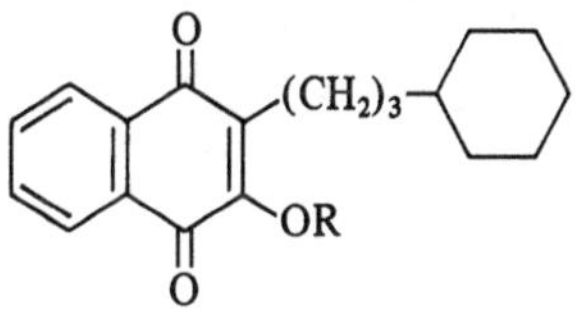

XXXI R = CH_3CO
XXXII R = CH_3CH_2CO

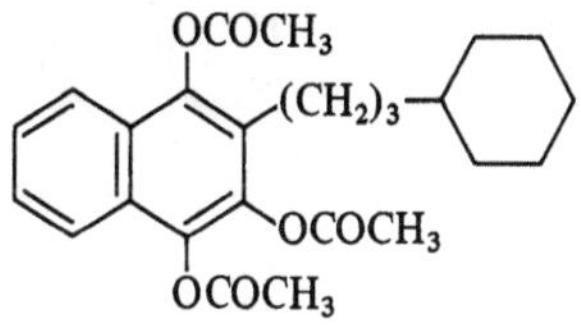

XXXIII

Fig. 11. Chemical structures XXX–XXXIII

In hindsight this practice can be argued to have been somewhat presumptuous. The antimalarial pamaquine, like the hydroxynaphthoquinones, rapidly disappears from blood following intravenous administration – after 15 min only 5% of the initial dose could be found in circulating blood (ZUBROD et al. 1948). Likewise the blood levels of mepacrine are misleading as the drug is concentrated in tissues hundreds of times greater than in plasma (FAIRLEY 1945). Thus it may be that the hydroxynaphthoquinones are similarly tissue concentrated. In support of this these compounds have been shown to be far more effective against tissue stages of malaria than against the erythrocytic forms (BERBERIAN and SLIGHTER 1968; BERBERIAN et al. 1968).

In an extension of the pharmacokinetic studies carried out in man the bioavailability and metabolism of lapinone (II) and the cyclohexylpropyl analogue (VIII) were also examined in various avian and mammalian species (FIESER et al. 1948 b). Both drugs were very rapidly metabolised in dogs, cats and rabbits but in monkeys and ducks they persisted for considerable periods without any signs of oxidative degradation being seen. In mice, however, both II and VIII were observed to persist in blood and suffer metabolic degradation as in man. The quinones were also shown to be metabolised in rats and chickens as in man although in these species the process was much slower and occurred to a lesser extent (FIESER et al. 1948 a).

The suitability of the mouse as a model for predicting the pharmacokinetic behaviour of hydroxynaphthoquinones in man probably had little impact on the early quinone antimalarial studies. However, when the *P. berghei*-mouse assay was introduced (THURSTON 1950), this must have been seen as the ideal test system for the hydroxynaphthoquinones and provided a stimulus for the work in which menoctone was synthesised (FIESER et al. 1967 a). It was rationalised that a highly lipophilic quinone such as menoctone (III) should be metabolised in man (and presumably mouse) to a cyclocarbinol (XXXIV) which should have potent antimalar-

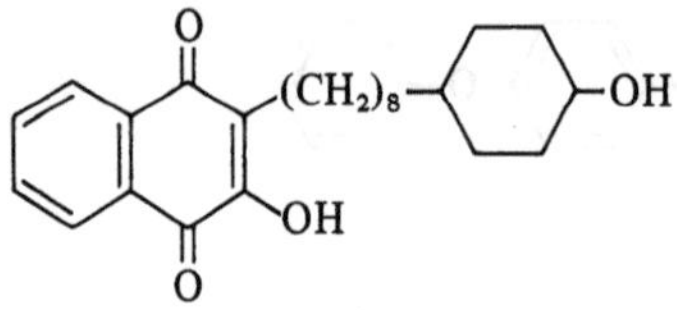

XXXIV

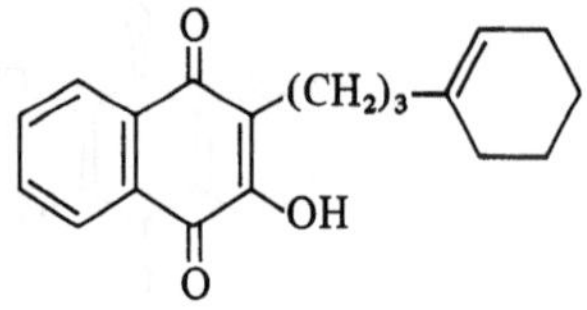

XXXV

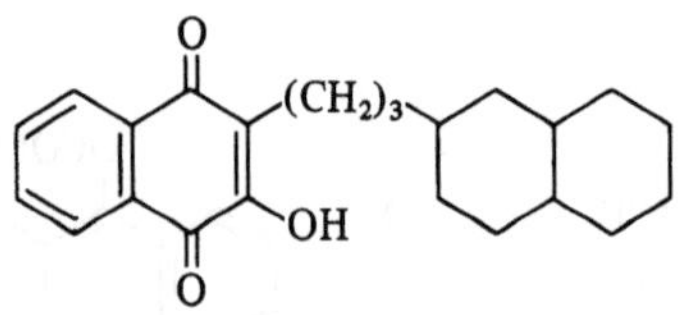

XXXVI

Fig. 12. Chemical structures XXXIV–XXXVI

ial activity and be fairly resistant to metabolism. Unfortunately no pharmacokinetic studies on the metabolic fate of menoctone in any species have been reported and it is not known whether a metabolite such as XXXIV contributed significantly to the activity observed against *P. berghei* (FIESER et al. 1967 b).

In addition to studies on the metabolic fate of the hydroxynaphthoquinones work has been carried out on their interaction with plasma proteins. The efficacy of these compounds against *P. lophurae* in vitro was shown to be antagonised by plasma proteins (WENDEL 1946). Dialysis experiments established that the affinity of plasma from various species for the hydroxyquinones was in general in the order human > monkey > duck (HEYMANN and FIESER 1948 b). The cyclohexylpropylquinone VIII was shown to be 25 times less potent against *P. lophurae* in vitro when the assay was conducted in human serum rather than duck serum (WENDEL 1946). The highly active 4′-cyclohexylcyclohexyl analogue (V) was, however, equipotent against *P. lophurae* in either duck or human serum (HEYMANN and FIESER 1948 b).

The possibility of serum protein-binding influencing the bioavailability of the hydroxynaphthoquinones in vivo is yet another variable factor which must be taken into account when attempting to predict antimalarial activity in man on the basis of results obtained in other species. The extrapolation of results obtained from in vitro drug-protein binding studies to an in vivo situation is, however, fraught with difficulty. For instance the degree of binding of drugs with serum proteins is temperature variable and less binding occurs at body temperature than at ambient temperature (VALLNER 1977). Furthermore, plasma represents only a small portion of the actual volume available for drug distribution in man and, in order to reduce significantly the quantity of free drug available, exceptionally stable protein-drug complexes must be formed (MEYER and GUTTMAN 1968). It is not clear from the work carried out on the interaction of hydroxynaphthoquinones with serum proteins whether the observed binding was exceptionally strong. Consequently the claim that the hydroxynaphthoquinones are valueless clinically because of strong serum protein-binding (WEBB 1966) must be regarded as suspect.

E. Toxicity

In view of the potent effects of the hydroxyquinones on mammalian mitochondrial enzymes (see Sect. C, p. 350) it might expected that these compounds would be toxic to man. However, to date at least five hydroxynaphthoquinones (I, II, III, VII, and VIII) have been evaluated in malaria-infected patients (WISELOGLE 1946; FIESER et al. 1948 a; FAWAZ and HADDAD 1951; WHO 1973) and some 18 other in non-infected patients (FIESER et al. 1948 c) at fairly high doses (orally and parenterally) without any serious toxicity being reported. A tendency of several of the compounds (I, VII, and VIII) to induce nausea, anorexia, and a pink skin coloration was observed in some patients (WIESELOGLE 1946). Haemorrhagic effects in rats were also noted but these were preventable by coadministration with vitamin K (SMITH et al. 1946; SMITH 1947). The toxic effects of some 25 naphthoquinones have been examined in mice (FIESER et al. 1948 b). Striking variations of toxicity with structure were apparent and several quinones were revealed to be fairly toxic, e.g. XXXV.

F. Deployment

The efficacy of the hydroxynaphthoquinones and their hetero analogues from results to date suggests that, as proposed by BERBERIAN and SLIGHTER (1968), the greatest value of these drugs would be as causal prophylactics and, when used in conjunction with other antimalarials, as agents for effecting radical cures. In the latter connection it is of interest to note that the antimalarial effects of menoctone have been shown to be potentiated by coadministration with cycloguanil (PETERS 1970), while pamaquine enhances the activity of the *cis-β*-decalylpropyl analogue (XXXVI) (THOMPSON et al. 1953; WALKER and RICHARDSON 1948).

G. Drug Resistance

No reports have appeared on any species of *Plasmodium* developing resistance to the hydroxynaphthoquinones. However, in cross-resistance studies the activity of menoctone and the *cis-β*-decalylpropyl analogue (XXXVI) have been examined for blood schizontocidal activity against various drug-resistant strains of *P. berghei* in mice (PETERS et al. 1975 a).

Only against the cycloguanil-resistant strain was menoctone significantly less active. XXXVI was, however, equally effective against this strain and the one deemed drug-sensitive. Both quinones were shown to have good causal prophylactic activity against the rodent parasite *P. yoelii nigeriensis* (PETERS et al. 1975 b), which is considered a good model for chloroquine-resistant *P. falciparum*.

H. Future Prospects

The quinones evaluated in malaria-infected patients have all been selected on the basis of their activity against model *Plasmodium* in model hosts. Consequently structure-activity relationships must not only have been affected by parasite species differences but probably to an even greater extent by varying bioavailability factors. The recent development of an in vitro antimalarial screen employing cultures of a human parasite, *P. falciparum* (TRAGER and JENSEN 1976; TRAGER 1979), now offers a tremendous opportunity to perform definitive structure-activity studies on the hydroxyquinones. Since the assay involves cultivation of the parasite in human blood, any detrimental effects resulting from serum protein binding should be reflected in the observed activity of the compounds. Activity in this test system will, of course, only reflect efficacy against the blood stages of *P. falciparum*. However, once this has been optimised, secondary testing, albeit using model host/parasite systems, should give some insight into the potential curative and causal prophylactic properties of selected compounds. Pharmacokinetic studies could then be carried out in mice in view of the apparent similarity of this species to man in metabolising the hydroxynaphthoquinones (see Sect. D, p. 353). Special attention should be paid not only to drug plasma levels but also to the quinone concentrations in tissues. In this manner compounds could be selected for detailed evaluation in man with some confidence of them achieving their desired antimalarial effects.

References

Aviado DM, Will DH (1969) Pharmacology of naphthoquinones with special reference to the antimalarial activity of lapinone (WR 26,041). J Trop Med Hyg 18:188–198

Ball EG, Anfinsen CB, Cooper O (1947) The inhibitory action of naphthoquinones on respiratory processes. J Biol Chem 168:257–270

Beaudoin RL, Strome CPA, Clutter WG (1969) Tissue culture system for the study of drug action against the tissue phase of malaria. Milit Med 134:979–985

Berberian DA, Slighter RG (1968) The schizonticidal activity of hydroxynaphthoquinones against *Plasmodium berghei* infections in mice. J Parasitol 54:999–1005

Berberian DA, Slighter RG, Freele HW (1968) Causal prophylactic activity of menoctone (a new hydroxynaphthoquinone) against sporozoite-induced *Plasmodium berghei* infection in mice. J Parasitol 54:1181–1189

Bogentoft C, von Klaudy A, Folkers K (1972) Antimetabolites of coenzyme Q.17. Improved synthesis of 5-hydroxy-1,4-benzoquinone analogs and their indices. J Med Chem 15:1135–1138

Bowman CM, Skelton FS, Porter TH, Folkers K (1973a) Antimetabolites of coenzyme Q. 14. Quinolinequinone analogs which inhibit mitochondrial DPNH-oxidase and succinoxidase. J Med Chem 16:206–209

Bowman CM, Wikholm RJ, Boler J, Bogentoft CB, Folkers K (1973b) Synthesis and inhibitory activity of new ethylenedioxyquinones as analogs of coenzyme Q. J Med Chem 16:988–991

Catlin JC, Daves GD, Folkers K (1971) New substituted 2,3-dimethoxy-1,4-benzoquinones as inhibitors of coenzyme Q systems. J Med Chem 14:45–48

Crane FL (1960) Quinones in electron transport. I. Coenzymatic activity of plastoquinones, coenzyme Q and related natural quinones. Arch Biochem Biophys 87:198–202

Crane FL, Hatefi Y, Lester RL, Widmer C (1957) Isolation of a quinone from beef heart mitochondria. Biochim Biophys Acta 25:220–221

Crane FL, Widmer C, Lester RL, Hatefi Y, Fechner W (1959) Studies on the electron transport system. XV. Coenzyme Q (Q 275) and the succinoxidase activity of the electron transport particle. Biochim Biophys Acta 31:476–489

Dauben WG, Adams RE (1948) The synthesis of 2-hydroxy-3-[3′-*cis*(4-hydroxycyclohexyl)-propyl]-1,4-naphthoquinone. J Am Chem Soc 70:1759–1762

Fairley NH (1945) Chemotherapeutic suppression and prophylaxis in malaria. Trans R Soc Trop Med Hyg 38:311–365

Fawaz G, Haddad FS (1951) The effect of lapinone (M-2350) on *P. vivax* infection in man. Am J Trop Med Hyg 31:569–571
Fieser LF, Heymann H (1948) Naphthoquinone antimalarials. XXII. Relative antirespiratory activities (*Plasmodium lophurae*). J Biol Chem 176:1363–1370
Fieser LF, Richardson AP (1948) Naphthoquinone antimalarials. II. Correlation of structure and activity against *P. lophurae* in ducks. J Am Chem Soc 70:3156–3165
Fieser LF, Berliner E, Bondhus FJ, Chang FC, Dauben WG, Ettlinger MG, Fawaz G, Fields M, Fieser M, Heidelberger C, Heymann H, Seligman AM, Vaughan WR, Wilson AG, Wilson E, Wu MI, Leffler MT, Hamlin KE, Hathaway RJ, Matson EJ, Moore EE, Moore MB, Rapala RT, Zaugg HE (1948 a) Naphthoquinone antimalarials. I–XVII. J Am Chem Soc 70:3151–3244
Fieser LF, Heymann H, Seligman AM (1948 b) Naphthoquinone antimalarials. XX. Metabolic degradation. J Pharmacol Exp Ther 94:112–124
Fieser LF, Chang FC, Dauben WG, Heidelberger C, Heymann H, Seligman AM (1948 c) Naphthoquinone antimalarials. XVIII. Metabolic oxidation products. J Pharmacol Exp Ther 94:85–96
Fieser LF, Schirmer JP, Archer S, Lorenz RR, Pfaffenbach PI (1967 a) Naphthoquinone antimalarials. XXIX. 2-Hydroxy-3-(ω-cyclohexylalkyl)-1,4-naphthoquinones. J Med Chem 10:513–517
Fieser LF, Nazer MZ, Archer S, Berberian DA, Slighter RG (1967 b) Naphthoquinone antimalarials. XXX. 2-Hydroxy-3-[ω-(1-adamantyl)alkyl]-1,4-naphthoquinones. J Med Chem 10:517–521
Friedman MD, Stotter PL, Porter TH, Folkers K (1973) Synthesis of alkyl-4,7-dioxobenzothiazoles with prophylactic antimalarial activity. J Med Chem 16:1314–1316
Gutman M, Kliatchko S (1976) Mechanisms of inhibition by ubicidin: inhibitor with piericidin ring structure and ubiquinone side chain. FEBS Lett 67:348–353
Gutman M, Singer TP (1970) Studies on the respiratory chain linked reduced nicotinamide adenine dinucleotide dehydrogenase. XVII. Reaction sites of piericidin A and rotenone. J Biol Chem 245:1992–1997
Gutteridge WE, Dave D, Richards WHG (1979) Conversion of dihydroorotate to orotate in parasitic protozoa. Biochim Biophys Acta 582:390–401
Hendlin D, Cook TM (1960) The reversible inhibition of succinoxidase by naphthoquinones. Biochem Biophys Res Comm 2:71–75
Heymann H, Fieser LF (1948 a) Naphthoquinone antimalarials. XXI. Antisuccinate oxidase activity. J Biol Chem 176:1359–1362
Heymann H, Fieser LF (1948 b) Naphthoquinone antimalarials. XIX. Antirespiratory study of protein binding. J Pharmacol Exp Ther 94:97–111
Hooker SC (1936) Lomatiol. Part II. Its occurrence, constitution, relation to, and conversion into lapachol. Also a synthesis of lapachol. J Am Chem Soc 58:1181–1190
Howells RE, Peters W, Fullard J (1970) The chemotherapy of rodent malaria. XIII. Fine structural changes observed in the erythrocytic stages of *Plasmodium berghei berghei* following exposure to primaquine and menoctone. Ann Trop Med Parasitol 64:203–207
Jaffe JJ (1980) Filarial folate-related metabolism as a potential target for selective inhibitors. In: Van den Bossche H (ed) The host invader interplay. Elsevier/North-Holland Biomedical, Amsterdam, p 605–614
Jaffe JJ, Gutteridge WE (1974) Purine and pyrimidine metabolism in protozoa. Actual Protozool 1:23–35
Klingenberg M (1968) The respiratory chain. In: Singer TP (ed) Biological oxidations. Wiley Interscience, New York, p 3–55
Meyer MC, Guttman DE (1968) The binding of drugs by plasma proteins. J Pharm Sci 57:895–918
Olenick JG (1979) 2-Hydroxy-3-alkyl-1,4-naphthoquinones. In: Hahn FE (ed) Mechanism of action of antieukaryotic and antiviral compounds, vol 2. Springer, Berlin Heidelberg New York, p 214–222
Olenick JG, Hahn FE (1974) Bactericidal action of a 2-hydroxy-3-alkyl-1,4-naphthoquinone: blockade of metabolite permeation across the membrane. Ann NY Acad Sci 235:542–552

Peters W (1970) A new type of antimalarial drug potentiation. Trans R Soc Trop Med Hyg 64:462–464

Peters W, Portus J, Robinson BL (1975a) The chemotherapy of rodent malaria. XXII. The value of drug-resistant strains of *P. berghei* in screening for blood schizontocidal activity. Ann Trop Med Parasitol 69:155–171

Peters W, Davies EE, Robinson BL (1975b) The chemotherapy of rodent malaria. XXIII. Causal prophylaxis, Part II: Practical experience with *Plasmodium yoelii nigeriensis* in drug screening. Ann Trop Med Parasitol 69:311–328

Porter TH, Folkers K (1974) Antimetabolites of coenzyme Q. Their potential application as anti-malarials. Angew Chem (Engl) 13:559–569

Porter TH, Skelton FS, Folkers K (1971) Synthesis of new 5,8-quinolinequinones as inhibitors of coenyzme Q and as antimalarials. J Med Chem 14:1029–1033

Porter TH, Bowman CM, Folkers K (1973) Antimetabolites of coenzyme Q. 16. New alkylmercaptoquinones having antimalarial curative activity. J Med Chem 16:115–118

Razdan RK, Bruni RJ, Mehta AC, Weinhardt KK, Atkinson ER (1971) Synthesis of new antimalarial drugs. Derivatives of benzothiopyrans, derivatives of menoctone. US Nat Tech Inform Serv, AD Rep. No 728829

Rietz PJ, Skelton FS, Folkers K (1967) Occurrence of ubiquinones -8 and -9 in *Plasmodium lophurae*. Int J Vitam Nutr Res 37:405–411

Roberts H, Choo WM, Smith SC, Marzuki S, Linnane AW, Porter TH, Folkers K (1978) The site of inhibition of mitochondrial electron transfer by coenzyme Q analogues. Arch Biochem Biophys 191:306–315

Schnell JV, Siddiqui WA, Geiman QM, Skelton FS, Lunan KD, Folkers K (1971) Biosynthesis of coenzymes Q by malarial parasites. 2. Coenzyme Q synthesis in blood cultures of monkeys infected with malarial parasites (*Plasmodium falciparum* and *P. knowlesi*). J Med Chem 14:1026–1029

Sherman IW (1979) Biochemistry of *Plasmodium* (malarial parasites). Microbiol Rev 43:453–495

Skelton FS, Lunan KD, Folkers K, Schnell JV, Siddiqui WA, Geiman QM (1969) Biosynthesis of ubiquinones by malarial parasites. I. Isolation of ^{14}C ubiquinones from cultures of rhesus monkey blood infected with *Plasmodium knowlesi*. Biochemistry 8:1284–1287

Skelton FS, Rietz PJ, Folkers K (1970) Coenzyme Q. CXXII. Identification of ubiquinone-8 biosynthesized by *Plasmodium knowlesi, P. cynomolgi* and *P. berghei*. J Med Chem 13:602–606

Skelton FS, Porter TH, Littarru GP, Folkers K (1973) Antimetabolites of coenzyme Q. XV. Inhibition of mitochondrial reductase systems by naphthoquinone and quinolinequinone analogs. Int J Vitam Nutr Res 43:150–164

Smith CC (1947) Antagonism of the hemorrhagic syndrome induced by derivatives of 3-hydroxy-1,4-naphthoquinone. Proc Soc Exp Biol Med 64:45–47

Smith CC, Fradkin R, Lackey MD (1946) A haemorrhagic syndrome induced by derivatives of 3-hydroxy-1,4-naphthoquinone. Proc Soc Exp Biol Med 61:398–403

Thompson PE, Reinertson JW, Bayles A, Moore AM (1953) The curative action of antimalarial drugs against *Plasmodium lophurae* in chicks. J Infect Dis 92:40–51

Thurston JP (1950) The action of antimalarial drugs in mice infected with *Plasmodium berghei*. Br J Pharmacol 5:409–416

Trager W, Jensen JB (1976) Human malaria parasites in continuous culture. Science 193:673–675

Trager W (1979) *Plasmodium falciparum* in culture: improved continuous flow method. J Protozool 26:125–129

Tullar BF, Lorenz RR (1972) (3,3,5-Trimethylcyclohexyl)alkylcarboxylic acids-inters for antimalarial agents. US Patent 3, 682, 991

Vallner JJ (1977) Binding of drugs by albumin and plasma protein. J Pharm Sci 66:447–465

Walker HA, Richardson AP (1948) Potentiation of the curative action of 8-aminoquinolines and naphthoquinones in avian malaria. J Nat Malaria Soc 7:4–11

Wan YP, Porter TH, Folkers K (1974) Antimalarial quinones for prophylaxis based on a rationale of inhibition of electron transfer in *Plasmodium*. Proc Natl Acad Sci USA 71:952–956

Webb JL (1966) In: Webb JL (ed) Enzyme and metabolic inhibitors, vol III. Academic Press, New York, p 581

Wendel WB (1946) The influence of naphthoquinones upon the respiratory and carbohydrate metabolism of malarial parasites. Fed Proc 5:406–407

WHO (1973) Chemotherapy of malaria and resistance to antimalarials; Report of a WHO Scientific Group. WHO Tech Rep Ser 529:70

Wiselogle FY (ed) (1946) A survey of antimalarial drugs 1941–1945, vol I. Edwards, Ann Arbor

Zubrod CG, Kennedy TJ, Shannon JA (1948) Studies on the chemotherapy of the human malarias. VIII. The physiological disposition of pamaquine. J Clin Invest [Suppl] 27:114–120

CHAPTER 12

4-Aminoquinolines and Mannich Bases

T. R. SWEENEY and R. O. PICK

A. Introduction

The antimalarial 4-aminoquinolines and Mannich bases have been compiled and/or discussed in a number of compendia and reviews. These reviews have, for the most part, considered only those drugs or compounds that have shown an activity sufficient to focus broad attention upon them. Because established drugs are discussed elsewhere in this volume (see Chap. 1), much of the discussion in this chapter will centre on research and development efforts to obtain new 4-aminoquinoline- or Mannich base-type antimalarials. The various efforts described are based upon reasonable medicinal chemical rationales, but the research was exploratory and the synthesis of compounds competitive with chlorquine or amodiaquine would not necessarily be immediately anticipated.

Many years ago the Mannich base antimalarial compounds were considered to be amino derivatives of *ortho* cresol (BURCKHALTER et al. 1946). However, when a search for 4-aminoquinolines superior to chloroquine led to the incorporation of a 4-aminoquinoline moiety into a Mannich base to produce amodiaquine and related compounds (BURCKHALTER et al. 1948) the structural relationship to the 4-aminoquinolines was apparent. This fact, coupled with an outstanding antimalarial activity similar to that of thc 4-aminoquinolines, led to the dominance of the quinoline-type Mannich bases and to their being considered by most workers as 4-aminoquinolines. It thus seemed logical to review the 4-aminoquinolines and Mannich bases in the same chapter, although they will be considered as distinct classes.

In the present discussion of recent developments in these two classes of drugs, it has arbitrarily been decided to include discussions of quinoline ring modifications, such as the azaquinolines, and tricyclic fused ring quinolines. The results of studies of side chain modifications will also be considered. However, recent developments involving established drugs such as chloroquine, hydroxychloroquine, amodiaquine, amopyroquine and mepacrine are not discussed because they are considered elsewhere in this volume. Only those compounds actually tested for antimalarial activity have been selected for discussion from among the many presented in the various references. Most of the compounds discussed have not, and probably will not, reach the stage of preclinical pharmacological or clinical testing. Antimalarial data on numerous structural modifications of the established 4-aminoquinoline and Mannich base antimalarials have been compiled elsewhere (WISELOGLE 1946, COATNEY et al. 1953).

B. 4-Aminoquinolines

I. Exploratory Work

1. Quinoline Ring Modifications

a) 1,5-Naphthyridines

Shortly after the end of World War II, a number of azaquinoline (1,2-, 1,3- and 1,5-naphthyridine) modifications of chloroquine or related 4-aminoquinolines were reported. More recently McCAUSTLAND and CHENG (1970) synthesized several 1,5-naphthyridine congeners of chloroquine (I–IV). Compound II, 5-azachloroquine, was comparable to chloroquine in activity when screened for blood schizontocidal activity in the *P. berghei*-mouse model; it was, however, much less toxic than chloroquine. No acute toxicity was noted at a dose of 640 mg/kg whereas chloroquine was 100% lethal at a dose of 320 mg/kg. Compounds I and III were inactive when tested in the same model. It should be noted that I–IV are also 1,5-naphthyridine congeners of the 8-aminoquinoline, pamaquine.

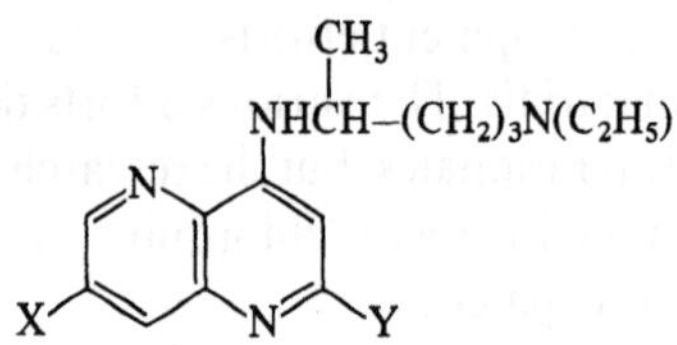

I X = Cl, Y = OCH_3
II X = Cl, Y = H
III X = H, Y = OCH_3
IV X = Y = H

Fig. 1. 1,5-Naphthyridines (I–IV)

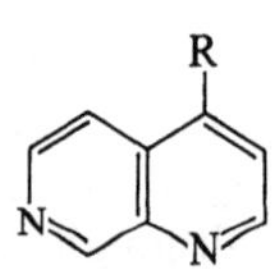

V R = $NHCH(CH_3)(CH_2)_3N(C_2H_5)_2$

VI R = $NH(CH_2)_3N(C_2H_5)_2$

VII R = NH–
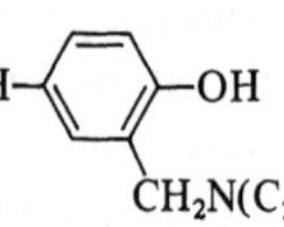

Fig. 2. 1,7-Naphthyridines (V–VII)

b) 1,7-Naphthyridines

CHIEN and CHENG (1968) reasoned that the electron-withdrawing effect produced by the Cl substituent in the chloroquine molecule may also be produced by a nitrogen in the ring in place of the C-Cl group. If so, the 1,7 naphthyridine analogues of the 4-aminoquinolines may retain similar antimalarial activity. To test this hypothesis they synthesised the 7-aza congeners of chloroquine (V, VI) and an amodiaquine-related analogue (VII). When evaluated for blood schizontocidal activity in the *P. berghei*-mouse model VI was devoid of activity and V and VII produced only a slight extension in survival time of the treated mice compared with the untreated controls. Neither V nor VII approached the potency of chloroquine or amodiaquine.

c) Pyrido[2,3-b]pyrazines

To assess the effect on antimalarial activity when the chloroquine molecule was modified by the addition of (a) ring nitrogens, (b) exocyclic groups containing electron-rich centres and (c) groups capable of hydrophobic bonding to the quinoline ring, TEMPLE et al. (1968, 1970a) synthesised for antimalarial screening a large series of substituted pyrido[2,3-b]pyrazines, including a series of 8-[4.diethylamino)-1-methylbutyl]amino pyrido[2,3-b]pyrazines in which substituents in the 6-position were NH_2 or $NHCOOC_2H_5$ and substituents in the 2- and 3-positions were H, CH_3 or substituted phenyl. The most potent of the series, when screened in the *P. berghei*-mouse model for blood schizontocidal activity, was VIII, giving 100% cures at a dose of 640 mg/kg and 60% cures at a dose of 160 mg/kg; activity below the 160-mg/kg dose was not reported. Compound VIII was less acutely toxic and much superior to chloroquine in this model. Other very active compounds were IX and X. It was concluded that the 4-(diethylamino)-1-methylbutyl (noval) group in the 8-position was necessary for activity, but that other groups influenced the degree of activity. When $R_3 = H$, activity was present in the 3-phenyl derivatives (R_2=phenyl) but not in the unsubstituted, the 3-alkyl or 2,3-bis (*p*-chlorophenyl) derivatives. In contrast to the *para*-substituted phenyl compounds VIII and IX, the corresponding *ortho*-substituted compounds were completely inactive. This fact and the inactivity of the 2,3-bis-*p*-chlorophenyl derivative suggests steric interaction and the necessity of coplanarity between the phenyl and pyrazine rings. Thus both the electron-withdrawing effect of the phenyl substituents and the coplanarity may play a role in the activity. It is interesting that, if the 6-position of IX is left unsubstituted, the compound is more active than IX (TEMPLE et al. 1970b). While the purpose of the investigations of the substituted pyrido[2,3-b] pyrazines was to compare their blood schizontocidal activity with that of chloroquine, it should be noted that the former are also structural modifications of the 8-aminoquinoline, pamaquine. The prophylactic or radical curative activity, if any, of the pyrido[2,3-b]pyrazines was, apparently, not determined.

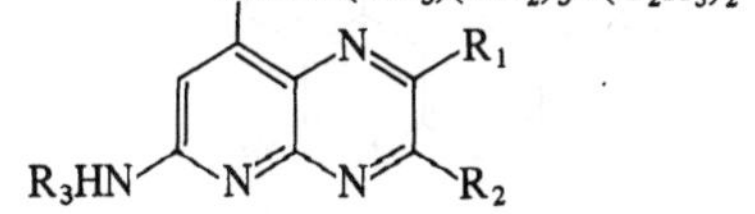

VIII $R_1 = R_3 = H$, $R_2 = 4\text{–}CF_3C_6H_4$
IX $R_1 = R_3 = H$, $R_2 = 4\text{–}ClC_6H_4$
X $R_1 = R_3 = H$, $R_2 = 4\text{–}FC_6H_4$

Fig. 3. Pyrido[2,3-b]pyrazines (VIII–X)

d) 2,3-Dihydro-2,2-dimethylbenzofurans

The isomeric 4-, 5-, 6- and 7-(1-diethylamino-4-pentylamino)-2,3-dihydro-2,2-dimethylbenzofurans and the isomeric 4-, 5-, 6- and 7-(1-amino-4-pentylamino)-2,3-dihydro-2,2-dimethylbenzofuran XI and XII were synthesised by CRUICKSHANK et al. (1970) as potential antimalarials. These compounds were devoid of blood schizontocidal activity when tested in the *P. berghei*-mouse model.

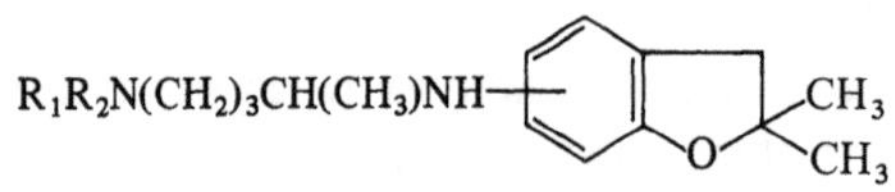

XI $R_1 = R_2 = C_2H_5$
XII $R_1 = R_2 = H$

Fig. 4. Benzofuran derivatives (XI, XII)

2. Tricyclic Congeners

a) Tetrahydropyrimido[5,4-c]quinolines

It was postulated by NASR et al. (1978) that tetrahydropyrimido[5,4-c]quinolines of the type XIII–XV may have a dual mode of antimalarial action in that the flat quinoline ring might be expected to intercalate with DNA in the manner of chlorquine, and the tetrahydropyrimidine moiety might be expected to exhibit antifolate activity in the manner of pyrimethamine. It was also felt that the acyclic tertiary nitrogen might serve as a conductophoric grouping analogous to the terminal nitrogen in the side chain of chloroquine although, unlike the terminal nitrogen in the chloroquine side chain, it would not be able to reach the phosphate groups of DNA. The 3-chloroanilino group was introduced to see if a free hydrogen at that position was essential for activity. The introduction of a styryl group, XV, was considered a desirable modification in that it would increase the area of planarity and remove the 2-methyl group, which was viewed as dystherapeutic in the 4-aminoquinaldines. When tested in the *P. berghei*-mouse model for blood schizontocidal activity XIII–XV were inactive at a dose of 640 mg/kg.

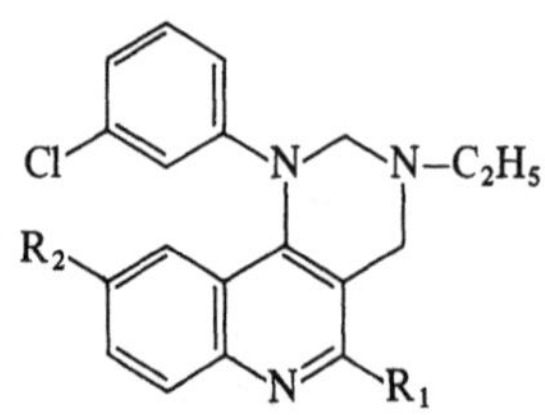

XIII $R_1 = CH_3$, $R_2 = CH_3$
XIV $R_1 = CH_3$, R_2 OCH_3
XV $R_1 = CH{=}CHC_6H_5$, $R_2 = OCH_3$

Fig. 5. Tetrahydropyrimidino [5,4-c] quinolines (XIII–XV)

b) 1H-Pyrazolo[3,4-b]quinolines

Because of the wide spectrum of biological activity of pyrazole derivatives, it was of interest to combine the features of the pyrazole ring, a substituted quinoline and an "antimalarial"-type side chain in one molecule for antimalarial testing (STEIN et al. 1970). Towards this end a series of 1*H*-pyrazolo[3,4-b]quinolines related to chloroquine and amodiaquine, XVI–XVIII, were synthesised and tested for blood schizontocidal activity in the *P. berghei*-mouse model. Congeners with diamino chains other than the noval chain were also synthesised and tested. None of the compounds had appreciable activity.

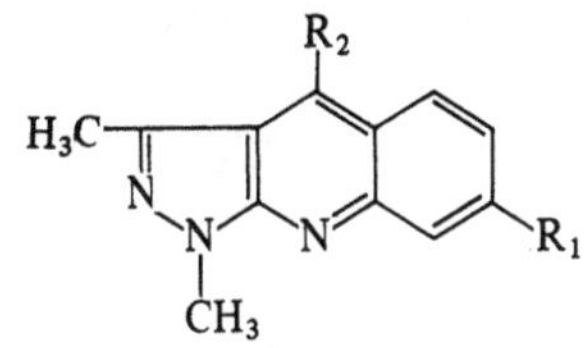

XVI R_1 = H, R_2 = $NHCH(CH_3)(CH_2)_3N(C_2H_5)_2$

XVII R_1 = Cl, R_2 = $NHCH(CH_3)(CH_2)_3N(C_2H_5)_2$

XVIII R_1 = Cl, R_2 = NH–

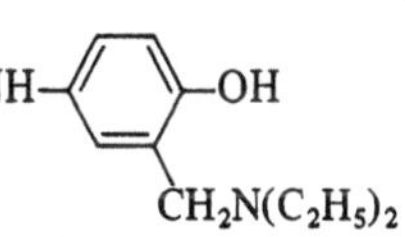

Fig. 6. 1*H*-Pyrazolo[3,4-b]quinolines (XVI–XVIII)

c) 2,3-Dihydrofuroquinolines

A series of isomeric 2,3-dihydro-2,2-dimethylfuroquinolines, XIX–XXII, representing modifications of the chloroquine structure, and other aminoalkylamino-chain congeners in the three ring systems were synthesised by CRUICKSHANK et al. (1970) as potential antimalarial agents. The compounds showed very little or no activity when screened in the *P. berghei*-mouse model and were generally toxic. Compounds with the [2,3-g] ring system (XXI) were significantly more toxic than the others.

d) Benzo[g]quinolines

The 4-(aminoalkylamino)benzo[g]quinolines, XXIII and XXIV, were reported to have a better chemotherapeutic coefficient than chloroquine against the erythrocytic forms of *P. berghei* in mice (BEKHLI et al. 1977). The *N*-oxide of XXIII, in contrast, had a chemotherapeutic coefficient of 0.25 (chloroquine = 1) and the *N*-oxide of XXIV was inactive (KOZYREVA et al. 1979). A variety of 4-dialkylamino-(hetero)alkylaminobenzo[g]quinolines were also synthesised and tested. Most were inactive; the best had a chemotherapeutic coefficient of less than 1.

$ArNHCH(CH_3)(CH_2)_3N(C_2H_5)_2$

XIX Ar =

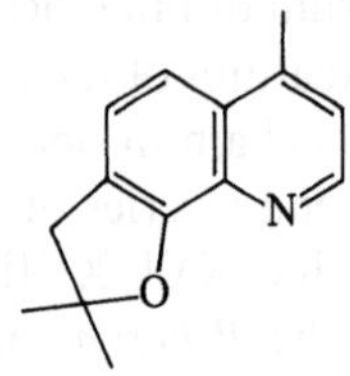

XX Ar =

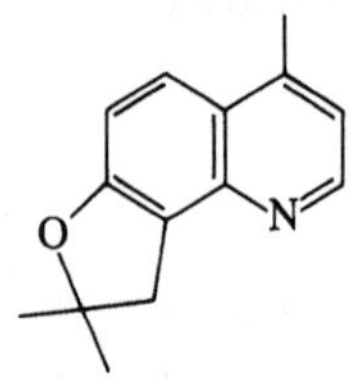

XXI Ar =

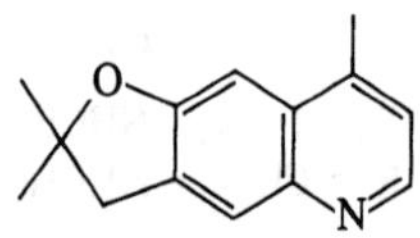

XXII Ar =

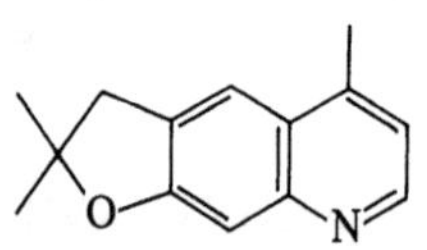

Fig. 7. 2,3-Dihydrofuroquinolines (XIX–XXII)

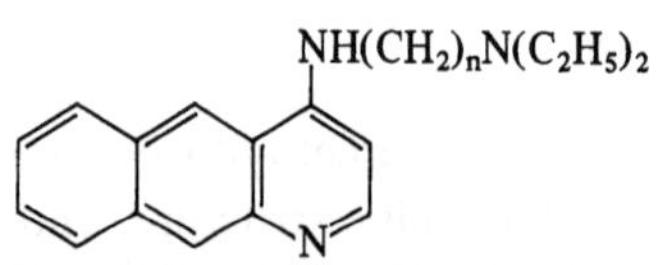

XXIII n = 2
XXIV n = 3

Fig. 8. Benzo[g]quinolines (XXIII, XXIV)

3. Side Chain Variations

a) Hydrazino Congeners

SINGH et al. (1969a) prepared a number of "proximal" hydrazino congeners of chloroquine as potential antimalarials. It seemed possible to these workers that such compounds might be effective against chloroquine-resistant malaria in view of the fact that, in contrast to the parent amines, resistance did not develop to drugs bearing a hydrazino moiety, e.g. α-methylphenylhydrazine. The congeners synthesised were hydrazine derivatives of the type $QNHNR_1R_2$ where Q is a 7-chloro-4-quinolyl group, R_1 is H, CH_3 or C_2H_5 and R_2 is a dialkylaminoalkyl group

(XXVI–XXIX). Also synthesised were congeners in which the terminal amino function was heterocyclic as in the piperidino (XXX) and 3-pyridyl (XXXI) analogues and hydrazones of the type QNHN=CHR where R is a dialkylamino-alkyl, piperidinomethyl, 3-pyridyl or 4-dialkylaminophenyl group. When the hydrazines were tested for blood schizontocidal activity in the *P. berghei*-mouse model the parent compounds, 7-chloro-4-hydrazinoquinoline (XXV), was acutely toxic. Compounds containing a cyclic moiety in the side chain, e.g. XXX and XXXI, were inactive. The *N* isostere of chloroquine, XXVI, was disappointing in that it was acutely toxic at doses of 320 mg/kg and above and had no appreciable activity below this dose. The homologues XXVII–XXIX, however, were curative at doses of 320 and 640 mg/kg with no acute toxicity and showed activity at lower doses; thus they were distinctly superior to chloroquine in this model.

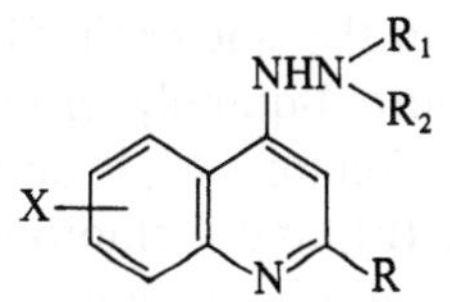

XXV $R = R_1 = R_2 = H$, $X = 7\text{–}Cl$
XXVI $R = H$, $R_1 = CH_3$, $R_2 = (CH_2)_3N(C_2H_5)_2$, $X = 7\text{–}Cl$
XXVII $R = H$, $R_1 = CH_3$, $R_2 = (CH_2)_2N(CH_3)_2$, $X = 7\text{–}Cl$
XXVIII $R = H$, $R_1 = C_2H_5$, $R_2 = (CH_2)_2N(CH_3)_2$, $X = 7\text{–}Cl$
XXIX $R = H$, $R_1 = CH_3$, $R_2 = (CH_2)_3N(CH_3)_2$, $X = 7\text{–}Cl$
XXX $R = R_1 = H$, $R_2 = CH_2CH_2N(CH_2)_5$, $X = 7\text{–}Cl$
XXXI $R = R_1 = H$, $R_2 = CH_2(3\text{–}C_5H_4N)$, $X = 7\text{–}Cl$
XXXII $R = CH_3$, $NR_1R_2 = N(CH_2CH_2)_2O$, $X = 6\text{–}OCH_3$
XXXIII $R = H$, $NR_1R_2 = N(CH_2CH_2)_2O$, $X = 7\text{–}Cl$
XXXIV $R = H$, $NR_1R_2 = N(CH_2CH_2)_2NCH_3$, $X = 7\text{–}Cl$
XXXV $R = CH_3$, $NR_1R_2 = N(CH_2)_6$, $X = 6\text{–}OCH_3$

Fig. 9. "Proximal" hydrazino congeners (XXV–XXXV)

In a related study, ELSLAGER et al. (1969a), in developing an earlier antischistosomal lead with XXXII, synthesised a group of proximal hydrazine analogues of chloroquine in which one nitrogen of the hydrazino moiety is incorporated in a heterocyclic ring (XXXII–XXXV). These copounds were tested for blood schizontocidal activity in mice against a normal, drug-sensitive strain of *P. berghei*. The compounds were administered continuously in the diet for 6 days. Compound XXXV was inactive. Compound XXXII was active but less potent than quinine and considerably less potent than chloroquine. Compound XXXIII was slightly more potent than quinine but much less potent than chloroquine. Compound XXXIV, however, was comparable in potency to chloroquine and amodiaquine.

The one proximal hydrazino analogue of mepacrine that was synthesised and tested by ELSLAGER et al. (1969a), viz 6-chloro-2-methoxy-9(4-methyl-1-piperazinylamino) acridine, LV, was about twice as potent as quinine but considerably less potent than mepacrine or chloroquine.

When the side chain of chloroquine was replaced with the hydroxylamino moiety, $NH\text{-}O(CH_2)_2N(R)_2$ (ELSLAGER et al. 1969a), the resulting methyl

Table 1. Generic structures based on Q=7-chloro-4-quinolyl

a) Q-$NHCH(CH_3)(CH_2)_nN(R)NH_2$
b) Q-$NHN(CH_2CH_2)_2NNHR$
c) Q-$N(CH_2CH_2)_2NR$
d) Q-$NHCH(CH_3)CH_2CH{=}NN(R)_2$

analogue ($R{=}CH_3$) was inactive but the ethyl analogue ($R{=}C_2H_5$) was about two-thirds as potent as quinine. When the side chain of mepacrine was replaced with the NH-$O(CH_2)_2N(CH_3)_2$ chain, the compound was devoid of activity.

In addition to the 7-chloro-4-substituted quinolines with a "proximal" hydrazino function in the side chain, SINGH et al. (1971a) also prepared analogues with a "distal" hydrazino function in the side chain (Table 1). These had the generic structure (a) where Q is a 7-chloro-4-quinolyl group, *n* is 1 or 2, and R is alkyl or benzyl. Also synthesised were 7-chloro-4-[(4-substituted amino)-1-piperazinylamino]-quinolines, generic type (b), and 7-chloro-4-(4-substituted-1-piperazinyl)-quinolines, generic type (c). Several hydrazones of type (d) where R is alkyl, or $N(R)_2$ is piperazinyl or substituted piperazinyl, were prepared as intermediates and also tested for antimalarial activity. When tested for blood schizontocidal activity in the *P. berghei* mouse model the hydrazones were, as a class, very toxic. Compounds of generic structure (a) where n is 2 and R is benzyl or substituted benzyl gave only slight extensions in survival time at toxic doses. In the ge-

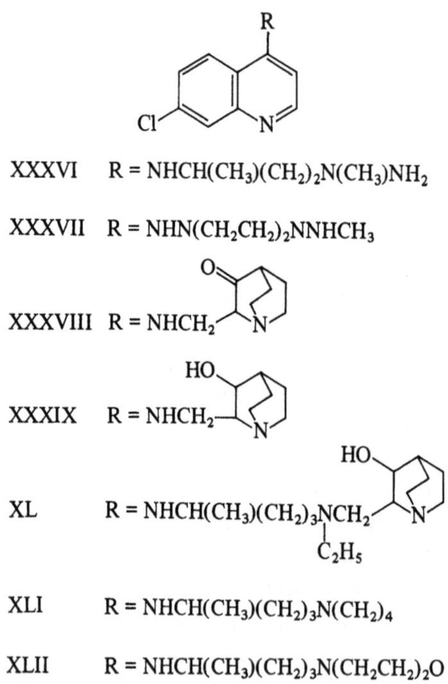

Fig. 10. "Distal" hydrazino congeners (XXXVI–XLII)

Table 2. Blood schizontocidal activity against *P. berghei* in mice[a] of chloroquine analogues with unsaturated side chains (SINGH et al. 1969b)

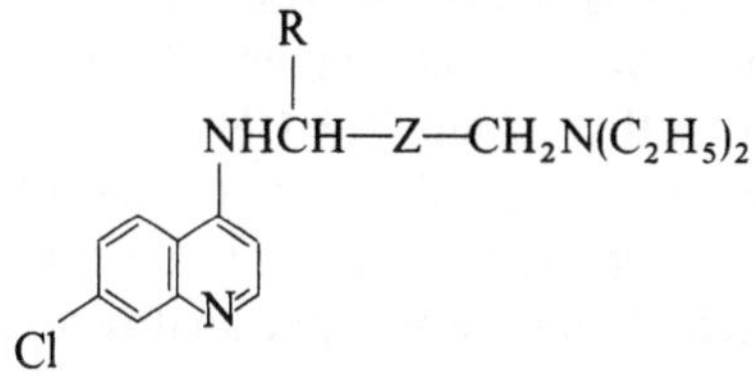

Z	MTD[b] (mg/kg)		MAD[c] (mg/kg)		MCD[d] (mg/kg)	
	R=H	R=CH$_3$	R=H	R=CH$_3$	R=H	R=CH$_3$
C≡C	>640	>640	320	20	>640	160
H H C=C (H, H on the same side)	320	160	80	20	640	40
H C=C H (H, H on opposite sides)	>640	80	40	10	160	20
CH$_2$CH$_2$ (Chloroquine)		40		20		NC[e]

[a] Interfections were blood induced. Compounds administered in single dose, subcutaneously to five mice at each dose level. Doses were 640, 320, 160, 80, 40, and 20 mg/kg
[b] MTD, maximum tolerated dose, the highest dose that resulted in no toxic deaths
[c] MAD, minimum active dose
[d] MCD, minimum curative dose, the minimum dose that cured at least one of five treated mice
[e] NC, not curative; all treated mice died from compound toxicity before a curative level was reached

neric class (a) compounds, XXXVI was active at 40 mg/kg, curative at 160 mg/kg but toxic at higher doses; acetylation or methylation of the terminal amino group reduced both activity and toxicity. The most active and least toxic compounds were those of generic group (b). Type (c) gave little or no extension in survival time and was toxic at high doses. Some of the generic group (b) compounds, for example XXXVII, which was curative at 160 mg/kg and active at 40 mg/kg, had therapeutic indices superior to chloroquine in the *P. berghei*-mouse model. The best of the compounds was the bis-piperazine (b, R = Q), which was curative at a dose as low as 40 mg/kg.

b) Unsaturated Side Chains

In an exploration of the effect of a double or triple bond on antimalarial activity, SINGH et al. (1969b) synthesised an interesting series of six chloroquine analogues (Table 2) with unsaturated side chains. Unsaturation was in the form of *cis* and *trans* ethylenic and acetylenic bonds. Blood schizontocidal activities for the six compounds have been summarised in Table 2. The data indicate that in the case of compounds with the ethylenic chains, both *cis* and *trans*, those having a 1-methyl group (R = CH_3) were more acutely toxic than those without the methyl group (R = H), but all of the ethylenic compounds were less toxic than chloroquine.

Furthermore, when $R=H$, the *trans* isomer is less toxic than the *cis* whereas the reverse is true when $R=CH_3$. Compounds with an acetylenic bond in the chain were the least toxic of the series; a relative toxicity of the $R=H$ analogue compared with the $R=CH_3$ analogue was not determined. The data also show that analogues with chains bearing a 1-methyl group ($R=CH_3$), regardless of the nature of the unsaturation, are more potent than those analogues lacking the 1-methyl group ($R=H$). In addition, the *trans* isomers are more potent than the *cis* and the ethylenic analogue more potent than the acetlyenic analogues regardless of the presence of the 1-methyl group in the chain.

The ethylenic analogues, *cis* and *trans*, $R=CH_3$, compared favourably with chloroquine in both potency and toxicity. Although SINGH et al. (1969b) felt that the data were insufficient to draw concrete conclusions, they suggested that, since the additive bond distances between the two *N* atoms in the side chain varied from that of chloroquine, the greatest at 7.56 Å, through that of the ethylenic compounds (*cis* and *trans*, $R=CH_3$) at 7.35 Å, to that of the acetylenic compound, the shortest ($R=CH_3$) at 7.22 Å, the difference between the longest and shortest separations, 0.34 Å, may not be sufficiently significant to account for the differences in activity. If the mode of action of chloroquine involves intercalation and adjustment of the side chain between the phosphate groups of the complementary strands of DNA across the minor groove (O'BRIEN and HAHN 1965) the actual distance between the N atoms may be more important than the additive bond distances, since the actual distance can vary more widely to make necessary adjustments than can the additive bond distance. Thus the data indicate that configuration differences in the side chains of chloroquine analogues may be important and that the relationship of side chain geometry to antimalarial activity may involve complexities greater than just additive bond distances between the *N* atoms.

Because of promising pharmacological properties exhibited by certain compounds containing the 1,2,3,6-tetrahydropyridyl moiety and the lower toxicity with improved antimalarial activity observed when unsaturation was introduced into the side chain of chloroquine (SINGH et al. 1969b), SING et al. (1969c) synthesised three side chain-modified chloroquines containing both a cyclic and an unsaturated feature in the form of a 1-alkyl-1,2,3,6-tetrahydropyridyl moiety (XLIII–XLV). When tested for blood schizontocidal activity in the *P. berghei*-mouse model XLIII was curative only at a toxic level, 640 mg/kg. However, XLIV was curative at 160 mg/kg and above, and active at a dose as low as 20 mg/kg; compound XLV had essentially the same activity. Thus all three compounds were less toxic than chloroquine and two were more potent.

BAILEY (1969) synthesised several analogous compounds containing a fully saturated ring in the side chain (XLVI–XLVIII). Compounds XLVI and XLVIII cured blood-induced infections of *P. berghei* in mice at doses of 10 and 12.5 mg/kg per day administered for 5 days; XLVII and chloroquine were curative at a dose of 5 mg/kg per day administered for 5 days.

c) Quinuclidine Congeners

The quinuclidine moiety, present in the cinchona alkaloids that have antimalarial activity, was incorporated by SINGH et al. (1969d) in several side chain modifi-

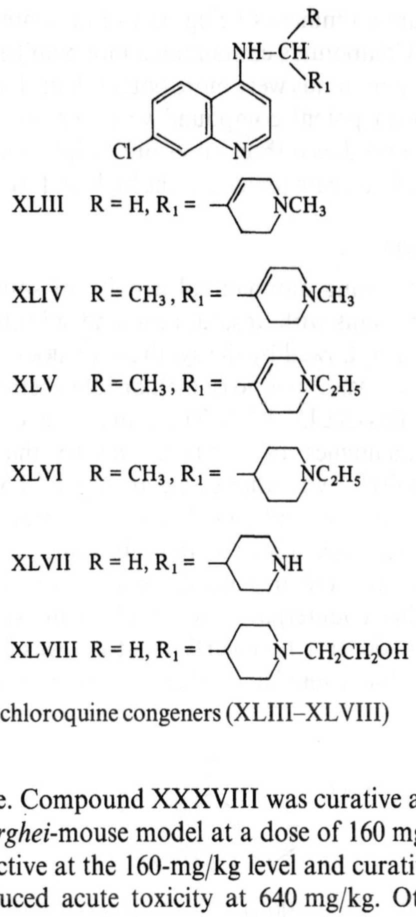

Fig. 11. Other side chain chloroquine congeners (XLIII–XLVIII)

cations of chloroquine. Compound XXXVIII was curative against blood-induced infections in the *P. berghei*-mouse model at a dose of 160 mg/kg and above; compound XXXIX was active at the 160-mg/kg level and curative at 640 mg/kg. Neither compound produced acute toxicity at 640 mg/kg. Other compounds synthesised were inactive and toxic including XL, which contained a substituted chloroquine chain.

d) Heterocyclic Congeners

IBER and BOONE (1967) synthesised two chloroquine analogues in which the terminal $N(C_2H_5)_2$ moiety on the side chain was replaced by a pyrrolidino and a morpholino moiety (XLI, XLII). The antimalarial data reported were incomplete. The compounds were only slightly active as blood schizontocides against *P. berghei* infections in mice at the doses administered, viz. 40 mg/kg for XLI and 160 mg/kg for XLII. Apparently no acute toxicity was noted at these doses.

SINGH et al. (1971 b) reported the synthesis of 41 7-chloro-4-substituted quinolines as potential antimalarial agents. Some of the 4-position substituents were side chains analogous to that of chloroquine with the general structure $NHCH(CH_3)(CH_2)_3NR_1R_2$, where R_1 and/or R_2 were H, alkyl, benzyl, substituted benzyl, or cycloalkyl or where NR_1R_2 constituted a heterocyclic system. Also synthesised were 7-chloro-4-substituted quinolines in which the 4-substituent was a heterocyclic moiety or in which it was a simple alkyl or substituted alkyl amine. Twenty-seven of the compounds exhibited blood schizontocidal activity when screened in the *P. berghei*-mouse model. The active compounds all had diamine-type side chains, the amino moieties being part of an aminoalkylamino chain or part of a heterocycle. Compounds containing a monoamine side chain were inactive. A number of the compounds were more potent than chloroquine in the mouse model. Perhaps the most potent compound was 7-chloro-4-(4-methylpyrazinyl) aminoquinoline, which produced three cures out of five treated animals at a dose of 40 mg/kg and showed no acute toxicity at the highest dose tested, 640 mg/kg.

e) Mepacrine Congeners

The synthesis and interesting antimalarial activity of some of the chloroquine analogues having side chains with unsaturation and side chains with "proximal" hydrazino functions was followed by the synthesis (TARA et al. 1973) of a number of mepacrine analogues, viz. 2-methoxy-6-chloro-9-substituted-amino acridines, bearing similar side chains (XLIX–LIV). These analogues correspond to the unsaturated chloroquine analogues of Table 2, and to the proximal hydrazino analogues, XXVI–XXVIII. Two other cyclic analogues, LV, LVI, were also synthesised. All of these analogues had good blood schizontocidal activity against *P. berghei* infections in mice when administered subcutaneously. They were all more potent than mepacrine but were, in general, less potent than their 7-chloro-4-substituted aminoquinoline counterparts. Most of them were more potent than chloroquine and less toxic. It is noteworthy that LV was found to be less potent than mepacrine when administered in the diet (ELSLAGER et al. 1969 a).

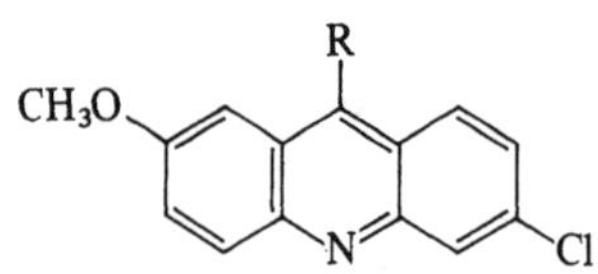

XLIX $R = NHCH(CH_3)CH{=}CHCH_2N(C_2H_5)_2$ (cis)
L $R = NHCH(CH_3)CH{=}CHCH_2N(C_2H_5)_2$ (trans)
LI $R = NHCH(CH_3)C{\equiv}CCH_2N(C_2H_5)_2$
LII $R = NHN(CH_3)CH_2CH_2N(CH_3)_2$
LIII $R = NHN(CH_3)(CH_2)_3N(CH_3)_2$
LIV $R = NHN(C_2H_5)CH_2CH_2N(CH_3)_2$
LV $R = NHN(CH_2CH_2)_2NCH_3$

LVI R = NH–
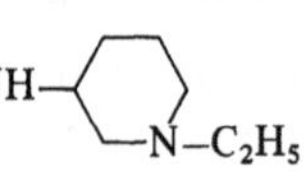

LVII $R = NH(CH_2)_2NHCH_2CH_2OH$

Fig. 12. Mepacrine congeners (XLIX–LVII)

f) Repository Congeners

In a search for repository antimalarials, ELSLAGER et al. (1969 b) synthesised a number of ester and amide congeners of hydroxychloroquine (LVIII), oxychloroquine (LIX) and related substances. The acetate, heptanoate and palmitate esters of LVIII and the acetate, heptanoate and cyclopentylpropionate of LIX were prepared. Esters (C_1,C_5,C_8,C_{11},C_{15}) of the mepacrine congener LVII were also synthesised. The drugs were tested for repository activity by administering a single dose of 400 mg/kg (base equivalent) subcutaneously to mice and subsequently challenging the treated mice with *P. berghei* trophozoites at weekly or biweekly intervals. The esters conferred slight to moderate protection against the challenge with *P. berghei* ranging from 2 to 4 weeks. Amide esters, formed by acetylation of the amine esters, were without significant repository effect.

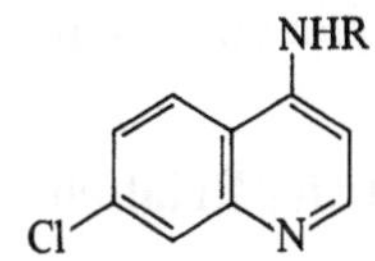

LVIII R = $CH(CH_3)(CH_2)_3N(C_2H_5)CH_2CH_2OH$
LIX R = $CH_2CHOHCH_2N(C_2H_5)_2$
LX R = $(CH_2)_3N(C_2H_5)_2$
LXI R = $CH_2CHOHCH_2N(C_2H_5)_2$

Fig. 13. Esters and amides (LVIII–LXI)

II. Molecular Biology

In an effort to learn more about the nature of the interaction of the side chains of 4-aminoquinolines with DNA according to the mode suggested earlier (HAHN et al. 1966; O'BRIEN and HAHN 1965), MARQUEZ et al. (1974) synthesised a number of chloroquine analogues with polyamine side chains of various length, comformation and number of basic groups. It was desired to determine whether or not antimalarial activity could be explained in terms of an extension of the type of intercalation suggest by HAHN. Interaction of calf thymus DNA with the 4-aminoquinolines and the polyamines corresponding to the side chains alone was investigated by measuring changes in melting temperature (Tm). The inhibition of DNA function as a template for *E. coli* RNA polymerase and changes in ultraviolet spectra brought about by the interaction of the 4-aminoquinolines was also investigated. The Tm data indicated that the stabilisation of DNA was a function of the length and number of basic groups in the side chain; the same trend was seen with the polyamines alone. The data also indicated that the side chain makes a greater contribution to the binding energy of the complex than does the ring. Inhibition of *E. coli* RNA polymerase by the 4-aminoquinolines increased with increasing chain length. Since the polyamines themselves were non-inhibitory it appears that ring intercalation or some other type of ring interaction is necessary to bring about inhibition. Because of the inadequacy of the antimalarial data no correlation of activity with other data could be made.

The antimalarial drug fluoroquine, 4-(1-methyl-4-diethylaminobutylamino)-7-fluoroquinoline, the fluoro analogue of chloroquine, has been used in studies of interaction with DNA, tRNA and poly(A) (BOLTON et al. 1981). Since fluoroquine has about the same antimalarial potency as chloroquine it serves as a useful drug for study since most cells do not have endogenous fluorine and cellular samples will exhibit ^{19}F-nuclear magnetic resonance (NmR) signals from the drug. The interaction of fluoroquine was investigated by optical absorption, fluorescence, and ^{19}F-

NMR chemical-shift and relaxation methods. Measurements indicated that fluoroquine binds to nucleic acids in a manner similar to that of chloroquine. The NMR data are consistent with the intercalation of fluoroquine into DNA. At low drug-to-base pair ratios the binding of both drugs appears to be random. Both drugs bring about a similar elevation in melting temperature (Tm). The chemical shift for the ^{19}F resonance of free fluoroquine is dependent upon the isotopic composition of the solvent (D_2O vs H_2O). Binding to any one of the nucleic acids eliminates the solvent isotope shift, indicating that the F is not accessible to the solvent.

III. Quantitative Structure-Activity Relationships

Structure-activity studies (BASS et al. 1971) were carried out on several series of 4-aminoquinolines, using antimalarial data generated in an avian model by the World War II programme. The work was designed in part to quantify and test the DNA intercalation and electrostatic interaction mechanism of antimalarial action proposed by O'BRIEN and HAHN (1965). Three series of compounds were subjected to several regression equations involving the octanol-water partition coefficients, charge at position 7 of the quinoline ring and charge on the two nitrogen atoms of the diamino side chain; no steric parameters were used. With compounds of type LXII, regressions involving only the partition coefficient accounted for 30% of the variance in the biological data; the electronic parameter did not correlate well. No good correlations were obtained using compounds of type LXIII. The best correlation, obtained with compounds of type LXIV, involved both the partition coefficient and the charge on the terminal nitrogen, and accounted for 70% of the variance. This good correlation suggested a cooperative effect. No good correlations were obtained when series were combined. The results were, in general, consistent with the mechanisms of O'BRIEN and HAHN. The authors suggested, as a re-

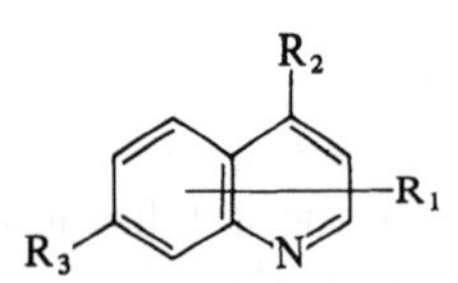

LXII $R_1 = H$
$R_2 = NHCH(CH_3)(CH_2)_3N(C_2H_5)_2$
$R_3 = H, Cl, Br, I, F, CF_3, OCH_3$ or CH_3

LXIII $R_1 = H, Cl, Br, OCH_3, CH_3, C_6H_5$, or NH_2; various positions
$R_2 = NHCH(CH_3)(CH_2)_3N(C_2H_5)_2$
$R_3 = H$ or Cl

LXIV $R_1 = H$
R_2 = various alkylamino- and dialkylaminoalkylamino chains

Fig. 14. Quinoline structures (LXII–LXIV)

finement of the O'BRIEN and HAHN (1965) model, that the size of the alkyl groups on the terminal nitrogen significantly moderates the ability of that nitrogen to participate in electrostatic binding to the phosphate groups and that such binding can be affected by drug-DNA orientations, which, in turn, are dictated by the nature of the substituent in the 7-position.

IV. Primate Studies

SCHMIDT et al. (1977) compared the antimalarial activity of chloroquine and several other drugs against chloroquine-susceptible and chloroquine-resistant strains of *P. falciparum* in owl monkeys. Two established Mannich base-type drugs were used in the study, viz. amodiaquine (LXVII) and amopyroquine, and a bis 4-aminoquinoline, dichloroquinazine. While the calculated ED_{90} values (the dose required to suppress, clear or cure infections in 90% of the treated animals) for chloroquine and the other drugs were essentially the same against infections with chloroquine-susceptible strains, the ED_{90} values obtained against chloroquine-resistant strains with amodiaquine, amopyroquine and dichloroquinazine were lower by a factor of 2–5 than the ED_{90} values achieved with chloroquine. However, the doses of the amodiaquine and amopyroquine required to cure 90% of the infections with the resistant strains were two to three times greater than those required for the susceptible strains.

The significance of these findings, in view of earlier clinical and laboratory results indicating that chloroquine-resistant infections were not susceptible to maximally tolerated doses of amodiaquine and amopyroquine, prompted the investigation of three old 4-aminoquinolines, one closely related to amodiaquine, SN 10274 (LXV) and two closely related to chloroquine, SN 9584 and SN 8137 (LX, LXI). Compounds LX, LXI were found to have about one-half of the activity of amodiaquine or amopyroquine against infections with a chloroquine-susceptible strain of *P. falciparum;* compound LXV was definitely less active than LX, LXI. Against infections with a chloroquine-resistant strain, LX, LX were found to be less effective than amodiaquine and amopyroquine but clearly superior to chloroquine. In view of these results, SCHMIDT et al. (1977) concluded that the reluctance of those concerned with the chemotherapy of malaria to continue to investigate 4-aminoquinolines as alternatives to chloroquine, because of the prevalence of chloroquine resistance, was not fully justified and that there may be merit in the continued evaluation of available and new 4-aminoquinolines. Despite the results obtained with

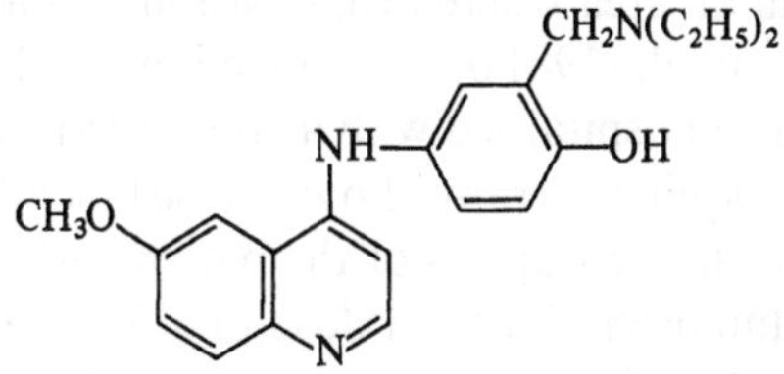

LXV

Fig. 15. SN 10274 (LXV)

amodiaquine under these experimental conditions, its use against chloroquine-resistant malaria was not recommended as a practical therapy except, possibly, under hospital conditions, because of the relatively high dosage that would be required.

V. Clinical Studies

A field study on a new bis 4-aminoquinoline, hydroxypiperaquine tetraphosphate, LXVI, has been reported by LI et al. (1981 a). Ninety-three patients with acute falciparum malaria were each treated with a total of 1.5 g (base) of the drug in three divided doses (0.6, 0.6, 0.3 g) on consecutive days. Chloroquine phosphate was used as a reference drug. In all cases fever was cleared within 72 h following the first dose. The mean $\pm$SE fever clearance time was 28.18 ± 1.62 h. The mean parasite clearance time was 50.24 ± 1.43 h. A follow-up of 60 of the patients for 3 weeks showed that only one recrudesced.

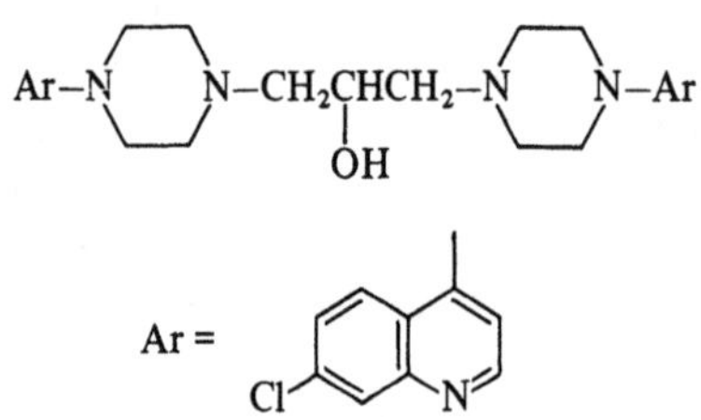

LXVI

Fig. 16. Hydroxypiperaquine (LXVI)

Infections in 7 of 28 patients receiving 1.5 g chloroquine phosphate were resistant to the drug. The dose, 1.5 g, was presumably calculated as the free base; the regimen was not described. Excluding four patients whose fevers had not returned to normal in 7 days, the mean fever clearance time for 24 patients was 41.96 ± 4.69 h. The mean parasite clearance time, excluding the seven patients with chloroquine-resistant infections, was 67.81 ± 4.65 h. Five of 19 patients who were followed after clearance recrudesced within 21 days. Five of the patients with the chloroquine-resistant infections were cured with 1.5 g hydroxypiperaquine phosphate.

Side effects from the hydroxypiperaquine were somnolence, nausea and dizziness, but these effects were milder than those produced by chloroquine.

The results of another field study conducted 4 years after the study described above and carried out in an area where drug-resistant malaria was common have also been reported by LI et al. (1981 b). The infections of slightly over one-half of 158 patients who had been hospitalised with acute falciparum malaria and had received "standard" chloroquine therapy showed resistance to the drug to various degrees (RI–RIII). From this group, 66 of the patients with RII or RIII levels of resistance were each administered a total dose of 1.5 g (base) of hydroxypiperaquine over three consecutive days. All were cured. Excluding 17 of these patients whose fever, but not parasitaemia, had been cleared after chloroquine administration, the mean fever clearance time for the 49 patients was 37.18 ± 2.37 h; the mean time for clearance of parasitaemia for the 66 patients was 52.36±2.33 h. After a 7-day observation period 64 of the patients were followed up weekly in the field for a period of 3 weeks. No protective measures against reinfection were taken. Recrudescences occurred in three of the patients.

C. Mannich Bases

The Mannich base (α-aminocresol)-type antimalarials were extensively investigated during the World War II antimalarial drug development programme and reported shortly thereafter (BURCKHALTER et al. 1946; WISELOGLE 1946). The established drug from this class of compounds, amodiaquine (LXVII) (BURCKHALTER et al. 1948), is discussed in detail elsewhere in this volume (see Chap. 1). The present section, therefore, is limited to relatively recent developments in the Mannich bases other than those concerned specifically with amodiaquine.

I. Exploratory Work

1. 2-(ω-Aminoalkyl)-4-*t*-butyl-6-phenylphenols

Prompted by the antimalarial activity of the α-aminocresols (BURCKHALTER et al. 1946; WISELOGLE 1946; COATNEY et al. 1953) and amodiaquine (BURCKHALTER et al. 1948), DUNCAN and HENRY (1969) synthesised a series of 2-substituted-4-*t*-butyl-6-phenylphenols in which the Mannich base side chain (one carbon atom) was replaced by longer dialkylaminoalkyl chains. Compounds LXVIII, LXIX showed slight blood schizontocidal activity in the *P. berghei*-mouse model at a dose that was toxic. When the methylene chain was extended to two, three or four carbon atoms all activity was essentially abolished. An analogue, LXX (WR 194965),

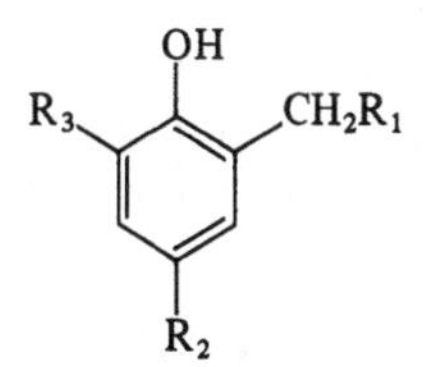

	R_1	R_2	R_3
LXVII	$N(C_2H_5)_2$	QNH	H
LXVIII	$N(CH_3)_2$	$C(CH_3)_3$	C_6H_5
LXIX	$N(C_2H_5)_2$	$C(CH_3)_3$	C_6H_5
LXX	$NHC(CH_3)_3$	$C(CH_3)_3$	$4\text{–}ClC_6H_4$
LXXI	$N(C_2H_5)_2$	$QNCH_3$	H
LXXII	$NHC(CH_3)_3$	QNH	$4\text{–}ClC_6H_4$

Q = 7–chloro–4–quinolyl

Fig. 17. 2-(ω-Aminoalkyl) 4-*t*-butyl-6-phenylphenols (LXVII–LXXII) (LXVII, amodiaquine; LXX, WR 194965; LXXII, WR 228258)

that was synthesised subsequently was very active and selected in the US Army antimalarial drug development programme for advanced studies.

2. Amodiaquine Derivatives

A bis amodiaquine derivative, LXXII (NASR and BURCKHALTER 1979), had blood schizontocidal activity against *P. berghei* infections in mice at a dose of 640 mg/kg, but was toxic at this level.

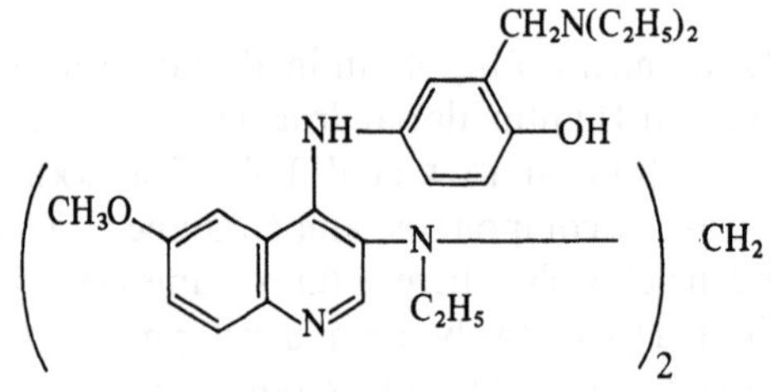

LXXIII

Fig. 18. Bis-amodiaquine derivative (LXXIII)

ELSLAGER et al. (1964) synthesised, for biological investigation, a number of *N*-oxides of amodiaquine, the 1-oxides of N^4-methylamodiaquine and *O*-methylamodiaquine and the 1-oxides of various 4-(7-chloro-4-quinolylamino)-α-dialkylamino-*o*-cresols. With the exception of the 1-oxide of amodiaquine, the antimalarial activity of the compounds was not reported. Amodiaquine 1-oxide was 3.4 times as potent as the free base against *P. berghei* infections in mice. The compound N^4-methylamodiaquine (LXXI) was six times as active as quinine (one-fifth as active as amodiaquine) against *P. lophurae* infections in chicks. This fact is interesting in that the N^4-methyl group would block tautomerism with a quinoid structure, a process postulated by SCHONHOFER (1942) to be associated with antimalarial activity.

In a current synthesis programme Werbel et al. (personal communication) has replaced the 4-*t*-butyl group in the 4-*t*-butyl-6-substituted-phenyl-α-aminocresols (e.g. LXX) with a 7-chloro-4-quinolylamino group to yield a very active series of compounds. An example of the class is WR 228258 (LXXII), which is discussed below.

II. Molecular Biology

A comparison has been made by MARQUEZ et al. (1972) of the complexing of amodiaquine, its methyl ether and a ring-closed analogue 3-chloro-8-methoxy-9-diethylaminomethyl-11*H*-indolo[3,2-c]quinoline (LXXIV). It was believed that the conformation of the two rings in the amodiaquine molecule might be of importance with respect to its interaction with DNA; furthermore, the conformation may lie between that of N^4-methylamodiaquine (LXXI), where, for steric reasons, the rings would be non-planar, and (LXXIV), a planar structure. From measurements of a) the changes in Tm of native DNA in the presence of the drugs, b) the sensitivity of these changes to changes in pH and c) the percentage inhibition of *E. coli* RNA polymerase by the drugs, it was concluded that the planarity of the molecules, or a possible planar transition state, is an important factor in their interaction with DNA and that, unlike the side chain of chloroquine, according to the model of O'BRIEN and HAHN (1965), the side chain of amodiaquine might be involved in the intercalation process along with the quinoline ring.

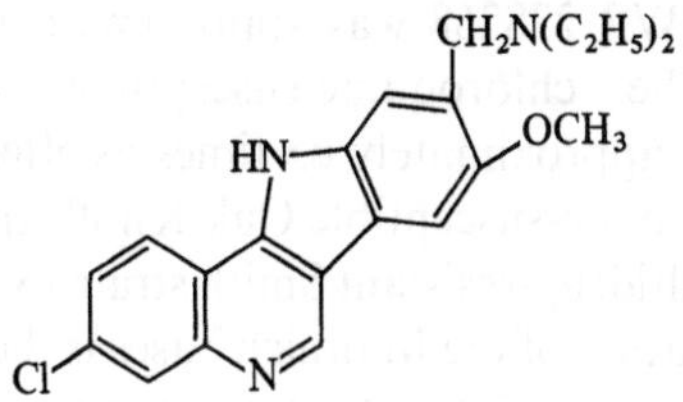

LXXIV

Fig. 19. Ring-closed amodiaquine derivative (LXXIV)

III. Primate Studies

Three of the Mannich base-type compounds were chosen from those synthesised in the US Army research programme for expanded evaluation in monkeys, viz. WR 194965 (LXX), WR 204165 (LXXV) and, somewhat later, WR 228258 (LXXII). Compounds LXX and LXXV (which may be cleaved to form LXX in vivo) showed no acute toxicity and were of approximately equal potency against *P. berghei* infections in mice; they were, however, somewhat less active than amodiaquine (LXVII). The lower activity, relative to amodiaquine, was surprising in view of subsequent activities obtained in monkey models. Against *P. cynomolgi* infections in rhesus monkeys the minimum consistently curative dose of LXX and LXXV was approximately 3 mg/kg per day for 7 days, one-tenth of the dose required for amodiaquine (SWEENEY et al. 1981). When tested against the multi-drug-resistant Smith strain of *P. falciparum* in the *P. falciparum*-owl monkey model, LXX and LXXV had similar activities, with CD_{90}s (dose required to cure 90% of the infections) of 27 mg/kg per day × 7 and 35 mg/kg per day × 7 respectively (SCHMIDT and CROSBY 1978). Against infections with the Vietnam Palo Alto strain of *P. vivax* in the owl monkey, a CD_{90} of 12 mg/kg per day × 7 was achieved with LXX. Thus the compound had greater activity against *P. vivax* infections than against *P. falciparum* infections; in addition, clearance of parasitaemia was more rapid with the former infection. Against Smith strain *P. falciparum* infections LXX was approximately ten times more potent than amodiaquine.

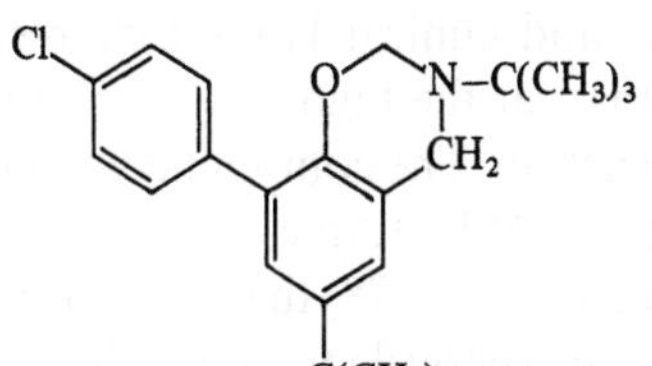

LXXV

Fig. 20. WR 204165 (LXXV)

Compound WR 228258 (LXXII) was the most potent of all of the Mannich bases tested. Against *P. berghei* infections in mice it was almost ten times as potent (CD_{50}) as amodiaquine and showed no acute toxicity at the highest tested dose, 640 mg/kg. Against *P. cynomolgi* infections in rhesus monkeys it was approximately 30 times more potent than amodiaquine. When tested against *P. falciparum* infections in owl monkeys WR 228258 was approximately 20 times as effective as amodiaquine against the chloroquine-susceptible, pyrimethamine-resistant Uganda Palo Alto strain, approximately 65 times as effective against the chloroquine-resistant, pyrimethamine-susceptible Oak Knoll strain and about 140 times as effective against the multidrug-resistant Smith strain (SWEENEY et al. 1981).

Another interesting feature of the Mannich bases is their relatively long biological half-life. Protection against *P. berghei* trophozoite or sporozoite challenge is obtained with WR 228258 for 30 days after drug administration. This long half-life produces false-positive results against sporozoite-induced infections in the *P. berghei*-mouse model. These compounds have, in fact, no causal prophylactic or radical curative activity against relapsing malarias.

IV. Toxicology

Both LXX and LXXII are being developed as potential drugs for clinical use in the US Army Programme. The acute oral LD_{50} of LXXII in male mice, female mice, male rats and male guinea pigs was 1481, 1546, 3465 and 490 mg/kg respectively (LEE et al. 1976a, 1977a). Oral doses of 15 or 45 mg/kg per day for 28 consecutive days did not cause any adverse effects in rats. Oral doses of 135 or 250 mg/kg per day caused weight depression, hair loss and discharge around the eyes and nose. These doses did not, however, cause any apparent changes in peripheral blood elements or clinical blood chemistry, nor did they produce any distinctive pattern of lesions. In dogs (LEE et al. 1976b, 1977b), single oral doses of 15 or 45 mg/kg produced no adverse signs or lesions in 72 h; 135 mg/kg caused mild reticulocytopaenia at 48 and 72 h. Repeated oral administration of 15 mg/kg per day for 28 consecutive days did not cause any adverse effects. At a dose of 45 mg/kg per day for 28 days atrophy of the gastrointestinal mucosa, cloudy swelling of the kidney and involution of the thymus was observed. At a dose of 135 mg/kg per day for 28 days, one of four dogs became moribund on day 21. Toxic signs included salivation, emesis, diarrhoea, muscular weakness, incoordination, anorexia and weight loss. More severe lesions were observed in the kidney and gastrointestinal mucosa while mild bone marrow depression was also observed. At a dose of 250 mg/kg per day for 28 days, two of four dogs survived; there were mild changes in peripheral blood elements and clinical laboratory results without any obvious lesions. It was suggested that, at the high dose, the adverse effects were due to a transient pharmacological action. The compound was not mutagenic (HODGSON et al. 1977) when assayed in the modified Ames test.

It has been shown (KORTE et al. 1978) that LXX produces cardiovascular alterations when administered intravenously to dogs. These included a dose-related decrease in mean arterial pressure and an increase in heart rate (cumulative decrease in heart rate) when administered as a bolus or in 1-min infusions. With longer infusion time, there was a delayed persistent decrease in heart rate. This was attenuated by vagotomy or pretreatment with atropine, hexamethonium or propranolol. Early clinical studies indicate that the drug is well tolerated orally up to doses of 1250 mg.

Subacute toxicity data on LXXII indicate that the dose-response toxicity curve is much less steep than those of traditional antimalarials. Publication of toxicological and clinical data on this compound are planned as the studies progress.

D. Conclusions

Within the past 2 decades a number of efforts have been made to develop new 4-aminoquinolines with antimalarial properties superior to chloroquine that would be effective against chloroquine-resistant strains of *P. falciparum*. Modifications of the quinoline ring system of chloroquine have been uniformly unrewarding. Modification of the side chain has produced some interesting and fairly potent compounds which, in murine models using chloroquine-sensitive strains of *P. berghei*, have distinctly better therapeutic indices than chloroquine. Results of the testing of such compounds in animal models using chloroquine-resistant laboratory strains of plasmodia, if undertaken, have not been reported. An expanded evaluation of such compounds may be justified.

The drug hydroxypiperaquine phosphate seems to be the only new 4-aminoquinoline antimalarial that has undergone clinical trials. Available reports suggest that it is superior to chloroquine and effective against chloroquine-resistant malaria at well-tolerated doses. This compound is a bis 4-aminoquinoline and, as such, may be metabolised differently from the established and available 4-aminoquinoline drugs. Nevertheless, the activity of this drug against chloroquine-resistant malaria constitutes additional evidence that the generally accepted concept of the universality of parasite cross-resistance involving chloroquine and other 4-aminoquinolines needs re-examination.

Much progress has also been made in the α-aminocresol-type antimalarials. Unfortunately clinical trials for the most promising compounds are some distance away; preclinical pharmacological and tolerance studies are yet to be completed. However, the activity of these compounds at well-tolerated doses against various drug-resistant strains of *P. falciparum* and *P. vivax* in primate models indicates that one or more very potent drugs will emerge in this class.

References

Bailey DM (1969) Quinoline antimalarials. Folded chloroquine. J Med Chem 12:184–185

Bass GE, Hudson DR, Parker JE, Purcell WP (1971) Mechanisms of antimalarial activity of chloroquine analogs from quantitative structure-activity studies. Free energy related model. J Med Chem 14:275–283

Bekhli AF, Kozyreva NP, Moshkovskii Sh D, Rabinovich SA, Maksakovskaya EV, Gladkikh VF, Lebedeva MN, Lychko ND, Soprunova N Ya (1977) Synthesis of benzo[g]-quinoline derivatives possessing antimalarial activity. Med Parazitol (Mosk) 46:71–72

Bolton PH, Mirau PA, Shafer RH, James TL (1981) Interaction of the antimalarial drug fluoroquine with DNA, tRNA, and poly A: ^{19}F-nmr chemical-shift and relaxation, optical absorption, and fluorescence studies. Biopolymers 20:435–449

Burckhalter JH, Tendick FH, Jones EM, Holcomb WF, Rawlins AL (1946) Aminoalkylphenols as antimalarials. II. Simply substituted α-aminocresols. J Am Chem Soc 68:1894–1901

Burckhalter JH, Tendick FH, Jones EM, Jones PA, Holcomb WF, Rawlins AL (1948) Aminolakylphenols as antimalarials. I. (Heterocyclic-amino)-α-amino-*o*-cresols. The synthesis of camoquin. J Am Chem Soc 70:1363–1373

Chien P-L, Cheng CC (1968) Synthesis and antimalarial evaluation of some 1,7-naphthyridines and 2,9-diazaanthracenes. J Med Chem 11:164–167

Coatney GR, Cooper WC, Eddy NB, Greenburg J (1953) Survey of antimalarial agents. In: Public health monograph No 9, U. S. Government printing office, Washington

Cruickshank PA, Lee FT, Lupichuk A (1970) Antimalarials. 1. Aminoalkylamino derivatives of 2,3-dihydrofuroquinolines. J Med Chem 13:1110–1114

Duncan WG, Henry DW (1969) 2-(ω-Aminoalkyl)-4-*t*-butyl-6-phenylphenols as antimalarial agents. J Med Chem 12:711–712

Elslager EF, Gold EH, Tendick FH, Werbel LM, Worth DF (1964) Amodiaquine *N*-oxides and other 7-chloro-4-aminoquinoline *N*-oxides. J Heterocycl Chem 1:6–12

Elslager EF, Tendick FH, Werbel LM, Worth DF (1969a) Antimalarial and antischistomal effects of proximal hydrazine and hydroxylamine analogs of chloroquine and quinacrine. J Med Chem 12:970–974

Elslager EF, Tendick FH, Werbel LM (1969b) Repository drugs. VIII. Ester and amide congenors of amodiaquine, hydroxychloroquine, oxychloroquine, promaquine, quinacrine and related substances as potential long-acting antimalarial agents. J Med Chem 12:600–607

Hahn FE, O'Brien RL, Ciak J, Allison JL, Olenick JG (1966) Studies on modes of action of chloroquine, quinacrine, and quinine and on chloroquine resistance. Milit Med [Suppl] 131:1071–1089

Hodgson JR, Kowalki MA, Goethem DV, Hainje M, Lee C-C (1977) Mutagenicity studies on 4-(*t*butyl)-2-(*t*-butylaminoethyl)-6-(4-chlorophenyl)phenol phosphate (WR-194,965.H_3PO_4). Interim report No. 130, U. S. Army medical research and development command No. DAMD-17-74-C-4036. Sept 9

Iber PK, Boone BJ (1967) 4-(1-Methyl-4-pyrrolidinobutylamino)-7-chloroquinoline and 4-morpholinobutylamino)-7-chloroquinoline as potential antimalarials. J Med Chem 10:509

Korte DW, Herman A, Neidig MH, Heiffer MH (1978) Cardiovascular activity of the candidate antimalarial drug 4-(*t*-butyl)-2-(*t*-butylaminomethyl)-6-(4-chlorophenyl) phenol phosphate (WR 194,965.H_3PO_4) in the dog. Pharmacologist 20:253

Kozyreva NP, Bekhli AF, Moshkovskii ShD, Rabinovich SA, Maksakovskaya EV (1979) Synthesis of derivatives of benzo[G]quinoline XIV. 4-Dialkylamino-(hetero)alkylamino-benzo[H]quinolines and their *N*-oxides. Pharmaceut Chem J 12:345–347. (Russian original Khimiko-Farmatsevticheskii Zhurnal 12(3): Part 1, 73–77, March 1978)

Lee CC, Kowalski JJ, Kintner LD, Hong C-B, Girwin JD, Ellis ER (1976a) Acute and subacute oral toxicities of 4-(*t*-butyl)-2-(*t*-butylaminomethyl)-6-(4-chlorophenyl)phenol phosphate, WR-194965.H_3PO_4, in rodents. Interim report No. 114, U. S. Army medical research and development command contract No. DAMD-17-74-C-4036, Oct 18

Lee CC, Kowalski JJ, Kintner LD, Hong C-B, Girvin JD, Ellis ER (1976b) Acute and subacute oral toxicities of 4-(*t*-butyl)-2-(*t*-butylaminomethyl)-6-(4-chlorophenyl)phenol phosphate, WR-194965.H_3PO_4, in dogs. Interim report No. 113, U. S. Army medical research and development command contract No. DAMD-17-74-C-4036, Oct 6

Lee CC, Kowalski JJ, Kintner LD, Hong C-B, Girvin JD, Ellis ER (1977a) Subacute oral toxicities of 4-(*t*-butyl)-2-(*t*-butylaminomethyl)-6-(4-chlorophenyl) phenol phosphate, WR-194965.H_3PO_4 in rodents. Supplement to interim report No. 114, U. S. Army medical research and development command contract No. DAMD-17-74-C-4036, Jan 27

Lee CC, Kowalski JJ, Kintner LD, Hong C-B, Girvin JD, Ellis ER (1977b) Subacute oral toxicity of 4-(*t*-butyl)-2-(*t*-butylaminomethyl)-6-(4-chlorophenyl)phenol phosphate. WR-194965.H_3PO_4, in dogs. Supplement to interim report No. 113, U. S. Army medical research and development command contract No. DAMD-17-74-C-4036, Feb 16

Li Y, Hu Y, Huang H, Zhu D, Huang W, Wu D, Qian Y (1981a) Hydroxypiperaquine phosphate in treatment of falciparum malaria. Chin Med J [Engl] 94:301–302

Li Y, Qin Y, Qu Y, Gong J (Kung CC) (1981 b) Hydroxypiperaquine phosphate in treating chloroquine resistant falciparum malaria. Chin Med J [Engl] 94:303–304
Marquez VE, Cranston JW, Ruddon RW, Kier LB, Burckhalter JH (1972) Mechanism of action of amodiaquine. Synthesis of its indoloquinoline analog. J Med Chem 15:36–39
Marquez VE, Cranston JW, Ruddon RW, Burckhalter JH (1974) Binding to DNA and inhibition of RNA polymerase by analogs of chloroquine. J Med Chem 17:856–862
McCaustland DJ, Cheng CC (1970) 1,5-Naphthyridines. Synthesis of 7-chloro-4-(4-diethylamino-1-methylbutylamino)-2-methoxy-1,5-naphthyridine and related compounds (1). J Heterocycl Chem 7:467–473
Mirau P, Shafer RH, James TL (1980) Studies on the binding of fluoroquine to tRNA, poly(A), and DNA by ^{19}F nmr. Fed Proc 39:1608
Nasr M, Burckhalter JH (1979) Bis-aminoquinolines as potential antimalarial agents and a novel fused ring system, pyrano[3,2-c:5,6-c']diquinoline. J Heterocycl Chem 16:497–500
Nasr M, Nabih I, Burckhalter JH (1978) Synthesis of pyrimido [5,4-c] quinolines and related quinolines as potential antimalarials. J Med Chem 21:295–298
O'Brien RL, Hahn FE (1966) Chloroquine structural requirements for binding to deoxyribonucleic acid and antimalarial activity. Antimicrob Agents Chemother – 1975 315–320
Schmidt LH, Crosby R (1978) Antimalarial activities of WR-194,965, an α-amino-*o*-cresol derivative. Antimicrob Agents Chemother 14:672–679
Schmidt LH, Vaughan D, Mueller D, Crosby R, Hamilton R (1977) Activities of various 4-aminoquinolines against infections with chloroquine-resistant strains of *Plasmodium falciparum*. Antimicrob Agents Chemother 11:826–843
Schonhofer F (1942) The importance of the quinoid bond for antimalarial action of quinoline compounds. Z Physiol Chem 274:1–8
Singh T, Stein RG, Biel JH (1969 a) Antimalarials. 4-"Proximal" hydrazino derivatives of 7-chloroquinoline. J Med Chem 12:801–803
Singh T, Stein RG, Biel JH (1969 b) Antimalarials. Unsaturation in chloroquine side chain and antimalarial activity. J Med Chem 12:368–371
Singh T, Stein RG, Biel JH (1969 c) Antimalarials. Chloroquine analogs with the 1,2,3,6-tetrahydropyridyl function in the side chain. J Med Chem 12:949–950
Singh T, Stein RG, Koelling HH, Hoops JF, Biel JH (1969 d) Antimalarials. Some quinuclidine derivatives of 7-chloro-4-aminoquinoline and 6-methoxy-8-aminoquinoline. J Med Chem 12:524–526
Singh T, Hoops JF, Biel JH, Hoya WK, Stein RG, Cruz DR (1971 a) Antimalarials. "Distal" hydrazine derivatives of 7-chloroquinoline. J Med Chem 14:532–535
Singh T, Stein RG, Hoops JF, Biel JH, Hoya WK, Cruz DR (1971 b) Antimalarials. 7-Chloro-4-(substituted amino) quinolines. J Med Chem 14:283–286
Stein RG, Biel JH, Singh T (1970) Antimalarials. 4-Substituted 1*H*-pyrazolo [3,4-b]quinolines. J Med Chem 1:153–155
Sweeney TR, Davidson DE, Nodiff EA, Saggiomo AJ, LaMontagne MP (1981) Recent developments in potential 8- and 4-aminoquinidine antimalarial drugs. In: Anand N, Sen AB Chemotherapy and immunology in the control of malaria, filariasis and leishmaniasis, Symposium, Lucknow, India, Feb 18–21, 1981
Tara, Stein RG, Biel JH (1973) Antimalarials. Some 9-substituted amino-6-chloro-2-methoxyacridines. J Med Chem 16:89–90
Temple Jr C, Rose JD, Elliott RD, Montgomery JA (1968) Synthesis of potential antimalarial agents. II 6,8 Disubstituted pyrido[2,3-b]pyrazines. J Med Chem 11:1216–1218
Temple C Jr, Rose JD, Elliott RD, Montgomery JA (1970 a) Synthesis of potential antimalarial agents V. Pyrido[2,3-b]pyrazines. J Med Chem 13:853–857
Temple C Jr, Rose JD, Montgomery JA (1970 b) Synthesis of potential antimalarial agents VI. Preparation of 3-(*p*-chlorophenyl)-8-[4-(diethylamino)-1-methylbutyl]amino pyrido[2,3-b]pyrazine. J Med Chem 13:1234–1235
Wiselogle FY (1946) A survey of antimalarial drugs. Edwards, Ann Arbor

CHAPTER 13

Triazines, Quinazolines and Related Dihydrofolate Reductase Inhibitors

P. MAMALIS and L. M. WERBEL

A. General Introduction

The level of basic information on the biochemistry of the malarial parasite has been severely limited until recently, and the mode of action of even the classic drugs remains unclear. However, substantial knowledge has been collected on the parasite folic acid cycle (see Part I, Chap. 2) and on those structures which exert their antimalarial effects via its inhibition. Thus the sulphonamides and the so-called antifolates act on the synthesis of folate cofactors by the enzymes of the parasite (see Chap. 5). We will deal in this chapter with the recent developments among the antifolates and, in particular, with those whose role involves the inhibition of plasmodial dihydrofolate reductase.

The classical structural types exhibiting this mode of action are the diaminopyrimidines of the pyrimethamine type, the dihydrotriazines and their biguanide precursors and, more recently, the diaminoquinazolines.

Little of interest has really appeared on the diaminopyrimidine class since the development of trimethoprim in the late 1960 s. The pyrimidines as a general class have been rather extensively explored since the early 1940 s when at the outset of the British wartime antimalarial programme it was decided to depart from the traditional quinoline and acridine structures. Although a variety of active structures resulted from these studies (THOMPSON and WERBEL 1972), no useful clinical agent has survived and, moreover, the mode of action of these types appears not to be the same as that of the diaminopyrimidines. Thus we have addressed in this chapter the classes of dihydrofolate reductase inhibitors most thoroughly explored in recent times, the dihydrotriazines and the diaminoquinazolines.

B. Dihydrotriazines

I. Introduction

The realisation of the potent antimalarial activity present in a wide range of 1-aryl substituted -2,4-diamino-1,2-dihydro-2,2-dimethyl-1,3,5-triazines (I) came with the finding that the prophylactic diguanide drug proguanil (chlorguanide) (II) was, in fact, a prodrug of the active dihydrotriazine (III) ($R = 4\text{-}ClC_6H_4$) later known as cycloguanil (see inter alia CARRINGTON et al. 1951, 1954; CROWTHER and LEVI 1953). The antimalarial activity of the triazines was confirmed by workers at the Children's Cancer Research Foundation, Boston, who independently synthesised some analogous 1-aryl-dihydrotriazines (MODEST et al. 1952), many of which, as well as showing activity against simian, avian and rodent malaria, showed activity against various microbiological systems, against chicken coccidiosis, and against experimental tumours. MODEST (1956, 1961) gives useful bibliographies. The isomeric dihydrotriazines such as IV, to which III could readily be converted, were inactive as antimalarials.

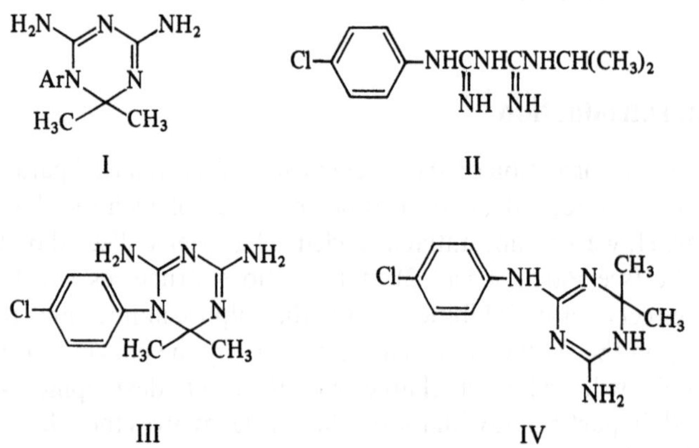

Fig. 1. Chemical structures I–IV

Despite the promising prophylactic antimalarial activity of this series of antifols and, in particular, that of cycloguanil, widespread clinical use has not occurred because of the ready emergence of resistant strains of *Plasmodium falciparum*. A number of general reviews which have included sections on antifol antimalarials since 1969 have given some account of the properties of the dihydrotriazines, particularly the clinical use of cycloguanil and its repository pamoate salt: see, for example, AVIADO (1969), ELSLAGER (1969 , 1974a, b), PETERS (1970, 1974), STECK (1972), ROZMAN (1973) and WHITE (1977) and, in particular, THOMPSON and WERBEL (1972).

Most reported work on antifol antimalarials since 1970 has dealt with diaminoquinazolines and pteridines. However, very recently a number of communications describing 1-arylalkoxy- and 1-aryloxylalkoxy-diaminodihydrotriazines V and VI have appeared indicating that, at least in rodent malaria, it was possible to obtain dihydrotriazines not showing cross-resistance with cycloguanil against triazine-resistant strains of *P. berghei* (MAMALIS 1971; KNIGHT and PETERS 1980; KNIGHT and WILLIAMSON 1980, 1981; KNIGHT et al. (1981). The 1-(dichlorobenzyloxy)-1,2-dihydrotriazine (VII) (WR 38839, clociguanil) showed activity against *P. falciparum* in man, both alone and synergistically with sulphadiazine (LAING 1974; CANFIELD and ROZMAN 1974; WILLERSON et al. 1974). Although showing drug potentiation (with sulphadiazine) against pre-erythrocytic stages of *P. falciparum* in man (RIECKMANN et al. 1971), clociguanil showed no marked advantages over pyrimethamine. Clociguanil cured infections of *P. cynomolgi* in the rhesus monkey (WALTER REED ARMY INSTITUTE OF RESEARCH 1968) and *P. falciparum* strains in the owl monkey (SCHMIDT 1978a). Most of this work was carried out between 1969 and 1971.

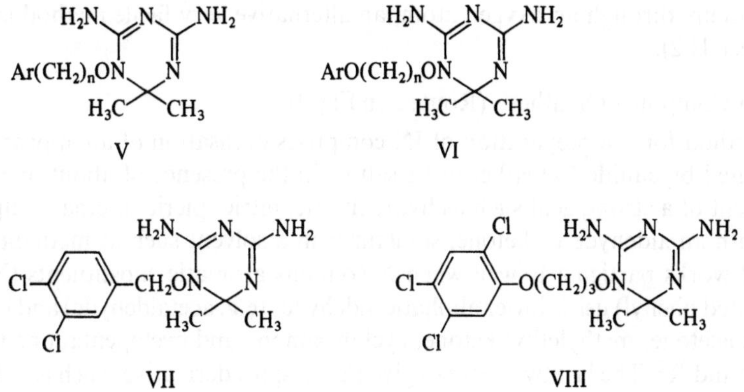

Fig. 2. Chemical structures V–VIII

The analogue VIII (VI; Ar = 2,4,5-$Cl_3C_6H_2$, $n = 3$) (BRL 6231, WR 99210) and its congeners showed in the mouse a very marked lack of cross-resistance to pyrimethamine- and cycloguanil-resistant strains of *P. berghei* (KNIGHT et al. 1981; KNIGHT and WILLIAMSON 1981).

II. Chemistry

1. 1-Substituted-2,4-diamino-1,2-dihydro-1,3,5-triazines

a) General

Ease of synthesis of diamino-dihydrotriazines depends very much on the nature of the substituents R, R^1 and R^2 in IX. Figure 3 indicates the most useful methods available for obtaining dihydrotriazines in which a carbon atom of group R is directly attached to the N^1 of the dihydrotriazine ring. When the attachment of R

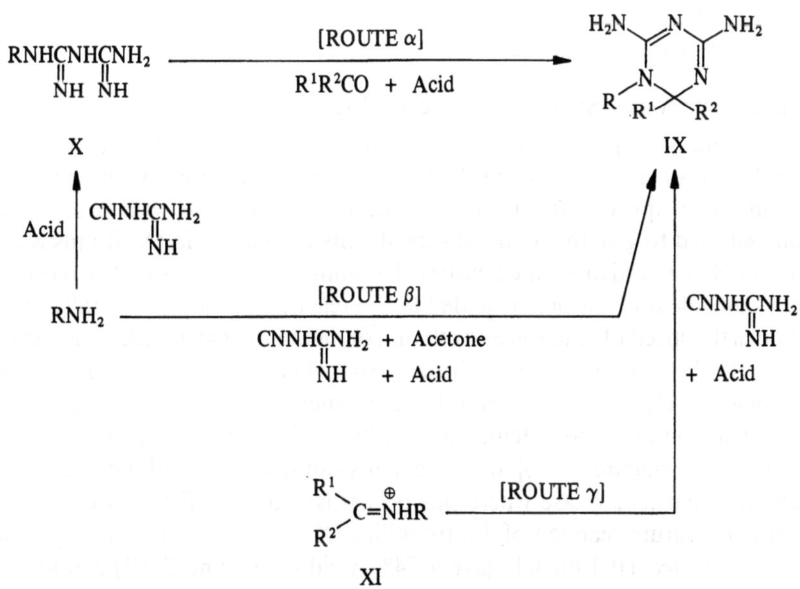

Fig. 3. Scheme including chemical structures IX–XI

to N^1 occurs through an oxygen atom, an alternative very facile method is available (Sect. II.2).

b) Two-Component Synthesis (Route α in Fig. 3)

This method for the preparation of IX comprises cyclisation of an appropriately substituted biguanide (X) either as its salt or in the presence of about one molar equivalent of a strong acid such as hydrochloric, nitric, picric or ethanesulphonic acid, with an aldehyde or ketone, sometimes in a solvent such as methanol. The method works particularly well when X contains aromatic substituents (X; R= substituted phenyl) using lower aliphatic aldehydes (e.g. acetaldehyde) and ketones such as acetone, methylethyl ketone, cyclohexanone and cyclopentanone to provide R^1 and R^2. The last two ketones give rise to spiro derivatives such as XII. The process is applicable to certain *N*-substituted biguanides such as XIII, giving rise, for example, to XIV on treatment with acetone (Modest and Levine 1956). Excellent preparative details may be found in papers by Crounse (1951), Modest et al. (1952), Carrington et al. (1954), Loo (1954), Modest and Levine (1956), Sen and Singh (1958, 1959, 1960, 1961), Schalit and Cutler (1959), Mamalis et al. (1962), Capps et al. (1968) and Rosowsky et al. (1973).

Groups R (in X) with electron-withdrawing substituents give acceptable yields only after long reaction times at room temperature. Use of acetic acid as the acid component, or reaction in the absence of an acid, gave rise to the isomeric anilinotriazines such as IV rather than IX (Modest and Levine 1956; Crounse 1951).

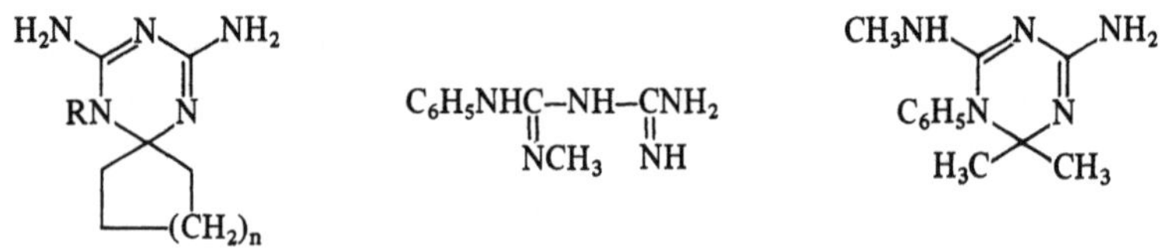

XII XIII XIV

Fig. 4. Chemical structures XII–XIV

c) Three-Component Synthesis (Route β in Fig. 3)

A convenient "one-pot" process developed by Modest (1956) from the original method of Basu et al. (1952) and Basu and Sen (1952) comprises stirring together a mixture of an appropriate aromatic amine, cyanoguanidine, with an aldehyde or ketone selected to give the required substituents R^1 and R^2 in IX. It fails with aliphatic aldehydes and aromatic ketones. The amine is used as its hydrochloride salt or one equivalent of the acid is added to the reaction mixture. Generally, heating facilitates the speed of reaction and ethanol or methanol may be added as a solvent. Acetone is the most reactive of all the carbonyl compounds used, giving rise to good yields of IX ($R^1=R^2=CH_3$). In cases where yields are poor when carrying out the reaction at elevated temperature [the yields of triazine (IX) decreasing at the expense of biguanide (X)], improvements can result by working at room temperature. A particular case where this occurs is shown in Fig. 5 (Modest 1956). Room temperature reaction of 4-nitroaniline (XV) with acetone, cyanoguanidine and concentrated HCl for 6 h gave a 74% yield of triazine (XVI) contaminated with traces of biguanide (XVII) from which it could be separated only with diffi-

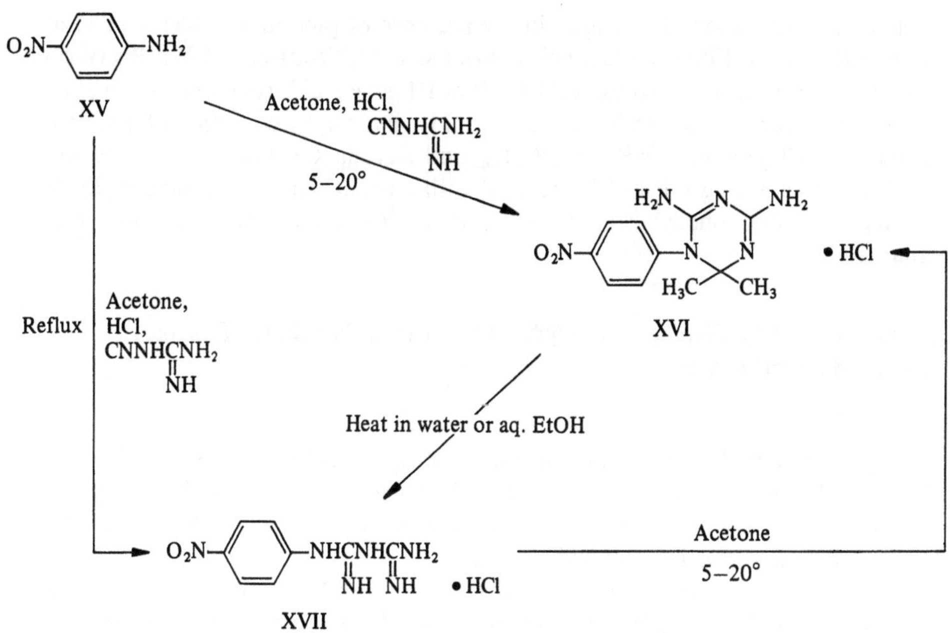

Fig. 5. Scheme including chemical structures XV–XVII

culty. Attempts to recrystallise (XVI) with heating led to recovery of biguanide (XVII). In fact the best method of obtaining pure XVII was to reflux the reaction mixture containing XV, when XVII free from XVI was isolated in high yield.

The method has been used by most of the workers noted under route α. Other papers of interest are those of ROTH et al. (1963) and FURUKAWA et al. (1961) and the numerous papers of BAKER (for example BAKER 1967; BAKER and LOURENS 1968).

d) Synthesis Through a Schiff Base (Route γ)

In this method the carbonyl component is present in situ as a Schiff base of the amine. Reaction fails to take place in the absence of acid, which suggests that cleavage of the anil occurs before the desired condensation and cyclisation (CARRINGTON et al. 1954; NEWMANN and MOON 1964).

e) Reaction of Dihydrotriazines (IX)

Cycloguanil hydrochloride (III-HCl) was a stable material at pHs below 5 or 6 but when neutralised or made basic in water with sodium hydroxide, the free base obtained was unstable and readily isomerised to the *p*-chloroanilino isomer IV, a compound devoid of antimalarial activity. Rearrangement of IX to analogues of IV appeared to be general, the proposed mechanism being equivalent to a Dimroth rearrangement (CARRINGTON et al. 1954). This instability explained why earlier workers (e.g. CROUNSE 1951) isolated IV as the metabolic triazine from animals dosed with proguanil rather than III. Heating III-HCl to its melting point on a small scale also afforded the rearranged triazine IV, and it could be obtained directly from II and acetone by heating in the presence of piperidine (BIRTWELL et al. 1948; CHASE et al. 1951) or acetic acid (CROUNSE 1951; CHASE et al. 1951; BIRTWELL 1952). Vigorous acid hydrolysis (3N-HCl) of III gave *p*-chloroaniline and acetone as the only identifiable products. Under milder hydrolytic conditions III gave *p*-chlorophenylbiguanide (X; R = *p*-ClC$_6$H$_4$) and acetone (CARRINGTON et al. 1954).

The two amino groups of IX reacted with reagents such as acetic anhydride, nitrous acid and phenyl isothiocyanate much less readily than did IV or its analogues.

2. O-Ethers of 4,6-diamino-1,2-dihydro-1-hydroxy-2-Substituted Triazines (*N*-Oxydihydrotriazines)

a) Synthesis

Compounds included within this category of structure XVIII have R = arylmethyl, heterocyclic methyl, aryloxyalkyl, arylthioalkyl, arylaminoalkyl, aralkyl, alkyl and alicyclicalkyl. Also included are bis-oxytriazines (XXI), in which X can be alkylene, alkoxyalkyl, alkylaminoalkyl and aryl.

Methods of synthesis differ somewhat from those for aryldihydrotriazines in Sect. II.1 since the "3-component" method fails. Thus, stirring together a mixture of benzyloxyamine hydrochloride XXII, cyanoguanidine, acetone and ethanol gave not the expected product XVIII (R = C$_6$H$_5$CH$_2$, R^1 = R^2 = CH$_3$) (XXVI) but amidinourea XXIII and the isopropylidene derivative XXIV. No trace of biguanide XX (R = C$_6$H$_5$CH$_2$) was detected at any time (MAMALIS et al. 1962).

Dihydrotriazines (XVIII) were readily obtained by cyclisation of biguanides XX (MAMALIS et al. 1960) in acid medium with an appropriate ketone or aldehyde as in Sect. II.

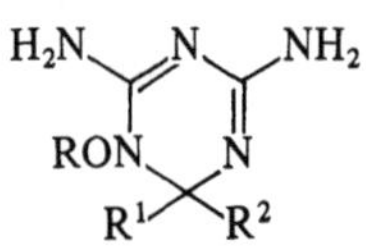
XVIII

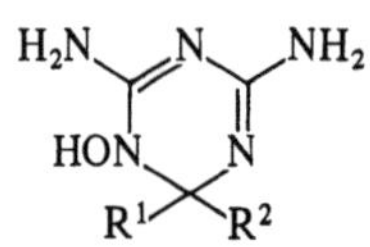
XIX

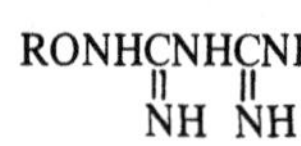
XX

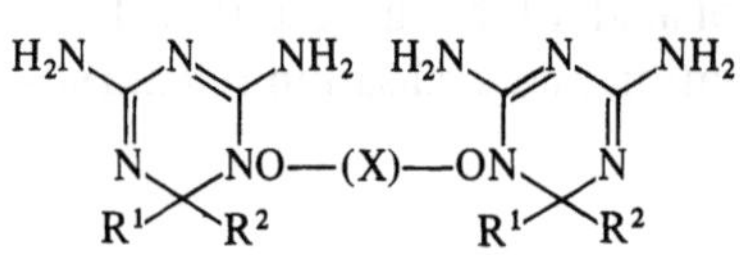
XXI

C$_6$H$_5$CH$_2$ONH$_2$ • HCl

XXII

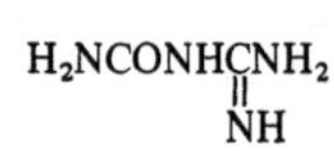
XXIII

C$_6$H$_5$CH$_2$ON=C(CH$_3$)$_2$

XXIV

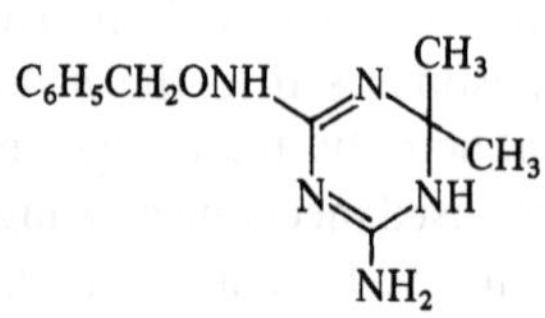
XXV

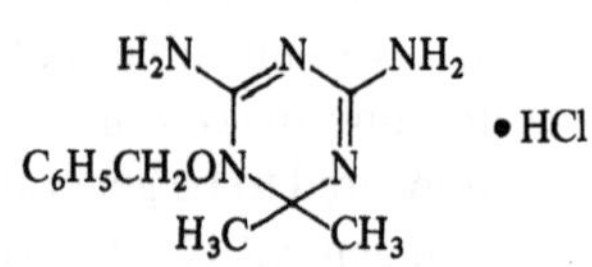
XXVI

Fig. 6. Chemical structures XVIII–XXVI

More conveniently, a method of broad applicability comprised alkylation of an *N*-hydroxytriazine XIX ($R^1 = R^2 = CH_3$ and $R^1R^2 = C_5H_{10}$ or $4\text{-}CH_3C_5H_{10}$) with a halide (RBr or RCl) in a solvent and in the absence of added base when the hydrohalide of the product XVIII was obtained directly and in good yield (MAMALIS et al. 1965a, b; VITAMINS LTD 1970a, b; BEECHAM GROUP LTD 1971, 1972). XIX was readily obtained by hydrogenation of the O-benzyl ethers. This method was applicable to all the groups R mentioned earlier in this section. The bis-compounds (XXI) were similarly prepared.

Reaction of XX (R = 2-naphthylmethyl) with acetone and formic acid gave the triazine formate of triazine XVIII ($R = 2\text{-}C_{10}H_7CH_2$, $R^1 = R^2 = CH_3$) whereas using acetic acid the acetate of biguanide (XX) ($R = 2\text{-}C_{10}H_7CH_2$) was obtained. In basic medium using piperidine, XX ($R = C_6H_5CH_2$) reacted with acetone to give the rearranged triazine XXV, also obtained by heating XXVI base in water or melting XXVI hydrochloride (MAMALIS et al. 1962).

b) Properties

As with the aryldihydrotriazines (IX), heating the bases with or without added inorganic base gave the rearranged triazine such as XXV. In a manner similar to the formation of XIX from its benzylic ethers, XXV could be hydrogenated catalytically to give the hydroxyamino derivative XXVII. Whereas the *N*-hydroxytriazines XIX were readily alkylated, no reaction took place on heating XXVII with benzyl bromide in dimethyl formamide (MAMALIS et al. 1965b).

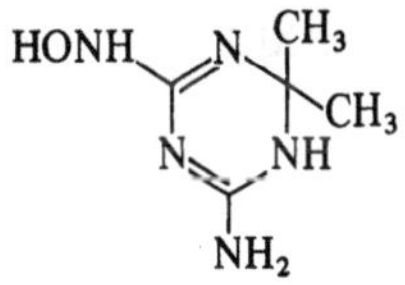

XXVII

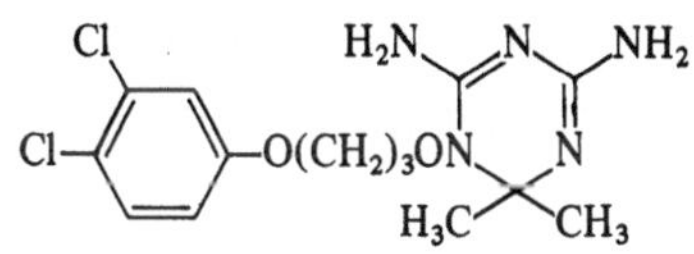

XXVIII

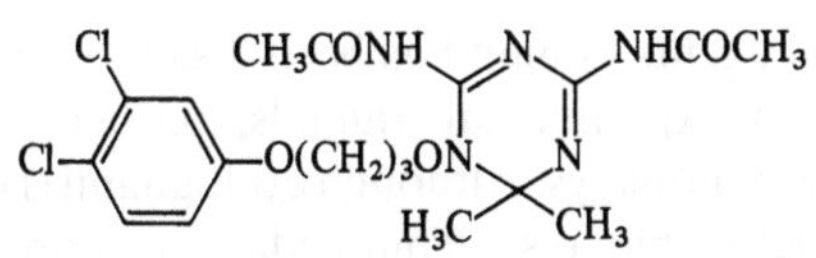

XXIX

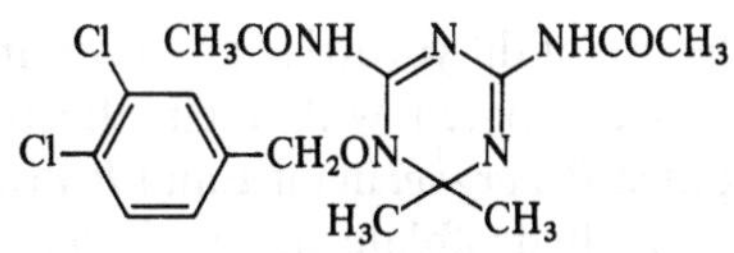

XXX

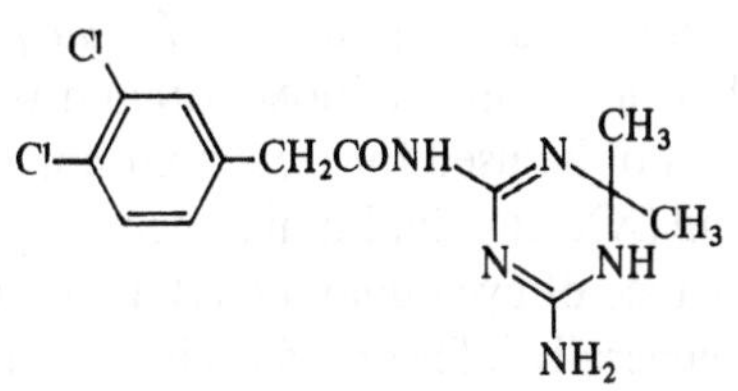

XXXI

Fig. 7. Chemical structures XXVII–XXXI

Rearranged cycloguanil IV on treatment with acetic anhydride gave an unspecified diacetyl derivative (CARRINGTON et al. 1954), while a monoacetyl derivative of IV (on the NH_2) was reported by CROUNSE (1951). Acetylation of cycloguanil itself has not been reported. The oxy-analogues of cycloguanil have been acylated to give products with improved antimalarial activity. Thus, XXVIII gave rise to a diacetyl derivative XXIX; clociguanil (XVIII; $R=3,4\text{-}Cl_2C_6H_3$, $R^1=R^2=CH_3$) also gave a diacetyl derivative (XXX), while its rearrangement product (XXXI) gave both a mono- and a di-acetyl derivative.

An X-ray crystallographic study of clociguanil (VII) was reported by AMMON and PLASTAS (1979b).

3. Miscellaneous Dihydrotriazines

In contrast to the wide variety of reported *N*-aryl- and *N*-aryl-alkoxydihydrotriazines, little is known of *N*-alkyl analogues. LOMBARDINO (1963) reported the preparation of IX with various substituents R^1 and R^2, and R = alkyl or 2-phenylethyl. Close control of reaction conditions in the condensation of the biguanide with a carbonyl compound was necessary. The "3-component" method failed. In contrast, NEWMAN and MOON (1965) found that benzylbiguanide (X; R = $C_6H_5CH_2$) reacted with acetone to give mixtures of XXXII and XXXIII, the proportion of XXXIII increasing with rise in reaction temperature.

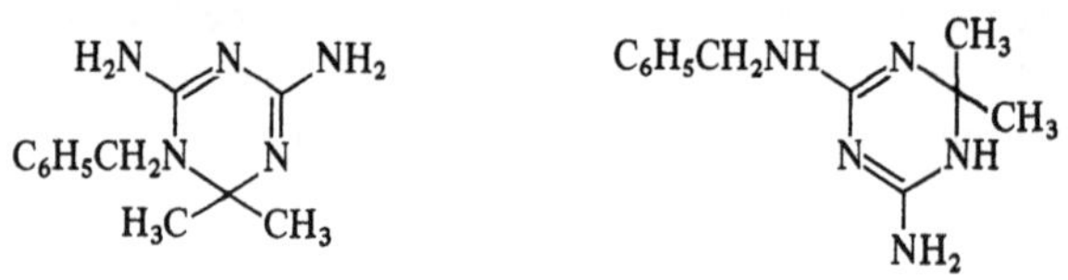

XXXII XXXIII

Fig. 8. Chemical structures XXXII and XXXIII

III. Structure-Activity Relationships

1. Cycloguanil Analogues

The use of dihydrotriazines as antimalarial agents in man has been disappointing when compared with their effectiveness in experimental animals, particularly against *P. berghei* in mice and *P. cynomolgi* in monkeys. Although cycloguanil (III) was a dihydrofolate antagonist with slow-acting blood schizontocidal and sporontocidal activity, it was clinically an effective, true causal prophylactic agent (ROBERTSON 1965). However, in practice it could only be used against chlorguanide- and pyrimethamine-sensitive strains of *P. falciparum* and suffered from possessing a very short half-life in man (THOMPSON and WERBEL 1972; SINGH et al. 1956). It could, therefore, not be used for treatment nor used alone for mass prophylaxis. Chlorcycloguanil (XXXIV) had similar general properties.

The superior performance of cycloguanil (III) in animals compared with proguanil (in contrast to its generally inferior effects in man) is shown in Table 1. This is, at least in part, a reflection of the rapid rate of excretion and metabolism of the dihydrotriazine in man. The same argument could be used to explain the relative

Table 1. Comparative activities of proguanil and cycloguanyl

Test (host)	Effect	Dose in mg/kg × days (route)		Reference
		Proguanil	Cycloguanil	
P. gallinaceum (chick)				
Sensitive strain	ED_{98}	5.0	0.5	RYLEY (1953)
Cycloguanide-resistant strain		> 60	> 140	
P. berghei (mouse)				
N-strain schizontocidal	ED_{50}	30 × 4 (s.c.)	0.25 × 4 (s.c.)	PETERS (1965a)
N-strain schizontocidal	ED_{90}		11 × 4 (s.c.)	PETERS et al. (1975b)
P. yoelii nigeriensis (mouse)				
Causal prophylaxis	ED_{100}	3–10 × 1 (s.c.)	1–2 × 1 (s.c.)	PETERS et al. (1975a)
P. cynomolgi (rhesus monkey)	ED_{100}	1.0 × 7 (p.o.)	6.0 × 7 (p.o.)	BASU and PRAKESH (1962) SINGH et al. (1956)

superior activity of cycloguanil compared with proguanil against *P. cynomolgi* in the rhesus monkey (*Macaca mulatta*) (BASU and PRAKESH 1962; SINGH et al. 1956).

The rapid excretion problem was overcome by the development of a long-acting pamoate salt of III (CI-501) (THOMPSON et al. 1963; LAING 1971; GUSMÃO and JUAREZ 1970; and review by ELSLAGER 1974a) which, in the rhesus monkey, provided, after a single deep intragluteal muscular injection at 50 mg/kg, protection from repeated sporozoite-induced challenge of *P. cynomolgi* for 6 months and more (SCHMIDT et al. 1963). Despite confirmation of prophylactic activity in man using the "Camolar" preparation (5 mg/kg CI-501 for non-immune patients) against both *P. falciparum* and *P. vivax*, side effects and poor protection against resistant strains have precluded its widespread adoption (see reviews by HALL 1969; THOMPSON and WERBEL 1972; ROZMAN 1973; and Chap. 7). A long-acting preparation of CI-501 plus acedapsone (CI-564) developed to overcome resistance problems gave variable results (ROZMAN 1973; THOMPSON et al. 1965a, b).

Very little fresh work has emerged on antimalarial properties of 1-aryl-dihydrotriazines in recent years although some new compounds and their antibacterial and other properties have been reported (Sect. III.3).

Some 1-(chloro-2-naphthyl) derivatives such as XXXV and XXXVI were prepared by ROSOWSKY et al. (1973). In the Rane test using *P. gallinaceum* in the chick, XXXV showed some activity in prolonging survival time by 115% at 80 mg/kg; the effect was dose related. Compound XXXVI suppressed sporozoite and oocyst development of *P. gallinaceum* in *Aedes aegypti* in the Gerberg mosquito screen when administered at 0.001% (GERBERG et al. 1966). Neither compound was acitve in the

Rane *P. berghei* test. PETERS (1971 b) confirmed earlier evidence of potentiation between cycloguanil and menoctone in blood schizontocidal tests in the mouse.

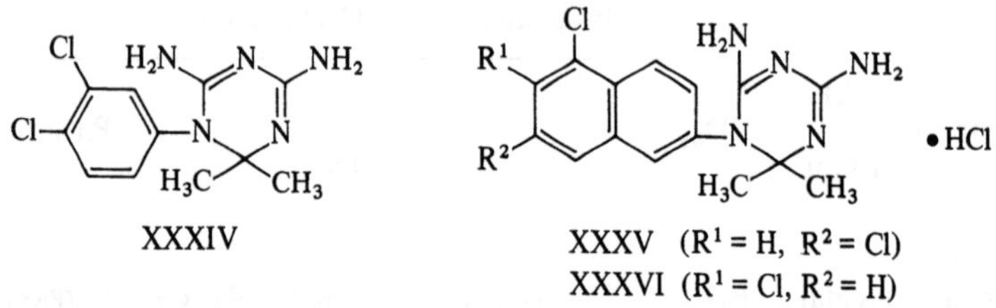

Fig. 9. Chemical structures XXXIV–XXXVI

An interesting structural feature common to several classes of antimalarial agents was pointed out by CHENG (1974). This is shown in structure XXXVII, where X^1, X^2 and X^3 are electronegative atoms such as nitrogen or oxygen containing a lone pair of electrons. Falling into this category are the 6-amino-8-methoxy- and the 8-amino-6-methoxy-quinolines [such as primaquine (XXXVIII)]. That this feature is at best only a partial explanation of antimalarial activity is shown by the activity of chloroquine and cycloguanil, which do not possess this feature. The *N*-oxydihydrotriazines (XXXIX) do, however, fall into the pattern.

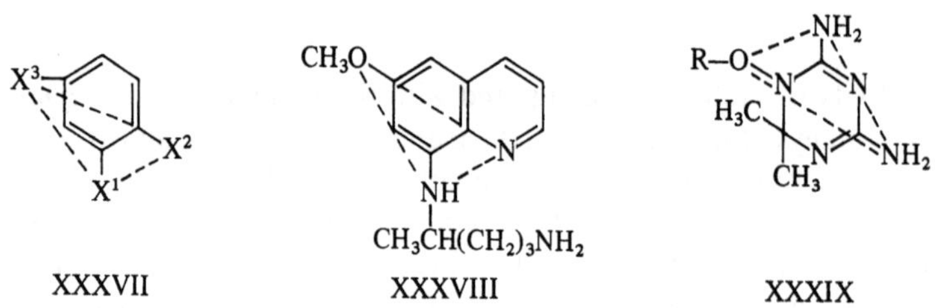

Fig. 10. Chemical structures XXXVII–XXXIX

2. Substituted *N*-Oxydihydrotriazines

The literature to 1970 on dihydrotriazines has been well covered in the monographs by THOMPSON and WERBEL (1972) and PETERS (1970). It is of interest to compare some of the experimental data obtained in mice and monkeys to show the antimalarial effects of substituents in aryl derivatives with corresponding effects in oxygen-containing analogues of the arylalkoxydihydrotriazines and related series.

a) Arylmethoxydihydrotriazines

These have the general structure XL. Rane survival time test results against infections of *P. berghei* in mice are given in Table 2 (KNIGHT and PETERS 1980) for some chlorobenzyloxydihydrotriazines, many of which showed prophylactic effects for 60 days. Clociguanil VII with 3,4-dichloro- substitution in the phenyl ring produced outstanding activity amongst this group under the conditions of the test.

Table 2. Antimalarial activity of some benzyloxydihydrotriazines including clociguanil against drug-sensitive *P. berghei* infections in mice (Rane test)

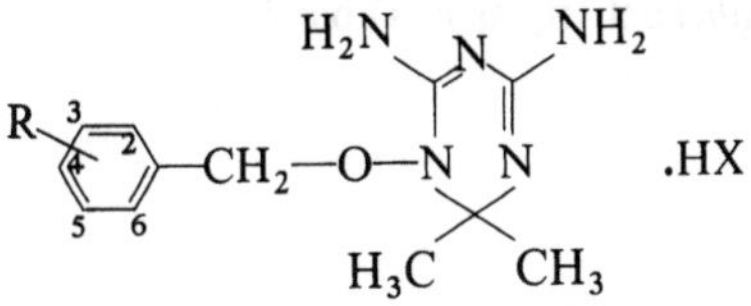

P. berghei activity
No. of survivors in groups of five on day 60 after infection
Dose levels in mg/kg sc x1 given on day 3 of infection

BRL	R	X	640	320	160	80	40	20
50470	2-Cl	Br	4	1	1	0	0	0
51004	3-Cl	Br	4[a]	0[b]	0[b]	0	0	0
50209	4-Cl	Cl	2[a]	4	4	2	0[b]	0[b]
51137	2,3-Cl_2	Cl	5	2	0	0	0	0
50984	2,4-Cl_2	Br	5	2	0	0	0	0
51108	2,5-Cl_2	Br	5	4	2	0[b]	0[b]	0[b]
50995	2,6-Cl_2	Br	2	0	0	0	0	0
50216[c]	3,4-Cl_2	Cl	5	5	5	5	3	1
50461	3,5-Cl_2	Cl	5	4	4	0[b]	0	0
51087	2,4,5-Cl_3	Br	5	5	4	2	1	0[b]

[a] Toxicity
[b] Prolongation of survival times over controls > 100%
[c] Clociguanil (VII)

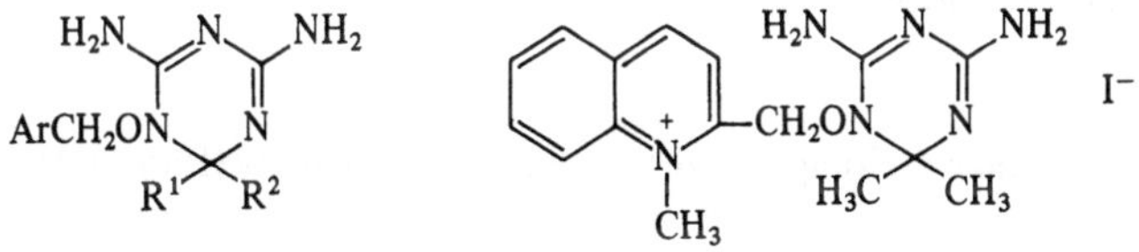

XL XLI

Fig. 11. Chemical structures XL and XLI

Table 3 (RANE 1970) shows that activity in this series was not restricted to the phenyl ring, nor to chloro- substituents. Thus, the chlorine-free analogue of clociguanil, benzyloxydihydrotriazine (BRL 50189), showed good activity but, as is sometimes the case, removal of the chlorine atoms resulted in increased mammalian toxicity. Introduction of nitro and sulphamyl groups (BRL 20242 and 50511) maintained activity but alkyl, alkoxy, alkoxycarbonyl and mixed chloronitro substituents resulted in all cases in reduction or complete loss of activity. These findings parallel the situation in the aryldihydrotriazine series (HEWITT et al. 1954). Table 3 also shows that optionally substituted polycarbocyclic ring systems (Ar = a fused-ring system) resulted in compounds with appreciable antimalarial activity (BRL 50208, 50239, 50386). Analogues in which R was reduced or partially reduced phenyl (BRL 51212, 51397, 51387) and a few heterocyclic derivatives such as BRL 50508 also retained activity Quaternising the pyridyl analogue BRL 50508 gave an inactive product XLI (BRL 50604).

Table 3. Antimalarial activity of some aryl methoxydihydrotriazines against drug-sensitive *P. berghei* in mice (Rane test)

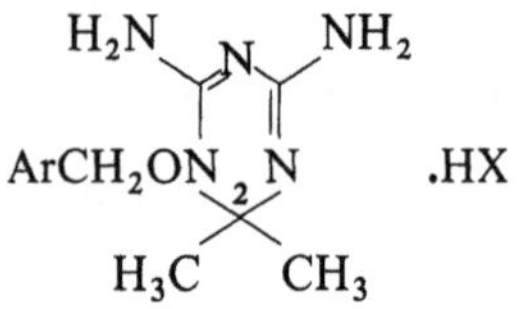

Dose and *P. berghei* activity as in Table 2

BRL	Ar	X	640	320	160	80	40	20
50242	4-$O_2NC_6H_4$	Cl	5	5	5	5	4	1
50239	1-Br-2-$C_{10}H_6$[a]	Cl	5	4	3	1	1	0[b]
50386	$C_{16}H_9$[c]	Br	5	5	5	4	3	1
50511	4-$H_2NSO_2C_6H_4$	Base	5	3	3	0[b]	0[b]	0[b]
50189	C_6H_5	Cl	1[d]	3[d]	5	5	0[b]	0[b]
51387	3,4-$Cl_2C_6H_9$[e]	Br	5	5	2	0[b]	0[b]	0
51212	C_6H_{11}[f]	Br	3[d]	3[d]	2	0[b]	0[b]	0
51397	Δ^3-C_6H_9[i]	Br	[j]	[j]	4	0[b]	0[b]	0[b]
50782	3-O_2N-4-ClC_6H_3	Br	1	0	0	0	0	0
50208	2-$C_{10}H_7$[g]	Cl	5	4	4	0[b]	0[b]	0[b]
50508	2-C_5H_4N[h]	Cl	4[d]	5	3	2	0[b]	0[b]

[a] 1-Bromo-2-naphthyl
[b] Prolongation of survival times over controls >100%
[c] 2-Pyrenyl
[d] Toxicity
[e] 3,4-Dichlorocyclohexyl
[f] Cyclohexyl
[g] 2-Naphthyl
[h] 2-Pyridyl
[i] Δ^3-Cyclohexenyl
[j] Not available

Table 4. Comparative mouse *P. berghei* activity (Rane test)

BRL No./compound	Dose and *P. berghei* activity as in Table 2					
	640	320	160	80	40	20
Cycloguanil	0–3[a]	–	4	–	0[b]	–
50209	2[a]	4	4	2	0[b]	0[b]
Chlorocycloguanil	–	0[a]	5	5	3	2
50216 (clociguanil)	5	5	5	5	3	1
50242	5	5	5	5	4	1

[a] Toxicity
[b] Prolongation of survival times over controls >100%

The 4-chlorobenzyloxydihydrotriazine BRL 50209 showed activity comparable to its direct *N*-aryl analogue cycloguanil. The aryl analogue of clociguanil, WR 62450, chlorocycloguanil I (Ar = 3,4-$Cl_2C_4H_3$) showed similar activity but greater toxicity (Table 4; RANE 1970).

Use of the blood schizontocidal test of PETERS (1965 b) with triazine-sensitive N-strain *P. berghei* in the mouse confirmed the greater activity of clociguanil

Table 5. Comparative antimalarial activity and acute toxicity of clociguanil, cycloguanil, and chloroquine against *P. berghei* N-strain in mice

Compound	Antimalarial activity[a]		Acute toxicity LD_{50} (mg/kg s.c.)	
	$ED_{50} \pm SE$	$ED_{50} \pm SE$	×1	×4
Clociguanil (as hydrochloride)	0.16±0.03	0.39±0.08	>2,500	>800
Cycloguanil hydrochloride	2.0 ±0.4	13.5 ±2.5	220	145
Chloroquine diphosphate	2.3 ±0.2	3.8 ±0.3	200	170
BRL 50242	0.1	0.34		

[a] Doses in mg/kg s.c. ×4 given days 0–3, blood films made on day 4

(>30×) compared with cycloguanil and also its superiority over chloroquine (10×) in this test. The therapeutic ratio for the mouse was greatest for clociguanil (Table 5; KNIGHT and PETERS 1980). The inactivity of some of the compounds in the Rane test was confirmed in all cases which were subjected to the blood schizontocidal test.

All modifications of the 2,2-gem-dimethyl group of clociguanil resulted in reduced activity in the Rane mouse survival time test. Structural modifications and their effects on survival time are shown in Table 6 (data from RANE 1970).

In a study of the effects of various cycloguanil salts on duration of activity in mice (EISLAGER and THOMPSON 1964) no mention was made of their toxicities rel-

Table 6. Effect of Structural changes at position 2 of clociguanil against drugsensitive *P. berghei* in mice (Rane test)

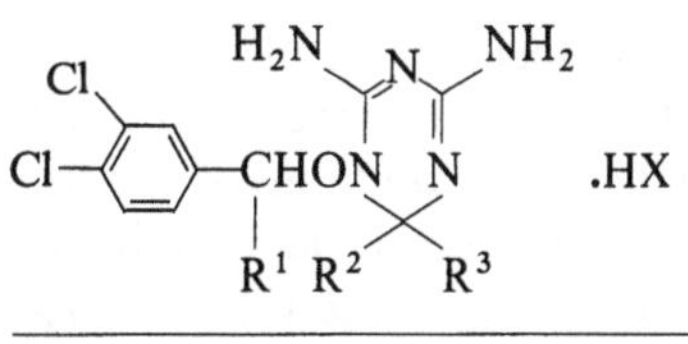

Dose and *P. berghei* activity as in Table 2

BRL	R^1	R^2	R^3	X	640	320	160	80	40	20
Clociguanil	H	CH_3	CH_3	Cl	5	5	5	5	3	1
50973	H	CH_3	C_2H_5	Cl	2[a]	4[a]	2	0[b]	0[b]	0
50974	H	$-(CH_2)_4-$		Cl	2[a]	1	0	0	0	0
50595	H	H	CH_3	Cl	1[a]	2	1	0	0	0
50593	H	H	C_2H_5	Cl	4[a]	3	3	2	0	0
50976	H	H	$4\text{-}CH_3OC_6H_4$	Cl	0	–	0	–	0	–
50997	CH_3	CH_3	CH_3	Br	0[a]	1	1	0[b]	0[b]	0
51026	CH_3	H	C_2H_5	Br	5	3	0[b]	0[b]	0	0
51028	CH_3	H	CH_3	Br	4[a]	5	1	0[b]	0[b]	0
50817	C_6H_{13}	$-(CH_2)_5-$		Br	0	–	0	–	0	–

[a] Toxicity
[b] Prolongation of survival times over controls >100%

Table 7. Effect of salts on antimalarial activity and toxicity of dihydrotriazines in the mouse

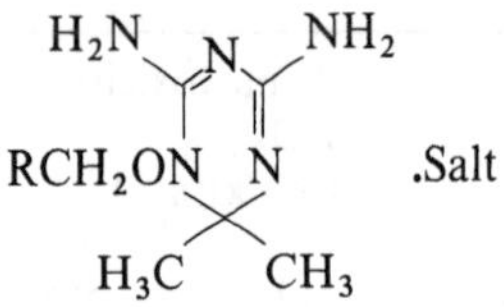

BRL	R	Salt	Dose and *P. berghei* activity as in Table 2					
			640	320	160	80	40	20
Clociguanil	3,4-$Cl_2C_6H_4$	HCl	5	5	5	5	3	1
50998	3,4-$Cl_2C_6H_4$	HBr	2	0[b]	0[b]	0[b]	0[b]	0
50697	3,4-$Cl_2C_6H_4$	Pamoate	1[a]	1[a]	2[a]	0[b]	0[b]	0
51025	3,4-$Cl_2C_6H_4$	Saccharinate	4	3	0[b]	0[b]	0[b]	0[b]
50912	C_9H_{19}	HBr[c]	0[a]	0[a]	3	1	1	0[b]
50538	C_9H_{19}	Saccharinate	4	4	3	2	1	0[b]
50202	1-$C_{10}H_7$	HCl	3	2	1	0[b]	0	0
50397	1-$C_{10}H_7$	Saccharinate	3	1	0[b]	0	0	0

[a] Toxicity
[b] Prolongation of survival times over controls >100%
[c] The hydrochloride had s.c. mouse LD_{50} 150 mg/kg
The acetate has s.c. mouse LD_{50} >500 mg/kg

ative to the more soluble hydrochloride. These workers reported that, while the least soluble salt, the pamoate (0.03 mg/ml at pH 7 in water), showed by far the longest protective effect against *P. berghei,* other salts of only slightly higher solubility (0.04–0.06 mg/ml) were very much less effective. In the oxyamino series, variations in salts were studied in three representative compounds. As the results in Table 7 show, results both for mouse antimalarial activity in the Rane test and for toxicity showed no clear trends (MAMALIS and OUTRED 1969). It must be presumed that differences in absorption due to solubility account for at least some of the observations made. The high toxicity of the pamoate of clociguanil and the greatly reduced toxicity of the saccharinate (BRL 50538) of BRL 50912 were unexpected.

The activity of clociguanil against sensitive and drug-resistant lines of *P. berghei* was investigated in the "4-day test" of blood schizontocidal activity in the mouse by KNIGHT and PETERS (1980). Considerable cross-resistance was observed towards a strain resistant to cycloguanil (B-strain), but not to one resistant to pyrimethamine (PYR-strain). Clociguanil was fully active (ED_{90} 0.6 mg/kg s.c.) against a chloroquine-resistant strain (RC) whilst the sulphaphenazole-resistant ORA line showed considerable hypersensitivity. Table 8 summarises the data and gives resistance indices.

Clociguanil was also shown by KNIGHT and PETERS (1980) to be a true causal prophylactic when mice infected i.v. with a sporozoite suspension of the NY S/149 strain of *P. berghei* from *Anopheles stephensi* were dosed 45 min later with 1 mg/kg drug s.c. Protection was obtained for at least 30 days after infection (patency in blood films taken as criterion). Similar results were shown by PETERS et al. (1975a), who reported minimum fully active doses of 1–3 mg/kg and 1–2 mg/kg s.c. ×1 for clociguanil HCl and cycloguanil HCl respectively.

Table 8. Clociguanil activity spectrum against sensitive and various drug-resistant lines of *P. berghei* in "4-day test" of blood schizontocidal activity in mice

P. berghei				Sensitivity to clociguanil[a]			
Parent strain	Resistant strain	Primary drug resistance	Resistance factor	$ED_{50} \pm SE$	$ED_{90} \pm ES$	I_{50}[c]	I_{90}[c]
NK 65		Sensitive	–	0.3 ±0.1	0.76 ± 0.15	1.0	1.0
	PYR	Pyrimethamine	>175	0.4 ±0.06	1.2 ± 0.15	1.33	1.6
N/NY		Sensitive	–	0.16 ±0.03	0.39 ± 0.08	1.0	1.0
	B	Cycloguanil	× 71	3.4 ±1.2	16.0 ± 6.0	21.0	41.0
			× 800[b]	12.5 ±7.7	41.5 ±20.0	78.1	106.0
	ORA	Sulphaphenazole	× 100	0.012±0.007	0.11 ± 0.05	0.1	0.28
	RC	Chloroquine	× 60	0.14 ±0.08	0.6 ± 0.4	0.9	1.5

[a] Milligrams per kilogram as single daily doses given subcutaneously on days 0, 1, 2, and 3
[b] Extrapolated graphically since above LD_{100}
[c] $\text{I, resistance index} = \frac{ED_{50} \text{ or } ED_{90} \text{ of resistant strain}}{ED_{50} \text{ or } ED_{90} \text{ sensitive strain}}$

Sporozoite suppression was obtained by GERBERG (1968) against *P. gallinaceum* in *Aedes aegypti* and oocyst suppression against *P. gallinaceum, P. vivax* and *P. falciparum* (Thai strain) in the same host.

The pattern of SAR in the arylmethoxydihydrotriazine series followed that found in the aryldihydrotriazines of MODEST (1956) tested by HEWITT et al. (1954), who dosed infected mice daily p.o. for 6 days measuring parasitaemias on the 6th or 7th day. His ED_{90} values for cycloguanil and chlorcycloguanil were 2 mg/kg × 6 and 0.4 mg/kg respectively for the sensitive KBG-173 strain of *P. berghei.* Table 8 shows that KNIGHT and PETERS (1980) obtained s.c. ED_{90} values of 0.76 mg/kg and 0.39 mg/kg for the NK65 and N/NY strains of *P. berghei* respectively for clociguanil. Unpublished results of KNIGHT et al. (1969) indicated an oral ED_{90} for clociguanil of ca. 3 mg/kg.

The arylmethoxydihydrotriazines in general showed considerable cross-resistance with cycloguanil against the cycloguanil-resistant B-strain (PETERS et al. 1975 b; KNIGHT et al. 1969). Nevertheless, three of the analogues had an s.c. ED_{90} against B-strain *P. berghei* of 10 mg/kg or less in the 4-day test (Table 9), one of these, BRL 51212, having an I_{90} of ca. 13, indicating reduced cross-resistance.

Experimental development of resistance to cycloguanil by *P. berghei* in the mouse was described by PETERS (1965 a). Indication of resistance by *P. berghei* to clociguanil has been reported and compared with that to cycloguanil under similar conditions (KNIGHT and WILLIAMSON 1980). Resistance to cycloguanil by *P. berghei* was rapidly obtained using both the relapse technique (PETERS 1970) and the stepwise dose increase technique. Resistance to clociguanil using the relapse method alone could not be achieved; a combination of the two methods, however, produced an index of resistance (I_{90}) of 194 after 77 passages. The resistant lines to both drugs were stable when serially passaged through mice 20 times in the absence of drug pressure.

Table 9. Response of B-strain resistant *P. berghei* to arylmethoxydihydrotriazines in 4-day blood schizontocidal test

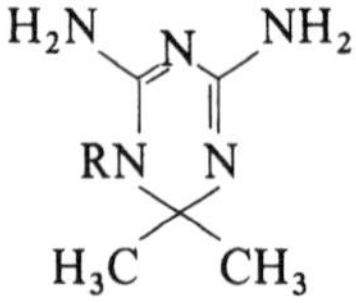		ED_{90} mg/kg s.c.		I_{90} [a]
		N-strain	B-strain	
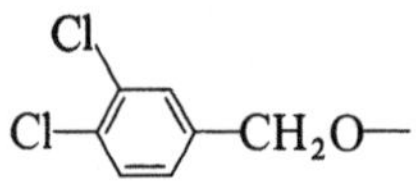	(Clociguanil)	0.35 [b]	ca. 100 [b]	ca. 286
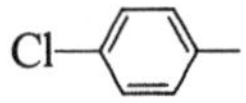	(Cycloguanil)	11 [b]	>1,500 [b]	>140
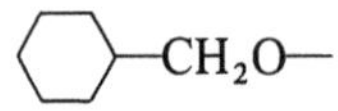	(BRL 51212)	0.3	ca. 4	ca. 13
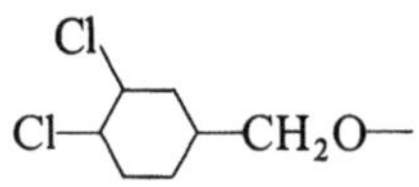	(BRL 51387)	< 0.1	10	>100
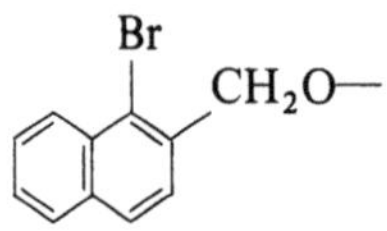	(BRL 50239)	NA [c]	5	–

[a] Index of resistance
[b] PETERS et al. (1975b). Other results from KNIGHT et al. (1969)
[c] Not available

Potentiation was obtained between clociguanil and sulphadimethoxine against the cycloguanil-resistant B-strain of *P. berghei*. At maximum potentiation the s.c. ED_{90} for the combination was approximately 25% that required for either drug alone (see Fig. 12; KNIGHT and PETERS 1980). This had previously been demonstrated by PETERS (1971c) and by many other workers for cycloguanil and sulphonamide in the mouse, and by SINGH et al. (1956) for cycloguanil and sulphadiazine against *P. cynomolgi* in the monkey.

Clociguanil cured infections of *P. cynomolgi* in the rhesus monkey with no detectable blood parasitaemias at 60 days, following splenectomy 30 days after dosing orally for seven consecutive days, 5 days after i.v. infection. Oral doses of 0.1–100 mg/kg and s.c. doses of 3–10 mg/kg were fully effective (WALTER REED ARMY INSTITUTE OF RESEARCH 1968). The rate of fall of parasitaemia was slow, a feature shown by other antifol antimalarials.

The schizontocidal activities of clociguanil and the trichloropropyloxydihydrotriazine HCl (WR 99210, BRL 6231) (XLII) in the owl monkey (*Aotus trivirgatus*) were reported by SCHMIDT (1978a). The owl monkey model was developed extensively by SCHMIDT (1970, 1978b, 1978c). Clociguanil and WR 99210 cured infections of the drug-sensitive Uganda Palo Alto strain of *P. falciparum* with a primary treatment comprising seven daily doses p.o. of 2.5 and 10–40 mg/kg respectively. Against the chloroquine-resistant Vietnam Monterey strain, the doses required for cure in primary treatment were 10–40 mg/kg for both drugs. Under the same con-

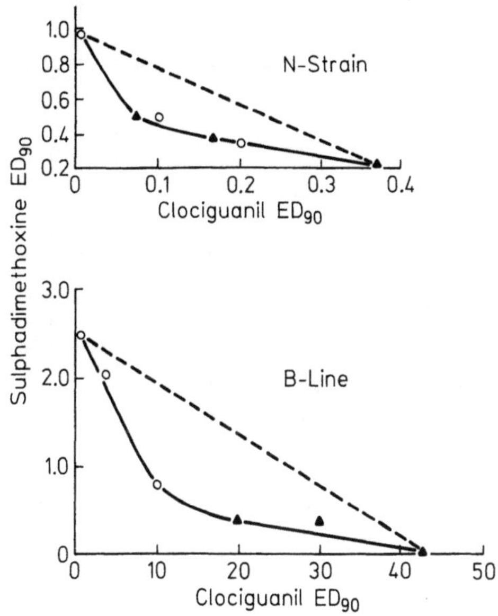

Fig. 12. Graph showing potentation of supressive action of clociguanil *triangles* and sulphadimethoxine *circles* in combination against *P. berghei* N-strain and the cycloguanil-resistant B-line (from KNIGHT and PETERS 1980)

Table 10. Comparative binding of various diaminoheterocycles including clociguanil by *P. knowlesi* and rat liver dihydrofolate reductases

DHF reductase	Molar concentration of drug required for 50% inhibition of dihydrofolate reductase activity			
	Clociguanil	Pyrimethamine	Trimethoprim	Cycloguanil
P. knowlesi	1×10^{-12}	1×10^{-9}	3×10^{-8}	1×10^{-12}
Rat liver	1×10^{-8}	7×10^{-7}	3×10^{-4}	3×10^{-7}

ditions (SCHMIDT 1978d), chloroquine failed to cure *P. falciparum* Monterey infections at 20 mg/kg × 7 p.o., while curing the Uganda strain at 10 mg/kg × 7. Pyrimethamine cured Monterey strain infections at 2.5 mg/kg × 7 but was ineffective at the highest tolerated dose (2.5 mg/kg × 7) against the Uganda strain.

Considerable selectivity was shown in the ability of clociguanil to inhibit the dihydrofolate reductase obtained from *P. knowlesi* compared with its ability to inhibit the corresponding enzyme from rat liver (KNIGHT and PETERS 1980). Table 10 shows that selectivity for pyrimethamine was considerably less than for the other drugs. MCCORMICK et al. (1971) studied the effect of antimalarial antifols on the in vitro rate of incorporation of [^{14}C]orotic acid into nucleic acids by *P. knowlesi.* The incorporation was stimulated by PABA and folic acid and inhibited by antifols such as pyrimethamine and trimethoprim. Of a number of compounds studied, clociguanil and pyrimethamine were the most potent. Another study of the in vitro activity of antimalarials was made by RIECKMANN (1968) and first reported by PETERS (1974). Results (Table 11) showed that clociguanil was more effective, in

Table 11. The in vitro activity of experimental antimalarial compounds against strains of *P. falciparum* with varying degrees of sensitivity to pyrimethamine and chloroquine. Data from RIECKMANN (1968)

Drug	Strain of *P. falciparum*[a]	Concentration (µg salt/litre blood)												
		2,500	1,000	500	250	100	50	25	10	5	2.5	1.0	0.5	0.25
Chloroquine diphosphate	Vietnam[a] (Marks)	+ + +[f]	+	0										
	Malaya[b] (Camp.)		+ + +	+ +	+	0								
	Uganda I[c]				+ + +	+	0							
Pyrimethamine isethionate	Vietnam (Marks)	0												
	Malaya (Camp.)		+ + +		+ +	+	0							
	Uganda I								+ + +	+ +	+	0		
Cycloguanil hydrochloride	Vietnam (Marks)				+ + +	+ +	+	0						
	Malaya (Camp.)					+ + +	+ +	+		0				
	Uganda I									+ + +		+ +	+	0
WR 38839[d]	Vietnam (Marks)						+ + +	+ +	+	0				
	Malaya (Camp.)							+ + +	+ +	+	0			
	Uganda I											+ + +	+ +	+
WR 99210[e]	Vietnam (Marks)										+ + +	+	0	
	Malaya (Camp.)										+ + +	+ +	+	0
	Uganda I										+ + +	+ +	+	0

[a] Chloroquine and pyrimethamine resistant
[b] Chloroquine susceptible, pyrimethamine resistant
[c] Chloroquine and pyrimethamine susceptible
[d] Clociguanil
[e] BRL 6231
[f] Percentage of schizonts affected: + + + >90, + + 50–90, + <50, 0 No effect

terms of concentration required, than cycloguanil, and that both were considerably less potent than WR 99210. In particular, they were most effective against the cloroquine- and pyrimethamine-resistant Marks strain of *P. falciparum*.

b) Aryloxy- and Arylalkyloxydihydrotriazines

The title compounds having structures XLIII (X=0, n=2–10, Ar=optionally substituted phenyl) and XLIV (n=0–8, R=H or C_1–C_8 alkyl, Ar=optionally substituted phenyl) were described by workers at the Beecham Group Laboratories some years ago (see Sect. II.2.a) and found to possess unexpectedly interesting antimalarial profiles in the mouse using resistant strains of *P. berghei*.

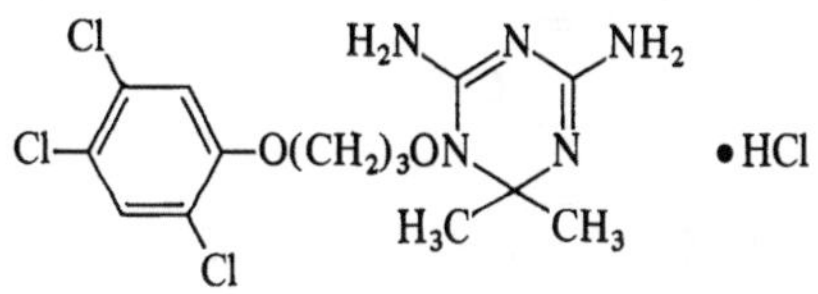

XLII

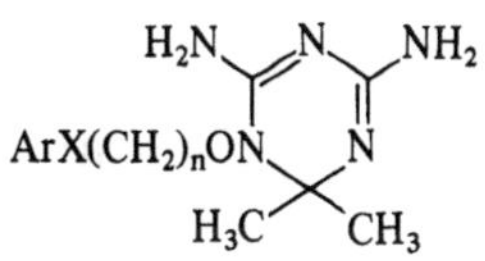

XLIII

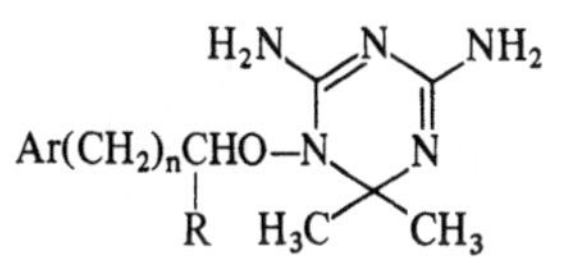

XLIV

Fig. 13. Chemical structures XLII–XLIV

Early results from the Rane survival time screen indicated that many of these analogues were effective prophylactics (MAMALIS and OUTRED 1969) against the cycloguanil-sensitive N-strain of *P. berghei* in the mouse. Some examples are given in Tables 12 and 13.

PETERS (1968) and PETERS et al. (1975b) reported that the trichlorophenoxy-propyl-dihydrotriazine BRL 6231 (WR 99210) (XLII), unlike clociguanil, showed only a low degree of cross-resistance with cycloguanil against the cycloguanil-resistant B-strain of *P. berghei* in the mouse 4-day test (Table 14). It was later reported (KNIGHT et al. 1982) that the s.c. activity found for WR 99210 against B-strain *P. berghei* extended to a number of other analogues of XLIII and XLIV (Table 15). ED_{90} values of 1–3 mg/kg × 4 were obtained with a number of the compounds. PETERS et al. (1975b) also reported results of a systematic study of activities of a number of dihydrotriazines against six resistant lines of *P. berghei:* RC, NS, P, B, PYR and ORA. Good activities were obtained.

PETERS (1968) and PETERS et al. (1975b) reported that the trichlorophenoxypro-pyl-dihydrotriazine BRL 6231 (WR 99210) (XLII), unlike clociguanil, showed on-

Activity in the mouse against *P. berghei* by the oral route was lower than by s.c. dosing, a reflection of lower blood levels. WR 99210 had an ED_{90} of ca. 50 mg/kg × 4 (over 4 days) against B-strain, compared with ca. 1.5 mg/kg s.c. Acetylation of the 2,4-diamino groups resulted in an improvement in oral ED_{90} with figures of 20 mg/kg × 4 for BRL 6548 (XLVI; R^1=H, R^2=Cl), and a similar trend was noted with some related analogues (Table 16; MAMALIS et al. 1971).

Table 12. Antimalarial activity of some aryloxyalkyloxydihydrotriazines and analogues against drug-sensitive *P. berghei* in mice (Rane test)

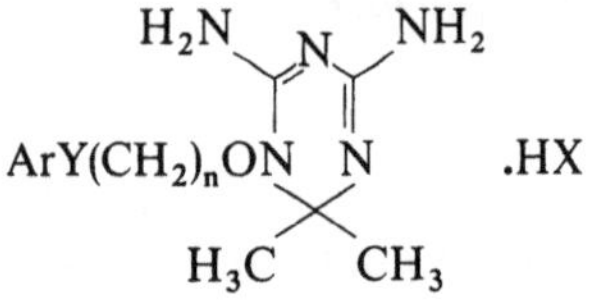

P. berghei activity
Nos. of survivors and doses as in Table 2

BRL	*n*	X	Y	Ar	640	320	160	80	40	20
6231	3	Cl	0	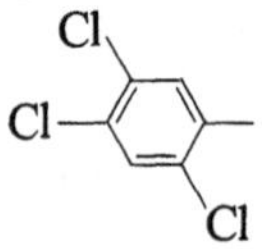	5	5	2	0[a]	0[a]	0[a]
51091	3	Br	0	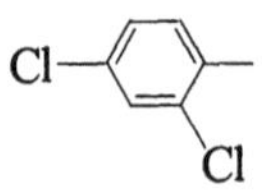	4[b]	5	3	3	2	1
51096	8	Br	0	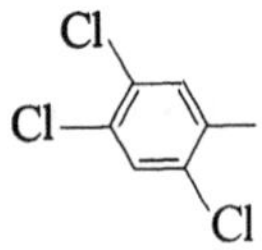	5	5	5	0[a]	0[a]	0
51157	3	Br	0	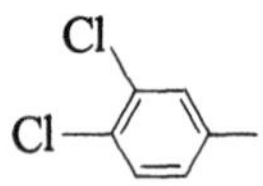	0[b]	0[b]	2[b]	1[b]	2	0[a]
51226	2	Br	S	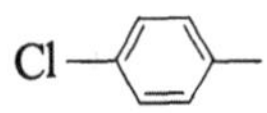	5	3	2	2	0	0
51231	2	Br	0	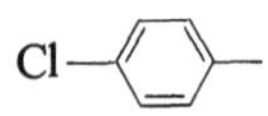	1[b]	3[b]	3	1	0[a]	0
51264	3	Br	S	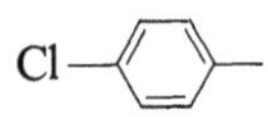	2	0[a]	0[a]	0	0	0
51266	2	Br	NH	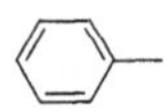	3[b]	2	0[a]	0[a]	0[a]	0

[a] Prolongation of survival time over controls > 100%
[b] Drug toxicity

The ability to decrease or eliminate triazine cross-resistance in the mouse by lengthening the side chain in XLIII and XLIV was not reported in the case of the analogous diaminopyrimidines, such as pyrimethamine XLV, by FALCO et al. (1951). There were, in fact, indications that activity might lessen as a side chain was inserted between the C(5) carbon of the pyrimidine and the 5-substituents. This is yet another example of the differences to be found in these heterocyclic antifols.

PETERS et al. (1975a) showed that WR 99210 was a causal prophylactic in mouse *P. yoelii nigeriensis* with a minimum effective dose of 1–3 mg/kg s.c. (× 1).

The superior therapeutic ratios of the acetylated derivatitves in the mouse against *P. berghei* were not observed in the owl monkey. Thus, the acetylated de-

Table 13. Antimalarial activity of some aralkyloxydihydrotriazines against drugsensitive *P. berghei* in mice (Rane test)

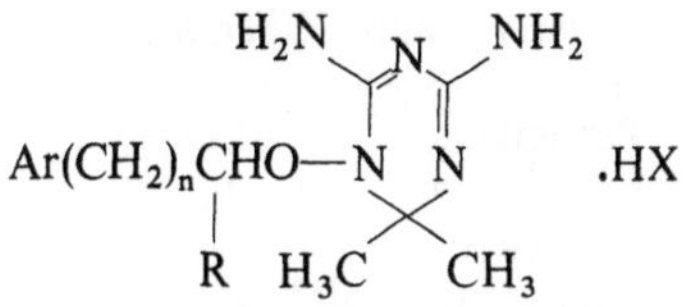

P. berghei activity
Nos. of survivors and doses as in Table 2

BRL	n	R	X	Ar	640	320	160	80	40	20
50827	5	H	Br	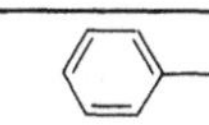	3[a]	4	5	0[b]	0[b]	0[b]
50818	0	C_6H_{13}	Br	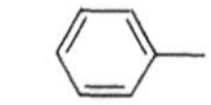	3[a]	1	0[b]	0	0	0
51080	2	H	Br	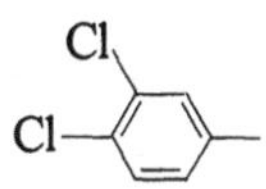	2[a]	2[a]	4	2	1	0[b]
51164	2	H	Br	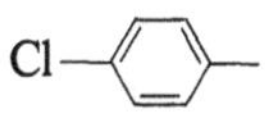	0[a]	2[a]	4[a]	3	3	2
50224	2	H	Cl	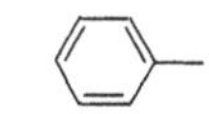	0[b]	0[b]	0[b]	0[b]	0	0

[a] Drug toxicity
[b] Prolongation of survival times over controls >100%

Table 14. Blood schizontocidal activity against various strains of *P. berghei* in mouse "4-day test"

Strain[b]	ED_{90} mg/kg (×4) p.o. Cpd.				
	Clociguanil	Cycloguanil	BRL 6231[a]	Pyrimethamine	Chloroquine
N	0.35	11	0.5	(0.44 (i.p.) (0.25[c]	3.3
B	ca. 100	> 1,500	1.5	3.4	2.6
PYR	0.6	> 330	0.3	48	3.6
RC	1.0	7	0.6	0.6	640
ORA	0.2	–	0.6	1.1	–
P	–	> 140	0.7	0.75	2.3

[a] WR 99210
[b] N, sensitive strain; B, cycloguanil resistant; PYR, pyrimethamine resistant; RC, chloroquine resistant; ORA, sulphonamide resistant; P, primaquine resistant
[c] SCHNEIDER et al. (1949)

rivative WR 169627 (BRL 7638) (XLVI; $R^1 = Cl$, $R^2 = H$) showed good activity against the Malayan Camp-CH/Q and Vietnam Oak Knoll strains of *P. falciparum* in the owl monkey and was more active than its unacetylated parent WR 99209 (BRL 51091) and WR 99210. It had, however, an unacceptably low therapeutic index in the owl monkey (SCHMIDT 1972). Using a daily dose of 2.5 mg/kg p.o. for

Table 15. Blood schizontocidal activity of extended chain oxydihydrotriazines against drug-sensitive and -resistant *P. berghei* in mouse "4-day test" (s.c. dosing)

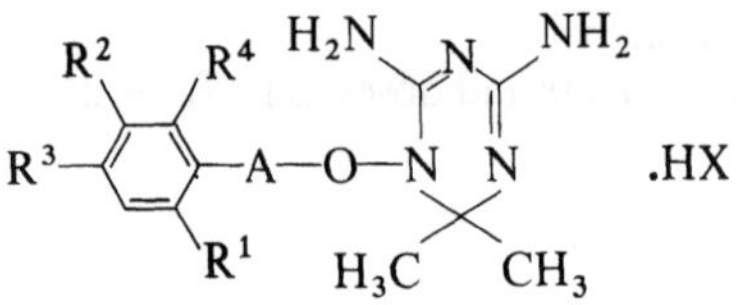

BRL	R^1	R^2	R^3	R^4	A	X	Activity against *P. berghei*: Percentage parasitaemias relative to undosed controls[a] [dose 1 mg/kg s.c. (×4)] N-strain	Percentage parasitaemias B-strain	ED_{90}[b] (mg/kg s.c.) B-strain
51079	H	Cl	Cl	H	$(CH_2)_2$	Br	0.1	6.9	
51157	H	Cl	Cl	H	$O(CH_2)_3$	Br	NA[c]	1.1	0.95
51091	Cl	H	Cl	H	$O(CH_2)_3$	Br	NA	6.8	2.7
6231	Cl	Cl	Cl	H	$O(CH_2)_3$	Cl	0	1.0	1.5
51162	H	Cl	Cl	H	$O(CH_2)_4$	Br	NA	16	
51163	Cl	H	Cl	H	$O(CH_2)_4$	Br	0.4	16	
51165	Cl	Cl	Cl	H	$O(CH_2)_4$	Br	NA	1.2	
51314	Cl	H	Cl	Cl	$O(CH_2)_4$	Br	0.4	1.8	
6548[d]	Cl	H	Cl	H	$O(CH_2)_3$	–			1.4
7368[e]	H	Cl	Cl	H	$O(CH_2)_3$	–			1.0

[a] KNIGHT et al. (1981)
[b] PETERS et al. (1975b)
[c] Not available
[d] Diacetyl derivative of BRL 51091
[e] Diacetyl derivative of BRL 51157

Table 16. Blood schizontocidal activity of extended chain oxydihydrotriazines against N- and B-strain *P. berghei* in mouse "4-day test" (oral)

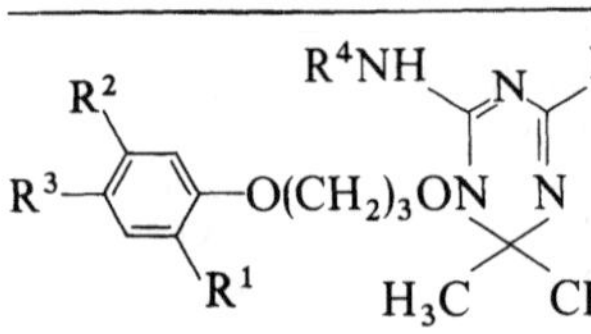

BRL	R^1	R^2	R^3	R^4	Activity against *P. berghei* ED_{90} mg/kg × 4 p.o. N-strain	B-strain
51296	H	H	Cl	H	NA[a]	46
1406	H	H	Cl	$COCH_3$	NA	17
51091	Cl	H	Cl	H	ca. 90	88
6548	Cl	H	Cl	$COCH_3$	7.7	21.5
51157	H	Cl	Cl	H	NA	87
7638	H	Cl	Cl	$COCH_3$	8.9	17
6231	Cl	Cl	Cl	H	23	60
6547	Cl	Cl	Cl	$COCH_3$	NA	38

[a] Not available

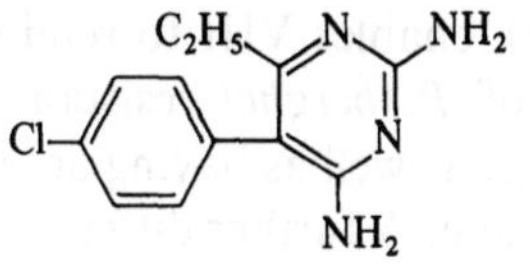

XLV

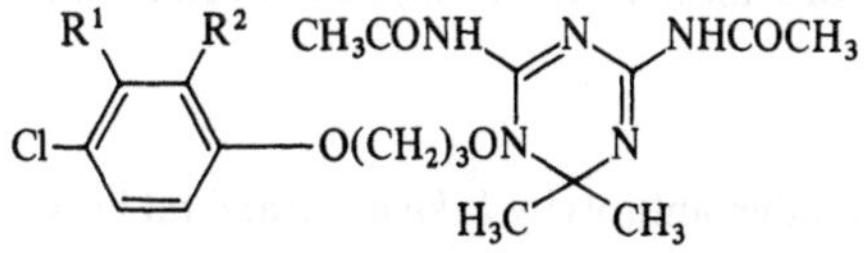

XLVI

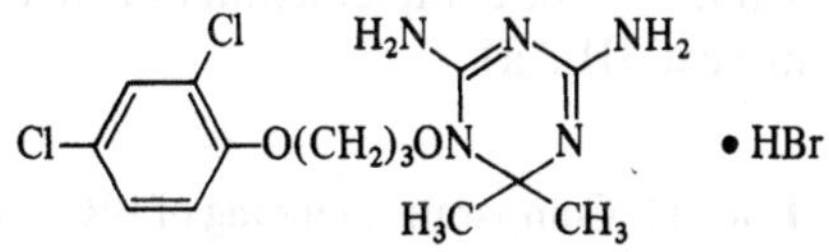

XLVII

Fig. 14. Chemical structures XLV–XLVII

7 days, BRL 7638 regularly cured infections of the two foregoing strains, the dose being 25% that required to effect a cure with WR 99210. The maximum tolerated dose was ca. 7.5–10 mg/kg p.o. The activity of these triazines was not compromised by either chloroquine or pyrimethamine resistance.

Good activity was observed with BRL 6231 (XLII) against *P. cynomolgi* infections in rhesus monkeys with a 7-day schedule of dosing beginning 4 days postinfection (WALTER REED ARMY INSTITUTE OF RESEARCH 1969). Subcutaneous doses of 0.3 and 1.0 mg/kg cured the blood-induced infections, with no evidence of parasitaemia 30 days after splenectomy (carried out 30 days after infection). The oral dose required to effect a cure was 10–32 mg/kg × 7, and the i.m. dose 1 mg/kg × 7. KNIGHT et al. (1982) demonstrated causal prophylaxis against a sporozoite-induced infection of the Langur strain of *P. cynomolgi*, obtained from *A. stephensi*, dosing s.c. from day 1 before infection to day +8. Splenectomy was carried out 37 days after infection and the experiment was run to day 69.

A blood-induced infection of *P. knowlesi* in the rhesus monkey was suppressed by two successive daily doses of BRL 51084 (the hydrobromide of BRL 6231) at 1 mg/kg s.c., but not by two oral doses of the drug at 10 mg/kg.

Unlike the cases of cycloguanil and clociguanil, resistance by *P. berghei* to BRL 6231 was comparatively difficult to induce (PETERS 1969). After 35 stepwise passages of *P. berghei* through the mouse, the ED_{90} of the N-stain, originally 0.8 mg/kg × 4, rose to 5.1 mg/kg × 4, a resistance factor of ca. 6.

The 4-day dosing method was used by KNIGHT and WILLIAMSON (1982) in groups of five mice following a stepwise technique for 24 passages, followed by 26 passages using the relapse technique. After 50 passages the ED_{90}, originally 0.34 mg/kg (N-strain *P. berghei*), had risen to 4.2 mg/kg, an I_{90} of 12. The resistance to BRL 6231 appeared to be stable. This BRL 6231-resistant line was cross-resistant to cycloguanil and pyrimethamine but not to chloroquine or sulphadimethoxine. It was hypersensitive to primaquine.

The foregoing reports highlight the unexpected findings that introduction of a longer side chain into an *N*-oxytriazine such as VII (clociguanil) to give, for example, VIII HBr (BRL 51084), enables VIII to retain its activity, at least in the mouse model, against lines of *P. berghei* resistant to other antifols such as cycloguanil and pryimethamine, as well as having activity against strains resistant to chloroquine and sulphonamide. A further difference between VII und VIII lies in the potent inhibiton of dihydrofolate reductase isolated from *P. knowlesi* by VIII as compared with that from rat liver reductase, the $IC_{50}S$ being respectively 10^{-18} *M* and 10^{-9} *M* (KNIGHT, personal communication). Results are given in Table 17. The complementary in vitro results of RIECKMANN (1968) have been given in Sect. III.2.a).

Table 17. Comparative binding of BRL 51084 and other antifols by *P. knowlesi* and rat liver dihydrofolate reductases

Origin of reductase	Molar concentration required for 50% inhibition of dihydrofolate reductase IC_{50}				
	BRL 51084	Clociguanil	Cycloguanil	Pyrimethamine	Trimethoprim
P. knowlesi	1×10^{-18}	1×10^{-12}	1×10^{-12}	1×10^{-9}	3×10^{-8}
Rat liver	1×10^{-9}	1×10^{-8}	1×10^{-7}	7×10^{-7}	3×10^{-4}

3. Miscellaneous Dihydrotriazines

Dihydrotriazines in general possess a very wide range of biological properties including antimicrobial, antiparasitic and antitumour, as mentioned in Sect. I. One group of triazines devoid of antimalarial properties were the bis-triazines (XXI). These, as well as being antibacterials (MAMALIS et al. 1965a), showed good activity against murine trypanosomiasis but not against *P. berghei* in the mouse (KNIGHT and PONSFORD 1982). Antimalarial activity has not been claimed for the few 1-aralkyldihydrotriazines such as XXXII so far reportes (LOMBARDINO 1963; NEWMAN and MOON 1965). 1-Hydroxytriazines XIX are also devoid of antimalarial (or any other) properties.

Following on some earlier work (HITCHINGS et al. 1952) with 6-substituted-3,5-diamino-as-triazines, it was confirmed by REES et al. (1972) that the 6-(3,4-dichlorophenyl)-*as*-triazine XLVIII was the most potent of a series of analogues in the Rane mouse-*P. berghei* test system using a triazine-sensitive strain. The much lower activity of XLVIII against *P. gallinaceum* in the chick was also confirmed.

The 6-(3-trifluorophenyl)-analogue XLIX was almost as active as XLVIII against the drug-sensitive *P. berghei* KBG 173 strain. In tests using a strain of *P. berghei* made 100-fold resistant to cycloguanil with the drug XLIX given in feed, ED_{90} for the parent strain was 4 mg/kg per day and 38 mg/kg per day for the resistant strain, an index of resistance (I_{90}) of ca -10. This may be compared with I_{90} values (Table 14) of 100 for clociguanil and 1.5 for BRL 6231 (WR 99210). These compounds were also described by AMERICAN HOME PRODUCTS CORPORATION (1973).

It was not found possible to synthesise the potentially interesting 6-benzyl analogues

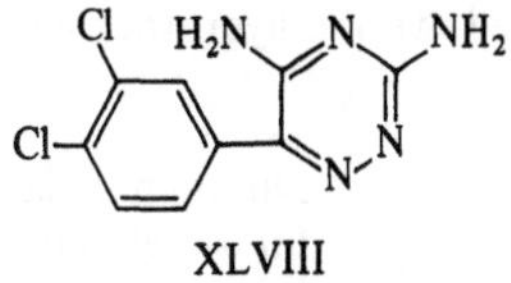

XLVIII

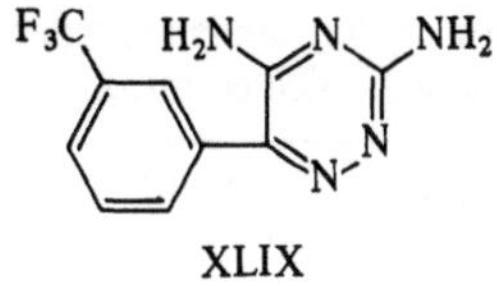

XLIX

Fig. 15. Chemical structures XLVIII–XLIX

4. Repository Formulations

The use of silicone rubber implants for sustained release of prophylactic antimalarial drugs was proposed by POWERS (1965), who investigated the use of pyrimethamine-containing implants i.p. or s.c. in chicks. Blood-induced infections of *P. gallinaceum* were applied 12 days after implantation. The s.c. implanted chicks failed to become patent 30 days after exposure. The principle of controlled release was taken further by FU et al. (1973a, b), who used flexible silicone rubber-epoxy drug capsules containing pyrimethamine, and silicone rubber discs containing chloroquine diphosphate for in vitro release rate experiments, when more or less steady release was obtained during 2–4 months.

JUDGE and HOWELLS (1979) used Silastic medical grade discs containing 3% pyrimethamine as implants for mice which were challenged at 4-weekly intervals with N-strain *P. berghei* over a 3-month period without becoming infected. A low concentration of drug (0.5%) was effective for 5–6 months. Formulations containing cycloguanil HCl and sulphonamides were also effective, although the former gave rise to local tissue necrosis. Chloroquine was ineffective by this technique.

Mice and rhesus monkeys were used as models for prophylactic experiments using a dual antimalarial mixture (WISE et al. 1979). The polymer used for the two drugs employed was a biodegradable polylactate-polyglycolate copolymer and the drugs (used in 10:1 ratio) were sulphadiazine and 2,4-diamino-6-(2-naphthylsulphonyl)quinazoline (WR 158122). No significant delay in rate of release of sulphadiazine occurred with the polymer formulation dosed s.c. compared with that of intact drug. A slower release was, however, obtained using the polymer formulation of WR 158122. It is important to develop individual polymer materials for each drug in a mixture in order to obtain parallel release rates. This work followed on from experiments with individual drug polymer mixtures (WISE et al. 1976, 1978) where good release rates were obtained.

HOWELLS and JUDGE (1977) reported mouse experiments on silicone rubber implants containing 5% dihydrotriazines of type L. Mice were infected with N-strain *P. berghei* on the day of implantation and blood parasite counts were made daily. Mice negative for *P. berghei* were reinfected at 14-day intervals. Results are given in Table 18. The most effective compound was Brl 7638 (L; $R^1 = H$, $R^2 = R^3 = Cl$,

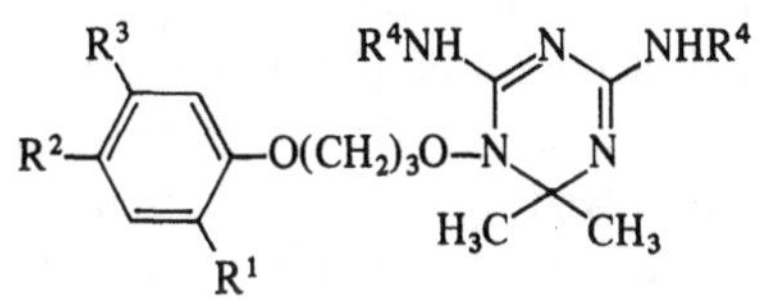

L

Fig. 16. Chemical structure L

Table 18. Duration of antimalarial effect obtained with dihydrotriazine silastic rubber implants in *P. berghei* – infected mice

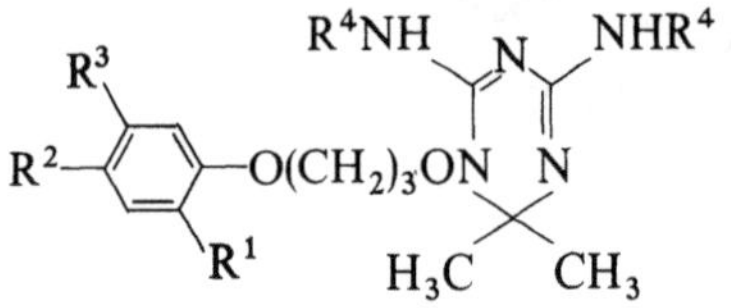

BRL	R^1	R^2	R^3	R^4	Duration in days following implant[a]: Days prepatent (range)	Days survival (range)
51084	Cl	Cl	Cl	H	5.1 (2–12)	21 (18–26)
6231	Cl	Cl	Cl	H	10 (NA)[b]	23.6 (22–27)
6547	Cl	Cl	Cl	$COCH_3$	8.4 (7–10)	23.6 (21–26)
51091	Cl	Cl	H	H	9.6 (8–10)	17.6 (14–25)
6548	Cl	Cl	H	$COCH_3$	25.8 (22–30)	46 (40–50)
7638	H	Cl	Cl	$COCH_3$	>60	>70 (72–>119)

[a] Implants (suprascapular) size 5 × 10 × 3 mm containing 5% drug
[b] Not available

$R^4 = COCH_3$), which protected mice for over 70 days. This compound had earlier shown activity in the owl monkey-*P. falciparum* model (SCHMIDT 1972) and was a diacetyl derivative. A second diacetyl derivative BRL 6548 (L; $R^1 = R^2 = Cl$, $R^3 = H$, $R^4 = COCH_3$) was less active, while the remaining compounds gave no prolongation of protection. All behaved similarly in the standard 4-day test.

IV. Clinical Properties

1. Aryldihydrotriazines

a) Normal Formulations

Drugs including the aryldihydrotriazine, cycloguanil pamoate (embonate), available for prophylaxis and chemotherapy were reviewed by PETERS (1971a). The author suggested that an antifol-sulphonamide combination might prove a most useful prophylactic in the future. This idea has yet to be adopted on any scale and clinical work on aryldihydrotriazines has been noticeably lacking in recent years. Triazine research appears to have been largely replaced by work on quinoline- and phenanthrene-methanols such as mefloquine.

b) Repository Formulations

Repository preparations containing cycloguanil pamoate (CI-501) alone or in combination (CI-564) with acedapsone (CI-556) were comprehensively reviewed by ELSLAGER (1969) (see also Chap. 7). Results from a number of field trials using CI-501 and CI-564 were reviewed by CLYDE (1969) and four situations were suggested for use of the formulations at 4-monthly intervals. These included use as a causal prophylactic for non-immune visitors to malarious areas and in the consolidation phase of eradication programmes. The discomfort in some subjects from the injections and the possibility of induction of resistance appear, in practice, to have retricted their use, despite the fact that CI-564 had some activity against resistant strains.

GUSMÃO and JUAREZ (1970) conducted trials with CI-564 alone or with amodiaquine (10 mg/kg) in 600 children in the Amazon valley of Brazil and concluded that CI-564 could be a practical malaria prophylactic in suitable situations. The dose provided 7.5–7.9 mg/kg CI-564 given i.m. in benzyl benzoate/castor oil. LAING (1971) in trials in the Gambia using CI-564 at similar dose rates found that concomitant oral amodiaquine at the time of each injection (4-monthly intervals) did not materially increase the period of protection. *P. falciparum* suppression was achieved in 90% of the subjects after the first and second injections, and in 100% after the third injection. As there were many refusals for the third round of treatment, its use as a mass prophylactic was considered to be unsuitable.

2. Arylmethoxy- and Aryloxyalkoxy-dihydrotriazines

RIECKMANN et al. (1971) investigated the use of WR 38839 (clociguanil) alone and admixed with sulphadiazine to control the pre-erythrocytic stages of the chloroquine-resistant Vietnam (Marks) strain of *P. falciparum* in human volunteers. Either of the drugs alone failed to prevent development of patent parasitaemia (0.84 g/day WR 38839 and 2 g/day sulphadiazine) 11 days after infection. However, a mixture of 0.28 g WR 38839 and 2 g sulphadiazine prevented the development of parasitaemia during a 60-day follow up period. These findings suggested that a causal prophylactic effect might occur as a result of potentiation between these two drugs.

LAING (1974) conducted hospital trials with clociguanil in Gambian children suffering from acute *P. falciparum* infections. While single oral doses and two daily doses of 3 mg/kg were not fully effective, three daily doses of 3 mg/kg p.o. eradicated asexual parasitaemias within 2 or 3 days, with no toxic side effects. Two daily doses of 0.3 mg/kg clociguanil in conjunction with sulphadimethoxine or sulphafurazole at 3 mg/kg rapidly eliminated asexual parasitaemias. Sulphadimethoxine alone at 3–6 mg/kg was ineffective. There was a sporontocidal effect against *P. falciparum* with the combinations. *P. malariae* trophozoites were sensitive to the drug alone or in combination with a sulphonamide. It was concluded that clociguanil was as effective as pyrimethamine or proguanil, but that rapid excretion precluded single-dose therapy.

CANFIELD and ROZMAN (1974) reported similar findings from unpublished work of Rieckmann and noted that WR 99210 (BRL 6231, XLII), an antifol dihydrotriazine not significantly cross-resistant with pyrimethamine in animal systems, would undergo human trials in 1974. Results of any tests conducted have not been published.

As part of a comprehensive study on the susceptibility of the chloroquine-resistant Vietnam (Marks) strain of *P. falciparum* to a number of antimalarial drugs, WILLERSON et al. (1974) investigated WR 38839 (clociguanil) alone or with sulphadiazine. Treatment for 3 days with doses up to a total of 3.8 g clociguanil in immune or partially immune subjects elicited, at best, RI responses (i.e. clearance of parasitaemia followed by recrudescence). A combination of 0.28 g clociguanil and 2 g sulphadiazine daily for 3 days in five non-immunes resulted in two cures and three RI responses. One partially immune subject was cured. Similar responses were obtained with pyrimethamine plus sulphalene or sulphadiazine.

V. Pharmacology

1. Toxicity and Cardiovascular Effects

Dihydrotriazines are potent inhibitors of folate and dihydrofolate reductases and, as such, may block the conversion of folic acid to its reduced forms vital, inter alia. to the life of bacteria, malaria parasites and mammals. Selective toxicity, therefore, becomes of paramount importance and undue mammalian toxicity can impose severe constraints on the use of what could otherwise be very useful drugs. Concise accounts of the enzyme systems involved are given by ELSLAGER (1974a) and ELSLAGER and DAVOLL (1974).

Repeated oral doses of WR 38839 (clociguanil) to beagle dogs at 5 mg/kg per day for 28 days produced no untoward effects, but higher doses (15–45 mg/kg per day) produced a pattern of toxicity common to other antifols. The toxic effects could be eliminated by simultaneous i.m. administration of folinic acid but not of folic acid (LEE et al. 1976).

A comparison of acute oral toxicities of a number of *N*-oxytriazines using a 4 × daily dose schedule in mice showed that clociguanil was the least toxic (unpublished work from BEECHAM PHARMACEUTICALS). Single-dose oral LD_{50}s in the mouse followed a similar pattern, being >4.6 g/kg for clociguanil, 480 mg/kg for BRL 6231 (XLII), 480 mg/kg for BRL 6547 (diacetyl XLII) and 120 mg/kg for BRL 6548 (L; $R^1 = R^2 = Cl$, $R^3 = H$, $R^4 = COCH_3$). Clociguanil was tolerated by human volunteers at 1440 mg/day for 3 days. Much toxicological information was obtained for this series of compounds (to be published).

NETTLETON et al. (1974) studied the cardiovascular effects of clociguanil and BRL 6231 in dogs and cats. Both compounds showed sympathomimetic effects. BRL 6231 caused a rise in blood pressure and tachycardia, while clociguanil produced a direct effect on adrenoreceptors. Clociguanil showed quinidine-like antiarrhythmic activity, an activity also noted with this compound by workers at the WALTER REED ARMY INSTITUTE OF RESEARCH (unpublished). Pyrimethamine does not exhibit sympathomimetic effects.

RUIZ et al. (1971) reported toxicities for cycloguanil in the mouse, rat and dog. It was more toxic than clociguanil and increased cardiac output in dogs. Like clociguanil, cycloguanil showed antiarrhythmic activity against chloroform-induced arrhythmias in mice. CHEBOTAR (1974), showed that cycloguanil dosed orally to pregnant rats at 25–50 mg/kg on day 1 or 7–13 of gestation produced no embryotoxic or teratogenic effects. It inhibited development of ova during cleavage.

2. Blood Levels

The rapid excretion of clociguanil from man (Sect. IV.2) is paralleled to some extent in the mouse. The longer chain oxydiaminodihydrotriazines BRL 51084 (VIII HBr) and BRL 51091 (XLVII) elicited much lower mouse blood levels than did clociguanil. BRL 6548, however, the diacetyl derivative of BRL 51091, gave rise to improved blood levels similar to those of clociguanil, an effect attributed to the acetylated structure. Table 19 MIZEN (1970) gives blood levels following oral dosing with a couple of s.c. dosing levels for comparison.

Table 19. Concentrations in whole blood following administration of 200 mg/kg drug to mice

BRL	Route	Concentrations in μg/ml – hours after dosing[a]						
		0.25	0.5	1.0	2	4	6	24
50216	p.o.	1.2[b]	0.7	3.7	5.7		3.3	< 0.15
51084	p.o.	0.8[b]	0.58	0.55	1.1		1.4	< 0.1
51091	p.o.	0.38	0.88	0.67	1.8		1.2	< 0.1
51091	s.c.	3.9	4.5	3.4	2.5		2.45	1.6
6548	p.o.	1.12	1.67	4.8	3.7	1.9	1.39	2.48
6548	s.c.	1.33	1.94	3.3	5.4	4.5	5.3	12.8

[a] Microbiological plate assay using *Streptococcus pyogenes* A
[b] 0.17 h after dosing

VI. Other Biological Activities Shown by Dihydrotriazines

The wide variety of biological effects produced by dihydrotriazines has been reviewed by CAPPS et al. (1968). An update of more recent findings is not without interest.

KNIGHT (1981) reported that a number of antimalarial dihydrotriazines of type VI showed excellent activity against *Babesia rodhaini* in mice whereas the closely related arylalkoxy analogues V showed little activity (and, incidentally, little activity against B-strain *P. berghei*). BRL 51091 (XLVII) was particularly active, being 100% effective at 2.5 mg/kg s.c. × 4 in a 4-day suppression test and 99%–100% effective at 1 mg/kg × 4. BRL 51157 (L; $R^1=R^4=H$, $R^2=R^3=Cl$) was very effective down to 2.5 mg/kg s.c. × 4 but the analogue V ($Ar=3,4\text{-}Cl_2C_6H_3$, $n=4$) was totally inactive at 25 mg/kg s.c. × 4.

TAKEDA (1973) claimed that the cycloguanil isomer LI was effective in the therapy of and prophylaxis against *Leucocytozoon* infections in poultry.

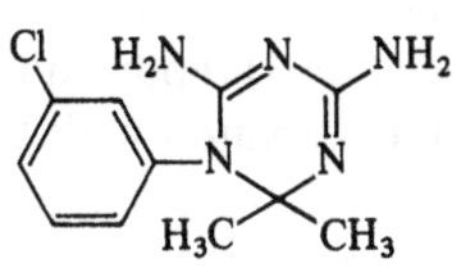

LI

Fig. 17. Chemical structure LI

Good activity against trypanosomiasis in the mouse was reported for a number of bis-dihydrotriazines (XXI), in particular XXI [$X=(CH_2)_6$] as the pamoate salt (BRL 6202). Thus, single doses of 5–12.5 mg/kg s.c. protected mice from *T. brucei* and *T. congolense* infections when given at the time of infection. A single dose of 100 mg/kg protected mice from a *T. congolense* challenge completely at 2 weeks and partially at 6 weeks. BRL 6202, however, provided no prophylactic effects to zebu cattle in a Uganda field trial when exposed to *T. vivax* and *T. congolense* infection (KNIGHT and PONSFORD 1981). It was stated by JAFFE et al. (1969) that dihydrofolate reductase inhibitors did not exert effective antitrypanosomal activity in vivo. This is clearly no longer the case in the light of the foregoing mouse results. McCORMACK and JAFFE (1969) reported that aryldihydrotriazines such as cycloguanil (III) were less active as inhibitors of *T. equiperdum* dihydrofolate reductase than against rat liver reductase. Results from GUTTERIDGE and TRIGG (1969) using a dihydrofolate reductase isolated from *T. rhodesiense* tended to confirm these observations.

KIM et al. (1980) attempted to make a quantitative correlation between the structures of some aryldihydrotriazines (I) (Ar = substituted phenyl), with inhibition of dihydrofolate reductases from bovine liver and murine L5178YR-L_3 tumour cells. Although correlations were deduced, significant deviations were found for some compounds. A comparable study by STEPAN et al. (1977) used a Walker 256 rat tumour reductase.

The antibacterial properties of the aryldihydrotriazines (I) have long been known. WALSH et al. (1977) prepared a series of analogues of I and correlated their in vitro antibacterial activity against *Staphylococcus aureus* and *Escherichia coli* with the physical properties of the various substituted triazines. They reported high parabolic dependence on partition with no significant contribution from electronic or steric terms. The concept was taken further by WOOLDRIDGE (1980) and equations were calculated to fit the results. MAMALIS et al. (1962, 1965a, b) found that many benzyloxydihydrotriazines exhibited improved antimicrobial activity over their corresponding phenyl analogues.

SMITH and his colleagues have continued their attempts to correlate folic acid antagonism and antimicrobial activity with antimalarial activity. Dihydrotriazines clociguanil and BRL 6231 (XLII) were found to behave in a widely different manner from cycloguanil and pyrimethamine (GENTHER and SMITH 1977; GENTHER et al. 1977). A microbiological assay of these compounds using *Streptococcus faecium* was described by SMITH and GENTHER (1976).

One of the antiparasitic activities claimed for cycloguanil is the treatment of cutaneous leishmaniasis (oriental sore). Earlier work was summarised by ELSLAGER (1969). Typical of these studies was the use of the repository pamoate to cure *Leishmania braziliensis* in Panama using a single i.m. dose of 350 mg (WALTON et al. 1968). KURBAN et al. have since (1969) reported improvements in 60% of cases of *L. tropica* infections in Syria and Lebanon with the same drug, while SALEM et al. (1969) observed a 50% cure rate of *L. tropica* in Iraq.

MATTOCK and PETERS (1975) showed that all of the seven substituted *N*-oxytriazines tested were active against *L. mexicana* in a tissue culture model. One of these, BRL 6548 (XLVI; $R^1 = H$, $R^2 = Cl$) was also active against *L. tropica* major P, but not against *L. donovani* HV3. Tissue culture experiments using *L. infantum* LV9 were reported by PETERS et al. (1980a) using a large number of "standard" compounds. Cycloguanil HCl was effective in this test but not clociguanil. PETERS et al. (1980b) showed that some, but not all, antifols were markedly active, unlike sulphonamides and sulphones, against *L. mexicana amazonensis* and *L. major* in tissue culture. Although neither cycloguanil nor clociguanil were active in this system the acetylated dihydrotriazine BRL 6548 showed some activity.

C. Quinazoline and Related Dihydrofolate Reductase Inhibitors

I. 2,4-Diaminoquinazolines

In an effort to develop novel folate antagonists with minimal toxicity and cross-resistance liability, attention was directed in the Parke-Davis laboratories to the synthesis of classical and non-classical quinazoline analogues of folic acid (LII). It was reasoned that the absence of N-5 in reduced forms of such compounds would preclude the formation and interconversion of one-carbon units analogous to the known tetrahydrofolate coenzymes.

The classical quinazoline analogues of folic acid (LIII) (DAVOLL and JOHNSON 1970; BIRD et al. 1970) tested as antimalarials all lacked significant activity with one notable exception. Compound LIII ($X=OH$, $R=CH_3$, $x=2$), which was also the most powerful inhibitor

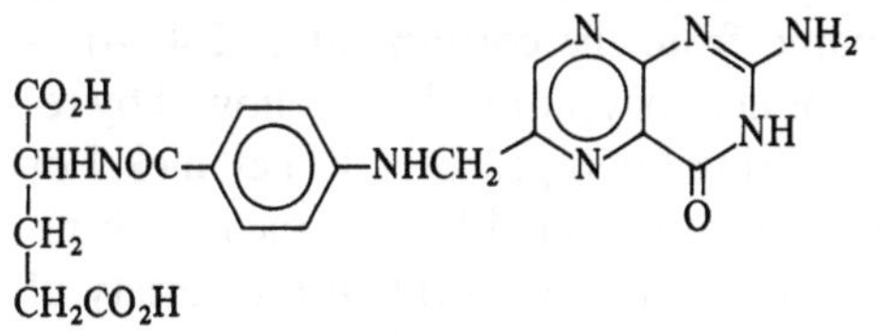

LII

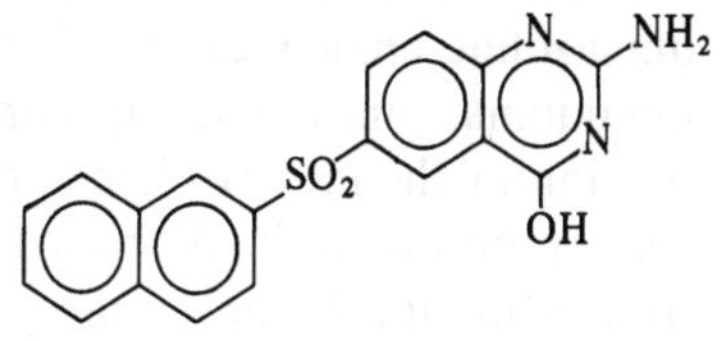

LIV

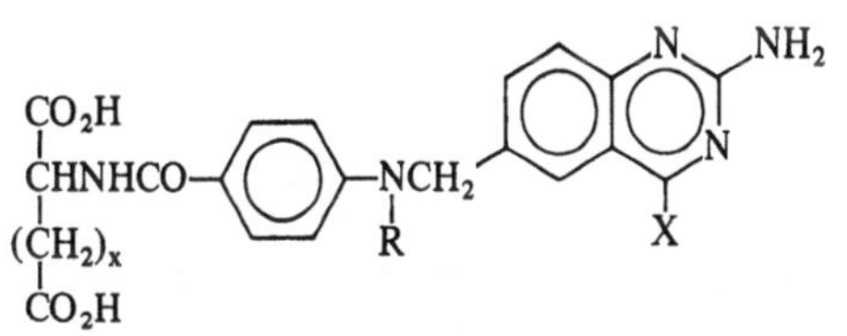

LIII x = 1, 2
R = H, CH_3
X = OH, NH_2

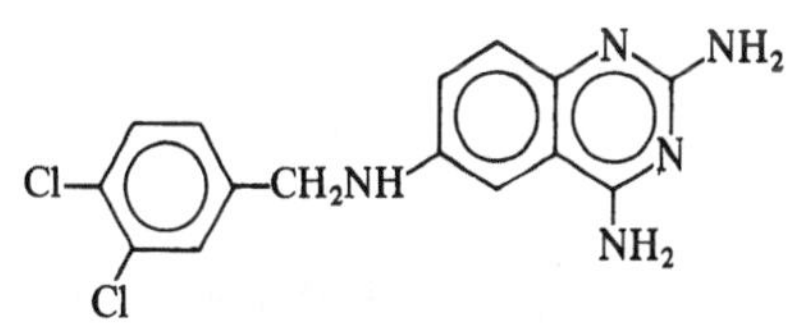

LV

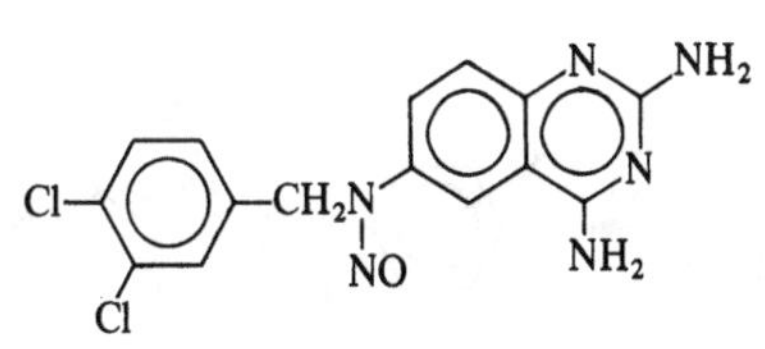

LVI

Fig. 18. Chemical structures LII–LVI

of thymidylate synthetase, showed good oral activity against *P. berghei* infections in mice ($SD_{90}=26$ mg/kg per day, Q=3.0[1]).

When the non-classical quinazoline analogues detailed below were identified 2-amino-4hydroxy and 2-amino-4-mercapto analogues of the prodigious 2,4-diamino-6-thioquinazoline antimalarials were also prepared (HYNES et al. 1974), in the

1 SD_{90} = dose causing a suppression of parasitaemia of 90%. Q = quinine equivalent (the ratio of the SD_{90} of guinine hydrochloride to the SD_{90} of the test substance under comparable experimental conditions)

hope that such configurations would confer greater inhibitory action upon tetrahydrofolate-dependent enzymes such as thymidylate synthetase. Only 2-amino-4-hydroxy-6-(2-naphthylsulfonyl)quinazoline (LIV) possessed appreciable antimalarial effects (curative at 160–640 mg/kg vs *P. berghei* in mice) and it was markedly less active than its 4-amino counterpart.

1. 6-Benzylamino Analogues

One of the early non-classical prototypes (LV) displayed strong antimalarial activities in a variety of experimental infections and was, moreover, effective against lines of *P. berghei* that were 30- to greater than 300-fold resistant to chloroquine, cycloguanil, pyrimethamine or 4,4′-sulphonyldianiline. A variety of synthetic analogues of this system were then prepared (DAVOLL et al. 1972a).

The secondary 2,4-diamino-6-{[benzyl and (heterocyclic)-methyl]amino} quinazoline analogues of LV were prepared from the corresponding 2,4,6-triaminoquinazoline and the appropriate aryl or heterocyclic aldehyde followed by reduction of the intermediate Schiff base utilising hydrogen over Raney nickel or sodium borohydride, N^6-nitroso analogues were prepared by treatment with nitrous acid, and N^6-acyl analogues were available by treatment with a variety of acylating agents. The N^6-alkyl congeners of LV were not available by direct alkylation, and were prepared via the general synthetic route for the diaminoquinazolines as shown in Fig. 19.

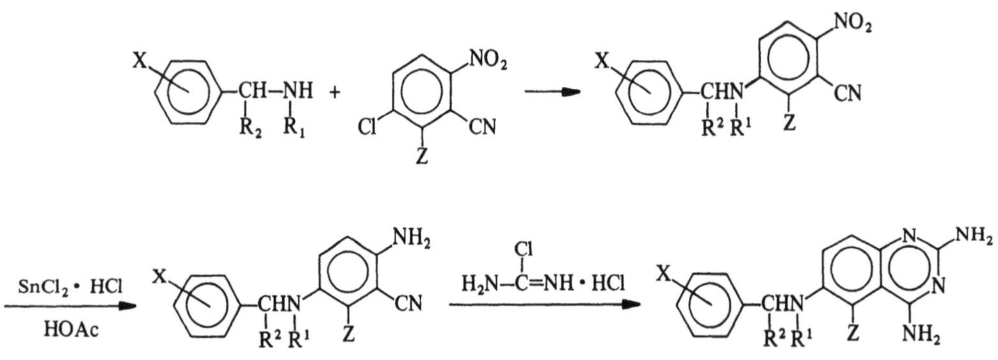

Fig. 19. Scheme

The antimalarial effects of selected analogues are summarised in Table 20 (ELSLAGER and DAVOLL 1974; THOMPSON et al. 1969). The oral antimalarial potency of LV is increased 2- to 12-fold by the insertion of a Cl or CH_3 substituent at position 5. Activity is increased 4- to 70-fold with the introduction of CHO, CH_3 or NO groups at N^6. Model compounds including 2,4-diamino-6-[(3,4-dichlorobenzyl)nitrosamino]quinazoline (LVI) and *N*-(2,4-diamino-6-quinazolinyl)-*N*-(3,4-dichlorobenzyl)formamide were essentially fully as active against chloroquine-, cycloguanil-, and DDS-resistant lines of *P. berghei* in mice as against the parent drug-sensitive lines.

Table 20. Antimalarial and antimetabolite effects of 2,4-diamino-6-[(3,4-dichlorobenzyl) amino] quinazolines

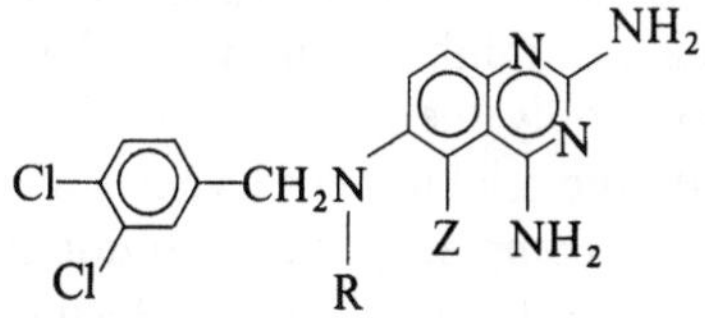

R	Z	*P. berghei* in mice D×6, SD_{90}, mg/kg/day	Quinine equiv.	SC×1 MAD, mg/kg	*S. faecalis* R MIC, FA[a]	ng/ml 5-CHO-FAH_4[a]
H	H	8.5	8.8	40	6	112
H	CH_3	5.1	15	40	2	3
H	Cl	0.7	110	–	1	3
CHO	H	2.1	36	20	8	108
CH_3	H	0.16	470	10	0.3	2
NO	H	0.12	620	10	4	88
CHO	CH_3	0.77	97	30	0.9	18
$(CH_2)_2CH_3$	CH_3	1.7	44	20	–	–
NO	CH_3	2.7	28	20	1	6
Pyrimethamine		0.28	270	10	4	3,100
Trimethoprim		120	0.6	>640	12	70
Cycloguanil · HCl		2.1	35	20	8	11,400

[a] 0.4 ng/ml

The nitroso analogue LVI was approximately 40 times as effective as the parent LV in suppressing infections with the parent sensitive strain of *P. berghei* and approximately ten times as effective in suppressing and curing infections with blood schizonts of *P. cynomolgi*. In addition the repository action of LVI was remarkable, a single intramuscular 50 mg/kg dose providing full protection for at least 105 days against repeated challenges with trophozoites of the simian parasite *P. cynomolgi* (THOMPSON et al. 1970).

Further studies with LVI (SCHMIDT and ROSSAN 1979) showed that its efficacy was compromised by high levels of pyrimethamine resistance and that resistance to the drug developed rapidly. These observations and the results of subacute toxicity studies which showed that LVI produced significant lesion in the adrenals, lymphoid tissue and bone marrow of rats and beagle dogs led to abandonment of further studies with this agent, but stimulated the extensive studies for the search for potent non-toxic analogues described below.

In an effort to clarify the antimetabolite nature of these compounds their inhibitory effects on a bacterial system *S. faecalis* R were examined. This organism is capable of using folic acid (FA) as well as various reduced folates. It is unable to synthesise folate, however, and requires preformed folate, thus allowing precise knowledge of the quantity of folate available to the organism. Inhibition using folic acid as the substrate indicates the overall strength of the inhibitor without providing information as to the nature of the inhibition. The use of 5-formyl tetrahydrofolate (5-CHO-FAH_4) provides some information as to the nature of the inhibition. Successful overcoming of inhibition using the latter substrate may indicate that the inhibition involves only the reduction of folate, or that the inhibition blocks the entry of FA into the cell but permits entry of 5-CHO-FAH_4. Failure of the reduced folate to reverse completely the inhibition may mean (a) that the inhibitor is acting on a site other than reductase, which could be further along the folate pathway or unrelated to folate, or (b) that the inhibitor is blocking transport enzymes necessary for the entry of 5-CHO-FAH_4 into the cell. These triaminoquinazolines exhibited strong inhibitory effects against *S. faecalis* R. The compounds inhibit one or both reduction stages and are competitive with folic acid and 5-formyl-tetrahydrofolate. With folic acid as a substrate, activity was comparable or superior to pyrimethamine, cycloguanil hydrochloride and trimethoprim. Moreover, activity against *S. faecalis* R was only partly reversed by 5-formyltetrahydrofolate, suggesting that these quinazolines, like trimethoprim, function not only as dihydrofolate reductase inhibitors, but also have significant effects either on the folate transport mechanism or elsewhere in the folate cycle. In addition, unlike trimethoprim and cycloguanil hydrochloride, many of the triaminoquinazolines retain some inhibitory effects against *S. faecalis* R even in the presence of 5-formyltetrahydrofolate, adenosine and thymidine, suggesting that they may also exert some activity outside the folate cycle.

2. 6-Benzylamino-5,6,7,8-tetrahydro Analogues

The corresponding 5,6,7,8-tetrahydro quinazoline analogues of LV were prepared from the 2,4,6-triamino-5,6,7,8-tetrahydroquinazolines, which were obtained by direct hydrogenation of the 2,4,6-triaminoquinazolines. The analogue of LV, i.e. LVII, was considerably less potent against *P. berghei* infections than LV. By anal-

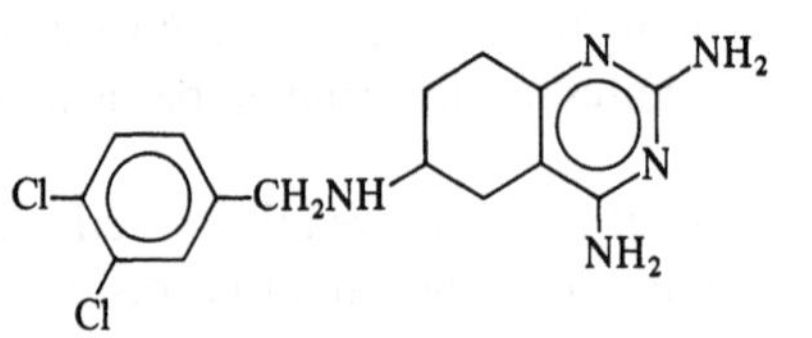

LVII

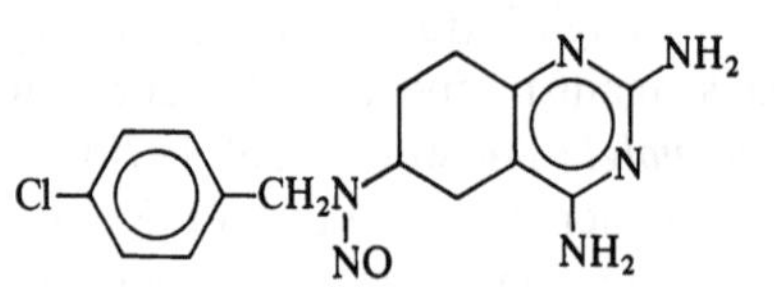

LVIII

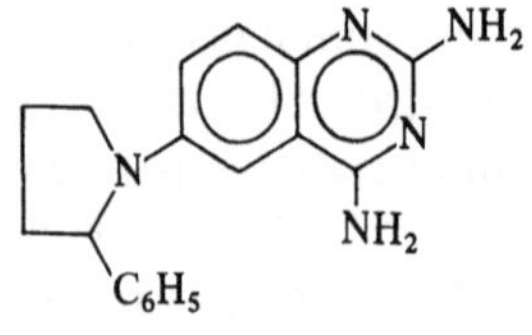

LIX

Fig. 20. Chemical structures LVII–LIX

ogy with the 6-benzyl-aminoquinazolines, antimalarial potency was markedly increased by N^6-nitroso or N^6-acyl substitution. For example LVIII was 910 times as potent as quinine orally and compared favourably with pyrimethamine when given subcutaneously (ELSLAGER and DAVOLL 1974).

3. 2,4-Diamino-6-(heterocyclic)quinazolines

A series of 2,4-diamino-6-(heterocyclic)quinazolines was prepared (ELSLAGER et al. 1972 a) proceeding from the reaction of 5-chloro-2-nitrobenzonitrile and the requisite saturated heterocycle to the corresponding 5-(heterocyclic)-2-nitrobenzonitrile. Reduction then provided the 2-amino-5-(heterocyclic)benzonitriles which were cyclised with chloroformamidine hydrochloride to the 2,4-diamino-6-(pyrrolidinyl), piperidino and piperazinyl) quinazolines. Optimal oral antimalarial activity in this series was observed with LIX, which was 213 times as potent as quinine.

4. N[1]-(Quinazolinyl)-N,N-Dialkylformamidines as Solubilised 2,4-Diaminoquinazoline Antimalarials

Many of the 2,4-diaminoquinazoline antimalarials are relatively insoluble in aqueous systems, and there are indications that some of these agents are poorly absorbed when administered orally. In an effort to develop more soluble derivatives with advantageous absorption properties it was discovered that certain *N'*-[6-(benzylamino)quinazolinyl]-*N,N*-dimethylformamidines not only exhibited improved solubility characteristics but also retained potent antimalarial properties. For example LX proved to be approximately 392 times as active as quinine ($SD_{90} = 0.19$ mg/kg per day) against *P. berghei* infections by the drug-diet technique. Representative formamidine derivatives of several of the most promising 2,4-diamino-6-thioquinazolines (Sect. I.7) were also prepared and each exhibited potent antimalarial activity in mice, although none was more potent than the parent 2,4-diaminoquinazolines (ELSLAGER and WERBEL, to be published).

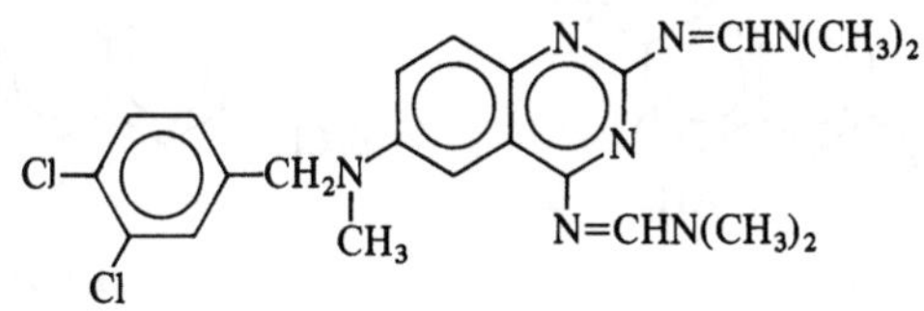

LX

Fig. 21. Chemical structure LX

5. 2,4-Diamino-6-[(anilino)methyl]quinazolines

These so-called reverse analogues of LV were prepared with the idea that replacement of the highly polar *N*-(*p*-aminobenzoyl)-L-aspartic acid moiety of the classical

Table 21. Antimalarial and antimetabolite effects of 2,4-diamino-6-[(*p*-chloroanilino)methyl]-quinazolines

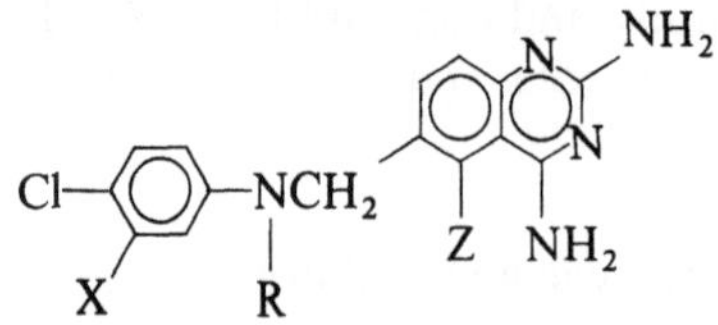

X	R	Z	*P. berghei* in mice: D × 6, mg/kg/day	*P. berghei* in mice: Quinine equiv.	*P. berghei* in mice: SC × 1, mg/kg MCD	*P. berghei* in mice: SC × 1, mg/kg MAD	*S. faecalis* R MIC, ng/ml FA[a]
H	H	H	1.9	39	160	40	3
H	H	Cl	–	–	20	2.5	–
H	H	CH_3	0.088	846	10	5	–
Cl	H	H	0.92	81	80	40	1
Cl	H	Cl	–	–	20	10	–
Cl	H	CH_3	0.33	226	10	2.5	–
Cl	NO	H	0.25	298	160	20	1
Cl	NO	Cl	–	–	80	20	–
Cl	NO	CH_3	1.15	65	10	5	–
Cl	CHO	Cl	–	–	20	5	–
Cl	CHO	CH_3	–	–	20	10	–
Cl	CH_3	H	–	–	80	40	–
Pyrimethamine			0.28	270	40	10	4

[a] 0.4 ng/ml

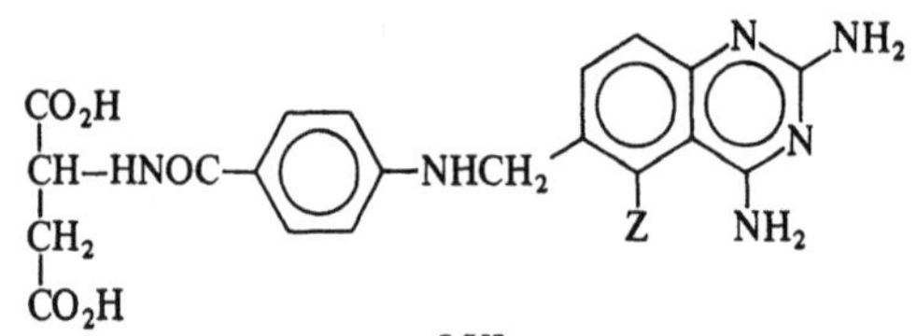

LXI

Z = H, CH_3, Cl

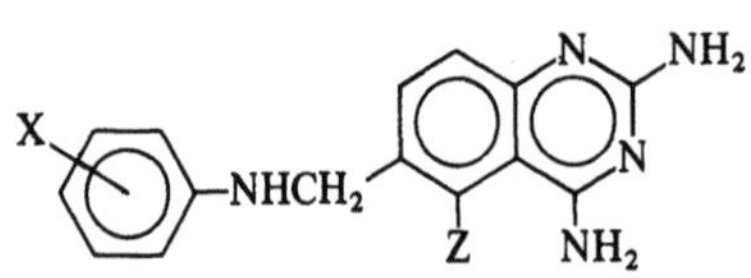

LXII

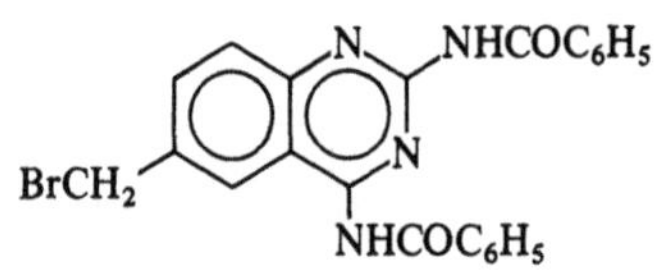

LXIII

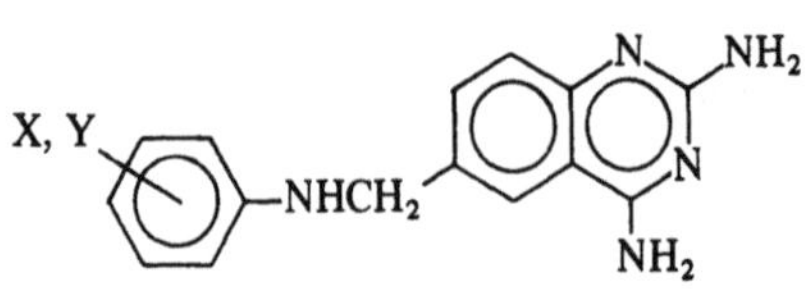

LXIV

a) X, Y = 4–Cl
b) X, Y = 3, 4–Cl_2

Fig. 22. Chemical structures LXI–LXIV

quinazoline antifolates such as LXI with more lipohilic substituents might confer useful antimalarial properties.

Reductive alkylation of the corresponding 2,4-diamino-6-cyanoquinazoline provided LXII, which were converted to the *N*-nitroso and *N*-acyl analogues. The corresponding *N*-alkyl analogues were more difficult and were finally obtained via the blocked 6-bromomethyl derivative LXIII. As a class the 2,4-diamino-6-[(anilino)methyl]quinazolines displayed striking antimalarial activity. Selected analogues are shown in Table 21 (ELSLAGER 1974a).

Among them LXIVa, b, were four to nine times as active as LV orally against *P. berghei* in mice. Again antimalarial potency was enhanced by 5-CH_3 or N-NO substitution, and three such analogues ranged from 226–846 times as potent as quinine.

6. 2,4-Diamino-6-(aryloxy)quinazolines

Oxygen and sulphur bioisosteres of LV such as LXV and LXVI had much reduced antimalarial activity. Potent antimalarial activity was, however, restored when the methylene bridge in LXV was removed. Although several of these aryloxyquinazolines possessed noteworthy antimalarial properties, none was markedly superior to LV (ELSLAGER et al. 1972b).

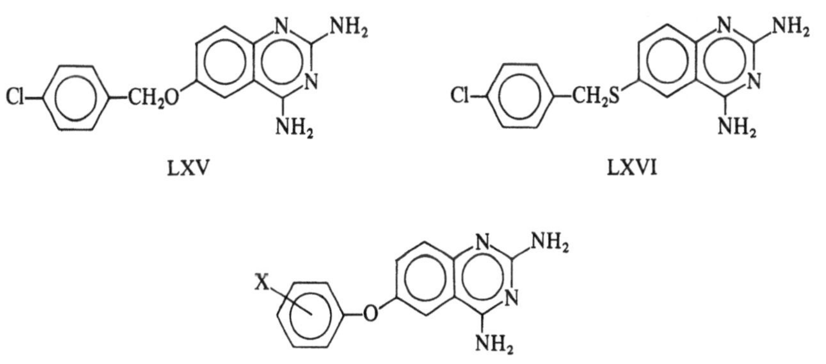

LXV LXVI LXVII

Fig. 23. Chemical structures LXV–LXVII

7. 6-Arylthio, Sulphinyl and Sulphonyl Analogues

Replacement of the oxygen in LXVII with sulphur led to a series of compounds with exceptional antimalarial properties (ELSLAGER et al. 1978, 1979, 1980). A veriety of 2,4-diamino-6[(aryl and heterocyclic)thio, sulphinyl and sulphonyl]-quinazolines (LXVIII) were more potent than quinine against a normal drug-sensitive strain of *P. berghei* in mice. The vast majority displayed, moreover, activity comparable with or superior to cycloguanil or pyrimethamine. Generally the correlation of the oxidation state of the sulphur with potency was $SO_2 > S \geqq SO$. In the 2,4-diamino-5-chloro-6-[(2-naphthyl)thio, sulphinyl and sulphonyl]-quinazoline series, however, this phenomenon was reversed, and potency decreased markedly as the oxidation state increased, possibly due to excessive steric hindrance.

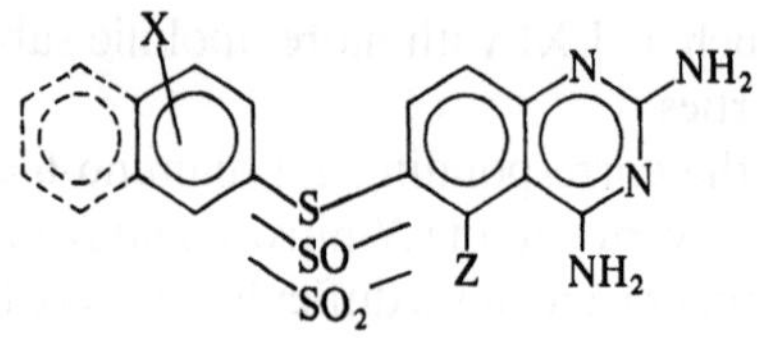

LXVIII

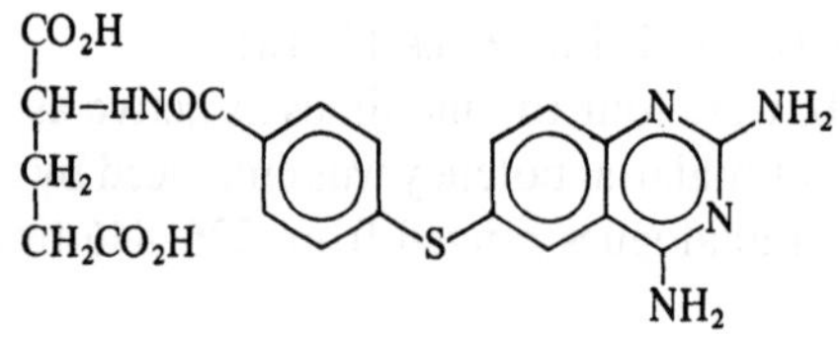

LXIX

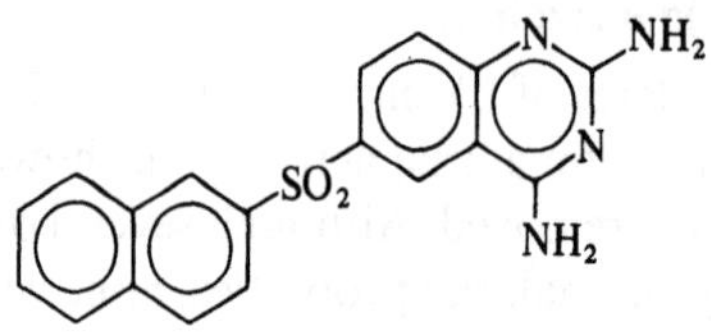

LXX

Fig. 24. Chemical structures LXVIII–LXX

Table 22. Oral effects of 2,4-diamino-6-thioquinazolines against sensitive and drug-resistant lines of *P. berghei* in mice

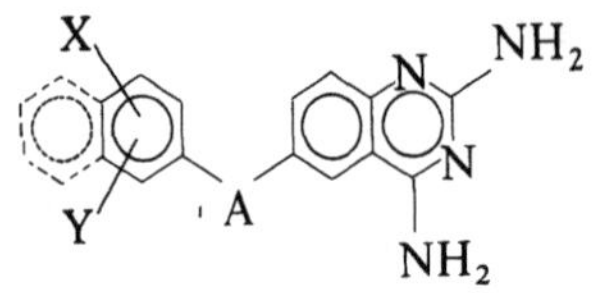

X, Y-Ar	A	Regimen	Q (SD_{75})	SD_{90}, mg/kg/day P	C	T	S	Cross-resistance C	T	S
4-ClC_6H_4	S	D×6	493	0.4	0.3	–	2.2	0	–	6
		D×6	150	0.6	–	2.3	–	–	4	–
3,4-$Cl_2C_6H_3$	S	G×3	482	0.2	<0.4	<0.4	0.8	0	0	4
4-$(CH_3)_2NC_6H_4$	S	G×3	188	0.8	<1.6	–	–	0	–	–
		G×3	169	0.8	–	0.9	1.1	–	0	<2
4-BrC_6H_4	S	G×3	>174	<0.4	<1.6	<1.6	<1.6	<4	<4	<4
4-BrC_6H_4	SO_2	G×3	>256	<0.4	<1.6	<1.6	<1.6	<3	<3	<3
4-FC_6H_4	SO_2	G×3	723	0.2	0.1	–	–	0	–	–
		G×3	830	0.2	–	0.6	1.0	–	3	6
2-$C_{10}H_7$	S	G×3	155	1.2	<1.6	<1.6	2.3	0	0	2
		G×3	352	0.6	–	–	2.8	–	–	5
2-$C_{10}H_7$	SO	G×3	152	0.8	0.2	0.1	–	0	0	–
		G×3	214	0.7	–	–	2.1	–	–	3
2-$C_{10}H_7$	SO_2	G×3	60	2.2	<1.6	2.4	2.9	0	0	<2
			250	0.8	<1.6	–	–	0	–	–

Table 23. Curative effects of 2,4-diamino-6-(thio sulphinyl, and sulphonyl) quinazolines against resistant *P. falciparum* in the *Aotus* monkey

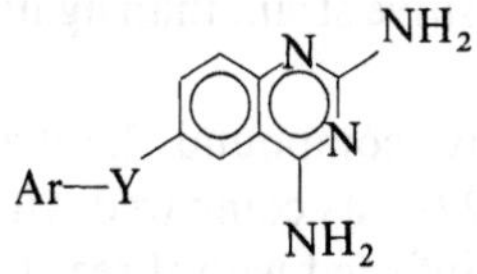

Ar	X	Y	mg/kg/day × 7 required for > 50% cures of infections with strains:	
			Malayan Camp-CH/Q; C–S, PYR–R	Vietnam Oak Knoll; C–R, PYR–S
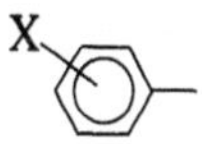	4-Cl	-S-	5.0	0.31
	4-N$(CH_3)_2$	-S-	2.5	1.25
WR 159412	3-CF_3	-S-	0.39	0.098
	3-CF_3	-SO_2-	1.56	0.39
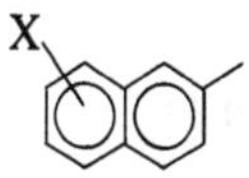	H	-S-	3.125	1.56
	H	-SO-	0.78	0.39
WR 158122	H	-SO_2-	0.39	0.025
Quinine			80	40
Chloroquine			5.0	> 20
Pyrimethamine			> 2.5[a]	0.6

[a] MTD

The analogous classical antagonist LXIX lacked appreciable antimalarial effects in mice (WERBEL et al. 1980).

The 2,4-diamino-6-[(aryl)thio, sulphinyl and sulphonyl]-quinazolines displayed potent activity when given orally by gavage for 3 or 4 days or continuously by drug-diet for 6 days to mice infected with a normal drug-sensitive strain of *P. berghei*. Among them, 15 compounds produced 70%–90% suppression of parasitaemia at daily oral doses of 0.08–2.2 mg/kg, thus ranging from 60 to 830 times as potent as quinine hydrochloride (Table 22)
The compounds also proved to be phenomenal folate antagonists, causing 50% inhibition of *S. faecalis* R at drug concentrations ranging from 0.2–2.0 ng/ml. Nine thioquinazolines which had demonstrated outstanding activity against normal drug-sensitive strains of *P. berghei* in mice were examined against drug-resistant lines. They displayed little or no cross-resistance with chloroquine, negligible cross-resistance with cycloguanil and < 2–6-fold cross-resistance with DDS.

Seven of the thioquinazolines were evaluated against the chloroquine-susceptible, pyrimethamine-resistant Malayan Camp-CH/Q and the chloroquine-resistant, pyrimethamine-susceptible Vietnam Oak Knoll strains of *P. falciparum* in the *Aotus trivirgatus* owl monkey model (SCHMIDT 1979 a) (Table 23).

All but one demonstrated high activity against infections with both strains. However, each compound was significantly more active against infections with the pyrimethamine-sensitive strain than against infections with the pyrimethamine-resistant strain.

The most active compound, 2,4-diamino-6-(2-naphthylsulphonyl)-quinazoline LXX (WR 158122) was compared with quinine, chloroquine and pyrimethamine in owl monkeys infected with three strains of *P. falciparum* and two strains of *P. vivax* (Table 24). Against *P. falciparum* infections, the CD_{90} of LXX for each of

Table 24. Curative effects of quinine, chloroquine, pyrimethamine, and WR 158122 against sensitive and drug-resistant strains of *P. falciparum* and *P. vivax* in owl monkeys

Strain	Curative dose – mg base/kg body wt. administered orally once daily for 7 days			
	Quinine	Chloroquine	Pyrimethamine	WR 158122
P. falciparum				
Malayan Camp-CH/Q	>20; <40 R I	>5; <10 R I	>2.5[a] R III	0.39
Vietnam Oak Knoll	80 R III	>2×20 R III	ca. 0.15 S	0.098
Vietnam Smith	>80 R III	>20 R III	>2.5[a] R III	>6.25
P. vivax				
New Guinea Chesson	40 S	2.5 S	0.625 S	0.39
Vietnam Palo Alto	40 S	2.5 S	>2.5[a] R III	6.25

[a] MTD

the three strains was: Vietnam Oak Knoll (pyrimethamine-sensitive, chloroquine-resistant), 0.098 mg/kg per day; Malayan Camp-CH/Q (chloroquine-sensitive, pyrimethamine-resistant), 0.39 mg/kg per day; and Vietnam Smith (quinine-, chloroquine- and pyrimethamine-resistant), >6.25 mg/kg per day. Against *P. vivax* the drug cured the pyrimethamine-susceptible New Guinea Chesson strain at 0.39 mg/kg per day and the pyrimethamine-resistant Vietnam Palo Alto strain at 6.25 mg/kg per day.

As with other folate antagonists including cycloguanil and pyrimethamine resitance to WR 158122 is easily induced. A rapid evolution of resistance to the drug occurred, for example, when infections with the Malayan Camp and Oak Knoll strains of *P. falciparum* and the Chesson and Palo Alto strains of *P. vivax* were exposed to subcurative doses. Recent observations utilising the related 2,4,6-triaminoquinazolines showed that they act synergistically with sulphones and sulpho-

Table 25. The influence of sulphadiazine on the capacity of WR 158122 to cure established infections with various strains of *P. falciparum* and *P. vivax* in owl monkeys

Strain	CD_{90} WR 158122 daily oral dose (mg/kg × 7)	
	Alone	With 5 mg/kg sulphadiazine × 7 [a]
P. falciparum		
Malayan Camp-CH/Q	0.39	0.025
Vietnam Oak Knoll	0.098	0.00156
Vietnam Smith	> 6.25	0.39
P. vivax		
New Guinea Chesson	0.39	–
Vietnam Palo Alto	6.25	0.098

[a] No development of resistance in > 200 monkeys

namides, and that the likelihood of resistance development is diminished when combination therapy is utilised. Therefore the effect of adding sulphadiazine to the WR 158122 regimen was examined in monkeys infected with the Malayan Camp, Vietnam Oak Knoll and Vietnam Smith strains of *P. falciparum* and the Vietnam Palo Alto strain of *P. vivax* (SCHMIDT 1979 b) (Table 25).

Dose levels of sulphadiazine of 0.31, 1.25, 5 and 20 mg/kg administered once daily for seven consecutive days were studied in the combination regimens. Control studies showed that even doses of 80 mg/kg of this sulphonamide alone effected no more than a transitory depression of the parasitaemia. However, when used in combination, optimal benefits were achieved with 5-mg/kg doses. The data are summarised in Table 25. The activity of the quinazoline against infections with the various strains of parasite is increased from 16- to 64-fold by the addition of 5 mg/kg sulphadiazine. Of greatest note is the effect of the combination regimen on treatment of infections with strains such as the Smith, which are fully resistant to treatment with the normally tolerated doses of pyrimethamine, chloroquine and quinine and cannot be cured regularly with the maximally tolerated dose of pyrimethamine, 2.5 mg/kg daily, combined with sulphadiazine in daily doses of 5.0 mg/kg. SCHMIDT has indicated that infections with this strain present perhaps the greatest challenge to new blood schizontocidal drugs of any strain of *P. falciparum* examined in the owl monkey model.

Moreover, the administration of sulphadiazine with WR 158122 completely blocked emergence of parasites resistant to the quinazoline. This was accomplished at a dose less than 1/50th that employed for treatment of acute bacterial infections in man when compared on a milligram per kilogram basis, so that human tolerance should not be questioned.

The outstanding properties of WR 158122 in experimental models strongly suggested that it should be tested in man. Thorough evaluation of acute and subacute toxicities in rats and beagle dogs showed acceptable levels of tolerability in both hosts. Tolerance evaluation in normal human volunteers indicated that the drug in doses up to 1.3 g daily for 3 days produced no untoward reactions. The therapeutic activity of WR 158122 was studied in eight subjects infected with a fully drug-susceptible Uganda I strain of *P. falciparum*. The drug was given for three consecutive days. Daily doses of 20.0 mg in one subject and 75.0 mg in two were without effect on parasitaemia. Daily doses of 250 mg resulted in temporary clearance of parasitaemia in three of three patients, with recrudescences 9, 11 and 16 days post-treatment. Daily doses of 1,000 mg cured one patient and resulted in temporary clearance of parasitaemia with recrudescence in 11 days in another. Thus WR 158122 was significantly less active in man infected with a drug-susceptible strain of *P. falciparum* than would have been anticipated from the performance of the drug in primates (see SCHMIDT 1979 b).

Brief studies utilising a microbiological assay for blood levels of WR 158122 indicated poor and erratic absorption from the gastrointestinal tract of humans. Further studies to substantiate this shortcoming and to address its solution have not appeared. Such an effort is required to determine whether the remarkable activity of this agent against human plasmodial infections in experimental models can be replicated in man.

8. 6-Arylthio-5,6,7,8-tetrahydro Analogues

The tetrahydro analogue LXXI of LXX has been prepared (Shapiro, unpublished data) and has been demonstrated to be a potent antimalarial agent as well as a potent folic acid antagonist. It was shown that, when administered with LXX, greater than additive chemotherapeutic effects of the two drugs was evident in mice with *P. berghei* infections (KINNAMON et al. 1976). The drugs were presumed to be acting synergistically by affecting two different sites in the folic acid metabolic pathway. Furthermore, both sites are believed to be at a location other than the incorporation of PABA into folic acid.

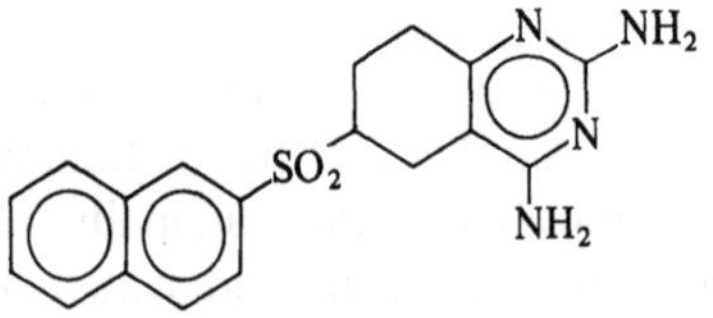

LXXI

Fig. 25. Chemical structure LXXI

9. 2,4-Diamino-6-quinazolinesulphonamides

Replacement of the -CH_2NH- linkage of the 2,4-diamino-6-[(benzyl)amino]-quinazolines with a variety of alternative biospacers such as -NH-, -CH_2CH_2-, -CH=CH-, -CONH-, -S-N=N-, -SO_2NH-, -N=N- and -NHCSNH- generally resulted in a marked lowering or complete loss of antimalarial activity. The 2,4-diamino-6-quinazolinesulphonamides, yowever, were an exception to the rule (ELSLAGER et al., to be published).

Table 26. Antimalarial and antimetabolite effects of 2,4-Diaminoquinazoline-6-sulphonamides

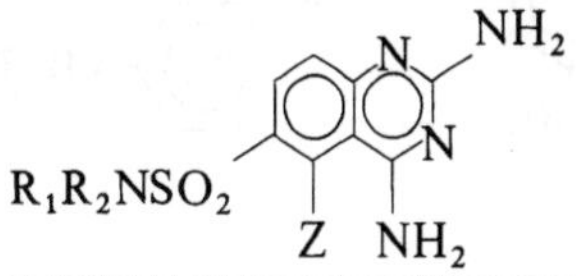

R_1R_2N	Z	*P. berghei* in mice: Route × days	Quinine equiv.	SC × 1, mg/kg: MCD	MAD	*S. faecalis* R MIC, ng/ml FA
NH_2	H	D × 6	0.5	> 640	> 640	1,720
$N(CH_3)_2$	H	SC × 4	11	320	20	2
$N(CH_3)_2$	Cl	–	–	160	40	–
$N(C_2H_5)_2$	H	G × 4	> 7.4	80	80	2
$N(C_2H_5)_2$	Cl	–	–	160	160	–
$N[(CH_2)_2CH_3]_2$	H	D × 6	0.5	> 640	> 640	8
$NH(CH_2)_3CH_3$	H	D × 6	6.9	–	–	14
NHC_6H_3-3, 4-Cl_2	H	–	–	320	80	–
$NCH_3CH_2C_6H_5$	H	D × 6	4.3	–	–	2

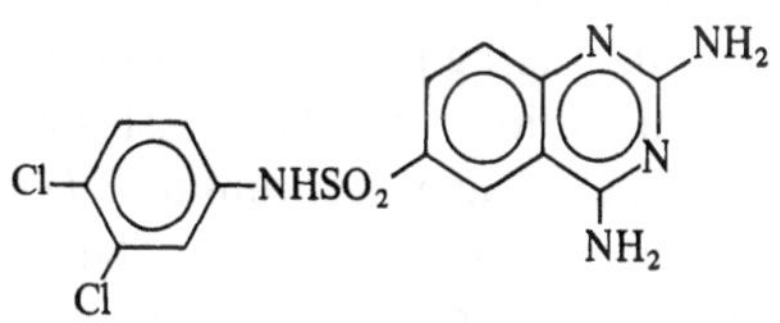

LXXII

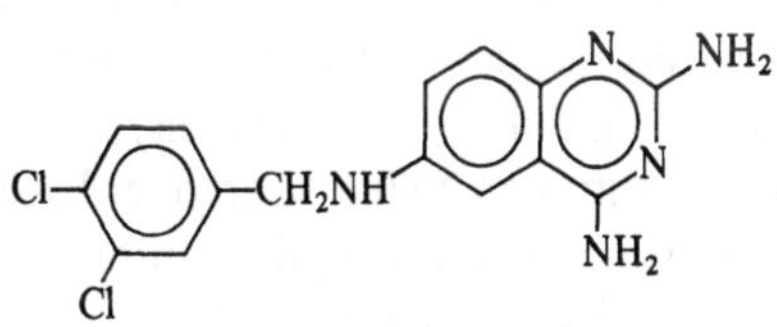

LXXIII

Fig. 26. Chemical structures LXXII and LXXIII

Strangely, antimalarial and antimetabolite effects within this series were quite the antithesis of those observed with the 2,4-diamino-6[(benzyl)amino]quinazolines (Table 26). Thus oral and parenteral antimalarial potency was optimal among lower *N*-mono and *N,N*-dialkyl derivatives (Q = 6.9–11; MAD = 20–160 mg/kg) and diminished with 5-substitution. Moreover, LXXII, a bioisostere of LXXIII proved to be less active than the simple *N,N*-dimethyl-6-quinazolinesulphonamides.

Although as a class the *N*-substituted-2,4-diaminoquinazoline-6-sulphonamides were highly active against *S. faecalis* R (MIC = 2–14 ng/ml), these results could not be correlated with antimalarial potency.

10. Pyrrolo[3,2-f]quinazoline-1,3-diamines

Based on the hypothesis that the activity of the quinazoline types against cycloguanil and pyrimethamine-resistant plasmodia may be related to the inhibition of tetrahydrofolate coenzymes within the interconversion cycle, further structural modifications were sought which would mimic the structure of these coenzymes and forestall the formation and interconversion of one-carbon derivatives al-

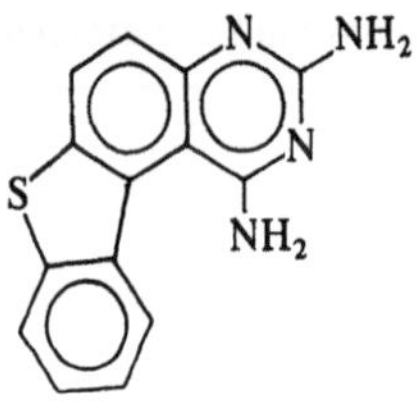

LXXIV

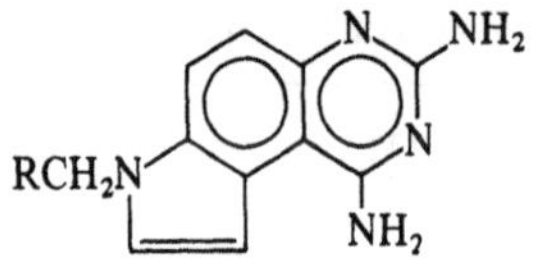

LXXV

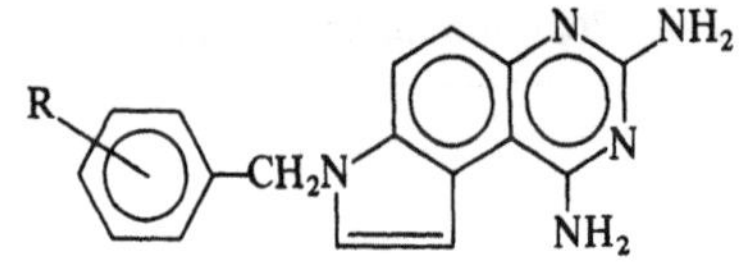

LXXVI

R
a) H
b) 4–OCH_3
c) 2, 5–diCH_3

Fig. 27. Chemical structures LXXIV–LXXVI

lied with the tetrahydrofolate coenzymes. The fused prototype [1] benzothieno [3,2-f]quinazoline-1,3-diamine (LXXIV) and the corresponding sulphone were prepared based on this rationale and found, however, to be devoid of antimalarial activity (JOHNSON et al. 1977).

In view of this, the preliminary reports of antimalarial activity among a series of pyrrolo[3,2-f]quinazoline-1,3-diamines (LXXV) are indeed exciting.

In particular LXXVI a–c were shown to be active against *P. cynomolgi* infection in rhesus monkeys at CD_{50} doses respectively of 0.1 mg/kg per day, 0.316 mg/kg per day and 1.0 mg/kg per day upon oral administration for 7 days (AMERICAN HOME PRODUCTS 1978). Moreover LXXVI a, c were active against strains of *P. berghei* resistant to chloroquine, sulphones, cycloguanil and pyrimethamine. The data reported also indicate a rather narrow spread between toxic dose and antimalarial active dose mice, and it will be most interesting to note whether future efforts can separate satisfactorily these factors to achieve a useful drug.

II. Ring Aza Analogues

1. 2,4-Diaminopyrido[2,3-d]pyrimidines

Byanalogy with the 2,4-diaminoquinazolines, the absence of N-5 in reduced forms of the pyrido[2,3-d]pyrimidines was considered as a potential block to the formation and interconversion of one-carbon derivatives allied with the FAH_4 coenzymes. Thus the non-classical 2,4-diamino-6[(benzyl)amino]pyrido[2,3-d]pyrimidine antifolates were prepared utilising the scheme outlined in (Fig. 28) (DAVOLL et al. 1972b).

Neither NH analogue (LXXVII showed significant antimalarial activity. The nitroso derivative LXXVIII, however, displayed oral activity against *P. berghei* infections in mice (Q = 6.2), but the active dose was 100 times greater than the SD_{90} of the 8-deaza analogue, i.e. 2,4-diamino-6-[(3,4-dichlorobenzyl)nitrosamino]-quinazoline. The pyrido[2,3-*d*]-pyrimidines LXXVII and LXXVIII were also less potent inhibitors of *S. faecalis* R (MIC = 29–50 ng/ml) than the corresponding quinazolines (MIC = 4–13 ng/ml), but this relatively small potency differential could not explain the large variation in antimalarial effects.

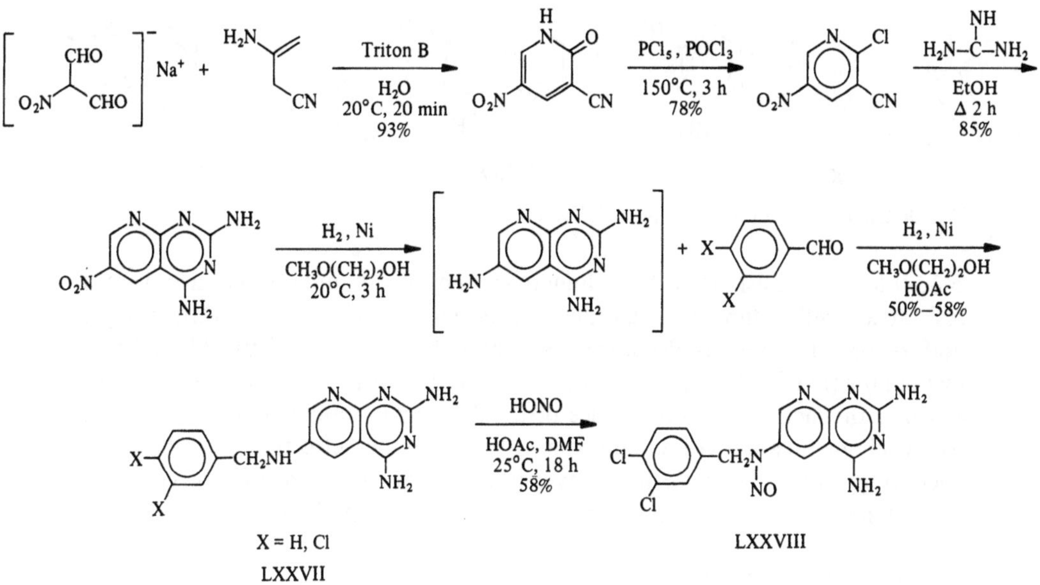

Fig. 28. Scheme including chemical structures LXXVII and LXXVIII

The corresponding 2,4-diamino-6-[(anilino)methyl]pyrido[2,3-*d*]-pyrimidines LXXIX were also prepared but, unlike their deaza (quinazoline) analogues, no appreciable activity against *P. berghei* infections in mice was apparent upon single s.c. administration of 40–60 mg/kg.

2. 2,4-Diaminopyrido[3,2-d]pyrimidines

The 2,4-diaminopyrido[3,2-d]pyrimidine ring system (the 5-aza-quinazoline) was also substituted for the 2,4-diaminoquinazoline moiety in the quinazoline antifolate structures. Several of the 2,4-diamino-6-[(aryl)thio, pyrido[3,2-d]pyrimidines (LXXX) exhibited strong suppressive activity against *P. berghei* infections in mice in single s.c. doses of 20–640 mg/kg. The most potent analogue cured seven of ten mice at 80 mg/kg although, in general, potency was below that of the corresponding 2,4-diamino-6-[(aryl)thio]quinazolines. Strangely, oxidation of the sulphur to the sulphinyl and sulphonyl analogues markedly reduced antimalarial efficacy (ELSLAGER 1974 b).

The 2,4,6-triaminopyrido[3,2-d]pyrimidines (LXXXI), however, exhibited generally high antimalarial activity and several compounds, including 2,4-diamino-6-[3,4-dichlorobenzyl)methylaminol]pyrido[3,2-d]pyrimidine, *N*-(2,4-diaminopyrido[3,2-d]pyrimidin-6-yl)-*N*-(3,4-dichlorobenzyl)formamide, and 2,4-diamino-6-[(p-chlorobenzyl)-isopropylamino]pyrido[3,2-d]pyrimidine, were more active against trophozoite-induced *P. berghei* in mice than the corresponding quinazoline analogues.

In tests orally against sensitive and drug-resistant lines of *P. berghei* in mice 2,4-diamino-6-[(*p*-chlorobenzyl)propylamino]pyrido-[3,2-*d*] pyrimidine (LXXXI, X= 4-Cl, R=Pr) was fully active against the chloroquine-resistant line, but showed

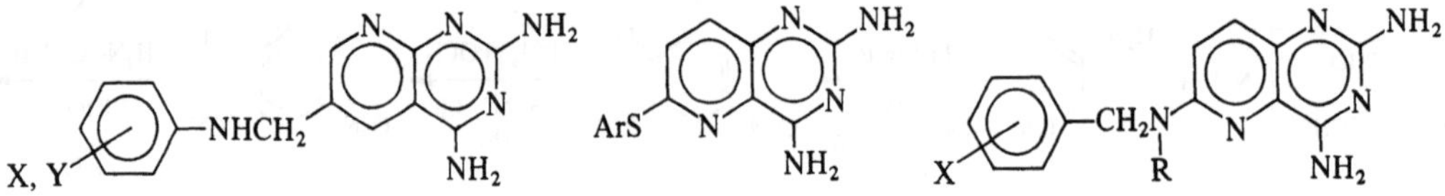

LXXIX LXXX LXXXI

Fig. 29. Chemical structures LXXIX–LXXXI

> 13-fold cross-resistance with cycloguanil and pyrimethamine and fourfold cross-resistance with dapsone. 2,4-Diamino-6-[(*m*-bromobenzyl)methylamino]pyrido[3,2-d]-pyrimidine was also cross-resistant with cycloguanil (fourfold) and pyrimethamine (fivefold). These results were believed to be in accord with the hypothesis that the lack of cross-resistance of the 2,4-diaminoquinazoline antimalarials with cycloguanil and pyrimethamine may be due to their effects against the FAH_4 coenzymes within the folate interconversion cycle. Such one-carbon units could be formed in the case of the 2,4,6-triaminopyrido[3,2-d]pyrimidine.

3. 2,4-Diamino-6-(benzyl and pyridylmethyl)-5,6,7,8-tetrahydropyrido[4,3-d]pyrimidines

A variety of 2,4-diamino-6-(benzyl and pyridylmethyl)-5,6,7,8-tetrahydropyrido[4,3-d]pyrimidines related to the 2,4-diamino-5,6,7,8-tetrahydroquinazolines (LVII) and the 2,4-diaminopyrido[2,3-d]pyrimidines (LXXVII) were prepared in a three-step sequence from *N*-cyanoethyl-*N*-cyanopropylamine (ELSLAGER et al. 1972c). Eight of these were more active than quinine when administered orally to mice infected with *P. berghei*. The most promising member of the series (LXXXII), was approximately 19 times as active as quinine and twice as potent as LV. This structural class also showed moderate to strong inhibotory effects against *S. faecalis R*. Structure LXXXII as well as the 3-chlorophenyl and 2,6-dichlorophenyl analogues produced 50% inhibition at concentrations fo 1–16 ng/ml, and were thus equipotent with or more potent than pyrimethamine, trimethoprim, cycloguanil hydrochloride and LV.

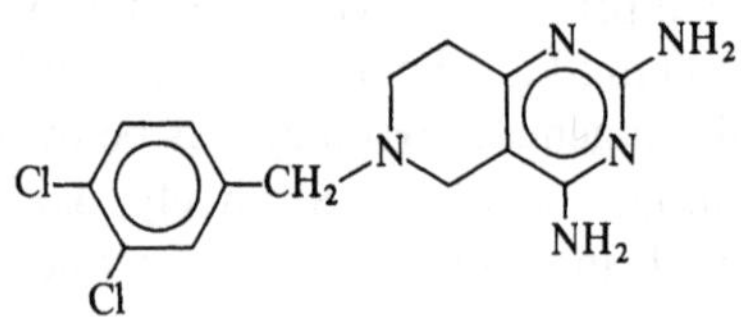

LXXXII

Fig. 30. Chemical structure LXXXII

4. 2,4-Diaminopteridines

A variety of non-classical pteridine-2,4-diamine antifolates, such as 6,7-diphenyl-2,4-pteridinediamine, 6,7-bis(1-methylethyl)-2,4-pteridinediamine and 6-(2-methylphenyl)-2,4,7-pteridinetriamine, possess appreciable activity against experimental malaria infections (THOMPSON and WERBEL 1972). However, cross-resistance with cycloguanil and pyrimethamine is generally present among this class of antimetabolites.

Moreover, tetrahydrohomopteroic acid (LXXXIII), an analogue of folic acid acontaining the pteridine ring but not the glutamic acid side chain, has been reported to be effective against both pyrimethamine-sensitive and -resistant strains of *P. cynomolgi* in rhesus monkeys (KISLIUK et al. 1967).

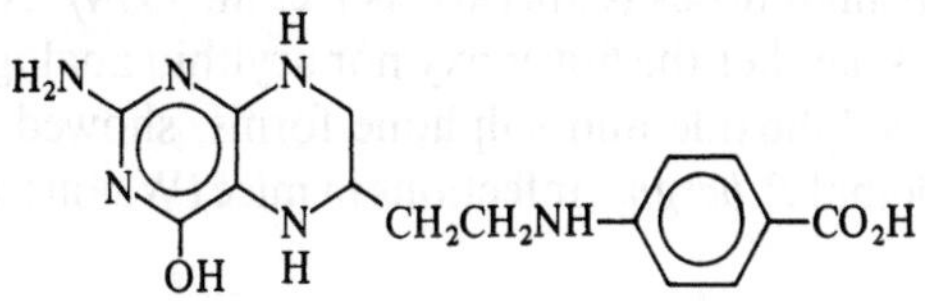

LXXXIII

Fig. 31. Chemical structure LXXXIII

A series of 6[[(aryl and aralkyl)amino]methyl]-2,4-pteridine-diamines (LXXXIV), the direct pteridine analogues of the potent quinazoline antifols, was therefore prepared for antimalarial evaluation (WORTH et al. 1978). The synthetic route is depicted in Fig. 32.

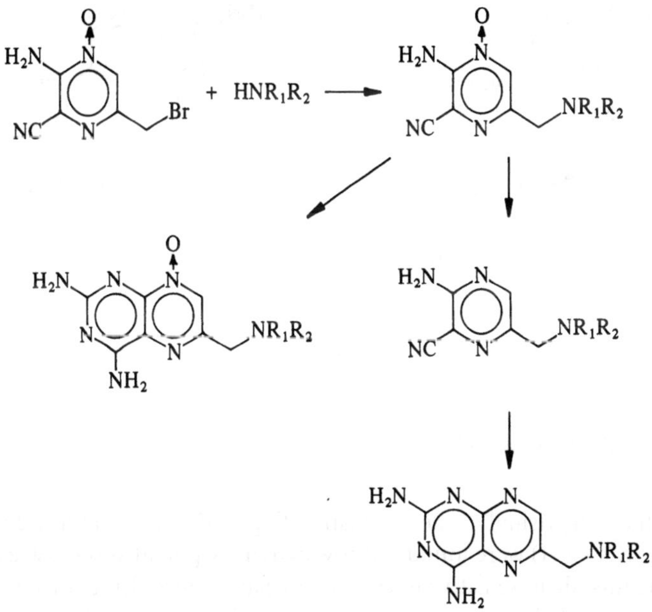

LXXXIV

Fig. 32. Scheme including chemical structure LXXXIV

In contrast to the quinazoline analogues the pteridines, when examined against trophozoite-induced *P. berghei* infections in mice, were at best poorly active. None of the *N*-oxides exhibited significant activity, while among the pteridines the best activity was noted with the 3,4,5-trimethoxyphenyl analogue which cured five of five mice at 320 mg/kg and showed strong suppressive activity at 160 mg/kg, and the 1-naphthalenyl analogue which cured five of five mice at 320 mg/kg and showed suppressive activity down to 40 mg/kg.

Interestingly, analogue LXXXV prepared earlier, which did not contain the large non-polar groups possibly needed for passive cellular transport, lacked significant activity even at high doses (CHAYKOVSKY et al. 1974). Not unexpectedly in view of these findings, neither the 6-aryloxy nor arylthio analogues (LXXXVI), as well as the oxidised sulphoxide and sulphone forms, showed significant activity when tested against lethal *P. berghei* infections in mice (WERBEL et al. 1978).

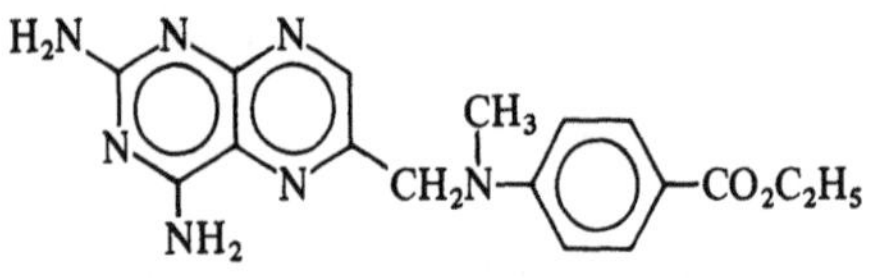

LXXXV

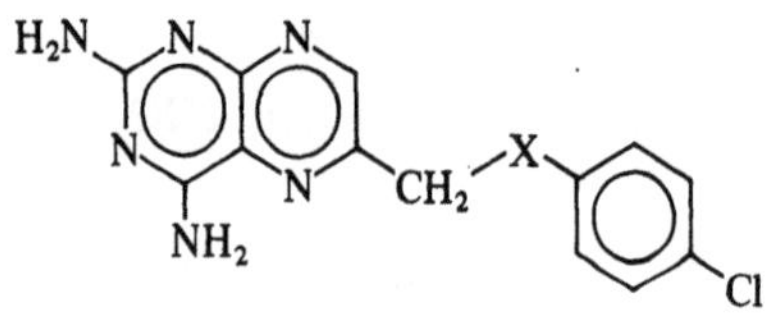

LXXXVI

a) X = O
b) Y = S, SO, SO_2

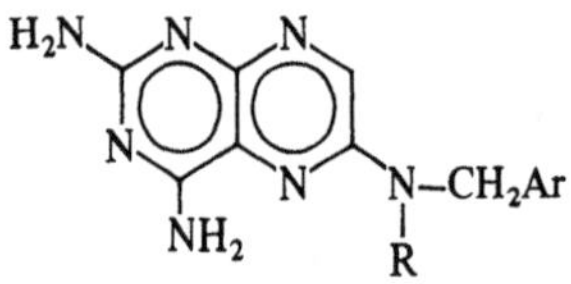

LXXXVII

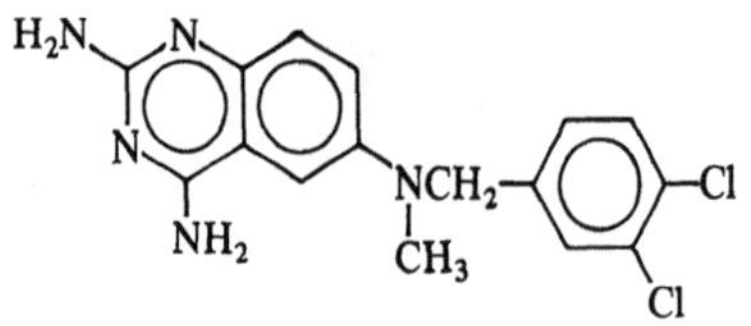

LXXXVIII

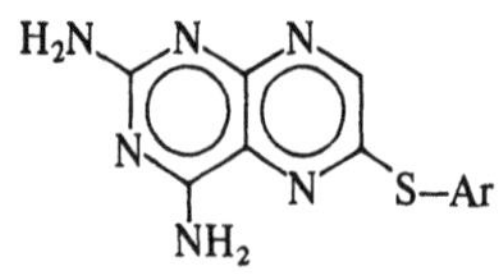

LXXXIX

Fig. 33. Chemical structures LXXXV–LXXXIX

Somewhat surprisingly, the corresponding 6-[(aralkyl)amino)-2,4-diaminopteridines (LXXXVII) were found to show extremely potent suppressive antimalarial effects against drug-sensitive lines of *P. berghei* in mice (ELSLAGER et al. 1981 a). The most active of the compounds, N^6-methyl-N^6-(l-naphthalenylmethyl)-2,4,6-pteridinetriamine (LXXXVIII), was even more potent than the corresponding quinazoline, being completely curative through 20 mg/kg, curing four of five at 10 mg/kg and two of five at 5 mg/kg. It was also curative at 3.16 mg/kg in a single oral dose against *P. cynomolgi* in the rhesus monkey. This material was shown to be effective against a chloroquine-resistant line of *P. berghei* in the mouse, but showed cross-resistance to a pyrimethamine-resistant strain.

The 2,4-diamino-6-[arylthio]pteridines (LXXXIX) corresponding to the highly active quinazolines were also prepared and were inactive against *P. berghei* infections in mice (ELSLAGER et al. 1981 b).

Acknowledgements. Dr. P. MAMALIS acknowledges permission from the Liverpool School of Tropical Medicine to reproduce Figure 1 from the Annals of Tropical Medicine and Parasitology (1980) vol. 74, p. 402; from Professor W. PETERS to use a considerable amount of unpublished data on Beecham antimalarial compounds (from work carried out during his tenure at the Liverpool School of Tropical Medicine); from the Walter Reed Army Institute of Research to use the rodent antimalarial results [OSDENE TS, RUSSELL PB, RANE L (1967) J Med Chem vol. 10, p. 431–434], and to use various pharmacological and toxicological results supplied by Colonel C. J. CANFIELD, Dr. E. J. GERBERG, Dr. D. P. JACOBUS, Dr. K. H. RIECKMANN, Major R. O. PICK, Dr. R. S. ROZMAN, Colonel W. E. ROTHE, Dr. L. H. SCHMIDT, Dr. C. C. SMITH and Dr. T. R. SWEENEY; and from Mr. D. J. KNIGHT of Beecham Pharmaceuticals Research Division to use much unpublished rodent data.

References

American Home Products Corporation (1973) 3,5-Diamino-1,2,4-triazines. British Patent 1,318,645

American Home Products (1978) US Patent 4,118,561

Ammon HL, Plastas LA (1979a) A reinvestigation of the structure of chlorguanide hydrochloride. J Med Chem 16:169–170

Ammon HL, Plastas LA (1979b) Structure of 1-[(3,4-dichlorophenyl)methoxy]-1,6-dihydro-6,6-dimethyl-1,3,5-triazine-2,4-diamine hydrochloride. Acta Crystollog Sect B 35:3106–3109

Aviado DM (1969) Parasitological Reviews: Chemotherapy of *Plasmodium berghei* including bibliography on *P. berghei*. Exp Parasitol 25:417–419

Baker BR (1967) Design of active-site-directed irreversible enzyme inhibitors. Wiley, New York

Baker BR, Lourens GJ (1968) Irreversible enzyme inhibitors CIX. Candidate irreversible inhibitors of dihydrofolic reductase derived from 4,6-diamino-1,2-dihydro-2,2-dimethyl-1-phenyl-*s*-triazine III. J Med Chem 11:26–33

Basu CP, Prakesh S (1962) The course of parasitaemia of *P. c. bastianelli* in *Macaca mulatta* monkeys: its sensitivity to different antimalarials. Indian J Malar 16:321–326

Basu UP, Sen AK (1952) Preparation of 2,4-diamino-1-*p*-chlorophenyl-1,6-dihydro-6,6-dimethyl-1,3,5-triazine. J Sci Ind Res (India) 11B:312

Basu UP, Sen AK, Ganguly AK (1952) Triazines from sulfa compounds. Science and culture (India) 18:45–46

Beecham Group Ltd (1971) 1-Phenylalkyloxy-2,4-diamino-1,2-dihydro-1,3,5-triazines. British Patent 1,250,531

Beecham Group Ltd (1972) 1-Aryloxy-2,4-diamino-1,2-dihydro-1,3,5-triazines. British Patent 1,270,881

Bird OD, Vaitkus JW, Clarke J (1970) 2-Amino-4-hydroxyquinazolines as inhibitors of thymidylate synthetase. Mol Pharmacol 6:573–575

Birtwell S (1952) Attempts to prepare a possible metabolite of "Paludrine" (Proguanil) and related 1,3,5-triazines. J Chem Soc 1279–1286

Birtwell S, Curd FHS, Hendry JA, Rose FL (1948) Synthetic antimalarials part XXX: Some N^1-aryl-N^4,N^5-dialkyldiguanides and observations on the conversion of guanylthioureas into diguanides. J Chem Soc 1645–1657

Canfield CJ, Rozman RS (1974) Clinical testing of new antimalarial compounds. Bull WHO 50:203–212

Capps DB, Bird OD, Elslager EF, Gavrilis ZB, Roush JA, Thompson PE, Vaitkus JW (1968) 1-Aryl-4,6-diamino-1,2-dihydro-s-triazines. Contrasting effects on intestinal helminths, bacteria and dihydrofolic reductase. J Heterocyclic Chem 5:335–369

Carrington HC, Crowther AF, Davey DG, Levi AA, Rose FL (1951) A metabolite of "Paludrine" with high antimalarial activity. Nature 168:1080

Carrington HC, Crowther AF, Stacey GJ (1954) Synthetic anti-malarials part XLIX. The structure and synthesis of the dihydrotriazine metabolite of proguanil. J chem Soc 1017–1031

Chase BH, Thurston JP, Walker J (1951) Antimalarial activity in 2,4-diamino-5-aryl-pyrimidines. Some reactions of α-formylphenylacetonitrile. J Chem Soc 3439–3444

Chaykovsky M, Rosowsky A, Papathanosopoulos N, Chen KKN, Modest EJ, Kisliuk RL, Goumont Y (1974) Methotrexate analogs. 3. Synthesis and biological properties of some side-chain altered analogs. J Med Chem 17:1212–1214

Chebotar NA (1974) Embryotoxic and teratogenic action of proguanil, chlorproguanil, and cycloguanil in rats. Biull Eksp Biol Med 77:56–57

Cheng CC (1974) Novel common structural feature among several classes of antimalarial agents. J Pharm Sci 63:307–310

Clyde DF (1969) Field trials of repository antimalarial compounds. J Trop Med Hyg 72:81–85

Crounse NN (1951) Isolation and identification of a metabolite of chlorguanide. J. Org Chem 16:492–500

Crowther AF, Levi AA (1953) Proguanil – the isolation of a metabolite with high antimalarial activity. Br J Pharmacol 8:43–97

Davoll J, Johnson AM (1970) Quinazoline analogues of folic acid. J Chem Soc C:997–1002

Davoll J, Johnson AM, Davies HJ, Bird OD, Clark J, Elslager EF (1972a) Folate antagonists. 2. 2,4-diamino-6-{[aralkyl and (heterocyclic)-methyl]amino}quinazolines, a novel class of antimetabolites of interest in drug-resistant malaria and Chagas disease. J Med Chem 15:812–826

Davoll J, Clarke J, Elslager EF (1972b) Folate antagonists. 4. Antimalarial and antimetabolite effects of 2,4-diamino-6-[(benzyl)amino]-pyrido[2,3-d]pyrimidines. J Med Chem 15:837–839

Elslager EF (1969) Progress in malaria chemotherapy Part I. Repository antimalarial drugs. Prog Drug Res 13:179–188, 197–198

Elslager EF (1974a) New vistas for folate antagonists in the chemotherapy of parasitic infections. In: Maas J (ed) Proc 4th Int Symp Med Chem. Elsevier, Amsterdam, p 227–231

Elslager EF (1974b) New perspectives on the chemotherapy of malaria, filariasis, and leprosy. Prog Drug Res 18:99–172

Elslager EF, Davoll J (1974) Synthesis of fused pyrimidines as folate antagonists. In: Castle RN, Townsend LB (eds) Lectures in heterocyclic chemistry. Hetero, Orem, Utah, p s97–s133

Elslager EF, Thompson PE (1964) Repository antimalarial drugs. Rep 9th Med Chem Symp Amer Chem Soc 6a–6z

Elslager EF, Werbel LM (to be published) N^1-(Quinazolinyl)-N^1-dialkylformamidines as solubilized 2,4-diaminoquinazoline antimalarials. J Med Chem

Elslager EF, Clarke J, Werbel LM, Worth DF, Davoll J (1972a) Folate antagonists. 3. 2,4-Diamino-6-(heterocyclic) quinazolines, a novel class of antimetabolites with potent antimalarial and antibacterial activity. J Med Chem 15:827–836

Elslager EF, Clarke J, Johnson J, Werbel LM, Davoll J (1972b) Folate antagonists. 5. Antimalarial and antibacterial effects of 2,4-diamino-6-(aryloxy and aralkoxy)quinazoline antimetabolites. J Heterocyclic Chem 9:759–773

Elslager EF, Clarke J, Jacob P, Werbel LM, Willis JD (1972c) Folate antagonists. 7. Antimalarial, antibacterial, and antimetabolite effects of 2,4-diamino-6-(benzyl and pyridylmethyl)-5,6,7,8-tetrahydropyrido[4,3-d]pyrimidines. J Heterocyclic Chem 9:1113–1122

Elslager EF, Jacob P, Johnson J, Werbel LM, Worth DF, Rane L (1978) Folate antagonists. 13. 2,4-diamino-6-[(α,α,α-trifluoro-*m*tolyl)thio]-quinazoline and related 2,4-diamino-6[(phenyl- and naphthyl)thio]-quinazolines, a unique class of antimetabolites with extraordinary antimalarial and antibacterial effects. J Med Chem 21:1059–1070

Elslager EF, Hutt MP, Jacob P, Johnson J, Temporelli B, Werbel LM, Worth DF (1979) Folate antagonists. 15. 2,4-diamino-6-(2-naphthylsulfonyl)quinazoline and related 2,4-diamino-6-(phenyl and naphthyl)-sulfinyl and sulfonyl quinazolines, a potent new class of antimetabolites with phenomenal antimalarial activity. J Med Chem 22:1247–1257

Elslager EF, Jacob P, Johnson J, Werbel LM (1980) Folate antagonists. 16. Antimalarial and antibacterial effects of 2,4-diamino-6-(heterocyclic)-thio, sulfinyl, and sulfonyl quinazolines. J Heterocyclic Chem 17:129–136

Elslager EF, Johnson JL, Werbel LM (1981a) Folate antagonists. 18. Synthesis and antimalarial effects of N^6-(arylmethyl)-N^6-methyl-2,4,6-pteridinetriamines and related N^6,N^6-disubstituted-2,4,6-pteridinetriamines. J Med Chem 24:140–145
Elslager EF, Johnson JL, Werbel LM (1981b) Folate antagonists. 19. Synthesis and antimalarial effects of 6-arylthio-2,4-pteridinediamines. J Med Chem 24:1001–1003
Elslager EF, Davoll J, Dickinson J, Johnson AM, Johnson J, Werbel LM (to be published)
Falco EA, Goodwin LG, Hitchings GH, Rollo IM, Russell PB (1951) 2,4-Diamino pyrimidines, a new series of antimalarials. Br J Pharmacol 6:185–200
Fu JC, Kale AK, Moyer DL (1973a) Diffusion of pyrimethamine from silicone rubber and flexible epoxy drug capsules. J Biomed Mater Res 7:193–200
Fu JC, Kale AK, Moyer DL (1973b) Drug-incorporated silicone discs as sustained release capsules. I. Chloroquine diphosphate. J Biomed Mater Res 7:71–78
Furukawa M, Seto Y, Toyoshima S (1961) Synthesis of compounds related to guanidine and their inhibitory action on growth of HeLa cells. Chem Pharm Bull 9:914–921
Genther CS, Smith CC (1977) Antifolate studies. Activities of 40 potential antimalarial compounds against sensitive- and chlorguanide triazine resistant-strains of folate-requiring bacteria and *E. coli*. J Med Chem 20:237–243
Genther CS, Schoeny RS, Loper JC, Smith CC (1977) Mutagenic studies of folic acid antagonists. Antimicrob Agents Chemother 12:84–92
Gerberg EJ (1968) Unpublished report to Walter Reed Army Institute of Research on WR 38839 (BRL 50216) WRAIR, Washington, DC
Gerberg EJ, Richard LT, Poole JB (1966) Standardized feeding of *Aedes aegypti* (L) mosquitoes on *Plasmodium gallinaceum* Brumpt-infected chicks for mass screening of antimalarial drugs. Mosquito News 26:354–363
Gusmão HH, Juarez E (1970) A trial of CI-564 (Dapolar), a repository antimalarial for prophylaxis in Amapá, Brazil. Am J Trop Med Hyg 19:394–400
Gutteridge WE, Trigg PI (1971) Action of pyrimethamine and related drugs against *Plasmodium knowlesi in vitro*. Parasitology 62:431–444
Hall SA (1969) Malaria treatment and prevention. East Afr Med J 46:553–563
Hewitt RI, Wallace WS, Gumble A, White E, Williams JH (1954) Antimalarial activity of dihydrotriazines. Am J Trop Med 3:225–231
Hitchings GH, Maggiolo A, Russell PB, Vanderwerff H, Rollo IM (1952) 3,5-Diamino-*as*-triazines as inhibitors of lactic acid bacteria and plasmodia. J Am Chem Soc 74:3200–3201
Howells RE, Judge B (1977) Sustained release/antimalarial activity of dihydrotriazine compounds in a silicone rubber matrix. Unpublished report to Beecham Pharmaceuticals Research Division from Liverpool School of Tropical Medicine
Hynes JB, Ashton WT, Merriman HG III, Walker FC (1974) Synthesis of analogs of 6-arylthio-6-arylsulfonyl-2,4-diaminoquinazolines as potential antimalarial agents. J Med Chem 17:682–684
Jaffe JJ, McCormack JJ, Gutteridge WE (1969) Dihydrofolate reductases within the genus *Trypanosoma*. Exp Parasitol 25:311–318
Johnson J, Elslager EF, Werbel LM (1977) Synthesis and antimalarial effects of [1] benzothieno [3,2-f]quinazoline-1,3-diamine. J Heterocyclic Chem 14:1209–1214
Judge BM, Howells RE (1979) The use of drug polymer mixture implants for sustained antimalarial effects in mice. Parasitology 79:ii–iii Br Soc Parasitology, Spring Meeting, Keele, 1979
Kim KH, Dietrich BW, Hansch C, Dolnick BJ, Bertino JR (1980) Inhibition of dihydrofolate reductase 3. 4,6-Diamino-1,2-dihydro-2,2-dimethyl-1-(2-substituted-phenyl)-*s*-triazine inhibition of bovine liver and mouse tumor enzymes. J Med Chem 23:1248–1251
Kinnamon KE, Lager A, Orchard RW (1976) *Plasmodium berghei:* Combining folic acid antagonists for potentiation against malaria infections in mice. Exp Parasitol 40:95–102
Kisliuk RL, Friedkin M, Schmidt LH, Rossan RN (1967) Antimalarial activity of tetrahydrohomopteroic acid. Science 156:1616–1617
Knight DJ (1981) *Babesia rodhaini* and *Plasmodium berghei* A highly active series of chlorophenoxy alkoxy-substituted diamino-dihydrotriazines against experimental infections in mice. Ann Trop Med Parasitol 75:1–6

Knight DJ, Peters W (1980) The antimalarial activity of *N*-benzyloxydihydrotriazines Part I. The activity of clociguanil (BRL 502169) against rodent malaria, and studies on its mode of action. Ann Trop Med Parasitol 74:393–404

Knight DJ, Ponsford RJ (1982) Trypanocidal activity and prophylaxis evaluation of a series of bis-oxydihydro-triazines in mice. Ann Trop Med Parasitol 76:589–594

Knight DJ, Williamson P (1980) The antimalarial activity of *N*-benzyloxydihydrotriazines Part II. The development of resistance to clociguanil (BRL 50216) and cycloguanil by *P. berghei*. Ann Trop Med Parasitol 74:405–413

Knight DJ, Williamson P 1982 The antimalarial activity of *N*-benzyloxydihydrotriazines Part IV. The development of resistance to BRL 6231 [4,6-diamino-1,2-dihydro-2,2-dimethyl-1-(2,4,5-trichlorophenoxypropyloxy-1,3,5-triazine hydrochloride] by *P. berghei*. Ann Trop Med Parasitol 76:9–14

Knight DJ, Mamalis P, Peters W (1982) The antimalarial activity of *N*-benzyloxidihydrotriazines Part III. The activity of 4,6-diamino-1,2-dihydro-2,2-dimethyl-1-(2,4,5-trichloropropyloxy)-1,3,5-triazine-hydrobromide (BRL 51084) and hydrochloride (BRL 6231). Ann Trop Med Parasitol 76:1–7

Kurban AK, Malok JA, Farah FS, Siage J, Jallad M (1969) Treatment of cutaneous leishmaniasis (oriental sore) with a new repository antimalarial. J Trop Med Hyg 72:86–88

Laing ABG (1971) The suppression of malaria with Dapolar: a trial of 4-monthly doses in a village community in the Gambia West Africa. Trans R Soc Trop Med Hyg 65:560–573

Laing ABG (1974) Studies in the chemotherapy of malaria III. Treatment of falciparum malaria in the Gambia with BRL 50216 alone and in combination with sulfonamides. Trans R Soc Trop Med Hyg 68:133–138

Lee CC, Heiffer MH, Kintner LD (1976) The effects of folic or folinic acid on the toxicity of 4,6-diamino-1,2-dihydro-2,2-dimethyl-1 (3,4-dichlorobenzyloxy)-1,3,5-triazine hydrochloride, an antifolate, in dogs. Toxicol Appl Pharmacol 38:29–37

Lombardino JG (1963) 4,6-Diamino-1-alkyl-1,2-dihydro-*s*-triazines. J Med Chem 6:213–214

Loo JL (1954) 1-*p*-Chlorophenyl-2,4-diamino-6,6-dimethyl-1,6-dihydro-1,3,5-triazine. J Am Chem Soc 76:5096–5099

Mamalis P (1971) Some biological properties associated with amino-oxy-containing compounds. Symposium on biological *N*-oxidation, Chelsea College, 22 December 1971 Xenobiotica 1:569–571 (Summary only)

Mamalis P, Outred DJ (1969) Unpublished Report, Beecham Pharmaceuticals, Research Division, Tadworth UK

Mamalis P, Green J, McHale D (1960) Amino-oxy derivatives Part II. Some derivatives of *N*-hydroxy diguanide. J Chem Soc 229–238

Mamalis P, Green J, Outred DJ, Rix M (1962) Amino-oxy derivatives Part III. Dihydrotriazines and related heterocycles. J Chem Soc 3915–3926

Mamalis P, Jeffries L, Price SA, Rix MJ, Outred DJ (1965 a) Amino-oxy derivatives IV. Antimicrobial activity of some *O*-ethers of 4,6-diamino-1,2-dihydro-1-hydroxy-2-substituted-1,3,5-triazines. J Med Chem 8:684–691

Mamalis P, Green J, Outred DJ, Rix MJ (1965 b) Amino-oxy derivatives Part V. Some *O*-ethers of 2-substituted-4,6-diamino-1,2-dihydro-1-hydroxy-1,3,5-triazines. J Chem Soc 1829–1843

Mamalis P, Knight DJ, Williamson P (1971) Comparative antimalarial activities of some chlorophenoxypropyloxy-diaminodihydrotriazines and their N,N^1-diacetyl derivatives. Report to Beecham Pharmaceuticals, Research Division, Tadworth, UK

Mattock NM, Peters W (1975) The experimental chemotherapy of leishmaniasis III. Detection of antileishmanial activity in some new synthetic compounds in a tissue culture model. Ann Trop Med Parasitol 69:449–462

McCormack JJ, Jaffe JJ (1969) Dihydrofolate reductase form *Trypanosoma equiperdum* II. Inhibition by 2,4-diaminopyrimidines and related heterocycles. J Med Chem 12:662–668

McCormick GJ, Canfield CJ, Willet GP (1971) *Plasmodium knowlesi: In vitro* evaluation of antimalarial activity of folic acid inhibitors. Exp Parasitol 30:88–93

Mizen L (1970) Unpublished Report, Beecham Pharmaceuticals, Research Division, Tadworth, UK
Modest EJ (1956) Chemical and biological studies on 1,2-dihydro-s-triazines II. Three-component synthesis. J Org Chem 21:1–13
Modest EJ (1961) *s*-Triazines In: Elderfield RC (ed) Heterocyclic compounds, vol 7. Wiley, New York, p 697–701
Modest EJ, Levine P (1956) Chemical and biological studies on 1,2-dihydro-s-triazines III. Two-component synthesis. J Org Chem 21:14–20
Modest EJ, Foley GE, Pechet MM, Farbers (1952) A series of new biologically significant dihydrotriazines. J Am Chem Soc 74:855–856
Nettleton MJ, Poyser RH, Shorter JH (1974) The cardiovascular effects of two new triazine antimalarials BRL 50216 (Clociguanil) and BRL 6231. Toxicol App Pharmacol 27:271–284
Newman H, Moon EL (1964) Reaction of Schiff bases with dicyandiamide – synthesis of 4,6-diamino-1,2-dihydro-*sym*-triazines. J Org Chem 29:2061–2063
Newman H, Moon EL (1965) Isomeric benzyldiaminodihydrotriazines. J Med Chem 8:702–704
Peters W (1965a) Drug resistance in *Plasmodium berghei*, Vincke and Lips 1948 II. Triazine resistance. Exp Parasitol 17:90–96
Peters W (1965b) Drug resistance in *Plasmodium berghei*, Vincke and Lips, 1948 I. Chloroquine resistance. Exp Parasit 17:80–89
Peters W (1968, 1969) Unpublished. Report on mouse *P. berghei* tests to Beecham Pharmaceuticals. Liverpool School of Tropical Medicine
Peters W (1970) Chemotherapy and drug resistance in malaria. Academic, London
Peters W (1971a) Chemoprophylaxis and chemotherapy (in malaria). Br Med J I:95–98
Peters W (1971b) Chemotherapy of rodent malaria drug action against exoerythrocytic stages and drug resistant strains. US Nat Techn Inform Serv AD Rep No. 726973
Peters W (1971c) The chemotherapy of rodent malaria XIV. The action of some sulphonamides alone or with folic reductase inhibitors against malaria vectors and parasites, part 4: The response of normal and drug-resistant strains of *Plasmodium berghei*. Ann Trop Med Parasitol 65:123–129
Peters W (1974) Recent advances in antimalarial chemotherapy and drug resistance. Adv Parasitol 12:69–112
Peters W, Davies EE, Robinson BL (1975a) The chemotherapy of rodent malaria XXIII Causal prophylaxis Part II. Practical experience with *Plasmodium yoelii nigeriensis* in drug screening. Ann Trop Med Parasitol 69:311–328
Peters W, Portus JH, Robinson BL (1975b) The chemotherapy of rodent malaria XXII The value of drug-resistant strains of *P. berghei* in screening for blood schizontocidal activity. Ann Trop Med Hyg 69:155–171
Peters W, Trotter ER, Robinson BL (1980a) The experimental chemotherapy of leishmaniasis V. The activity of potential leishmanicides against "*L. infantum* LV9" in NMRI mice. Ann Trop Med Parasitol 74:289–298
Peters W, Trotter ER, Robinson BL (1980b) The experimental chemotherapy of leishmaniasis VII. Drug responses of *L. major* and *L. mexicana amazonensis* with an analysis of promising chemical leads to new antileishmanial agents. Ann Trop Med Parasitol 74:321–335
Powers KG (1965) The use of silicone rubber implants for the sustained release of antimalarial and anti-schistosomal agents. J Parasitol [Suppl] 51:53
Rane L (1970) Unpublished data on mouse *P. berghei* screen to Beecham Pharmaceuticals. Walter Reed Army Institute of Research, Washington, DC
Rees RWA, Russell PB, Foell TJ, Bright RE (1972) Antimalarial activities of some 3,5-diamino-*as*-triazine derivatives. J Med Chem 15:859–861
Rieckmann KH (1968) Unpublished data on *in vitro* activity of antimalarial drugs against *P. falciparum*. Walter Reed Army Institute of Research, Washington, DC
Rieckmann KH, Willerson D, Carson PE (1971) Drug potentiation against pre-erythrocytic stages of *Plasmodium falciparum*. Trans R Soc Trop Med Hyg 65:533–535

Robertson GI (1957) Experiments with antimalarial drugs in man V Experiments with an active metabolite of proguanil and an active metabolite of 5943. Trans R Soc Trop Med Hyg 51:488–492

Roth B, Burrows RB, Hitchings GH (1963) Anthelmintic agents 1,2-Dihydro-*s*-triazines. J Med Chem 6:370–378

Rosowsky A, Chen KKN, St Amand R, Modest EJ (1973) Chemical and biological studies on 1,2-dihydro-*s*-triazines XVIII Synthesis of 1-(5,6- and 5,7-dichloro-2-naphthyl) derivatives and related compounds as candidate antimalarial and anti-tumor agents J Pharm Sci 62:477–479

Rozman RS (1973) Chemotherapy of malaria. Ann Rev Pharmacol 13:127–152

Ruiz R, Grigas EO, Aviado DM (1971) Cardiopulmonary effects of antimalarial drugs V. Cycloguanil and a new triazine compound (WR 99662). Toxicol Appl Pharmacol 18:487–497

Ryley JF (1953) The mode of action of proguanil and related antimalarial drugs. Br J Pharmacol Chemother 8:424–430

Salem HH, Elkomy HM, El-Allaf G (1969) The treatment of cutaneous leishmaniasis in Iraq with cycloguanil pamoate. Trans Soc Trop Med Hyg 63:388–392

Schalit S, Cutler RA (1959) New dihydrotriazines of chemotherapeutic interest. J Org Chem 24:573–576

Schmidt LH (1970) The use of *Aotus trivirgatus* as a tool for studies on the therapy of infections with *Plasmodium falciparum*. Interim Report (Jan–Mar 1970) to US Army Medical Research R & D Command

Schmidt LH (1972) The activities of BRL 7638 against infection with *Plasmodium falciparum* in the owl monkey (*Aotus trivirgatus*). Unpublished report to Beecham Pharmaceuticals Research Division, from Southern Research Institute Project No. 2843

Schmidt LH (1978a) *Plasmodium falciparum* and *Plasmoidum vivax* infections in the owl monkey (*Aotus trivirgatus*) III. Methods employed in the search for new blood schizonticidal drugs. Am J Trop Med Hyg 27:718–737

Schmidt LH (1978b) Experimental infections with human plasmodia in owl monkey – their contribution to development of new broadly active blood schizonticidal drugs. In: Adolphe M (ed) Advances in pharmacology & therapeuties, Proc. 7th int congr pharm, vol 10, chemotherapy. Pergamon Press, Oxford, p 71–90

Schmidt LH (1978c) *Plasmodium falciparum* and *Plasmodium vivax* infections in the owl monkey (*Aotus trivirgatus*) I. The courses of untreated infections. Am J Trop Med Hyg 27:671–702

Schmidt LH (1978d) *Plasmodium falciparum* and *Plasmodium vivax* infections in the owl monkey (*Aotus trivirgatus*) II. Responses to chloroquine, quinine, and pyrimethamine. Am J Trop Med Hyg 27:703–717

Schmidt LH (1979a) Studies on the 2,4-diamino-6-substituted quinazolines. II. Activities of selected derivatives against infections with various drug-susceptible and drug-resistant strains of *Plasmodium falciparum* and *Plasmodium vivax* in owl monkeys. Am J Trop Med Hyg 28:793–807

Schmidt LH (1979b) Studies on the 2,4-diamino-6-substituted quinazolines, III. The capacity of sulfadiazine to enhance the activities of WR-158,122, and WR-159,412 against infections with various drug-susceptible and drug-resistant strains of *Plasmodium falciparum* and *Plasmodium vivax* in owl monkeys. Am J Trop Med Hyg 28:808–818

Schmidt LH, Rossan RN (1979) Antimalarial activities of 2,4-Diamino-6-[(3,4-dichlorobenzyl)nitrosoamino]-quinazoline as exhibited in rhesus monkeys infected with the RO/PM strains of *Plasmodium cynomolgi*. Am J Trop Med 28:781–792

Schmidt LH, Rossan RN, Fisher KF (1963) The activity of a repository form of 4,6-diamoni-1-(p-chlorophenyl)-1,2-dihydro-2,2-dimethyl-*s*-triazine against infections with *Plasmodium cynomolgi*. Am J Trop Med Hyg 12:494–503

Schneider J, Decourt PH, Montézin G (1949) Sur l'utilisation d'un nouveau plasmodium (*P. berghei*) pour l'étude et la recherche de médicaments antipaludiques. Bull Soc Path Exot Filiales 45:29–33

Sen AB, Singh PR (1958) Search for new antimalarials: synthesis of some substituted 1,2-dihydro-*s*-triazines. J Indian Chem Soc 35:847–852

Sen AB, Singh PR (1959) Search for new antimalarials II. Synthesis of some new 1,2-dihydro-1,3,5-triazines. J Indian Chem Soc 36:260–262
Sen AB, Singh PR (1960) Search for new antimalarials VI. Synthesis of some new 1,2-dihydro-1,3,5-triazines. J Indian Chem Soc 37:643–644
Sen AB, Singh PR (1961) Search for new antimalarials VII. Synthesis of some new 1,2-dihydro-sym-triazines. J Indian Chem Soc 38:187–188
Shapiro HS (to be published)
Singh J, Nair CP, Ray AP (1956) Therapeutic effect of sulfadiazine and dihydrotriazines against blood-induced *P. cynomolgi* infection. Ind J Malariol 10:131–135
Smith CC, Genther CS (1976) Measurement of antibiotic drugs by microbiological assay. US NTIS, AD Rep. 1976. AD-AO 41193
Steck EA (1972) Chemotherapy of malaria. In: Chemotherapy of protozoan disease, vol III, p 23.226–23.238 US Gov. Printing Office, Washington DC
Stepan A, Badilescu IJ, Simon Z (1977) MTD Study of the structure-activity relationships of triazine derivatives inhibiting dihydrofolate reductase. Annals Univ Timisoara Ser. Stünte Fiz-Chim 15:61–71
Takeda Chem Ind. Ltd (1973) Veterinary composition for prophylaxis and treatment of leucozoon disease in poultry. British Patent 1328113
Thompson PE, Werbel LM (1972) Antimalarial agents, chemistry and pharmacology. Academic, London
Thompson, PE, Olszewski BJ, Elslager EF, Worth DF (1963) 4,6-Diamino-1-(*p*-chlorophenyl-1,2-dihydro-2,2-dimethyl-*s*-triazine pamoate (CI-501) as a repository antimalarial drug. Am J Trop Med Hyg 12:481–493
Thompson PE, Olszewski BJ, Waitz JA (1965a) Laboratory studies on the repository antimalarial activity of 4,4-diacetylamino-diphenylsulfone alone and mixed with cycloguanil pamoate (CI-501). Am J Trop Med Hyg 14:343–353
Thompson PE, Waitz JA, Olszewski BJ (1965b) The repository antimalarial activities of 4,4-diacetylaminodiphenylsulfone and cycloguanil pamoate (CI-501) in monkeys relative to local release following parenteral administration. J Parasitol 51:34–349
Thompson PE, Bayles A, Olszewski BJ (1969) PAM 1392 [2,4-diamino-6-(3,4-dichlorobenzylamino)quinazoline] as a chemotherapeutic agent: *Plasmodium berghei, P. cynomolgi, P. knowlesi* and *Trypanosoma cruzi*. Exp Parasitol 25:32–49
Thompson PE, Bayles A, Olszewski BJ (1970) Antimalarial activity of 2,4-diamino-6-[(3,4-dichlorobenzyl)nitrosamino]quinazoline, Laboratory studies in mice and rhesus monkeys. Am J Trop Med 19:12–26
Vitamins Ltd (1970a) 1-Benzyloxy-2,4-diamino-1,2-dihydro-1,3, 5-triazines. British Patent 1201825
Vitamins Ltd (1970b) 1-Benzyloxy-2,4-diamino-1,2-dihydro-1,3, 5-triazines. British Patent 1217415
Walsh RJA, Wooldridge KRH, Jackson D, Gilmour J (1977) The structure activity relationship of antibacterial substituted 1-phenyl-4,6-diamino-1,2-dihydro-2,2-dimethyl-*s*-triazines. Eur J Med Chem 12:495–500
Walter Reed Army Institute of Research (1968) Unpublished Report on WR 38839 (BRL 56216). W.R.A.I.R. Washington, DC
Walter Reed Army Institute of Research (1969) Unpublished Report on WR 99210 (BRL 6231). W.R.A.I.R. Washington, DC
Walton BC, Person DA, Ellman MH, Bernstein R (1968) Treatment of American cutaneous leishmaniasis with cycloguanil pamoate. Am J Trop Med Hyg 17:814–818
Werbel LM, Johnson J, Elslager EF, Worth DF (1978) Folate antagonists. II. Synthesis and antimalarial effects of 6-[(aryloxy- and arylthio-)-methyl]-2,4-pteridinediamines and -pteridinediamine 8-oxides. J Med Chem 21:337–339
Werbel LM, Newton L, Elslager EF (1980) Folate antagonists. 17. Synthesis and biological properties of a 2,4-diamino-6-thioquinazoline analog of aminopterin. J Heterocyclic Chem 17:497–500
White AI (1977) Antimalarials. In: Wilson CO, Jones E (eds) Wilson and Gisvolds textbook of organic medicinal and pharmaceutical chemistry. 7th edn. Lippincott, Philadelphia, p 247–261

Willerson D, Kass L, Frischer H, Rieckman KH, Carson PE, Richard L, Bowman JE (1974) Chemotherapeutic results in a multi-drug resistant strain of *P. falciparum* malaria from Vietnam. Milit Med 139:175–183

Wise DL, McCormick GJ, Willet GP, Anderson LC (1976) Sustained release of an antimalarial drug using a copolymer of glycolic/lactic acid. Life Sci 19:867–874

Wise DL, McCormick GJ, Willet GP, Anderson LC, Howes JF (1978) Sustained release of sulphadiazine. J Pharm Pharmacol 30:686–689

Wise DL, Gresser JD, McCormick GJ (1979) Sustained release of a dual antimalarial system. J Pharm Pharmacol 31:201–204

Wooldridge KRH (1980) A rational substituent set for structure-activity studies. Eur J Med Chem 15:63–66

Worth DF, Johnson J, Elslager EF, Werbel LM (1978) Folate antagonists. 10. Synthesis and antimalarial effects of 6-[(aryl and aralkyl)amino]methyl)-2,4-pteridinediamines and -pteridinediamine 8-oxides. J Med Chem 21:331–337

CHAPTER 14

Antibiotics

K. H. RIECKMANN

A. Introduction

The report by HINDLE and his associates, in 1945, that penicillin exerted no effects against malaria was followed, 4 years later, by the disclosure that another antibiotic, chlortetracycline, was effective against avian and human malaria parasites (COATNEY et al. 1949, COOPER et al. 1949). Reviewing the status of antibiotics up to 1952, COATNEY and GREENBERG pointed out that most of the 31 antibiotics tested had shown no appreciable activity against malaria parasites of birds or rodents. Penicillin, streptomycin, dihydrostreptomycin, and bacitracin were among the 22 compounds which showed no activity. Of the nine compounds which exhibited some antimalarial activity, only chlortetracycline, oxytetracycline, and chloramphenicol were considered sufficiently effective and non-toxic to be of potential therapeutic value. Although all three drugs were active against blood stages of the two avian and one rodent plasmodial species, chlortetracycline appeared to be somewhat more active than the other two compounds. The three drugs also exerted a causal prophylactic activity against sporozoite-induced infections of avian malaria. The two tetracyclines and chloramphenicol were the only antibiotics of those tested which were active against human infections with *Plasmodium vivax* and *P. falciparum* (COOPER et al. 1949; IMBODEN et al. 1950; RUIZ-SANCHEZ et al. 1951, 1952a, b). Subsequent studies with tetracycline (RUIZ-SANCHEZ et al. 1956) confirmed earlier findings that clearance of fever and parasitaemia after treatment with tetracyclines was slower than that observed with other antimalarials such as chloroquine. Antibiotics were, therefore, not considered to be of practical value in the treatment of malaria infections (WHO 1961).

The subsequent development and spread of drug-resistant falciparum infections prompted a reconsideration of the value of tetracyclines as antimalarial drugs. Tetracycline was shown to have a pronounced effect against both asexual erythrocytic and pre-erythrocytic stages of chloroquine-resistant strains of *P. falciparum* (RIECKMANN et al. 1971, 1972). In addition, two newer and more expensive tetracyclines, doxycycline and minocycline, were also shown to exert a marked activity against chloroquine-resistant falciparum malaria (CLYDE et al. 1971; WILLERSON et al. 1972). Both drugs could be administered less frequently (every 12–24 h) and at lower doses than other tetracyclines because of their more complete intestinal absorption and longer serum half-lives. Field studies carried out in Thailand confirmed the efficacy of tetracycline and minocycline in curing infections acquired in areas with chloroquine-resistant malaria (COLWELL et al. 1972a, b, 1973). In all these reports, it was emphasised that a rapidly acting schizontocide such as quinine or amodiaquine had to be administered in conjunction with the tetracyclines in order to ensure the rapid clearance of fever and parasites after initiation of treatment. The long duration of a course of treatment, lasting more than a week, is an obvious handicap in using the tetracyclines, particularly in developing countries with limited medical facilities.

The findings that a non-tetracycline antibiotic, clindamycin, was effective against a chloroquine-resistant strain of *P. falciparum* in *Aotus* monkeys (POWERS and JACOBS 1972) prompted clinical evaluation of this compound in persons infected with drug-resistant falciparum malaria (MILLER et al. 1974). The fact that 3-day courses of this drug, given in combination with quinine, were uniformly effective in curing these infections appeared to be an important advantage over the longer 7- to 10-day tetracycline regimens. Subsequent studies, however, have shown this more practicable drug regimen to be either too toxic or only partially effective in patients infected with other strains of *P. falciparum* (CLYDE et al. 1975; HALL et al. 1975).

Other antibiotics which have been reported to possess some antimalarial activity include the macrolide antibiotic, erythromycin (WARHURST et al. 1976; DUTTA and SINGH 1979), and the purine nucleoside antibiotic, cordycepin (TRIGG et al. 1971). Both these antibiotics do not appear to have been investigated for their action against human malaria parasites.

In this review, emphasis will be placed primarily on antibiotics which have demonstrated pronounced activity against human malaria parasites.

B. Chemistry

The principal antibiotics which have been reported to be active against human malaria parasites are the tetracyclines and clindamycin.

I. Tetracyclines

Tetracycline antibiotics were developed as the result of systematic screening of soil specimens from around the world for antibiotic-producing microorganisms. The first one to be discovered, chlortetracycline (Aureomycin), was produced by *Streptomyces aureofaciens*. Introduced in 1948, chlortetracycline was followed 2 years later by oxytetracycline (Terramycin), an antibiotic elaborated by *S. rimosus*. Definition of the chemical structure of these compounds led, in 1953, to the introduction of tetracycline, (Achromycin; Tetracyn), produced semisynthetically from chlortetracycline or oxytetracycline. Two other tetracyclines, the activities of which were evaluated against human malaria, were doxycycline (Vibramycin) and minocycline (Minocin); the former became available in 1966 and the latter in 1972. The tetracyclines are closely congeneric derivatives of the polycyclic naphthacenecarboxamide. Their structures are shown in Fig. 1.

The concentrations of tetracyclines in biological fluids have been estimated by conventional microbiological methods. Such methods are not entirely satisfactory because of the instability of tetracyclines in solution, etc. Although various earlier chromatographic procedures were rather laborious and not sufficiently sensitive or precise, a reverse-phase method using high-speed liquid chromatography appears

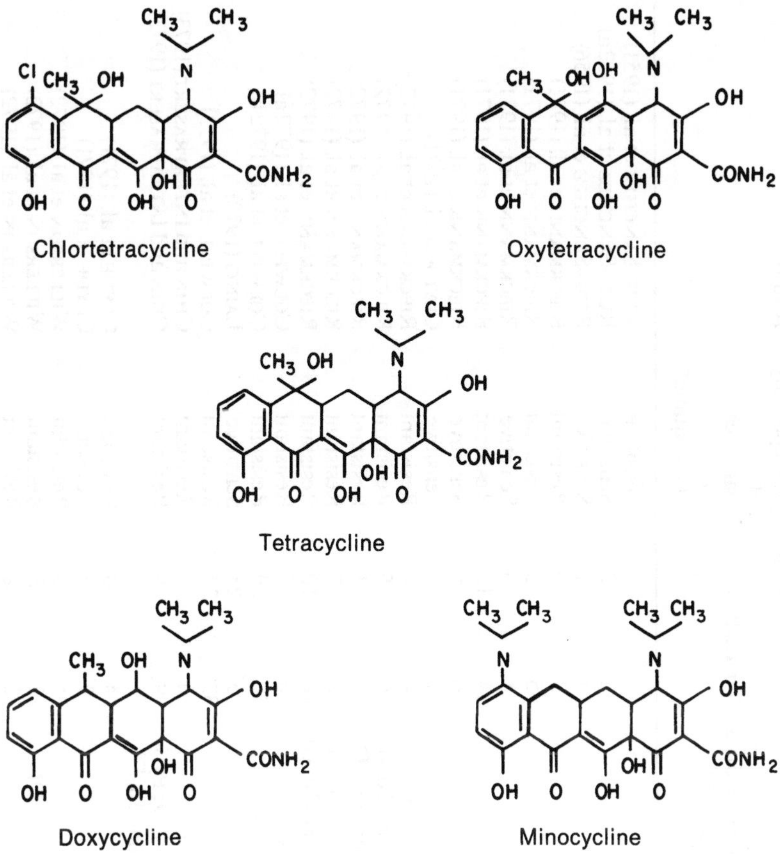

Fig. 1. Structural formulas of the tetracyclines

to offer quick and reliable quantitative microanalysis of tetracyclines in biological specimens (KNOX and JURAND 1975).

II. Clindamycin (7-Chlorolincomycin)

The parent compound of clindamycin is lincomycin, a water-soluble antibiotic that is very effective against gram-positive microorganisms. Clindamycin was produced

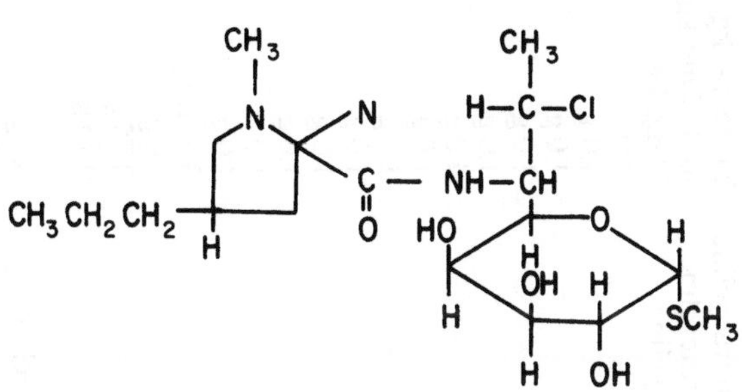

Clindamycin

Fig. 2. Structural formula of clindamycin

Table 1. Effects of various tetracyclines against asexual erythrocytic stages of *P. falciparum*. Legend see opposite page

Treatment[a]					No. of persons		Susceptibility of parasites to chloroquine[e]	Authors
Antibiotic	Daily dose	Doses per day	Duration (days)	Complementary drug[a] (duration, B or D)[b]	Treated[c]	Cured[d]		
Chlortetracycline	20–35 mg/kg			–			Sensitive	Ruiz-Sanchez et al. (1951)
Oxytetracycline	70–117 mg/kg	4	10–11	–	2	2	Sensitive	Ruiz-Sanchez et al. (1952a)
Tetracycline	50 mg/kg	3	10	–	1	1	Sensitive	Ruiz-Sanchez et al. (1956)
	1.0 g	4	$3^1/_4$	–	3	0	Resistant	Rieckmann et al. (1971)
	1.0 g	4	5	–	5	5	Resistant	Rieckmann et al. (1971)
	1.0 g	4	5	–	1	0	Sensitive	Rieckmann et al. (1971)
	1.0 g	4	7	–	14	13	Resistant	Rieckmann et al. (1971)
	1.0 g	4	7	–	6	6	Sensitive	Rieckmann et al. (1971)
	4.0 g	4	7	–	1	1	Sensitive	Clyde et al. (1971)
	1.0 g	4	10	Quinine (3d, B)	4	4	Resistant	Rieckmann et al. (1972)
	1.0 g	4	7	Amodiaquine (3d, B)	6	5	Resistant	Rieckmann et al. (1972)
	1.0 g	4	7	Amodiaquine (3d, D)	3	1	Resistant	Rieckmann et al. (1972)
	1.0 g	4	10	Amodiaquine (3d, B)	8	7	Resistant	Rieckmann et al. (1972)
	1.0 g	4	7	Amodiaquine (3d, D)	10	10	Resistant	Rieckmann et al. (1972)
	1.0 g	4	10	Quinine (3d, B)	28	27	Resistant	Colwell et al. (1972a)
	1.0 g	4	10	Quinine (3d, B)	30	29	Resistant	Colwell et al. (1972b)
	0.5–1.0 g	4	5	–	5[f]	?[g]	Sensitive	Laing (1972)
	1.0 g	4	7	Quinine (1d, D)	32	27	Resistant	Colwell et al. (1973)
	0.75 g	3	3	Quinine (3d, D)	6	4	Resistant	Chin and Intraprasert (1973)
	0.75 g	3	3	Quinine (3d, D; Pyrimethamine 1d, D)	9	6	Resistant	Chin and Intraprasert (1973)
Doxycycline	0.2 g	2	5	–	4	0	Resistant	Clyde et al. (1971)
	0.2 g	4	7	–	9	9	Resistant	Clyde et al. (1971)
Minocycline	0.4 g	2	7	–	5	5	Resistant	Willerson et al. (1972)
	0.4 g	4	7	Quinine (1–3d, D)	2	2	Resistant	Willerson et al. (1972)
	0.2 g	1	7	–	2	2	Resistant	Willerson et al. (1972)
	0.1 g	1	7	–	2	2	Resistant	Willerson et al. (1972)
	0.2 g	2	7	Quinine (3d, B)	28	27	Resistant	Colwell et al. (1972a)

by replacing the 7-hydroxyl group in lincomycin by chlorine. Clindamycin was absorbed more readily, produced higher blood concentrations and was more active against gram-positive bacteria than lincomycin (MAGERLEIN et al. 1967a, b). In contradistinction to its parent compound, clindamycin showed antimalarial activity against rodent malaria parasites (LEWIS 1968a). Further investigations showed that clindamycin and other chlorinated analogues, particularly *N*-demthyl-4^1-pentyl-7-chlorolincomycin, were also active against chloroquine and DDS-resistant strains of *P. berghei* (LEWIS 1968b). The structure of clindamycin is illustrated in Fig. 2.

The concentration of clindamycin in biological fluids has usually been estimated by microbiological assays using *Sarcina lutea* ATCC 9341 as the test organism (DEHAAN et al. 1972).

C. Modes of Action

I. Tetracyclines

The earlier and the more recently introduced tetracyclines have a broad spectrum of activity against different developmental stages of both *P. falciparum* and *P. vivax*. The tetracyclines which have been evaluated for their antimalarial activity include chlortetracycline, oxytetracycline, tetracycline, doxycycline, and minocycline.

The mode of action of tetracyclines against malaria parasites has not yet been established. In bacteria, the primary mechanism by which the tetracyclines exert their activity is through an inhibition of protein synthesis at the ribosomal level. Protein synthesis is arrested by tetracycline binding principally to the 30S subunits of ribosomes and specifically preventing the enzyme binding of aminoacyl-tRNA to the adjacent ribosomal acceptor site (CUNDLIFFE and MCQUILLEN 1967). It has been suggested that inhibition of protein synthesis in plasmodia may be compara-

---

[a] Except for the studies carried out by RUIZ-SANCHEZ et al. and LAING, a rapidly acting blood schizontocide was usually administered, just before or during treatment with a tetracycline, to persons with *acute* infections or parasite counts exceeding 15,000/mm^3

[b] Complementary drug was administered for 1–3 days immediately before (B) or during (D) treatment with antibiotic. Persons received 640–650 mg quinine salt three times a day or 900 mg amodiaquine base on the 1st day followed by 300 mg base on each of the next 2 days

[c] Treated individuals were at least 13 years old

[d] Persons were considered cured if asexual parasites did not recur during a follow-up period of a least 28 days after the start of treatment. Persons who where not cured of their infections invariably responded to treatment by initial clearance, but subsequent recrudescence, of parasitaemia

[e] The studies by RIECKMANN, CLYDE, and WILLERSON were carried out in non-endemic areas with strains of well-defined susceptibility to chloroquine and other drugs. The other studies were carried out in endemic areas where most of the parasites were presumed to be either sensitive or resistant to chloroquine

[f] Drug was administered to children 1½–5 years old

[g] No parasites were observed during the follow-up period of about 1 week after treatment

ble to that in bacteria since the overall protein-synthesising mechanisms of various organisms have been found to be very similar (LEWIS 1968 a).

In studies with *P. berghei*, neither tetracycline (WARHURST 1973) nor minocycline (KADDU et al. 1974) inhibited chloroquine-induced pigment clumping (WARHURST et al. 1972) in growing intraerythrocytic trophozoites in vitro; both drugs, however, exerted antimalarial activity against *P. berghei* in vivo. It was concluded that the drugs did not gain access to the growing trophozoites or that they did not affect cytoplasmic ribosomal protein synthesis in the organism (KADDU et al. 1974). By contrast, erythromycin, not a tetracycline antibiotic, did inhibit pigment clumping (WARHURST et al. 1976). Evaluation of the activity of antibiotics against *P. berghei* in vivo is complicated by the effects of antibiotics upon the intestinal flora of mice which, in turn, may affect the nutritional status of both the host and the parasite.

1. Chlortetracycline

This was the first tetracycline antibiotic discovered and the first one to be studied for its activity against human malaria parasites (COOPER et al. 1949). Significant antimalarial activity was observed in four individuals infected with vivax malaria. It was noted, however, that the response to treatment was far too slow to be of any practical value; fever and parasitaemia subsided only on the 5th or 6th day of treatment. This initial study and a subsequent one (IMBODEN et al. 1950) also showed that this drug significantly delayed the onset of parasitaemia when it was administered to volunteers for 6 days after they had been exposed to mosquitoes infected with *P. vivax* (Table 3). The findings suggested that this tetracycline inhibited, but did not prevent, the development of pre-erythrocytic schizonts. Relapses experienced after treatment showed that vivax infections could not be cured by this drug (Table 4). The studies by RUIZ-SANCHEZ et al. (1951) confirmed the effects of chlortetracycline against asexual erythrocytic forms of *P. vivax* and also demonstrated a similar activity against asexual parasites of *P. falciparum* (Table 1). Gametocytes of *P. falciparum*, however, persisted after treatment.

2. Oxytetracycline

Oxytetracycline was similar to chlortetracycline in its effects against erythrocytic stages of *P. vivax* and *P. falciparum* (RUIZ-SANCHEZ et al. 1952a; Table 1). No relapses of *P. vivax* were observed during a follow-up period of 3 months after treatment (Table 4).

In a later study, GARNHAM et al. (1971) found that oxytetracycline inhibited the normal maturation of exoerythrocytic schizonts in liver biopsy specimens taken from a chimpanzee infected with *P. vivax* (Table 3) and a rhesus monkey infected with *P. cynomolgi*. Although the prepatent period was lengthened by 4–12 days, both monkeys developed patent infections. The authors postulated that the prolonged period of incubation could be explained either by the release, on time, of a smaller than normal number of exoerythrocytic merozoites into the blood stream or by the delayed release of merozoites from "damaged" schizonts.

3. Tetracycline

In 1956, RUIZ-SANCHEZ and co-workers described the effects of tetracycline against one falciparum and 16 vivax infections. The response of these infections was similar to that described during earlier studies with chlortetracycline and oxytetracycline. Clearance of fever and parasitaemia was, in general, slower than that observed after treatment with other antimalarials such as chloroquine.

With the development of chloroquine-resistant strains of *P. falciparum*, a reappraisal of the value of some of the older antimalarials, including tetracycline, was carried out in the early 1970s. RIECKMANN et al. (1971, 1972) showed that 7–10 days of treatment with tetracycline cured most chloroquine-resistant infections and that it was equally effective against chloroquine-resistant and chloroquine-sensitive strains of *P. falciparum* (Table 1). Tetracycline had no effect on the parasite density or clinical condition of infected individuals during the first few days of treatment, but clearance of parasites and abatement of symptoms was usually observed within 4–7 days from the start of therapy. Because of the slow resolution of symptoms and the possible development of dangerously high levels of parasitaemia during the administration of tetracycline, rapidly acting blood schizontocides such as quinine or amodiaquine were given in conjunction with the tetracycline. Following the initial clinical studies (RIECKMANN et al. 1972), larger-scale studies in Thailand (COLWELL et al. 1972a, b) showed the value of using such drug combinations to achieve a rapid clinical response and radical cure in patients infected with chloroquine-resistant falciparum malaria (Table 1). When the course of treatment with tetracycline was reduced from 10 to 7 days (COLWELL et al. 1973) or to 3 days (CHIN and INTRAPRASERT 1973), 16%–33% of the patients showed a recrudescence of parasitaemia within 1 month of the start of treatment (Table 1).

The activity of tetracycline against *P. falciparum* is not limited to its asexual erythrocytic stages. Table 2 shows that the drug was also effective against the pre-erythrocytic tissue stages of chloroquine-resistant *P. falciparum*. All six non-immune volunteers who were bitten by heavily infected mosquitos on the 1st day of a 4-day course of tetracycline failed to develop malaria, whereas two untreated volunteers who were bitten by the same mosquitoes developed patent infections 11–12 days later. The causal prophylactic activity of the drug was confirmed by the fact that 3 days after the end of treatment, when the first asexual parasites might have been released into the peripheral blood stream, no tetracycline was detected in any of the blood samples collected at that time (RIECKMANN et al. 1972). As observed with the other tetracyclines, the drug has no effect upon the level of gametocytes of *P. falciparum*. It also exerts no sporontocidal activity against chloroquine-sensitive (CLYDE et al. 1971) or chloroquine-resistant (RIECKMANN et al. 1971) strains of *P. falciparum*.

The activity of tetracycline against *P. vivax* was studied by CLYDE and his co-workers (1971). They found that parasitaemia increased during the first 3 or 4 days of treatment, and that the subsequent clearance of fever and parasites were not related to the quantity of tetracycline administered nor to the initial parasite density. In two individuals who received 0.5 g tetracycline twice a day for 32 days after being bitten by infected mosquitoes, one developed a patent infection 14 days after completion of the drug course and the other showed no parasites during a post-

Table 2. Effects of two tetracyclines against pre-erythrocytic stages of *P. falciparum*

Treatment					No. of persons		Authors
Antibiotic	Daily dose	Doses per day	Duration (days)	Drug schedule[a]	Treated	Protected	
Tetracycline	1.0 g	4	4	0 to 3	6	6	RIECKMANN et al. (1972)
Minocycline	0.4 g	2	7	−1 to 5	3	3	WILLERSON et al. (1972)
	0.4 g	2	6	−1 to 4	3	3	WILLERSON et al. (1972)
	0.4 g	2	4	0 to 3	3	3	WILLERSON et al. (1972)
	0.2 g	1	7	−1 to 5	2	2	WILLERSON et al. (1972)
	0.1 g	1	7	−1 to 5	4	4	WILLERSON et al. (1972)
	0.1 g	1	2	0.3	2	2	WILLERSON et al. (1972)
	0.1 g	1	1	0	2	0	WILLERSON et al. (1972)

[a] Days indicated refer to the day before (−1), the day of (0) or the number of days after the person was bitten by infective mosquitoes

drug follow-up period of 45 days (Table 3). In 11 other persons who received 2–4 g/day for 7–14 days for treatment of their sporozoite-induced infections, a recurrence of parasitaemia was observed 21–44 days after the onset of drug therapy (Table 4). During another study by RIECKMANN (1971, personal observations), six patients showed a relapse of their vivax infections 43–85 days after receiving their first dose of tetracycline (Table 4). The delayed recurrence of parasites after treatment was probably due to the administration of a course of chloroquine in conjunction with 7–14 days of treatment with tetracycline.

4. Doxycycline

The effects of doxycycline against asexual erythrocytic stages of *P. falciparum* and *P. vivax* were similar to those observed with tetracycline (CLYDE et al. 1971). Clearance of fever and parasitaemia was slow and related to parasite density observed in the patients before the onset of treatment. Radical cure was observed in all patients who were treated with the drug twice a day for 7 days but not in those treated for 5 days (Table 1). The drug also showed no demonstrable effect against gametocytes, mosquitoes being able to transmit infections from one individual to another.

The effects of doxycycline against the exoerythrocytic stages of *P. vivax* were also studied by CLYDE et al. (1971). In two persons who were given the drug for 14 days after being exposed to infected mosquitoes, one developed parasitaemia 15 days after treatment and the other failed to develop a patent infection during a 7-month follow-up period (Table 3). Another two individuals who were treated for

Table 3. Effects of various tetracyclines against pre-erythrocytic stages of *P. vivax*

Treatment					No. of persons		Delay in onset of patency (days)[b]	Authors
Antibiotic	Daily dose	Doses per day	Duration (days)	Drug schedule[a]	Treated	Protected		
Chlortetracycline	8 g	8	7	0 to 6	2	0	16–19	COOPER et al. (1949)
Chlortetracycline	4 g	8	7	0 to 6	2	0	14–18	IMBODEN et al. (1950)
Chloramphenicol	4 g	8	7	0 to 6	2	0	4–11	IMBODEN et al. (1950)
Tetracycline	1.0 g	2	32	0 to 31[c]	2	1[d]	14[f]	CLYDE et al. (1971)
Doxycycline	0.1 g	1	14	0 to 13[c]	2	1[e]	15[f]	CLYDE et al. (1971)
Minocycline	0.4 g	2	6	– 1 to 4	2	0	20	RIECKMANN et al. (1971)
Oxytetracycline	35 mg/kg		2	3 to 4	1[g]	0	12	GARNHAM et al. (1971)

[a] Days indicated refer to the day before (– 1), the day of (0) or the number of days after individual was bitten by infective mosquitoes
[b] Delay represents the number of days after onset of parasitaemia in control individuals
[c] The drug may also have acted against the erythrocytic stages of *P. vivax* because drug administration was extended beyond the period required for development of the pre-erythrocytic stages
[d] Showed no relapse during a follow-up period of 45 days after the end of treatment
[e] Showed no relapse during a follow-up period of 7 months after the end of treatment
[f] Number of days after the end of treatment on which relapse was observed
[g] Drug administered to chimpanzees, not humans

Table 4. Effects of various tetracyclines against secondary exoerythrocytic stages of *P. vivax*

Treatment					No. of persons		Relapse [b] after start of treatment (days)	Authors
Antibiotic	Daily dose	Doses per day	Duration (days)	Complementary drug (dose)	Treated [a]	Cured		
Chlortetracycline	4–8 g	8	3–5	Quinine (14.0 g)	4	0	23–27	COOPER et al. (1949)
Chlortetracycline	4 g	8	7	Chloroquine (0.6 g)	2	0	32–36	IMBODEN et al. (1950)
Chloramphenicol	4 g	8	7	Chloroquine (0.6 g)	2	0	21–61	IMBODEN et al. (1950)
Chloramphenicol	50–75 mg/kg	3	6–10	–	13	13 [d]	–	RUIZ-SANCHEZ et al. (1952b)
Oxytetracycline	35–222 mg/kg	4	4–10	–	12 [c]	12 [e]	–	RUIZ-SANCHEZ et al. (1952b)
Tetracycline	40–50 mg/kg	3	8–11	–	16 [c]	16 [e]	–	RUIZ-SANCHEZ et al. (1971)
Tetracycline	2.0 g	4	7	–	4	0	23–44	CLYDE et al. (1971)
Tetracycline	2.0 g	4	14	–	1	0	32	CLYDE et al. (1971)
Tetracycline	4.0 g	4	7	–	6	0	21–29	CLYDE et al. (1971)
Tetracycline	1.0 g	4	7–10	Chloroquine (1.5 g)	2	0	43–57	RIECKMANN et al. (1971)
Tetracycline	1.0 g	4	14	Chloroquine (1.5 g)	4	0	44–85	RIECKMANN et al. (1971)
Minocycline	0.3 g	3	14	Chloroquine (1.5 g)	3	0	48–67	RIECKMANN et al. (1971)
Doxycycline	0.2 g	2	4–6	–	2	0	25–26	CLYDE et al. (1971)

[a] Treated individuals were at least 13 years old
[b] Number of days after start of treatment on which a recurrence of parasitaemia was observed
[c] Individuals included a few children
[d] Patients were followed up for 6–12 weeks after treatment
[e] Patients were followed up for 3–4 months after treatment

4–6 days during an acute episode of malaria showed a recurrence of parasitaemia 25–26 days after administration of the first dose of the drug (Table 4).

5. Minocycline

Various doses of minocycline, as low as 100 mg once a day for 7 days (Table 1), were effective in curing patients of their chloroquine-resistant falciparum infections (WILLERSON et al. 1972). The slow clearance of parasites and abatement of symptoms were characteristic of the response to treatment observed with other tetracyclines. The effects of the drug against pre-erythrocytic stages of *P. falciparum* were particularly striking; causal prophylaxis was achieved when 100 mg of the drug was administered on only two occasions, 4 h and 3 days after exposure to infected mosquitoes (Table 2). As observed with the other tetracyclines, minocycline did not prevent transmission of the infection to other individuals. Administration of this drug to patients in Thailand (COLWELL et al. 1972a) resulted in the radical cure of 96% of the infections (Table 1). As with other tetracyclines, minocycline should be used in combination with a rapidly acting blood schizontocide for treating acute infections of falciparum malaria. Later studies with *P. knowlesi* in Assamese monkeys also showed that minocycline was more effective at lower dosages than tetracycline (DUTTA and SINGH 1979).

Minocycline also exerted partial activity against the pre-erythrocytic stages of *P. vivax* (RIECKMANN 1971, personal observations). When drug administration to two volunteers was discontinued 4 days after they were bitten by infected mosquitoes, both developed a patent infection 30 days after sporozoite inoculation; an untreated volunteer exposed to the same mosquitoes showed parasites 10 days after sporozoite inoculation (Table 3). Minocycline was not effective, however, in curing vivax infections. When given in combination with chloroquine, it did not delay the onset of relapses; the time interval between treatment of an acute episode and reappearance of parasites was 48–67 days in patients who received minocycline combined with chloroquine and 47–65 days in patients who were treated with chloroquine alone (Table 4).

II. Clindamycin

Clindamycin and other chlorinated analogues, particularly *N*-demethyl-4′-pentyl-7-chlorolincomycin, were shown to have a marked activity against drug-sensitive and drug-resistant strains of *P. berghei* in rodents (LEWIS 1968a, b).

Evaluation of the activity of these compounds against blood-induced infections of *P. cynomolgi* in rhesus monkeys showed that, despite a very slow clearance of parasites, all monkeys were cured of their infections (POWERS 1969). During extensive studies with sporozoite-induced infections of *P. cynomolgi*, SCHMIDT and his co-workers (1970) confirmed the slow clearance of parasitaemia after administration of clindamycin or its *N*-demethyl analogue. Despite a marked increase in the interval between treatment and relapse, radical cures were only observed in a few animals receiving the highest doses of the *N*-demethyl analogue. The most interesting finding observed in these studies was the partial effect of both drugs against the pre-erythrocytic stages of *P. cynomolgi*. The onset of patent parasitaemia was usually delayed for 2–3 weeks when either one of the drugs was given at the time

Table 5. Effect of clindamycin against asexual erythrocytic stages of *P. falciparum*

Treatment				No. of persons		Susceptibility of parasites to chloroquine	Authors
Daily dose	Doses per day	Duration (days)	Quinine administration (B or D)[a]	Treated[b]	Cured		
1.80 g	4	7	B	4	4	Resistant	MILLER et al (1974)
1.80 g	4	3	B	8	8	Resistant	MILLER et al (1974)
1.80 g	4	3	D	5	5	Resistant	MILLER et al (1974)
1.35 g	3	3	–	11	6	Resistant	HALL et al. (1975)
32 mg/kg	3	3	–	1[c]	0	Resistant	HALL et al. (1975)
0.90 g	3	3	D	4	4	Resistant	HALL et al. (1975)
0.45 g	3	3	D[d]	5	3	Resistant	HALL et al. (1975)
1.35 g	3	3	–	2	2	Resistant	CLYDE et al. (1975)
1.35 g	3	3	–	1	1	Sensitive	CLYDE et al. (1975)
1.35 g	3	3	D	1	1	Sensitive	CLYDE et al. (1975)
1.35 g	3	3	D	4	2	Resistant	CLYDE et al. (1975)
0.60 g	1	3	D	2	1	Resistant	CLYDE et al. (1975)
0.60 g	1	3	–	1	0	Resistant	CLYDE et al. (1975)

[a] Quinine, 650–666 mg salt, was administered every 8 h for 3 days immediately before (B) or during (D) treatment with clindamycin
[b] Adult male individuals
[c] Twelve-year-old male weighing 28 kg
[d] Half dose of quinine administered every 8 h for 3 days

of sporozoite challenge and during the incubation period; in some animals which had received the *N*-demethyl analogue, patent infections never developed. Histological studies, carried out in animals which had received the *N*-demethyl analogue, showed a marked reduction in the number of pre-erythrocytic parasites found in their hepatic parenchyma. Although the causal prophylactic activity of the drug was complete in some cases, the fact that most monkeys eventually developed patent infections suggested that the injurious effects of the drug were at least partly reversible. In a study with *P. vivax*, the human counterpart of *P. cynomolgi*, clindamycin appeared to have no appreciable effect against exoerythrocytic schizonts (CLYDE et al. 1975). All four patients had a relapse of their infections 41–51 days after they were started on a 14-day course of clindamycin (450 mg every 6 h).

The activity of clindamycin and its *N*-demethyl analogue was subsequently demonstrated against chloroquine-resistant infections of *P. falciparum* in *Aotus* monkeys (Powers and Jacobs 1972). This prompted the evaluation of clindamycin in individuals infected with chloroquine-resistant and chloroquine-sensitive strains of *P. falciparum* (Table 5). Administration of 450 mg clindamycin every 6 h for only 3 days, given during or after a 3-day course of quinine, cured all 13 non-immune patients treated with such a drug combination (Miller et al. 1974). Quinine, given alone for 3 days, did not cure infections with these strains. Blood levels of clindamycin and quinine were similar whether individuals received these drugs alone or in combination with each other. Vomiting, diarrhoea or other evidence of toxicity were not observed in any of the volunteers. Severe upper gastrointestinal toxicity was observed, however, during the course of two subsequent studies in which patients were given these high doses of clindamycin and standard doses of quinine concurrently for 3 days (Hall et al. 1975; Clyde et al. 1975). In one of the studies (Hall et al. 1975), the dose of clindamycin administered to most patients was reduced from 450 mg to 300 mg or 150 mg every 8 h because of the toxicity of the drug; unacceptable upper gastrointestinal side effects were still apparent when clindamycin was given at the usually recommended adult dose of 150 mg every 6 or 8 h in combination with half the recommended doses of quinine. Whereas all four patients in this study treated with the higher drug doses were cured of their infections, two of the five patients treated with the lower standard doses showed a recrudescence of parasitaemia. In the other study (Clyde et al. 1975), two of the five patients receiving 450 mg clindamycin every 8 h in combination with quinine had a recrudescence of parasitaemia and two of the three patients who received a single daily dose of 600 mg clindamycin, alone or in combination with quinine, were also not cured of their infections. The results of these studies showed that clindamycin exerted a slow activity against asexual erythrocytic stages of *P. falciparum* and that, similar to the tetracyclines, it had to be given in combination with a quick-acting blood schizontocidal drug, such as quinine, for rapid clearance of fever and parasitaemia. The concurrent administration of clindamycin and quinine was, however, often associated with unacceptable upper gastrointestinal side effects which would appear to limit the value of this drug regimen in the treatment of chloroquine-resistant falciparum infections.

The effects of clindamycin and its *N*-demethyl analogue on the morphology of *P. knowlesi* were studied by Powers et al. (1976). The drugs had little effect on the course of infection in *P. knowlesi*-infected monkeys during the first 2 or 3 days of treatment. Although some drug effects were observed in the ribosomes during the first 24 h of treatment, morphological changes became more pronounced during the next two cycles of parasite development. The authors speculated that the morphological changes seen in the ribosomes could be the result of drug binding to parasites, thereby producing configurational changes or possibly activating intrinsic RNAase. The nuclear and mitochondrial changes observed in the malaria parasites appeared to be secondary to the ribosomal changes and were probably not directly related to the activity of these drugs. The progressive effect of clindamycin on the morphology of the parasites was not related to cumulative build-up of the antibiotics. The authors suggested that the most likely explanations for the effects of the drug being delayed until the second or third generations were (a) that the drug was bound to the ribosomes and transferred on these organelles to subsequent generations or (b) that the drug altered the DNA replication or repair process, thereby changing the normal transmission of genetic information from one generation to the next.

In bacteria, clindamycin inhibits protein synthesis and acts specifically on the 50S subunit of the ribosome, most likely by affecting the process of peptide chain initiation (REUSSER 1975). Since the mechanism of inhibition of protein synthesis by clindamycin may be similar in bacteria and plasmodia (see Sect. C.I) and since macrolide antibiotics also bind to the 50S subunit of the ribosome, it may be advisable not to use macrolide antibiotics, such as erythromycin, in combination with clindamycin.

D. Pharmacokinetics and Metabolism

I. Tetracyclines

1. Absorption

Chlortetracycline, oxytetracycline, and *tetracycline* are absorbed to a varying degree from the upper gastrointestinal tract. Whereas about 30% and 50% of the oral dose of *chlortetracycline* and *oxytetracyclines*, respectively, are absorbed, between 60% and 80% of a dose of *tetracycline* is absorbed when the stomach is empty. The percentage of drug that is not absorbed rises as the dose is increased. The serum half-life of tetracycline is 8–10 h and peak plasma levels of 3–4 µg/ml are reached when repeated doses of 250 mg of the drug are given every 6 h. Tetracycline administered in capsules appears to be better absorbed than from film-coated tablets (DAVIS et al. 1973). *Doxycycline* and *minocycline* are almost completely absorbed (90%–100%) from the gastrointestinal tract. As they also have longer serum half-lives (14–22 h), both drugs can be administered in lower doses and less frequently than the other tetracyclines. Whereas the recommended adult dose for *tetracycline* is 250–500 mg four times a day, the maintenance dose for *doxycycline* or *minocycline* is 100 mg of the drug taken once or twice a day. The absorption of tetracyclines is impaired by divalent and trivalent cations such as Ca^{++} (calcium), Al^{++} (aluminium), Mg^{++} (magnesium), and Fe^{++} or Fe^{+++} (iron), probably because the drugs form insoluble chelate complexes with these metals (ALBERT 1953; ALBERT and REES 1956; BESSMAN and DOORENBOS 1957; KUNIN and FINLAND 1961; SHILS 1962; KAKEMI et al. 1968; NEUVONEN et al. 1970). Therefore, tetracyclines should generally be administered on an empty stomach, and milk, milk products, antacids, and preparations containing iron, calcium or magnesium salts should be withheld for at least 2 h after the ingestion of tetracycline. Despite these considerations, it may sometimes be necessary to administer tetracyclines with a light meal to help overcome the gastric intolerance experienced by some patients. Antacid preparations containing only sodium bicarbonate can also interfere with the absorption of tetracyclines because the increased intragastric pH does not permit adequate dissolution of tetracycline capsules prior to absorption from the intestinal tract (BARR et al. 1971). Although the absorption of *doxycycline* and *minocycline* is less influenced by the ingestion of food or milk (ROSENBLATT et al. 1966;

MIGLIARDI and SCHACH VON WITTENAU 1967; KITAMOTO et al. 1969;; BROGDEN et al. 1975), the absorption of both these drugs can be adversely affected by the presence of iron, aluminium, calcium or magnesium (NEUVONEN et al. 1970; SCHACH VON WITTENAU and TWOMEY 1971; BRODGEN et al. 1975).

2. Distribution

After oral administration, the tetracyclines are widely distributed in human body tissues and fluids. The degree of cell and tissue penetration depends, to a large extent, on the lipid solubility of the drug. *Doxycycline* and *minocycline* are the most soluble of the tetraclines (ALLEN 1976) and this may account for their higher penetration into some organs (BARZA et al. 1975). Tetracyclines are taken up and stored by the reticuloendothelial cells of the liver, spleen, bone maroow, and in bone and the dentine and enamel of unerupted teeth (KUNIN and FINLAND 1961; MACDONALD et al. 1973). They also pass the placenta to reach the fetus and appear in the milk of lactating women (KUNIN and FINLAND 1961). With the exception of *oxytetracycline*, all the tetracyclines show a marked binding to serum proteins (KUNIN and FINLAND 1961; SCHACH VON WITTENAU and YEARY 1963; ROSENBLATT et al. 1966; MACDONALD et al. 1973). Between 50% and 90% of the tetracyclines form stable, though not irreversible, complexes with the proteins.

3. Metabolism and Excretion

Tetracyclines appear to be quite stable metabolically and, for the most part, are excreted unchanged in faeces and urine (KELLY et al. 1961; EISNER and WULF 1963; KELLY and KANEGIS 1967; STEIGBIGEL et al. 1968; SCHACH VON WITTENAU and TWOMEY 1971). Human studies carried out with *tetracycline* and with some of its earlier analogues showed that 50% or more of the drug was excreted in the urine and that patients with impaired renal function developed excessively high serum levels of these drugs. The lower urinary excretion of *doxycycline* and, probably, *minocycline* allows both drugs to be used in patients with renal disease whose renal function has not been severely impaired (LITTLE and BAILEY 1970; ALLEN 1976; APPEL and NEU 1977). The high concentrations of tetracyclines observed in the bile indicate that a considerable proportion of these antibiotics are concentrated in the liver and eliminated, by way of the bile, into the intestine from which they are partially reabsorbed (EISNER and WULF 1963; ISHIYAMA et al. 1969; MACDONALD et al. 1973). In addition, some tetracyclines are partly eliminated in the faeces by non-biliary excretion (ANDRÉ 1956; MAHON et al. 1970; SCHACH VON WITTENAU and TWOMEY 1971). *Doxycycline* is excreted in the faeces largely in an inactive form, possibly accounting for the minimal changes in intestinal flora observed after administration of this drug (HINTON 1970).

II. Clindamycin

1. Absorption

Clindamycin is almost completely absorbed from the gastrointestinal tract and peak serum levels of 2.5–3.0 μg/ml are attained within 1–2 h after oral administration of 150 mg of the drug (PEDDIE et al. 1975). Administration of 300 and 600 mg of the antibiotic results in peak levels of about 4 and 8 μg/ml, respectively (KEUSCH and PRESENT 1976). The half-life of clindamycin is about 2½ h. Absorption of clindamycin is not impaired by the presence of food in the stomach (MCGEHEE et al. 1968; WAGNER et al. 1968). Clindamycin palmitate, an oral preparation for use in children, is inactive per se. Its ester, however, is rapidly hydrolysed in vivo and its absorption is similar to that observed after administration of the parent compound.

2. Distribution

Clindamycin is widely distributed in body tissues and fluids. It crosses the placenta (PHILIPSON et al. 1973) and, as with lincomycin (MEDINA et al. 1964), is probably present in milk. Between 60% and 90% of the drug is bound to serum proteins (PANZER et al. 1972; PHILIPSON et al. 1973; EASTWOOD and GOWER 1974).

3. Metabolism and Excretion

Clindamycin is substantially metabolised and inactivated in the liver, presumably to *N*-demethylclindamycin and clindamycin sulphoxide. Much of the antibiotic is eliminated by biliary secretion (WILLIAMS et al. 1975). Patients with hepatic dysfunction show elevated serum levels of the drug (BRANDL et al. 1972; WILLIAMS et al. 1975; KEUSCH and PRESENT 1976), indicating that clindamycin-treated individuals should be carefully monitored in the event that a reduction in the dose becomes necessary. Clindamycin and its metabolites are excreted to a lesser extent in the urine (MCGEHEE et al. 1968). Consequently, serum levels are not significantly altered in patients with mild to moderate renal failure (EASTWOOD and GOWER 1974; PEDDIE et al. 1975) and modification of dosage is only required for individuals whose kidneys show very severe functional impairment (MALACOFF et al. 1975).

E. Toxicity

I. Tetracyclines

The use of tetracyclines after the first trimester of pregnancy and in babies up to 6 months of age may result in discoloration of the deciduous teeth (WEYMAN 1965; KUTSCHER et al. 1966). It may produce a similar effect in children from 2 months to 8 years of age during the calcification of their permanent teeth (STEWART 1973). Although this adverse reaction is more common during long-term administration, it has also been observed after repeated short-term courses of these antibiotics. The discoloration of teeth is permanent, but cosmetic improvement has been noted after bleaching with hydrogen peroxide (COHEN and PARKINS 1970). Tetracyclines may also interfere with normal development of enamel. In addition, they form a stable calcium complex in bone-forming tissues and can produce a marked depression of bone growth in premature infants (COHLAN et al. 1963). This effect can be readily reversed if the drug has only been given for a short period of time.

Administration of tetracyclines to individuals with impaired renal function may lead to excessively high serum levels and possible hepatic toxicity. Hepatotoxic effects are also observed in patients receiving large doses of tetracyclines orally or intravenously (LEPPER 1951). Pregnant and postpartum women are particularly susceptible to severe liver damage (SCHULTZ et al. 1963). Because of the antianabolic effect of the tetracyclines, patients with renal disease develop progressive azotaemia, hyperphosphataemia, and acidosis (POTHIER and ANDERSON 1966; PHILLIPS et al. 1974), which may be prevented by the use of anabolic steroids (SHILS 1963). Tetracycline-induced catabolic processes may also be responsible for the loss in body weight and negative nitrogen balance observed in malnourished individuals (GABUZDA et al. 1958).

Outdated or degraded *tetracycline* may have a toxic effect on the kidneys and result in a reversible Fanconci-like syndrome (GROSS 1963; FRIMPTER et al. 1963). It is unlikely that this complication will occur in the future because the acid excipient which led to degradation of the antibiotic during storage has been removed from current drug formulations.

Photosensitivity characterised by erythema in sun-exposed areas of the body can occur after treatment with the tetracyclines. Phototoxic reactions are most commonly observed with *democlocycline* and least with *minocycline*.

Gastrointestinal toxicity, usually dose related, can be induced by all tetracyclines. Side effects include abdominal discomfort, epigastric distress, nausea, vomiting, and diarrhoea. The symptoms often subside with continued medication and may be controlled by administering smaller doses of the drug at more frequent intervals. As gastrointestinal irritation may be controlled by administering tetracyclines with a meal, consideration should be given to using *minocycline* or *doxycycline* in sensitive individuals because the absorption of both drugs is influenced less by food than that of other tetracycline antibiotics. The diarrhoea caused by irritation of the gastrointestinal tract is characterised by frequent and fluid stools which do *not* contain blood or white cells. This type of diarrhoea must be distinguished from that caused by overgrowth of yeasts or bacteria resistant to the tetracyclines. Apart from the relatively benign suprainfections caused by *Candida* (SMITS et al. 1966) or *Escherichia coli* (BARTLETT et al. 1975), a serious but, fortunately, very rare result of treatment with tetracycline is staphylococcal enterocolitis (THAYSEN and ERIKSEN 1956). The infection is characterised by severe diarrhoea with liquid stools which frequently contain blood and leucocytes and always contain coagulase-positive staphylococci. Immediate cessation of tetracycline therapy, restoration of water and electrolyte balance, and treatment with vancomycin usually result in a rapid improvement of the patient's condition. Staphyloccal infections after the use of tetracyclines have been extremely rare during recent years and it is possible that earlier infections may, in fact, have been cases of pseudomembranous colitis (FEKETY 1979). Pseudomembranous colitis is seen more commonly after treatment with clindamycin and is described below (see Sect. E.II).

Hypersensitivity reactions to tetracyclines are rare. Urticaria, angioneurotic oedema, exfoliative dermatitis, and anaphylactoid reactions are among the allergic responses which have been reported. Cross-sensitisation among the different tetracyclines is common.

Intravenous administration of the tetracyclines is frequently followed by thrombophlebitis and intramuscular injections produce severe pain. However, there appear to be no indications for the parenteral administration of tetracyclines in the treatment of malaria.

The use of *minocycline* has been associated with a relatively high incidence of postural light-headedness, dizziness or vertigo, often with nausea and vomiting (ALLEN 1976). These symptoms, attributed to vestibular dysfunction, may disappear during therapy and always disappear after discontinuation of drug therapy. During studies to determine the effects of minocycline against falciparum infections, drug-related symptoms were observed in 7 out of 19 individuals who received 200 mg or more per day, but no symptoms were observed in six individuals who received 100 mg of the drug once a day (WILLERSON et al. 1972). On the other hand, 4 out of 47 patients with acne vulgaris stopped taking 100 mg minocycline once a day after 1–2 weeks of medication because they developed vestibular side effects (COSKEY 1976). In studies involving an additional 74 acne patients, no vestibular side effects were reported during the administration of 100 mg minocycline/day (50 mg twice a day) for 6–19 weeks (CULLEN and COHAN 1976; CULLEN 1978). Since preliminary evaluation of daily adult doses as low as 100 mg minocycline showed that they were effective in preventing and curing falciparum malaria (WILLERSON et al. 1972), it may not be necessary to use the higher doses (200 mg daily) recommended for the treatment of other infections, thereby reducing the incidence of vestibular side effects.

The long-term administration of low doses of tetracyclines to patients with acne vulgaris appears to have been associated with remarkably few side effects, despite the fact that about 10% of the tetracycline produced for human use in the United States is prescribed by dermatologists for the treatment of acne. The main complications which have been reported are *Candida vaginitis* and gram-negative folliculitis (BJORNBERG and ROUPE 1972; LEYDEN et al. 1973). In 1975, an AD HOC COMMITTEE ON THE USE OF ANTIBIOTICS IN DERMATOLOGY reviewed the experiences gained after treating acne vulgaris with systemically administered antibiotics over a period of a quarter of a century. The committee noted that "there have been no reports of overwhelming infections due to drug-resistant microorganisms in patients with acne who have received prolonged courses of systemic antibiotic treatment." After pointing out that "most patients with acne are otherwise healthy and are treated on an outpatient basis with low doses of antibiotics," that "therefore, inpatient experiences with seriously ill or immunologically compromised patients who constitute many of the drug-reaction cases cited in the literature, are inappropriate standards for comparison," and that "the most germane information concerning side-effects is that which has been derived from patients who have acne," the committee concluded that "*tetracycline* is a rational, effective, and relatively safe drug for use in the treatment of acne vulgaris when given in a dosage of 1 g or less per day for long-term therapy."

II. Clindamycin

The administration of a daily dose of 0.6–1.2 g clindamycin (in three or four divided doses) is sometimes associated with the development of severe enterocolitis and diarrhoea (COHEN et al. 1973; TEDESCO et al. 1974). The colitis induced by clindamycin is similar to that induced by other antimicrobial agents, the most frequently implicated ones being lincomycin, ampicillin, and various cephalosporins (W. L. GEORGE 1980). These drugs may alter the normal flora of the intestines, thereby interfering with the suppression of the growth of *Clostridium difficile;* the toxin produced by *C. difficile* has been implicated as the main cause of antimicrobial agent-associated pseudomembraneous colitis (W. L. GEORGE et al. 1978, BARTLETT et al. 1979). Diarrhoea may develop during antibiotic therapy or up to 3 weeks after it has been discontinued, and it usually resolves spontaneously within 1 or 2 weeks after cessation of therapy (TEDESCO 1976). The diarrhoea may be associated with nausea, vomiting, abdominal pain, cramps, and fever. More severe cases may develop intense pain and a pronounced fever and leucocytosis. Infrequent complications include toxic megacolon, colonic perforation and even death.

Treatment with oral vancomycin to eliminate *C. difficile* is usually recommended for the seriously ill patient after clindamycin therapy has been discontinued (TEDESCO et al. 1978). The disadvantages of vancomycin are its very high cost and its unavailability in many countries. Metronidazole, a relatively inexpensive drug and a possible alternative to vancomycin, has been used to treat several cases of antimicrobial-associated colitis (TRINH DINH et al. 1978; MATUCHANSKY et al. 1978; PASHBY et al. 1979). Other drugs which have been used include bacitracin (CHANG et al. 1980) and tetracycline (DEJESUS and PETERNEL 1978). Cholestyramine is an anion-exchange resin that binds *C. difficile* toxin in vitro (R. H. GEORGE et al. 1978). Since its effect in unpredictable in vivo (KEUSCH and PRESENT 1976), it has been recommended that this resin only be used in patients with mild to moderate symptoms (W. L. GEORGE et al. 1980). Since vancomycin can be bound to cholestyramine (R. H. GEORGE et al. 1978), the simultaneous administration of both agents should be avoided. Antiperistaltic agents, such as Lomotil and opiate derivates should also not be used.

Skin rashes have been reported in about 10% of patients treated with clindamycin. Rare side effects include exudative erythema multiforme (Stevens-Johnson syndrome) and anaphylactic reactions. Local thrombophlebitis may follow intravenous administration of the drug.

F. Deployment

The development of chloroquine-resistant strains of *P. falciparum* in South America and Southeast Asia led to the widespread use of sulfadoxine-pyrimethamine (Fansidar), alone or in combination with quinine, as the treatment of choice for falciparum infections acquired in these areas. This sulphonamide-pyrimethamine combination is also the most common chemoprophylactic used for protection against chloroquine-resistant falciparum malaria. Although such drug combinations have proven to be very useful against falciparum malaria, they sometimes fail to cure patients of their infections (CHIN et al. 1966) partly because of host erythrocytic factors (TRENHOLME et al. 1975). Under such circumstances, it may be necessary to use alternative drugs, e.g. the tetracyclines.

Recently, it has become increasingly obvious that sulfadoxine-pyrimethamine combinations are no longer capable of curing a high percentage of falciparum infections acquired in some areas where chloroquine resistance is prevalent (CENTER FOR DISEASE CONTROL 1980; HURWITZ et al. 1981; RIECKMANN 1981, personal observations). Previous experience in treating chloroquine-resistant infections with 7- to 14-day courses of quinine had already shown that cures were not achieved in a distressingly large number of patients, despite the fact that this drug was usually effective in bringing acute episodes of malaria under control (WHO 1973). This means, in effect, that the tetracyclines and clindamycin are the only known currently marketed drugs which are still capable of curing infections of *P. falciparum* that are resistant to chloroquine, quinine, and sulphonamide (or sulphone)-pyrimethamine combinations.

I. Treatment of Multidrug-Resistant Infections of *P. falciparum*

The tetracyclines are highly effective in curing patients of their falciparum infections, but they are slow in controlling fever and parasitaemia. It is, therefore, imperative that standard doses of a rapidly acting drug, such as quinine or amodiaquine, be administered in conjunction with the tetracycline for a period of 3 days. This leads to a prompt improvement in the clinical condition of the patient and prevents the development of dangerously high levels of parasitaemia in individuals with acute infections of the disease.

Many tetracycline antibiotics have been used to treat malaria, but the efficacy against chloroquine-resistant strains of *P. falciparum* has only been determined for tetracycline, doxycycline, and minocycline. All three tetracyclines cure the vast majority of patients when any of them are given orally over a period of 7–10 days. Parenteral administration of these drugs is not indicated in the treatment of malaria.

Tetracycline is administered every 6 h. The antimalarial dose is 1 g/day for adults and 25 mg/kg body wt. per day for children. *Doxycycline* and *minocycline* are administered less frequently. The usual adult dose for *doxycycline* is 200 mg on the 1st day of treatment followed by a maintenance dose of 100 mg/day. The dosage recommended for children is 4 mg/kg body wt. on the 1st day (in two equal doses) followed by 2 mg/kg once a day. The recommended adult dose for *minocycline* is 200 mg initially followed by a maintenance dose of 100 mg every 12 h. The dosage recommended for children is 4 mg/kg body wt. initially followed by 2 mg/kg every 12 h as the maintenance dosage.

Antimalarial studies with *doxycycline* and, to a lesser extent with *minocycline*, were performed with drug doses which are higher than those generally recommended at the present time. The results observed in a few patients who received low doses of *minocycline* suggest that this tetracycline, for one, might cure falciparum infections at lower-than-recommended doses; such doses also appear to lower the incidence of the bothersome, but reversible, vestibular disturbances noted with higher doses of the drug. As a general principle, patients should be treated with the minimal dosage of an antibiotic consistent with the desired therapeutic response because the incidence of side effects, e.g. gastrointestinal distress, colitis, etc., rises as the dose of the antibiotic is increased. Further studies are urgently needed to determine the minimum doses of *doxycycline* and *minocycline* needed to effect radical cure of falciparum infections. Until the results of such studies are available, it is advisable to use *tetracycline* for the treatment of such infections.

The potential advantages of eventually using *doxycycline* or *minocycline* are that these drugs can be taken less frequently than tetracycline, that they can be used in patients with renal disease and that they are absorbed more reliably than tetracycline in the presence of food. It has also been reported that *doxycycline* induces fewer changes in the intestinal flora than tetracycline and that *minocycline* is associatd with fewer phototoxic reactions than the other tetracyclines. The major disadvantage of both drugs is that a standard course of treatment is many times more expensive than that of tetracycline; the cost, however, may be reduced if lower doses of these drugs are shown to be effective against malaria infections.

In general, the use of tetracyclines during the latter half of pregnancy and during childhood (up to 8 years) should be avoided, primarily because of the effect of these drugs on the enamel of unerupted teeth. It should be noted that administration of the drug during pregnancy or during the first few months of life does not lead to discoloration of the permanent teeth. Although the routine use of tetracycline cannot be advocated in pregnant women and in children less than 8 years old, these drugs should be used unhesitatingly if the life of a malaria patient is threatened because of the lack of safe and effective, alternative drugs.

The use of clindamycin should probably be restricted, at present, to individuals who cannot be treated with the tetracyclines. Because of its slow effect against malaria parasites, clindamycin should be given in conjunction with a quick-acting blood schizontocide, such as quinine or amodiaquine. Since severe gastrointestinal toxicity has been noted during the combined administration of quinine and clindamycin, it is preferable to administer a rapidly acting drug for 3 days immediately prior to starting treatment with clindamycin.

Administration of oral clindamycin for 3 days has proven effective in curing a large proportion of individuals infected with chloroquine-resistant parasites of *P. falciparum*. As with doxycycline and minocycline, most studies involved doses which were two to three times higher than those recommended at present for the treatment of mild or moderate bacterial infections; the higher doses are now only recommended for the treatment of serious bacterial infections. The usual dose recommended is 150 mg every 6 h for adults and 8–16 mg/kg body wt. per day for children, given in three or four divided doses. The ester clindamycin palmitate hydrochloride is available as a suspension for administration to children.

The relatively high frequency of pseudomembranous colitis encountered after administration of clindamycin is a deterrent to current utilisation of this drug for the treatment of drug-resistant falciparum malaria. On the other hand, it does not produce many of the side effects noted with the tetracyclines and can be used in patients with mild to moderate impairment of renal function. Recent advances in understanding the aetiology of antimicrobial-associated colitis might lead to prevention of this condition (GEORGE et al. 1980) and, thereby, render clindamycin more acceptable for the treatment of falciparum malaria. Despite preliminary indications that a number of different agents are effective against antimcrobial-associated colitis, vancomycin is currently the drug of choice and the use of other potentially effective agents should await the results of further studies (GEORGE et al. 1980).

II. Prophylaxis Against Multidrug-Resistant *P. falciparum*

The failure of pyrimethamine-sulfadoxine to protect individuals against *P. falciparum* along the border between Thailand and Kampuchea has prompted consideration of the limited use of tetracyclines as prophylactic agents in these areas (CENTER FOR DISEASE CONTROL 1982). Although tetracycline was shown to exert a marked causal prophylactic activity against multidrug-resistant strains of *P. falciparum* over a decade ago (RIECKMANN et al. 1971), the widespread use of tetracyclines was not advocated for the prevention of chloroquine-resistant malaria. Since the tetracyclines are broad-spectrum antibiotics which were important in the clinical management and control of infections caused by many different microorganisms, it was felt (rightly so) that the use of tetracyclines in malaria prophylaxis would promote the development of tetracycline-resistant organisms. Furthermore, other drugs with fewer sideeffects were still able to provide effective protection against chloroquine-resistant falciparum malaria.

During the 1970s, indications for the use of tetracyclines in bacterial infections declined considerably due to (a) increased bacterial resistance to the tetracyclines resulting from extensive administration of these drugs to humans and animals and (b) the development of new antimicrobial agents which were more effective or less toxic for the treatment of specific infections. Over the same period of time, prolonged courses of low doses of tetracyclines were widely prescribed for the treatment of acne vulgaris. Long-term ingestion of these antibiotics, under minimal medical supervision, has apparently not been associated with serious side effects or overwhelming overgrowth of drug-resistant yeasts and bacteria (AD HOC COMMITTEE ON THE USE OF ANTIBIOTICS IN DERMATOLOGY 1975). Comparable administration of tetracyclines to individuals living in malarious communities may, however, be less innocuous; their overall status of health and nutrition would, in many instances, not be as good as that of acne patients, most of whom are otherwise healthy young people residing in non-malarious areas. The widespread use of tetracyclines in malarious areas can also not be recommended because of the demonstrated transfer, by R plasmids, of resistance (to tetracycline and other antibiotics) between organisms of the same or unrelated bacterial species.

In view of the unavailability of effective alternative drugs, the selective use of tetracyclines for chemoprophylaxis against falciparum malaria will probably be necessary in certain parts of the world. Their use should be limited, if possible, to personal prophylaxis by non-immune individuals visiting or working temporarily in areas with a high transmission of multidrug-resistant strains. Because of their long half-lives, it would be most convenient to use doxycycline or minocycline for this purpose. Adult doses of 100 mg, taken once a day, should be adequate in protecting individuals against *P. falciparum* malaria. As the tetracyclines suppress the blood stages of *P. vivax* and exert partial activity against the pre-erythrocytic stages of the species, it should not be necessary to use chloroquine for the suppression of vivax malaria. The tetracyclines are, however, not effective against the secondary exoerythrocytic stages of *P. vivax* and relapses can be expected after discontinuation of tetracycline prophylaxis. Since very limited studies have been undertaken to determine the efficacy of tetracyclines as prophylactic drugs against *P. falciparum* and *P. vivax*, the recommended doses should be regarded as preliminary and tentative. More definite recommendations with regard to the prophylactic use of tetracyclines can only be made following studies carried out to determine minimum effective drug doses and, in addition, side effects of these drugs among residents in malarious areas.

G. Drug Resistance

In view of the increasing scarcity of drugs which are still effective in the treatment and prophylaxis of multidrug-resistant strains of *P. falciparum,* it is important to investigate the rate at which parasites might develop resistance to antimalarial antibiotics, to explore the mechanisms involved in such a process and, if possible, to use these drugs in a manner which would prevent or delay the onset of resistance. The rate of development of resistance by *P. berghei* to minocycline or clindamycin was studied by JACOBS and KOONTZ (1976). Resistance to both antibiotics developed much slower than to the more conventional antimalarials such as chloroquine, quinine or pyrimethamine. Although *P. berghei* developed total resistance to the latter compounds in 9–12 treated passages in mice over a period of 60–85 days, development of total resistance to clindamycin required 42 passages over a period of 300 days and development of partial (not total) resistance to minocycline required 86 passages over a period of 600 days. The clindamycin-resistant strain showed normal susceptibility to minocycline and the strain which was partially resistant to minocycline showed normal susceptibility to clindamycin. The absence of cross-resistance suggested that the mode of action of these two antibiotics against *P. berghei* is different, the drugs conceivably inhibiting protein synthesis by different mechanisms. Resistance to clindamycin was stable during 51 drug-free passages in mice; the partial resistance to minocycline was unstable, the strain reverting to normal sensitivity during 16 drug-free passages. The findings observed in this study suggest that other plasmodial species, such as *P. falciparum,* might eventually develop resistance to the tetracyclines and clindamycin.

The mechanisms by which plasmodia might develop resistance to antibiotics have apparently not yet been investigated. In many Gram-negative bacteria, particularly those which are normal inhabitants of the gastrointestinal tract, resistance to tetracyclines may be acquired by transfer of R plasmids from one organism to another. Resistance may be transferred between organisms of the same or different species and it may be confined to the tetracyclines or may extend to other antibiotics. Although malaria parasites may acquire resistance to antibiotics by a process of conjugation, drug-resistant strains might emerge through genetic mutation and subsequent selection by drug pressure. If mutations were the predominant mechanism by which parasites acquired resistance to antibiotics, the use of suitable drug combinations might be an effective means of preventing or delaying the emergence of resistant strains. Drug combinations would be especially useful if it were demonstrated that the two agents acted synergistically against malaria parasites; the use of drugs which antagonised each other's antimalarial activity would obviously not be desirable. Before advocating the use of a particular drug combination, detailed investigations would have to be carried out to exclude the possibility of additive or supra-additive drug toxicities in the human host.

References

Ad Hoc Committee on the Use of Antibiotics in Dermatology (1975) Systemic antibiotics for treatment of acne vulgaris: efficacy and safety. Arch Dermatol III:1630–1636

Albert A (1953) Avidity of terramycin and aureomycin for metallic cations. Nature 172:201

Albert A, Rees CW (1956) Avidity of the tetracyclines for the cations of metals. Nature 177:433–434

Allen JC (1976) Minocycline. Ann Intern Med 85:482–487

André T (1956) Studies on the distribution of tritium-labelled dihydrostreptomycin and tetracycline in the body. Acta Radiol [Suppl] 142:1–89

Appel GB, Neu HC (1977) The nephrotoxicity of antimicrobial agents (second of three parts). N Engl J Med 296:722–728

Barr WH, Adir J, Garrettson L (1971) Decrease of tetracycline absorption in man by sodium bicarbonate. Clin Pharmacol Ther 12:779–784

Bartlett JG, Bustetter LA, Gorbach SL, Onderdonk AB (1975) Comparative effect of tetracycline and doxycycline on the occurrence of resistant *Escherichia coli* in fecal flora. Antimicrob Agents Chemother 7:55–57

Bartlett JG, Chang TW, Taylor NS, Onderdonk AB (1979) Colitis induced by *Clostridium difficile*. Rev Infect Dis 1:370–378

Barza M, Brown RB, Shanks C, Gamble C, Weinstein L (1975) Relation between lipophilicity and pharmacological behavior of minocycline, doxycycline, tetracycline, and oxytetracycline in dogs. Antimicrob Agents Chemother 8:713–720

Bessman S, Doorenbos N (1957) Chelation. Ann Intern Med 47:1036

Bjornberg A, Roupe G (1972) Susceptibility of infections during long-term treatment with tetracyclines in acne vulgaris. Dermatology 145:334–337

Brandl RC, Arkenau C, Simon C, Malercyk V, Eidelloth G (1972) Zur Pharmakokinetik von Clindamycin bei gestörter Leber- und Nierenfunktion. Dtsch Med Wochenschr 97:1057

Brogden RN, Speight TM, Avery GS (1975) Minocycline: a review of its antibacterial and pharmacokinetic properties and therapeutic use. Drugs 9:251–291

Center for Disease Control (1980) *Plasmodium falciparum* malaria contracted in Thailand resistant to chloroquine and sulfonamide-pyrimethamine. Illinois. Morbidity Mortality Weekly Report 29:493–495

Center for Disease Control (1982) Prevention of malaria in travelers 1981. Morbidity Mortality Weekly Report [Suppl] 30:15–285

Chang TW, Gorbach SL, Bartlett JG, Saginur R (1980) Bacitracin treatment of antibiotic-associated colitis and diarrhea caused by *Clostridium difficile* toxin. Gastroenterology 78:1584–1586

Chin W, Intraprasert R (1973) The evaluation of quinine alone or in combination with tetracycline and pyrimethamine against falciparum malaria in Thailand. Southeast Asian J Trop Med Public Health 4:245–249

Chin W, Contacos PG, Coatney GR, King HK (1966) The evaluation of sulfonamides, alone or in combination with pyrimethamine, in the treatment of multiresistant falciparum malaria. Am J Trop Med Hyg 15:823–829

Clyde DF, Miller RM, DuPont HL, Hornick RB (1971) Antimalarial effects of tetracycline in man. J Trop Med Hyg 74:238–242

Clyde DF, Gilman RH, McCarthy VC (1975) Antimalarial effect of clindamycin in man. Am J Trop Med Hyg 24:369–370

Coatney GR, Greenberg J (1952) The use of antibiotics in the treatment of malaria. Ann NY Acad Sci 55:1075–1081

Coatney GR, Greenberg J, Cooper WC, Trembley HL (1949) Antimalarial activity of aureomycin against *Plasmodium gallinaceum* in the chick. Proc Soc Exp Biol Med 72:586–587

Cohen LE, McNeill CJ, Wells RF (1973) Clindamycin-associated colitis. JAMA 223:1379–1380

Cohen S, Parkins FM (1970) Bleaching tetracycline-stained vital teeth. Oral Sur 29:465–471

Cohlan SO, Bevelander G, Tiamic T (1963) Growth inhibition of prematures receiving tetracycline. A clinical and laboratory investigation of tetracycline-induced bone fluorescence. Am J Dis Child 105:453–461

Colwell EJ, Hickman RL, Intraprasert R, Tirabutana C (1972a) Minocycline and tetracycline treatment of acute falciparum malaria. Am J Trop Med Hyg 21:144–149

Colwell EJ, Hickman RL, Kosakal S (1972b) Tetracycline treatment of chloroquine-resistant falciparum malaria in Thailand. JAMA 220:684–686

Colwell EJ, Hickman RL, Kosakal S (1973) Quinine-tetracycline and quinine-bactrim treatment of acute falciparum malaria in Thailand. Ann Trop Med Parasitol 67:125–132

Cooper WC, Coatney GR, Imboden CA Jr, Jeffrey GM (1949) Aureomycin in experimental Chesson strain vivax malaria. Proc Soc Exp Biol Med 72:587–588

Coskey RJ (1976) Acne: Treatment with minocycline. Cutis 17:799–801

Cullen SI (1978) Low-dose minocycline therapy in tetracycline-recalcitrant acne vulgaris. Cutis 21:101–105

Cullen SI, Cohan RH (1976) Minocycline therapy in acne vulgaris. Cutis 17:1208–1214

Cundliffe E, McQuillen K (1967) Bacterial protein synthesis: the effects of antibiotics. J Mol Biol 30:137–146

Davis CM, Vandersarl JV, Kraus EW (1973) Tetracycline inequivalence: the importance of 96-hour testing. Am J Med Sci 265:69–74

De Haan RM, Metzler CM, Schellenberg D, Van den Bosch WD, Masson EL (1972) Pharmacokinetic studies of clindamycin hydrochloride in humans. Int Z Klin Pharmakol 6:105–119

Dejesus R, Peternel WW (1978) Antibiotic-associated diarrhea treated with oral tetracycline. Gastroenterology 74:818–820

Dutta GP, Singh PP (1979) Blood schizontocidal activity of some antibiotics against *Plasmodium knowlesi* infection in Assamese monkey. Indian J Med Res [Suppl] 70:91–94

Eastwood JB, Gower PE (1974) A study of the pharmacokinetics of clindamycin in normal subject and patients with chronic renal failure. Postgrad Med J 50:710–712

Eisner HJ, Wulf RJ (1963) The metabolic fate of chlortetracycline and some comparisons with other tetracyclines. J Pharmacol Exp Ther 142:122–131

Fekety R (1979) Vancomycin. In: Mandell GL, Douglas RG, Bennet JE (eds) Principles and practice of infectious diseases. Wiley, New York, pp 304–307

Frimpter GW, Timpanelli AE, Eisenmenger WJ, Stein HS, Ehrlich LI (1963) Reversible "Fanconi syndrome" caused by degraded tetracycline. JAMA 184:111–113

Gabuzda GJ, Gocke TM, Jackson GG, Grigsby ME, Love BD Jr, Finland M (1958) Some effects of antibiotics on nutrition in man, including studies of the bacterial flora of the feces. AMA Arch Intern Med 101:476–513

Garnham PCC, Warren McW, Killick-Kendrick R (1971) The action of "terramycin" on the primary exoerythrocytic development of *Plasmodium vivax* and *Plasmodium cynomolgi ceylonensis*. J Trop Med Hyg 74:32–35

George RH, Youngs DJ, Johnson EM, Burdon DW (1978) Anion-exchange resins in pseudomembraneous colitis. Lancet 2:624

George WL (1980) Antimicrobial agent-associated colitis and diarrhea. West J Med 133:115–123

George WL, Sutter VL, Goldstein EJC, Ludwig SL, Finegold SM (1978) Aetiology of antimicrobial-agent-associated colitis. Lancet 1: 802–803

George WL, Rolfe RD, Finegold SM (1980) Treatment and prevention of antimicrobial agent-induced colitis and diarrhea. Gastroenterology 79:366–372

Gross JM (1963) Fanconi syndrome (adult type) developing secondary to the ingestion of outdated tetracycline. Ann Intern Med 58:523–528

Hall AP, Doberstyn EB, Nanakorn A, Sonkom P (1975) Falciparum malaria semi-resistant to clindamycin. Br Med J 2:12–14

Hindle JA, Rose AS, Trevett LD, Prout C (1945) The effect of penicillin on inoculation malaria. A negative report. N Eng J Med 232:133–136

Hinton NA (1970) The effect of oral tetracycline-HCl and doxycycline on the intestinal flora. Curr Ther Res 12:341–352

Hurwitz ES, Johnson D, Campbell CC (1981) Resistance of *Plasmodium* falciparum malaria to sulfadoxine-pyrimethamine (Fansidar) in a refugee camp in Thailand. Lancet 1:1068–1070

Imboden CA Jr, Cooper WC, Coatney GR, Jeffery GM (1950) Studies in human malaria. XXIX. Trials of aureomycin, chloramphenicol, penicillin, and dihydrostreptomycin against the Chesson strain of *P. vivax*. J Nat Malaria Soc 9:377–380

Ishiyama S, Sakabe T, Takahashi U, Kawakami K, Nakayama I, Iwamoto H, Oshima S, Takatore M, Suzuki H, Murakami F (1969) Minocycline in surgical field. Jpn J Antibiot 22:463–469

Jacobs RL, Koontz LC (1976) *Plasmodium berghei:* Development of resistance to clindamycin and minocycline in mice. Exp Parasitol 40:116–123

Kaddu JB, Warhurst DC, Peters W (1974) The chemotherapy of rodent malaria, IXI. The action of a tetracycline derivative, minocycline, on drug-resistant *Plasmodium berghei*. Ann Trop Med Parasitol 68:41–46

Kakemi K, Sezaki H, Ogata H, Nadai T (1968) Absorption and excretion of drugs. XXXVI. Effect of Ca^{++} on the absorption of tetracycline from the small intestine (1). Chem Pharm Bull (Tokyo) 16:2200–2205

Kelly RG, Kanegis LA (1967) Metabolism and tissue distribution of radio isotopically labelled minocycline. Toxicol Appl Pharmacol 11:171–183

Kelly RG, Kanegis LA, Buyske DA (1961) The metabolism and tissue distribution of radioisotopically labeled demethylchlortetracycline. J Pharmacol Exp Ther 134:320–324

Keusch GT, Present DH (1976) Summary of a workshop on clindamycin colitis. J Infect Dis 133:578–587

Kitamoto O, Fukaya K, Tomori G (1969) Studies on pharmacodynamics of antimicrobial agents – on minocycline. Jpn J Antibiot 22:435

Knox JH, Jurand J (1975) Separation of tetracyclines by high-speed liquid chromatography, J Chromatogr 110:103–114

Kunin C, Finland CM (1961) Clinical pharmacology of the tetracycline antibiotics. Clin Pharmacol Ther 2:51–69

Kutscher AH, Zegarelli EV, Tovell HMM, Hochberg B, Hauptman J (1966) Discoloration of deciduous teeth induced by administration of tetracycline antepartum. Am J Obstet Gynecol 96:291–292

Laing ABG (1972) The effect of tetracycline on *Plasmodium falciparum* in the Gambia. Trans R Soc Trop Med Hyg 66:956–957

Lepper MH (1951) Effect of large doses of Aureomycin on human liver. Arch Intern Med 88:271–283

Lewis C (1968a) Antiplasmodial activity of 7-halogenated lincomycins. J Parasitol 54:169–170

Lewis C (1968b) Antiplasmodial activity of halogenated lincomycin analogues in *Plasmodium berghei*-infected mice. Antimicrob Agents Chemother 1967:537–542

Leyden JJ, Marples RR, Mills OH Jr (1973) Gram-negative folliculitis: A complication of antibiotic therapy in acne vulgaris. Br J Dermatol 88:533–538

Little PJ, Bailey RR (1970) Tetracyclines and renal failure. NZ Med J 72:183–184

MacDonald H, Kelly RG, Allen ES, Noble JF, Kanegis LA (1973) Observations on the pharmacokinetic properties of a new tetracycline antibiotic – minocycline. Clin Pharmacol Ther 14:852–861

Magerlein BJ, Birkenmeyer RD, Kagan F (1967a) Chemical modification of lincomycin. Antimicrob Agents Chemother 1966:727–736

Magerlein BJ, Birkenmeyer RD, Kagan F (1967b) Lincomycin. VI. 4′ alkyl analogs of lincomycin. Relationship between structure and antibacterial activity. J Med Chem 10:355–359

Mahon WA, Wittenberg JVP, Tuffnel PG (1970) Studies on the absorption and distribution of doxycycline in normal patients and in patients with severely impaired renal function. J Can Med Assoc 103:1031–1034

Malacoff RF, Finkelstein FO, Andriole VT (1975) Effect of peritoneal dialysis on serum levels of tobramycin and clindamycin. Antimicrob Agents Chemother 8:574–580

Matuchansky C, Aries J, Maitre P (1978) Metronidazole for antibiotic associated pseudomembranous colitis. Lancet 2:580–581
McGehee RF Jr, Smith CB, Wilcox F, Finland M (1968) Comparative studies of antibacterial activity *in vitro* and absorption and excretion of lincomycin and clinimycin. Am J Med Sci 256:279–292
Medina A, Fiske N, Hjelt-Harvey I, Brown CD, Prigot A (1964) Absorption, diffusion, and excretion of a new antibiotic, lincomycin. Antimicrob Agents Chemother 1963:189
Migliardi JR, Schach von Wittenau M (1967) Pharmacokinetic properties of doxycycline in man. Proceedings 5th international congress of chemotherapy. Vienna, June–July 1967, 2:165–171
Miller LH, Glew RH, Wyler DJ, Howard WA, Collins WE, Contacos PG, Neva FA (1974) Evaluation of clindamycin in combination with quinine against multidrug-resistant strains of *Plasmodium falciparum*. Am J Trop Med Hyg 23:565–569
Neuvonen PJ, Gothoni G, Hackman R, Bjorksten K (1970) Interference of iron with the absorption of tetracyclines in man. Br Med J 4:532–534
Panzer JD, Brown DC, Epstein WL, Lipson RL, Mahaffrey HW, Atkinson WH (1972) Clindamycin levels in various body tissues and fluids. J Clin Pharmacol 12:259–262
Pashby NL, Bolton RP, Sherriff RJ (1979) Oral metronidazole in clostridium difficile colitis. Br Med J 1:1605–1606
Peddie BA, Dann E, Bailey RR (1975) The effect of impairment of renal function and dialysis on the serum and urine levels of clindamycin. Aust NZ J Med 5:198–202
Philipson A, Sabath LD, Charles D (1973) Transplacental passage of erythromycin and clindamycin. N Engl J Med 288:1219–1221
Phillips ME, Eastwood JB, Curtis JR, Gower PE, DeWardener HE (1974) Tetracycline poisoning in renal failure. Br Med J 2:149–151
Pothier AJ Jr, Anderson EE (1966) Tetracycline-induced azotemia. J Urol 95:16–18
Powers KG (1969) Activity of chlorinated lincomycin analogues against *Plasmodium cynomolgi* in rhesus monkeys. Am J Trop Med Hyg 18:485–490
Powers KG, Jacobs RL (1972) Activity of two clorinated lincomycin analogues against chloroquine-resistant falciparum malaria in owl monkeys. Antimicrob Agents Chemother 1:49–53
Powers KG, Aikawa M, Nugent KM (1976) *Plasmodium knowlesi:* morphology and course of infection in rhesus monkeys treated with clindamycin and its *N*-demethyl-4′-pentyl analog. Exp Parasitol 40:13–24
Reusser F (1975) Effect of lincomycin and clindamycin on peptide chain initiation. Antimicrob Agents Chemother 7:32–37
Rieckmann KH, Powell RD, McNamara JV, Willerson D Jr, Kass L, Frischer H, Carson PE (1971) Effects of tetracycline against chloroquine-resistant and chloroquine-sensitive *Plasmodium falciparum*. Am J Trop Med Hyg 20:811–815
Rieckmann KH, Willerson WD Jr, Carson PE, Frischer H (1972) Effects of tetracycline against drug-resistant falciparum malaria. Proc Helminth Soc Washington 39:339–347
Rosenblatt JE, Barrett JE, Brodie J, Kirby WMM (1966) Comparison of *in vitro* activity and clinical pharmacology of doxycycline with other tetracyclines. Antimicrob Agents Chemother 6:134–141
Ruiz-Sanchez F, Nieves M, Quezada M, Paredes M, Riebling R (1951) El tratamiento del paludismo con aureomicina. Medicina (B Aires) 31:183–188
Ruiz-Sanchez F, Casillas J, Paredes ME, Velasquez J, Riebeling R (1952a) Terramycin in the treatment of malaria. Antibiot Chemother 2:51–57
Ruiz-Sanchez F, Quezada M, Paredes M, Casillas J, Riebeling R (1952b) Chloramphenicol in malaria. Am J Trop Med Hyg 1:936–940
Ruiz-Sanchez F, Ruiz-Sanchez A, Naranjo-Grande E (1956) The treatment of malaria with tetracycline. Antibiot Med Clin Ther 3:193–196
Schach von Wittenau M, Twomey TM (1971) The disposition of doxycycline by man and dog. Chemotherapy 16:217–228
Schach von Wittenau M, Yeary R (1963) The excretion and distribution in body fluids of tetracyclines after intravenous administration to dogs. J Pharmacol Exp Ther 140:258–266

Schmidt LH, Harrison J, Ellison R, Worcester P (1970) The activities of chlorinated lincomycin derivatives against infections with *Plasmodium cynomolgi* in *Macaca mulatta.* Am J Trop Med Hyg 19:1–11
Schultz JC, Adamson JS Jr, Workman WW, Norman TD (1963) Fatal liver disease after intravenous administration of tetracycline in high dosage. N Engl J Med 269:999–1004
Shils ME (1962) Some metabolic agents of tetracyclines. Clin Pharmacol Ther 3:321–339
Shils ME (1963) Renal disease and the metabolic effects of tetracycline. Ann Intern Med 58:389–408
Smits BJ, Prior AP, Arblaster PG (1966) Incidence of *Candida* in hospital in-patients and the effects of antibiotic therapy. Br Med J 1:208–210
Steigbigel NH, Reed CW, Finland M (1968) Absorption and excretion of five tetracycline analogues in normal young men. Am J Med Sci 255:296–312
Stewart DJ (1973) Prevalence of tetracycline in children's teeth. II. A resurvey after five years. Br Med J 3:320–322
Tedesco FJ (1976) Clindamycin-associated colitis: Review of the clinical spectrum of 47 cases. Am J Digest Dis 21:26–32
Tedesco FJ, Barton RW, Alpers DH (1974) Clindamycin-associated colitis. A prospective study. Ann Intern Med 81:429–433
Tedesco F, Markham R, Gurwith M, Christie D, Bartlett JG (1978) Oral vancomycin for antibiotic-associated pseudomembraneous colitis. Lancet 2:226–228
Thaysen EH, Eriksen KR (1956) Staphylococcal enteritis following administration of the tetracyclines. In: Welch H, Marti-Ibãnez F (eds) Antibiot Ann 1955–1956, p. 867–874, Med Encyclopaedia Inc., New York
Trenholme GM, Williams RL, Frischer H, Carson PE, Rieckmann KH (1975) Host failure in treatment of malaria with sulfalene and pyrimethamine. Ann Intern Med 82:219–223
Trigg PI, Gutteridge WE, Williamson J (1971) The effects of cordycepin on malaria parasites. Trans R Soc Trop Med Hyg 65:514–520
Trinh Dinh H, Kernbaum S, Frottier J (1978) Treatment of antibiotic-induced colitis by metronidazole. Lancet 1:338-339
Wagner JG, Novak E, Patel NC, Chidester CG, Lummis WL (1968) Absorption, excretion and half-life of clinimycin in normal adult males. Am J Med Sci 256:25–37
Warhurst DC (1973) Chemotherapeutic agents and malaria research. In: Taylor AER, Muller R (eds) Chemotherapeutic agents in the study of parasites. Symposia of the british society for parasitology 11:1–28
Warhurst DC, Homewood CA, Peters W, Baggaley YC (1972) Pigment changes in *Plasmodium berghei* as indicators of activity and mode of action of antimalarial drugs. Proc Helminth Soc Washington [Suppl] 39:271–278
Warhurst DC, Robinson BL, Peters W (1976) The chemotherapy of rodent malaria, XXIV. The blood schizontocidal action of erythromycin upon *Plasmodium berghei.* Ann Trop Med Parasitol 70:253–258
Weyman J (1965) Tetracyclines and the teeth. Practitioner 195:661–665
Willerson D Jr, Rieckmann KH, Carson PE, Frischer H (1972) Effects of minocycline against chloroquine-resistant falciparum malaria. Am J Trop Med Hyg 21:857–862
Williams DN, Crossley K, Hoffman C, Sabath LD (1975) Parenteral clindamycin phosphate: pharmacology with normal and abnormal liver function and effect on nasal staphylococci. Antimicrob Agents Chemother 7:153–158
World Health Organization (1961) Chemotherapy of malaria. WHO Techn Rep Ser 226:16
World Health Organization (1973) Chemotherapy of malaria and resistance to antimalarials. WHO Techn Rep Ser 529:14

CHAPTER 15

Miscellaneous Compounds

D. WARBURTON

A. Introduction

The purpose of this chapter is to review work described in the recent chemical and biological literature on the miscellaneous compound types for which antiplasmodial activity is claimed, but which lie outside the main antimalarial series reviewed in the other chapters of this book. Most of the compounds described either have not been suitable for evaluation in man or have been insufficiently investigated for their activity in malaria to be definitively assessed. The chapter is divided into two sections, the first covering new work on established series for which the earlier data have already been adequately reviewed, and the second covering work on new series shown to have antiplasmodial activity. For most of the compounds discussed in this chapter only limited reports are available on their antimalarial properties, while some are found only as patent references for which testing details are often scanty.

B. Established Series with Antimalarial Activity

I. Amidinoureas

A series of papers has described work which explored the quantitative correlation between the antimalarial activity of arylamidinoureas and the physicochemical properties of the molecule. For a series of *meta-* and *para*-substituted analogues (I) the antimalarial activity in mice infected with *P. vinckei* was strongly influenced by the electron-withdrawing properties of the substituent (σ) and was also influenced to a lesser extent by its lipophilicity (π) (GOODFORD et al. 1973).

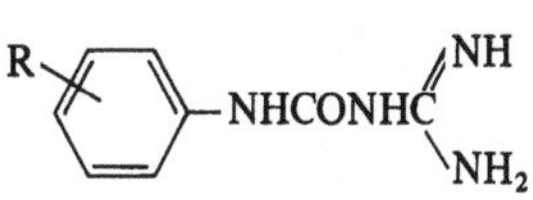

I

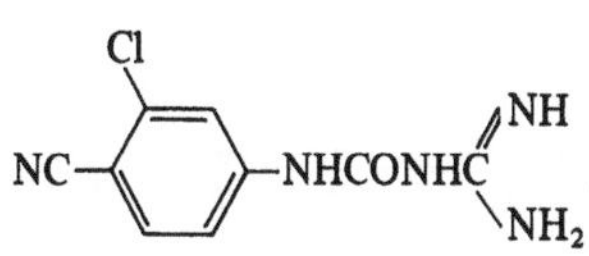

II

Fig. 1. Chemical structures I and II

As might be expected, correlation with these generalised parameters was reduced with *ortho-* substituted derivatives due to steric interaction between the substituents (GILBERT et al. 1975).

A similar study carried out using three separate types of infection, namely, *P. vinckei* in vivo in mice, *P. knowlesi* in vitro and *P. berghei* in vitro, showed that different regression equations and therefore correlations were obtained for each of the three test systems. This difference could well have been due in part to the differences in transport mechanisms operating in the in vivo and in vitro systems. Although it was not possible from the results available to predict which of the test systems mirrored most closely the human situation, the method did show that, for a given test system, it is possible to obtain a regression equation from the results on a few well-chosen substituents which then enables one to predict compounds with features favourable to high activity (CRANFIELD et al. 1974). It is a pity that this systematic approach to the design of new antimalarial agents with optimal activity does not appear to have been widely used in most of the antimalarial series being reviewed.

Further patents for (mainly) halogeno analogues of nitroguanil have appeared (WELLCOME FOUNDATION 1974a) where doses of 5–25 mg/kg were effective against infections of *P. berghei* in mice and *P. gallinaceum* in chicks. In vivo studies with the analogue II against *P. falciparum* in monkeys showed that, at an oral dose of 10 mg/kg per day for 3 days, this compound cleared the blood of asexual parasites as quickly as did chloroquine. The metabolic activity of the parasite, measured by in vitro uptake of tritiated leucine, was shown to be much reduced within 24 h of the initial dose, although there was no visible indication of parasite abnormality or reduction in numbers at that time (RICHARDS and WILLIAMS 1975).

II. Amidines

The binding of aryldiamidines to DNA is thought to be an important factor in the biological activity of these compounds. An examination of molecular models showed that in the most active compounds the amidine groups were usually separated by a distance of either 12 or 20 Å. To investigate further this relationship between activity and distance between the amidine groups, a series of furan diamidines and masked diamidines with the amidine groups held a distance of 12 Å apart were prepared and tested for antimalarial activity (DAS and BOYKIN 1977).

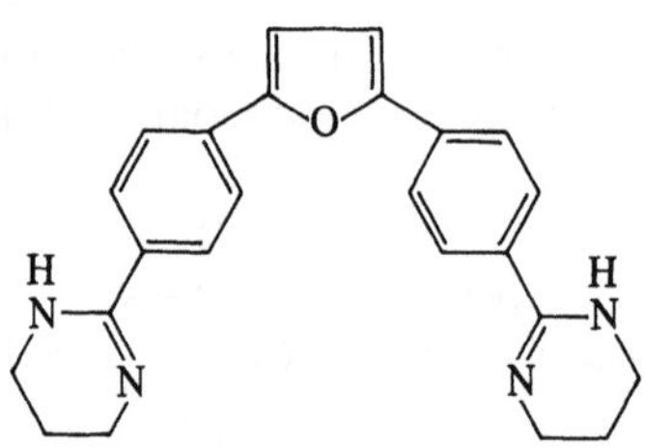

III

Fig. 2. Chemical structure III

The activity of these compounds was modest, with the most active compound (III) showing activity against *P. berghei* in mice at a dose of 320 mg/kg, while toxic symptoms were observed at a dose of 640 mg/kg. It is possible that the rigidity conferred by the ring system in compounds of the type prepared resulted in the compounds being unable to take up the conformation required to fit the receptor site, thus limiting their activity.

III. Biguanides

A small series of biguanide and amidinourea derivatives of chloromethyl sulphonylphenylamine have been prepared. Five of the compounds, including IV, showed slight activity against *P. berghei* in mice at the maximum tolerated dose (PETERS et al. 1975).

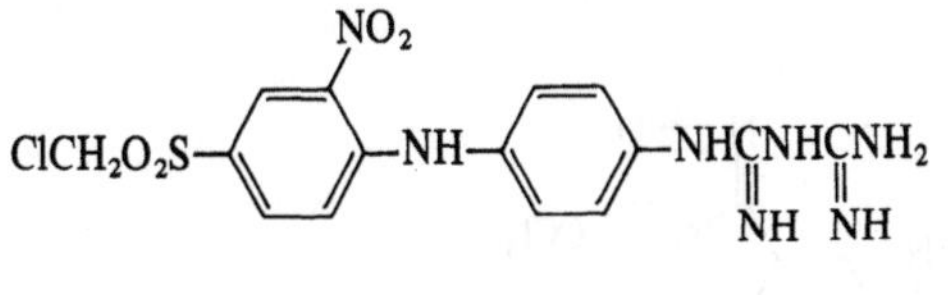

IV

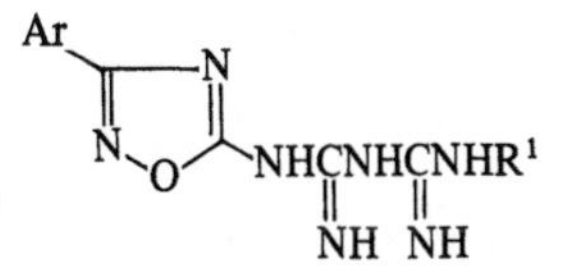

V

Fig. 3. Chemical structures IV and V

Patent claims for antimalarial and other activities have been made for biguanide derivatives (V) where R^1 is a basically substituted group and Ar is an optionally substituted phenyl ring (ARON SAMUEL 1973).

IV. Hydroxamic Acids

The in vitro inhibition of nucleic acid synthesis is a property shared by both arylhydroxamic acids and antimalarial agents such as quinine. A series of hydroxamic acids was synthesised and evaluated for antimalarial activity against *P. berghei* in mice. The level of activity found was disappointing, with only two compounds (VI a, VI b) showing a significant increase in survival time at a dose of 320 mg/kg (HYNES 1970).

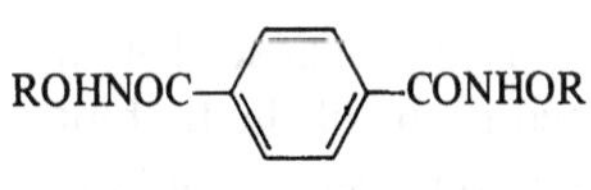

VI a) R = H; b) R = COC_6H_5

Fig. 4. Chemical structure VI

V. Oxa- and Thiadiazoles

A series of oxadiazoles containing the trichloromethyl group of Hetol (VII) was examined for antimalarial activity but no compound was as active as Hetol itself. The most active compound (VIII) cured 80% of mice infected with *P. berghei* at a dose of 640 mg/kg.

The analogue (IX) in which the substituted oxadiazole was attached to the benzene ring at its 5-position was slightly less active but significantly increased the survival time of mice infected with *P. berghei* at dose levels of 160–640 mg/kg (HYNES and GRATZ 1972).

The synthesis of a series of thiadiazoles which not only contained the trichloromethyl group of Hetol but also a basically substituted group such as oc-

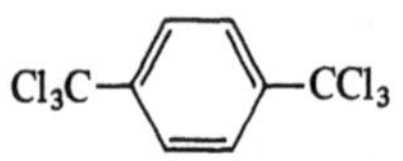

VII

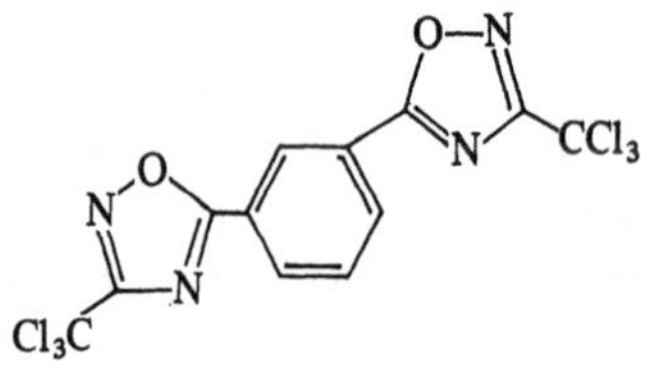

VIII

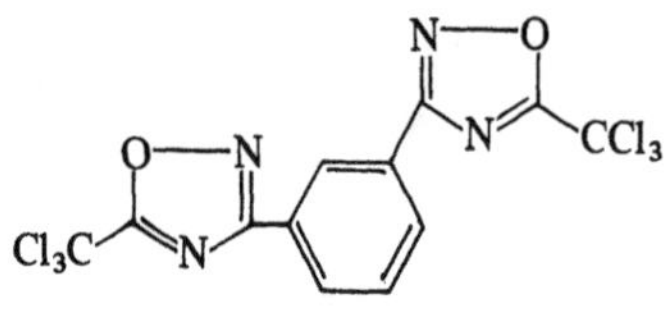

IX

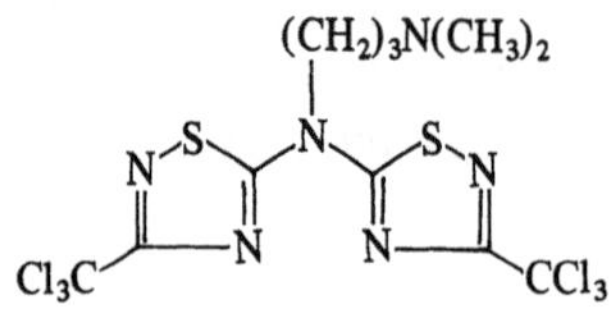

X

Fig. 5. Chemical structures VII–X

curs in many antimalarial compounds gave derivatives which were more active than the previously described oxadiazoles. A number of compounds were fully curative against *P. berghei* in mice at a single subcutaneous dose of 320 mg/kg, the most active compound (X) showing activity, as measured by a significant increase in survival time of the infected mice, at a dose of 80 mg/kg.

While activity was retained if one of the trichloromethyl groups was replaced by a 3,4-dichlorophenyl group, replacement of both trichloromethyl groups gave inactive analogues. In chicks, suppressive action against *P. gallinaceum* was shown by X at subcutaneous doses of 80–320 mg/kg (ELSLAGER et al. 1973).

VI. Quinolines and Deazaquinolines

Further studies have been carried out on compounds in which the basically substituted groups giving activity in the 4- and 8-aminoquinoline series have been introduced into the 6-position of the quinoline ring. It was found that, in such derivatives, substitution of the quinoline ring by methyl groups, especially at the 4-position, significantly reduced the toxicity encountered with earlier 6-aminoquinolines. While compounds of this type (XI a) showed good activity against *P. vinckei* in mice (NICKEL and FINK 1976), the activity of the 6-aminoquinoline derivatives against *P. berghei* in mice was less than that of the corresponding 4- or 8-substituted analogues. Thus, the 6-substituted analogue (XI b) of amodiaquine merely increased the survival time of mice infected with *P. berghei* by 5 days at a dose of 320 mg/kg (TEMPLE et al. 1974 a) as did the analogue XI c at 640 mg/kg (TEMPLE et al. 1974 b).

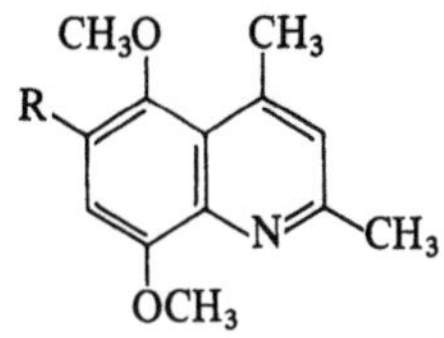

XI

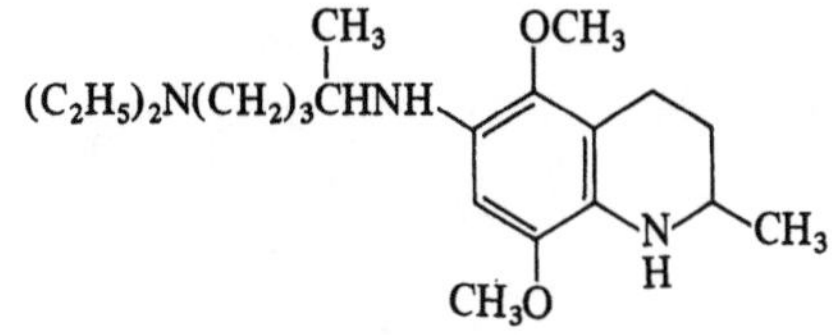

XII

a) R = $-NHCH(CH_3)(CH_2)_3N(C_2H_5)_2$

b) R =

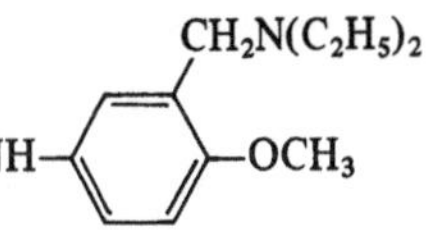

c) R = $-NH(CH_2)_2N(C_2H_5)_2$

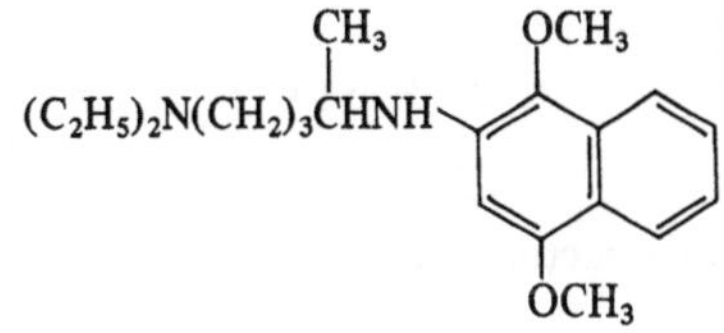

XIII

Fig. 6. Chemical structures XI–XIII

It is of interest to note that reduced derivatives XII retained some activity against *P vinckei* in the mouse, but the activity was much less than that of the corresponding quinoline (NICKEL and FINK 1972), while the deaza analogue XIII showed some activity in a sporozoite-induced mouse test at 10 mg/kg but was toxic at 160 mg/kg (McCAUSTLAND et al. 1973).

In another series of aminonaphthalenes, prepared as prodrugs for biotransformation to the *o*-quinone, as is believed to happen with the 8-aminoquinoline antimalarials, radical curative activity against *P. cynomolgi* in rhesus monkeys was obtained with two aminoalkylamino derivatives (XIV a, XIV b). These showed activity at dose levels of 3 mg/kg per day and 10 mg/kg per day respectively under the same conditions in which pamaquine was active at 1.3 mg/kg per day (ARCHER et al. 1980).

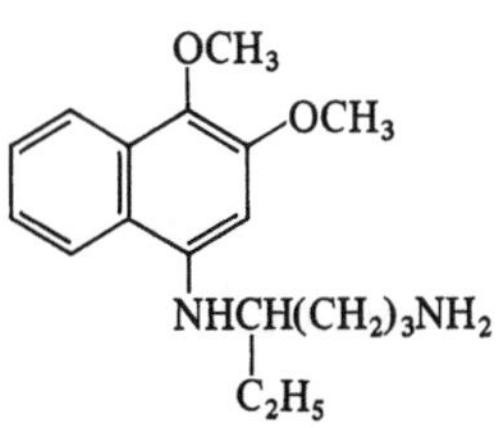

XIVa

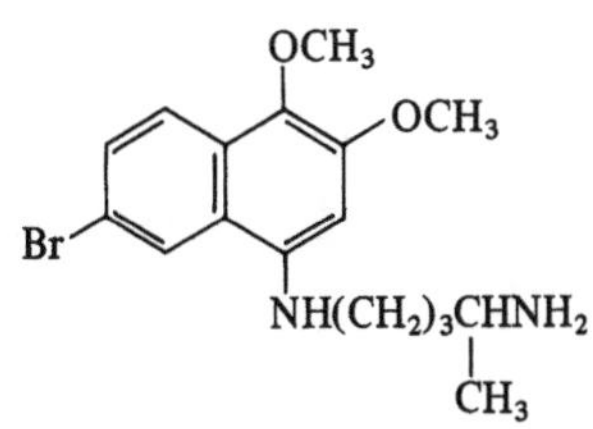

XIVb

Fig. 7. Chemical structures XIV a and XIV b

Antimalarial activity has been claimed for a small series of 5- or 8-nitroquinolines (XV), although no experimental details of the activity are given (SHOEB et al. 1978).

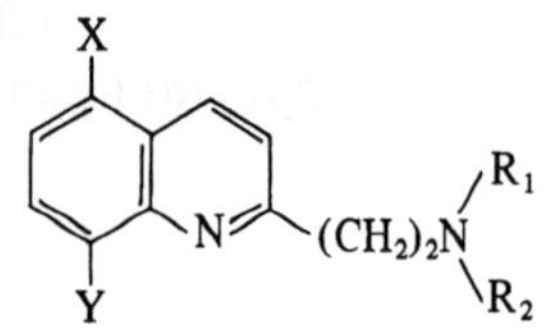

XV

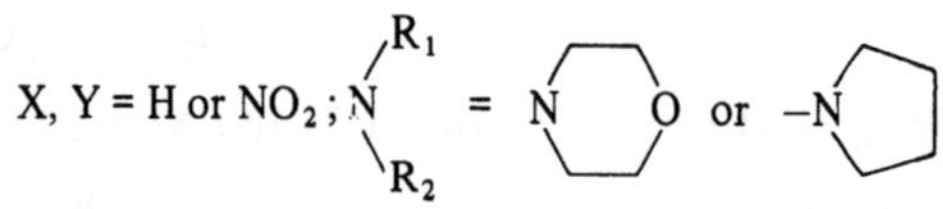

Fig. 8. Chemical structure XV

VII. Pyrocatechols, RC-12

A trial of the naphthalene disulphonate salt of RC-12 (XVI) against mosquito-induced *P. vivax* infection in man at oral doses of 10 mg (base)/kg per day for 7 days showed that the drug did not possess causal prophylactic activity nor did it prevent relapses (CLYDE et al. 1974).

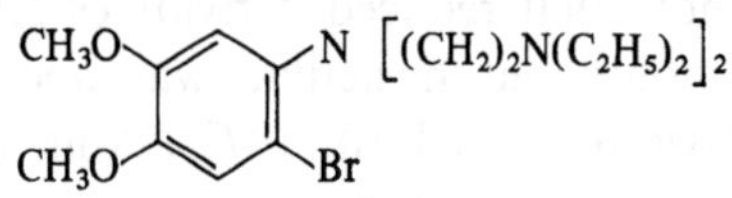

XVI

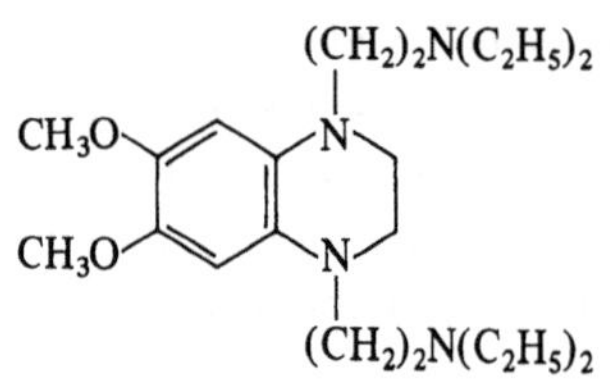

XVII

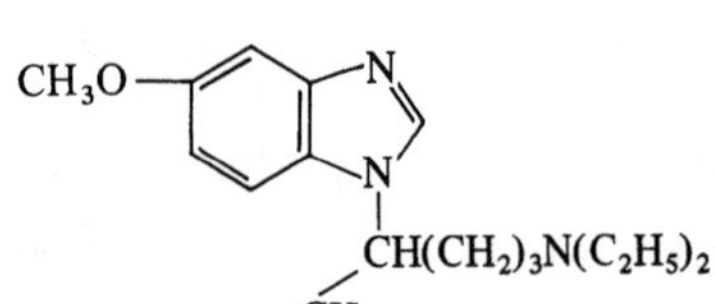

XVIII

Fig. 9. Chemical structures XVI–XVIII (XVI = RC 12)

In the monkey, RC-12 was equally effective against gametocytes and sporogony of *P. cynomolgi* at a dose (single or split) of 25 mg/kg per day. The onset of sporontocidal action was rapid and there was a marked decrease in infectivity to mosquitoes within a few hours of the initial treatment. Gametocytes disappeared from the peripheral blood 2–3 days after treatment began. This pattern of activity mirrors that of primaquine. Although the salivary glands of drug-treated mosquitoes displayed marked morphological changes, direct feeding of RC-12 to infected mosquitoes gave no discernable effects on either oocyst development or sporozoite production (OMAR and COLLINS 1974a).

A study of limited scope examined the possibility that, for basically substituted compounds exerting their antimalarial action by intercalation with DNA, the conformation of the group is more important than the nominal bond distances between the nitrogen atoms. Thus compounds were prepared in which the rotational and vibrational degrees of freedom of the basically substituted side chain were restricted by incorporation into rigid structures. Only a single compound (XVII) showed activity against *P. gallinaceum* in chicks at a dose of 120 mg/kg, but even this compound was inactive against *P. berghei*. It is probably of considerable significance that, of the compounds made and tested, the single active compound possessed the greatest degree of conformational mobility in the side chain (STOGRYN 1971).

A number of common structural features have been noted among different types of antimalarial agents and in one of these the stuctural feature consists of three electronegative atoms substituted at positions 1,2 and 4 of a benzene nucleus, this structural feature encompassing most of the antimalarial agents that participate in biological redox reactions. In a very limited investigation of this feature, a few benzimidazole and quinoxaline derivatives containing the novoldiamine chain (i.e. 4-diethylamino-1-methylbutylamino group) were prepared. Of these, only one compound (XVIII) showed activity against *P. gallinaceum* at a subcutaneous dose level of 50 mg/kg. The corresponding 5,6-dimethoxy analogue was less active (YAN et al. 1978).

VIII. Tetrahydrofurans

A structure-activity investigation into 2-(*p*-chlorophenyl)-2-(4-piperidyl) tetrahydrofuran (XIX) has shown that the structural requirements for antimalarial activity are more stringent than those for the aminoalcohols (see Chap. 9), to which they bear some structural resemblance.

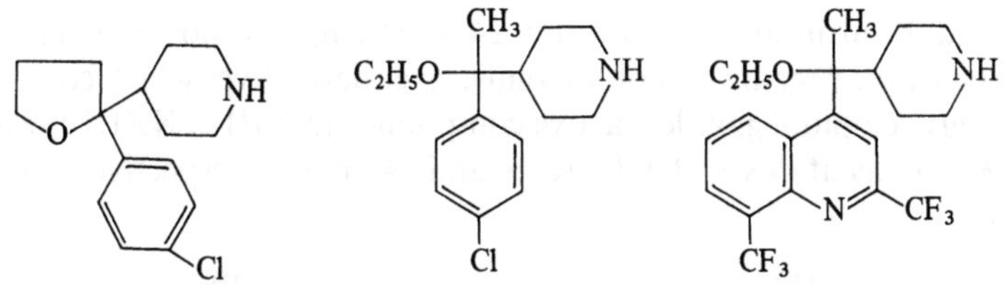

XIX XX XXI

Fig. 10. Chemical structures XIX–XXI

Only a few close analogues had activity comparable to that of XIX, the most active being the tetrahydrofuran ring opened analogue (XX), where a single subcutaneous dose of 320 mg/kg cured 40% of mice infected with *P. berghei*, while lower doses prolonged survival times. This compound was also active against *P. gallinaceum* in chicks at dose levels of 60–240 mg/kg. Alkylation of the piperidine nitrogen atom of XIX gave somewhat less active compounds. It was perhaps a pity that only a few non-systematic changes were made to replace the aromatic part of the molecule since the stuctural requirements for this part of the molecule were not defined. Of the analogues prepared, XXI showed activity against *P. gallinaceum* at dose levels of 40–160 mg/kg (MCCAUSTLAND et al. 1974).

C. Recently Described Antimalarial Series

I. Benzo(g)quinolines

A number of derivatives of benzo(g)quinoline were synthesised and tested against *P. berghei* in rodents and *P. gallinaceum* in chicks. The most active compound, dabequine (XXII), was found to be 2.5–5 times as active but only half as toxic as chloroquine (BEKHLI et al. 1977).

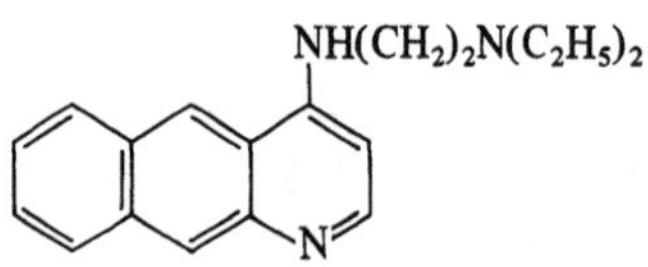

XXII

Fig. 11. Chemical structure XXII (dabequine)

II. Clopidol

Significant antimalarial activity has been claimed for the anticoccidial drug clopidol (XXIII a), where doses of 160 mg/kg given orally daily for 7 days were curative against *P. gallinaceum* and *P. cynomolgi* infections. Activity was also shown against *P. berghei* in mice and against a chloroquine-resistant strain of *P. falciparum* in man. However, the drug was rapidly excreted, over 90% being eliminated unchanged via the urine and faeces within 24 h. Attempts to slow down the excretion of the drug by the preparation of lipophilic ester derivatives which could hydrolyse in vivo to give clopidol gave less active compounds (XXIII b, XXIII c) with activity against *P. berghei* at doses of 320 mg/kg and 640 mg/kg respectively (MARKLEY et al. 1972).

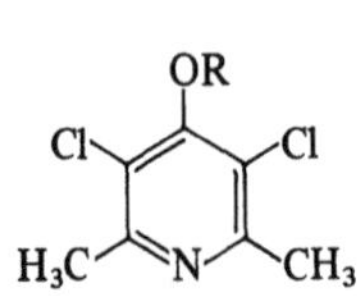

XXIII

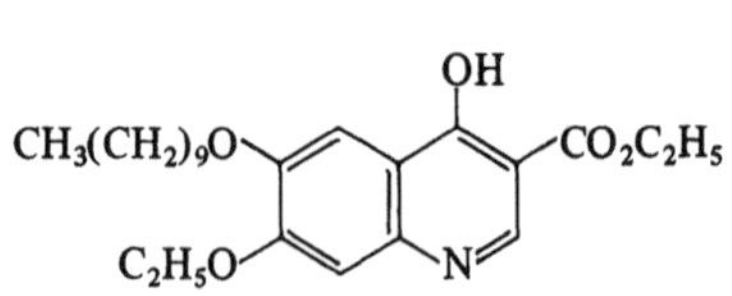

XXIV

a) R = H; b) R = COC_6H_5;
c) R = $SO_2(CH_2)_2Cl$

Fig. 12. Chemical structures XXIII and XXIV (XXIII a = clopidol; XXIV = decoquinate)

Synergistic combinations containing clopidol and decoquinate (XXIV) are claimed (WELLCOME FOUNDATION 1974b) where fractional doses of the combined drugs were effective in reducing the parasitaemia of *P. berghei* in mice.

III. Diazafluorenones

Patent claims have been made for a series of 9-oxime derivatives of 6,8-dibromo-1,3-diazafluorenes (XXV) as gametocytocidal or schizontocidal antimalarials with activity against *P. berghei* in mice and *P. knowlesi* and *P. falciparum* in monkeys.

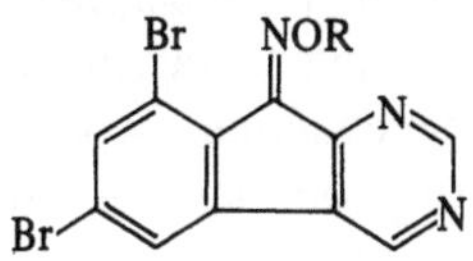

XXV

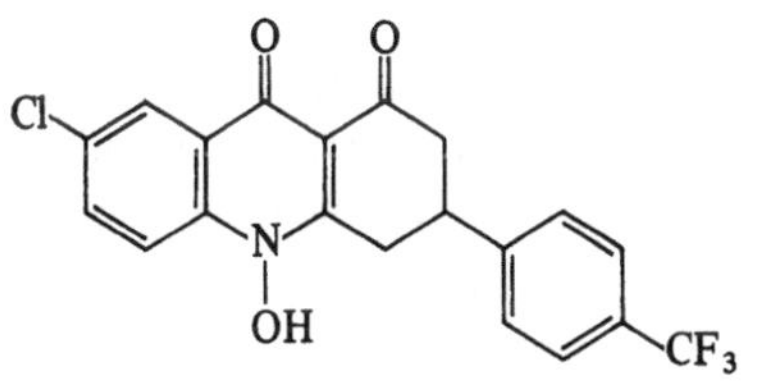

XXVI

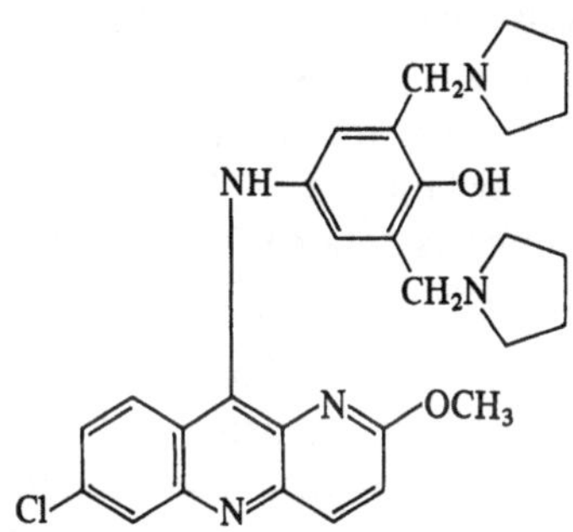

XXVII

Fig. 13. Chemical structures XXV–XXVII (XXVI = floxacrine; XXVII = pyronaridine)

The most active compounds are obtained when the group R is a 1-carboxy ethyl or propyl group or its alkali metal salt, a dialkylaminoalkylamide derived from the acid, or is a dialkylaminoalkyl group. Inactive compounds were obtained when the oxime oxygen atom was adjacent to a carbon atom with two alkyl substituents (CHRISTIAENS 1978).

IV. Floxacrine, Malaridine

Patents claiming antimalarial and anticoccidial activity for tetrahydroacridones have appeared (e.g. FARBWERKE HOECHST 1975) and one compound, 7-chloro-10-hydroxy-3(4-trifluoromethylphenyl)-3,4-dihydroacridine-1,9-(2H,1oH)dione, floxacrine (XXVI), was selected for more detailed studies, the first of which has now been published (RAETHER and FINK 1979).

These studies show that floxacrine is well tolerated and very effective against drug-sensitive and drug-resistant strains of *P. berghei*, with >90% curative active against drug-sensitive *P. berghei* at an oral dose of 7.5 mg/kg per day for 5 days and 5.0 mg/kg per day for subcutaneous doses. Similar results were obtained with strains resistant to chloroquine, mepacrine, pyrimethamine, sulphadoxine and dapsone. The same level of activity was given against *P. vinckei* in mice, rats and hamsters, indicating a very similar metabolic pathway for floxacrine in rodents. Studies in rhesus monkeys showed high activity against the asexual stages of *P. cynomolgi,* oral doses of 5–10 mg/kg per day for 7 days clearing the parasitaemia, but doses of 15–20 mg/kg were required to cure infections and prevent recrudescence. Oral dosing was again found to be less effective than intramuscular injection and the animals were cured by intramuscular doses of 1.25, 2.5 and 7.5 mg/kg daily for 7 days.

Resistance to floxacrine developed readily with strains of *P. berghei* and *P. cynomolgi* on repeated oral dosing at subeffective levels. While floxacrine was fully effective against a strain of *P. berghei* highly resistant to mepacrine, mepacrine was less effective against a floxacrine-resistant strain indicating some level of resistance, but supporting the assumption of a different mode of action of the two acridine derivatives. A search is being made for a combination drug to slow the development of resistant strains. A patent claim (Hoechst AG 1979) indicates that a synergistic effect is obtained with combinations of floxacrine and quinine, cycloguanil or trimethoprim.

The greater effect of parenteral over oral dosing is explained by the greater half-life of the drug after parenteral dosing. Subcutaneous dosing resulted in undissolved drug remaining at the site of injection for a considerable time, giving a depot effect. A single dose of 40 mg/kg in mice gave a half-life of 18 h on subcutaneous injection but only $2^3/_4$ h on oral dosing. Similar levels of half-life were seen in dogs and monkeys. Morphological changes seen in *P. berghei* after treatment with floxacrine included an early vacuolisation of their cytoplasm accompanied by damage to the cytoplasmic membrane, particularly at higher doses. This vacuolisation was not seen after treatment with either mepacrine or chloroquine. The latter drugs induced clumping of the pigment granules within 6 h but this effect was only observed after a longer time interval after treatment with floxacrine. While this early study indicated that floxacrine might have antimalarial properties suitable for its use as either a prophylactic or a therapeutic agent with an acceptable margin of safety between therapeutic and toxic doses, work by Schmidt in owl and rhesus monkeys indicated otherwise.

Thus Schmidt (1979) showed that, while the blood parasitaemia in owl monkeys infected with *P. falciparum* and *P. vivax* was cleared by floxacrine at a dose level of 1.25–2.25 mg/kg per day, much higher doses were needed to effect a cure. A similar result was obtained in rhesus monkeys infected with *P. cynomolgi*, where a dose level of 40 mg/kg per day not only failed to cure an established infection but also produced a haemorrhagic syndrome in some of the monkeys used in the study. This syndrome was indicative of vitamin K deficiency, since it was prevented by the simultaneous administration of menadiol sodium diphosphate. The owl monkeys used in Schmidt's experiments with *P. falciparum* and *P. vivax* were probably protected from this toxic effect by the menadiol sodium diphosphate routinely added to their diet and without this supplement they too would have succumbed.

The disparity between the prophylactic and curative activity shown in this study of floxacrine was attributed to the major differences between the morphology of developing tissue schizonts and that of mature tissue schizonts and the persisting tissue stages associated with relapse.

The toxicity, lack of curative activity, requirement for daily dosing as a prophylactic and the ready development of strains of *Plasmodia* resistant to floxacrine should prove insurmountable obstacles to the future development of this drug for use in man.

Brief mention has appeared of a new azaacridine derivative, Malaridine (pyronaridine) XXVII, which has been shown to have antimalarial activity. Animal and human studies are said to have revealed no evidence of cross-resistance to chloroquine (ZHENG et al. 1979).

V. Indolo(3,2-c)quinolines

Antimalarial properties are claimed for a series of basically substituted indolo(3,2-c)quinoline-*N*-oxides (XXVIII), where preventive activity was demonstrated against *P. berghei* in mice dosed at 100 mg/kg per day for 5 days while curative activity was demonstrated at doses of 25–100 mg/kg per day. A single sompound (XXIX) which lacked the *N*-oxide group showed suppressive activity (CM INDUSTRIES 1977).

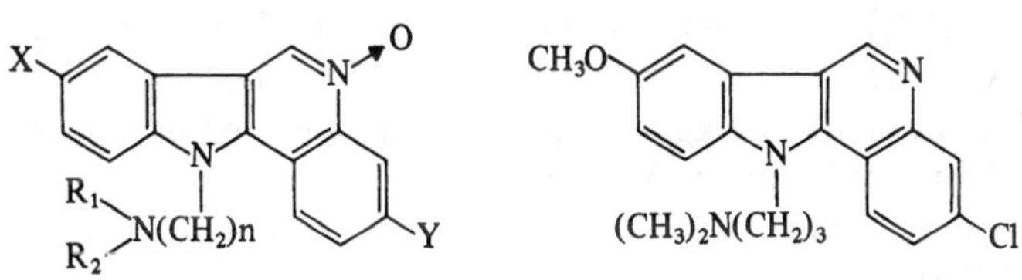

XXVIII XXIX

X = H, OCH_3; Y = H, Cl; R_1, R_2 = CH_3, C_2H_5

Fig. 14. Chemical structures XXVIII and XXIX

VI. Nitroheterocycles

Patent claims for antimalarial and other activities have been made for 2-aldehyde derivatives of 5-nitroheterocycles, for example 5-nitrofurans (XXX a) (CIBA GEIGY 1974) and (XXX b) (GEIGY SA 1972).

Activity against *P. berghei* in mice was demonstrated for 5-nitrothiophenes where the most active compounds (e.g. XXXI) were slightly more effective than quinine in prolonging survival time in infected mice. A single compound (XXXII) tested in rhesus monkeys at the maximum tolerated dose level of 100 mg/kg per day for 7 days showed activity against trophozoite-induced infections of *P. knowlesi* and *P. cynomolgi* (US SECRETARY OF THE ARMY 1973).

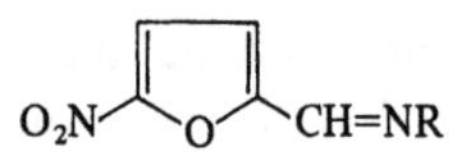

XXX

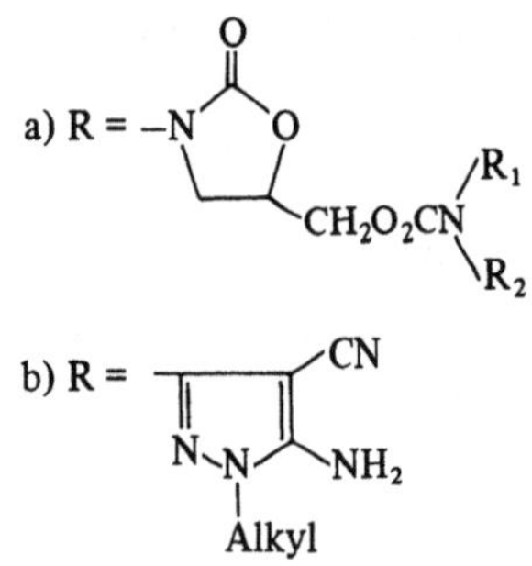

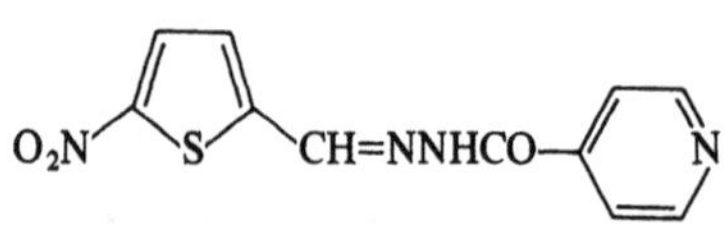

XXXI

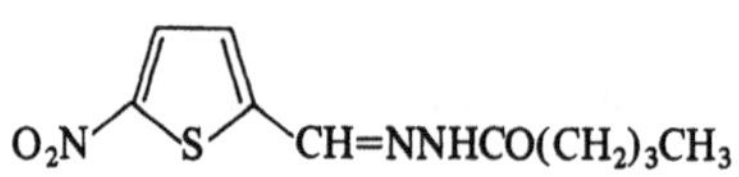

XXXII

Fig. 15. Chemical structures XXX–XXXII

VII. Oxadiazoles

A recent patent claims antimalarial activity for a series of 3-arylthiomethyl-1,2,4-oxadiazoles (XXXIII) and the corresponding dihydro derivatives. Activity against *P. berghei* was measured as a percentage inhibition of blood parasitaemia after seven oral doses of 100 mg/kg of compound administered over 4 days compared with that of untreated controls. While the best 3-substituted compound (XXXIII a) gave a 71% inhibition of parasitaemia, the corresponding 3,5-disubstituted compound (XXXIII b) gave a 99% suppression of parasitaemia under the same conditions.

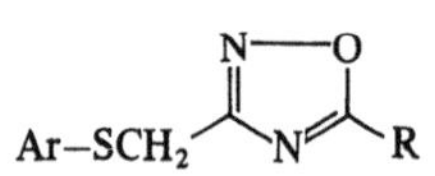

XXXIII

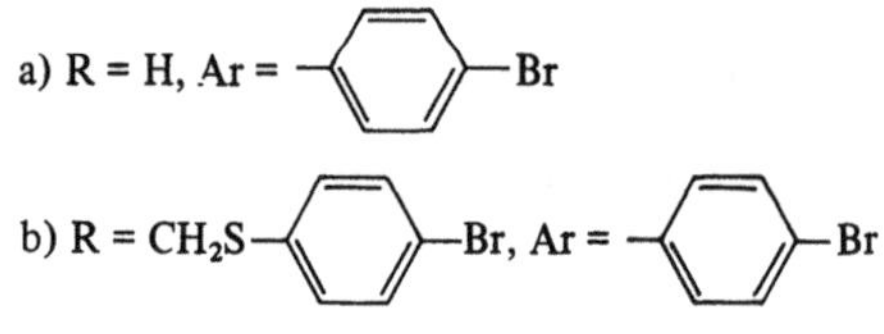

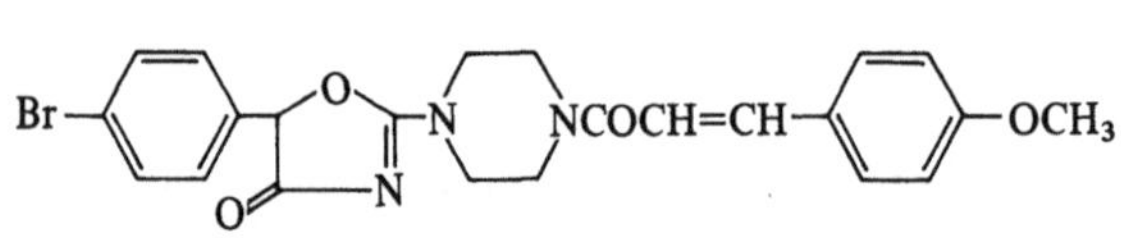

XXXIV

Fig. 16. Chemical structures XXXIII and XXXIV

Although the corresponding 3,5-bis(4-chlorophenylthiomethyl) derivative is claimed to show good activity, neither it, nor any other bis analogues apart from XXXI b are described and it is possible that more detailed investigation of this series would lead to more active compounds (WELLCOME FOUNDATION 1980).

VIII. Oxazolines

Activity against *P. berghei* in mice was demonstrated for a number of oxazolin-2-ylpiperazines, the most active compounds having the 4-methoxycinnamoyl substituent shown (XXXIV). Partial curative activity was shown for single subcutaneous doses of 320 and 640 mg/kg with activity, as measured by a significant increase in survival time, at a dose of 80 mg/kg (HERRIN et al. 1975). Patent claims have also been made for compounds in this series (ABBOTT 1974).

IX. Peptides, Amino Acids and Purines

Since haemoglobin is a poor source of L-isoleucine, an essential amino acid for the malaria parasite, this amino acid is thought to be obtained by the parasite from the plasma of the host. Antagonists of this amino acid could thus be selectively toxic to the malaria parasite. A study was carried out in which the L-isoleucine antagonist was contained in a short peptide chain where it could possibly be transported across the cell membrane more effectively before breakdown within the cell to release the antagonist. One of the three peptides investigated, *O*-methyl-L-threonyl-*O*-methyl-L-threonine (XXXV) had activity as measured by a significant increase in survival time of mice infected with *P. berghei* at a dose of 640 mg/kg (GERSHON and KRULL 1979).

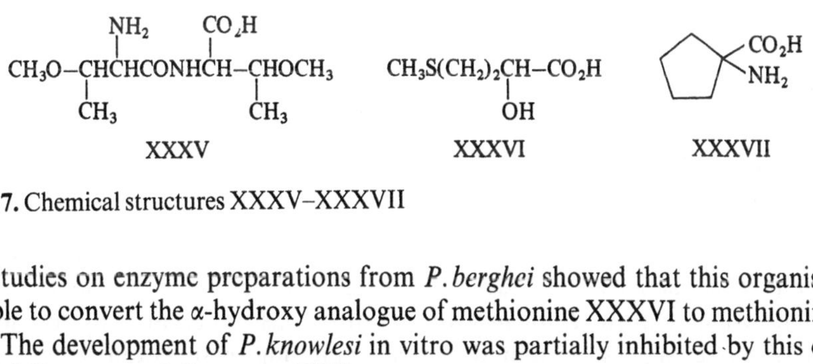

XXXV XXXVI XXXVII

Fig. 17. Chemical structures XXXV–XXXVII

Studies on enzyme preparations from *P. berghei* showed that this organism is unable to convert the α-hydroxy analogue of methionine XXXVI to methionine itself. The development of *P. knowlesi* in vitro was partially inhibited by this compound (LANGER and CANFIELD 1971).

Although 1-aminocyclopentane carboxylic acid XXXVII has sporontocidal action against *P. vivax* infection in monkeys, doses of 60–100 mg/kg per day given orally had no significant prophylactic activity against *P. cynomolgi* in monkeys (OMAR and COLLINS 1974b).

The intravenous injection of liposomes containing neutral glycolipids such as glucosyl, galactosyl or lactosyl ceramide prevented the appearance of erythrocytic forms of *P. berghei* in mice previously inoculated with sporozoites but did not inhibit infection when it was transmitted by injection of erythrocytic stages. The carbohydrate group was necessary for inhibition of the infection since other glycolipids which either did not contain one, or contained a modified one, were inactive. While most animals remained free of infection for the observation period of several weeks and were considered cured, some animals developed a patent infection despite treatment, the average prepatent period being similar to that for untreated mice. The reason why some mice failed to respond to treatment is unclear (ALVING et al. 1979).

The growth of *P. berghei* in vivo/in vitro, measured by uptake of labelled precursors into parasite protein and nucleic acid, was inhibited by enzymes which inhibit the breakdown of haemoglobin such as pepstatin, presumably by deprivation of the parasite to this source of essential amino acids (LEVY and CHOU 1975).

Claims that an immunostimulating glycopeptide from *Corynebacterium parvum* induces resistance to pathogens including malaria have been made (WELLCOME FOUNDATION 1977) while similar claims have been made for peptide sugar derivatives with activity against merozoites of *P. knowlesi* (CIBA GEIGY 1978).

A number of nucleic acid precursor analogues, including adenosines, were shown to inhibit the growth of *P. knowlesi* in vitro (MCCORMICK et al. 1974).

In vitro activity against *P. falciparum* has been demonstrated for some *S*-substituted adenosines, the most active compound (XXXVIII) being inhibitory at a concentration of 300 μg/ml (TRAGER et al. 1978).

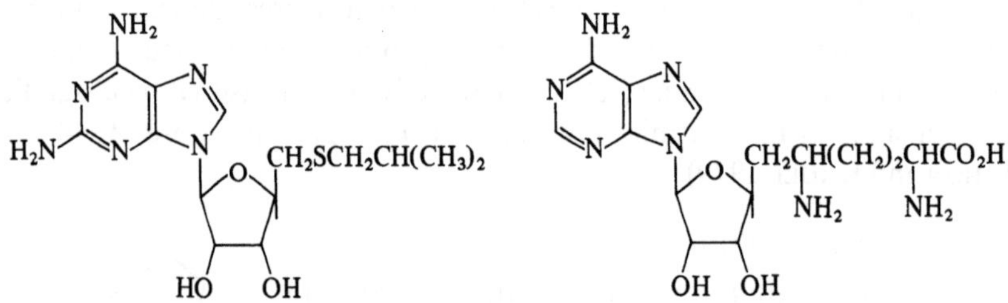

XXXVIII XXXIX

Fig. 18. Chemical structures XXXVIII and XXXIX (XXXIX = Sinefungin)

Other compounds known to inhibit methylation reactions gave similar effects. The inhibitory activity of 3-deazaadenosine and 5′-deoxy-5′-isobutylthio-3-deazaadenosine against *P. falciparum* in vitro was synergised by homocysteinethiolactone, suggesting that they were inhibiting methylation reactions indirectly via adenosylhomocysteinehydrolase. A third analogue, sinefungin (XXXIX), was much more active than the other two and gave complete inhibition at a concentration of 0.3 μ*M*. This compound is probably acting directly to inhibit methyl transferases (TRAGER et al. 1980).

X. Plant Extracts

The increasing prevalence of strains of *Plasmodium falciparum* which display resistance to chloroquine and the consequent increasingly important need to find compounds with new modes of action against the malaria parasite has led to renewed examination of folk remedies.

α) Agrimol. The preparation in the laboratory of somewhat simplified analogues of the active principle of Shian-Ho-Tsao (Agrimol, a group of structurally similar polyphenolic ketones) gave compounds XL a and XL b, which possessed a similar level of antimalarial activity to Agrimol itself (KAI et al. 1978).

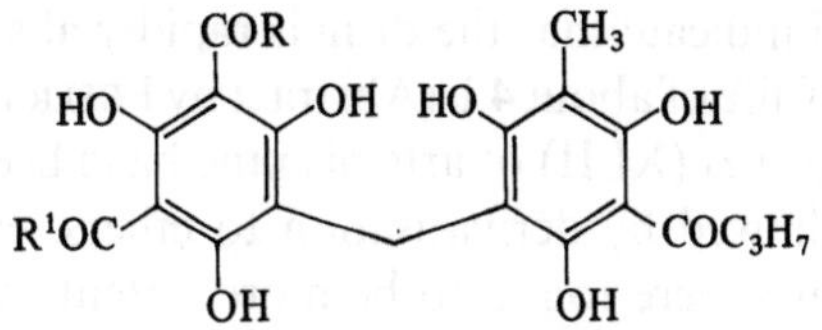

XL

a) $R = R^1 = C_2H_5$
b) $R = CH_3$; $R^1 = C_3H_7$

Fig. 19. Chemical structure XL

However, the presence of potentially toxic phenolic functions in these molecules would appear to make it unlikely that compounds of this type will be well tolerated and suitable for widespread use unless analogues can be found in which the phenolic groups are either masked or replaced with less toxic ones.

β) Artemisinine (Qinghaosu). The isolation and characterisation of artemisinine, the antipyretic principle of the plant *Artemesia annua*, has been accomplished and it has been shown to be an endoperoxide of a sesquiterpenoid lactone (XLI). This novel compound bears no structural resemblance to any other antimalarial agent.

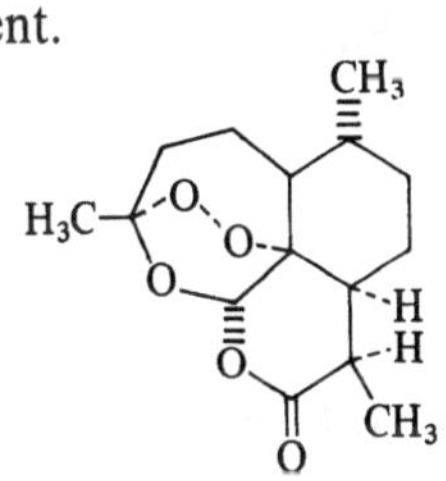

XLI

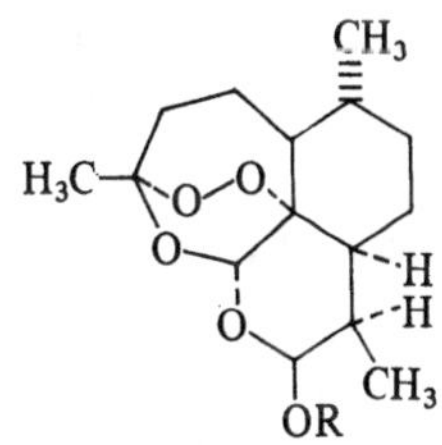

XLII

Fig. 20. Chemical structures XLI and XLII (XLI = Qinghaosu, artemisinine)

Artemisinine has been used in both animal studies and trials in man. Against *P. berghei* infections in mice, subcutaneous dosing was more effective than oral dosing, with oral ED_{50} values (total dose administered over 3 days) of ca. 140 mg/kg for a chloroquine-sensitive strain and ca. 450 mg/kg for a chloroquine-resistant strain, which indicates a slight degree of cross-resistance. A similar dosage regimen of 200 mg/kg cleared sporozoite-induced *P. cynomolgi* infection in rhesus monkeys but had no effect on the tissue stages. Tested in man against *P. vivax* (1,500 cases) and *P. falciparum* (500 cases) infections it was found to be at least as effective as quinine and better tolerated. Parenteral dosing was found to be more effective than oral dosing and produced a rapid clearance of parasitaemia even in patients whose infections did not respond to chloroquine medication. While clinical cures were effected, a relatively high recrudescence rate occurred. The recommended medication is a single intramuscular daily adult dose of 300 mg for three consecutive days. While little has been published on pharmacological data, pharmacokinetic studies using tritiated material indicate that the drug is rapidly absorbed and rapidly excreted with a serum half-life of about 4 h (Abstract by PETERS 1980).

A number of derivatives (XLII) of artemisinine have been prepared by reduction to the alcohol followed by derivatisation to ethers, esters and carbonates. Many of these analogues were found to be more potent than artemisinine itself against *P. berghei* in mice, possibly due to better absorption characteristics of the derivatives (LI et al. 1979).

γ) Dongoyaro. Although the structure of the active principle is not yet known, an aqueous extract of *Azadirachta indica*, a medicinal plant used in Nigeria, has been shown to have a definite schizontocidal action on chloroquine-sensitive *P. berghei* (EKANEM 1978).

δ) A chloroform extract of the plant *Brucea sumatrana* was partially purified by column chromatography and the first eluted fraction was shown to be more effective than chloroquine against a *P. berghei* infection in mice. Physical data indicated the presence of bruceolide (XLIII) in this fraction (THU et al. 1979).

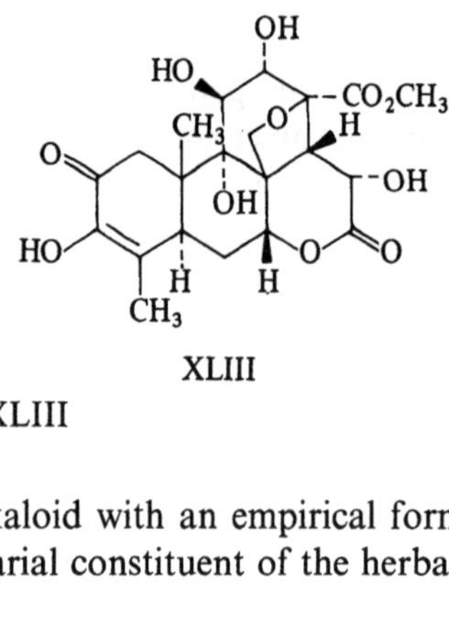

XLIII

Fig. 21. Chemical structure XLIII

ε) A pyrrolizidine alkaloid with an empirical formula $C_{18}H_{25}NO_5$ has been identified as the antimalarial constituent of the herbal medicine from *Gynura segetum* (TANG et al. 1980).

XI. Pyrazoles

A small series of 1,5-diphenyl-4-arylazopyrazole derivatives was prepared and tested against *P. berghei* in mice. The most active compound (XLIV) showed a significant increase in survival time at a dose of 320 mg/kg but the compound was toxic at this dose (GARG et al. 1973).

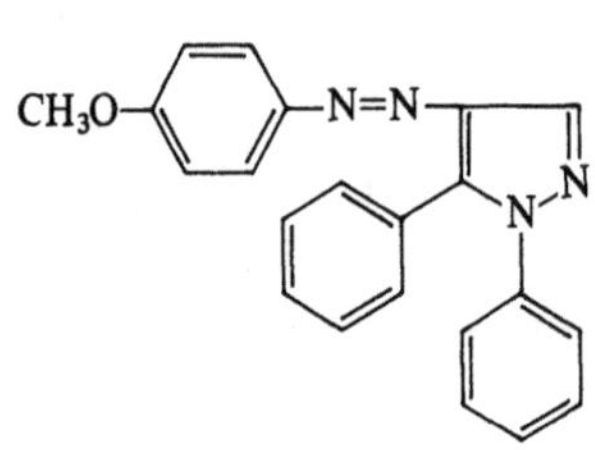

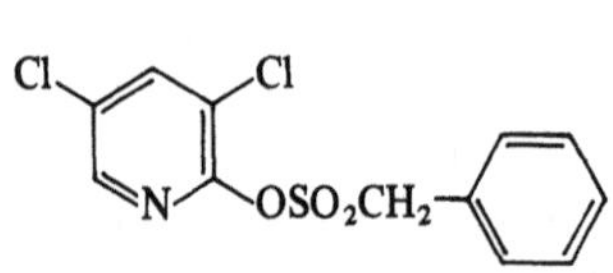

XLIV XLV

Fig. 22. Chemical structures XLIV and XLV

XII. Pyridyl-α-toluene Sulphonates

Of a series of 30 2-pyridyl-α-toluenesulphonates prepared for antimalarial testing only one XLV increased the mean survival time of *P. berghei*-infected mice by more than 100% at a dose of 640 mg/kg, although two other compounds with chlorine or methyl in the 4-position of the benzene ring did increase the survival time significantly but to a lesser extent (HAMER et al. 1975).

XIII. Riboflavin

A number of patent claims have been made for anticoccidial and antimalarial activity of riboflavin analogues where oral dosing of 100 1,000 mg/day for 1–10 days is effective against *P. falciparum* infections. Claims cover aza- (XLVI), deaza- (XLVII), and amino- (XLVIII) derivatives (MERCK 1976, 1977, 1978).

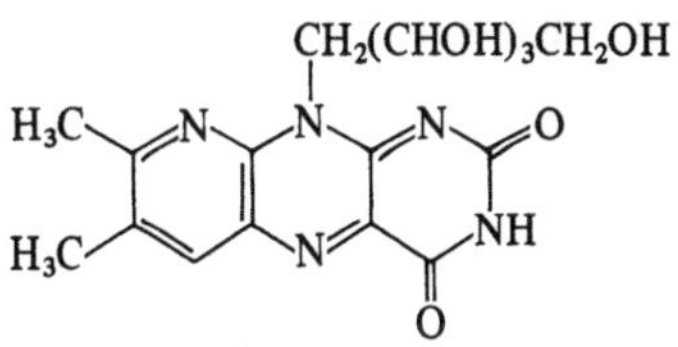

XLVI

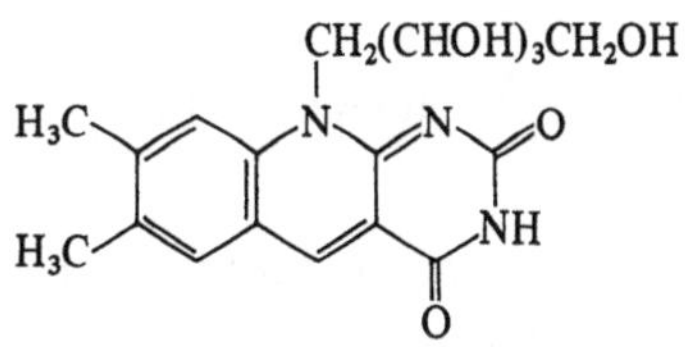

XLVII

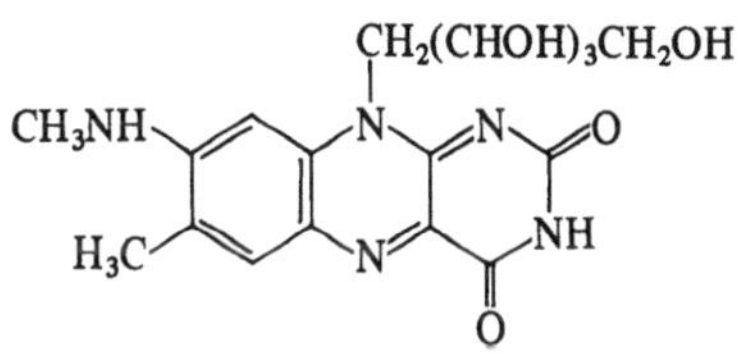

XLVIII

Fig. 23. Chemical structures XLVI–XLVIII

XIV. Robenidine

A series of patents claim anticoccidial and antimalarial activity for substituted guanidines related to the anticoccidial drug Robenidine (XLIX).

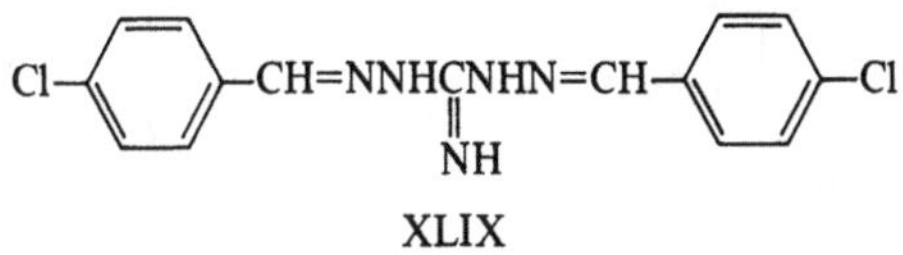

XLIX

Fig. 24. Chemical structure XLIX (Robenidine)

Separate patents claim direct (AMERICAN CYANAMID 1975), dihydrogenated (AMERICAN CYANAMID 1971) and tetrahydrogenated (AMERICAN CYANAMID 1973a) analogues. When used at a dose level of 150–300 mg/kg against *P. berghei* in mice the compounds show a similar level of activity to that of quinine.

XV. Tetrazines

Narrow-scope patent claims have been made (AMERICAN CYANAMID 1973b) for basically substituted tetrazines showing activity against *P. berghei* in mice at doses of 50–300 mg/kg per day. Other compounds (L) were later described which showed modest levels of antimalarial activity (WERBEL et al. 1979).

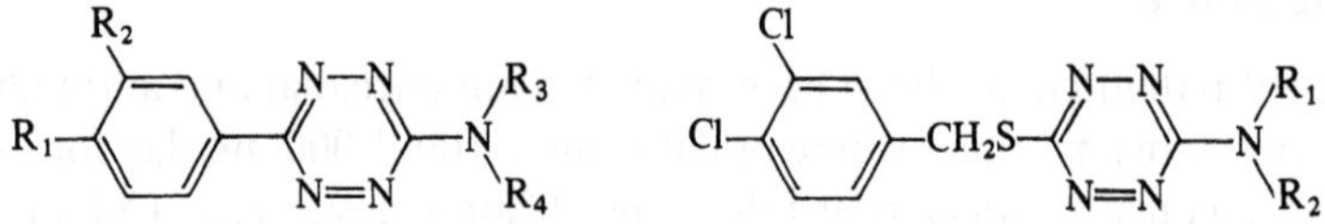

L

a) $R_1 = Cl; R_2 = R_3 = H; R_4 = CH_3$

LI

a) $R_1 = H; R_2 = CH_3$
b) $R_1 = R_2 = CH_3$

Fig. 25. Chemical structures L and LI

Further investigation into this series, when a heterocyclic spacer atom was introduced between the aryl group and the tetrazine moiety, did not yield compounds with greater activity. The two compounds (LIa, LIb) with the highest level of activity in mice gave an increase in survival time of 8–10 days at a single subcutaneous dose of 640 mg/kg given 72 h after infection with *P. berghei*, this activity being comparable to that of the lead compound (La) (JOHNSON et al. 1980).

XVI. Thienopyrimidines

Compounds in this series have been claimed to show activity against *P. berghei*, the most active compound (LII) bearing a dialkylaminoalkyl substituent (CIBA AG 1970).

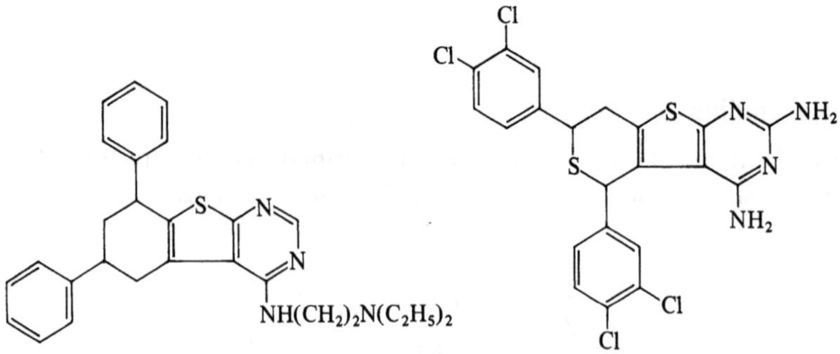

LII LIII

Fig. 26. Chemical structures LII and LIII

This thieno(2,3-d)pyrimidine ring system fused to a heterocyclic ring also features in a series of potential antifolates which showed only slight activity against

P. berghei in mice, with the most active compound (LIII) giving a significant increase in survival time only at a dose of 640 mg/kg (CHAYKOVSKY et al. 1973).

XVII. Thiopyrans

A limited series of 4-(dialkylaminoalkyl)benzthiopyrans was prepared following the discovery of activity in the lead compound LIV a. While the range of substituents was too small to make detailed comments on the structure-activity relationships, substitution of halogen in either the 6-position of the benzthiopyran or in the 4′-position of the 2-phenyl substituent gave compounds with enhanced activity. A further requirement for activity is the presence of a strongly basic nitrogen atom separated by three or four carbon atoms from the imino nitrogen atom on the 4-position of the benzthiopyran. The most active compounds exerted their effect at subcutaneous dose levels of 160–360 mg/kg against both *P. berghei* and *P. gallinaceum* with some curative activity at higher doses. Replacement of the ring sulphur atom by oxygen to give the flavone analogue did not affect the activity significantly (RAZDAN et al. 1978).

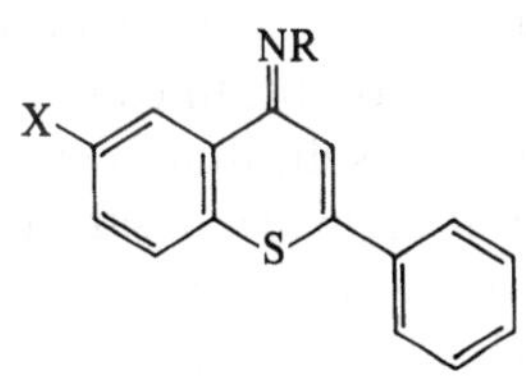

LIV

a) X = Cl; R = $(CH_2)_3N(CH_3)_2$

b) X = OCH_3; R = NHC(=NH)NH_2

Fig. 27. Chemical structrue LIV

Compounds containing the same ring system with the Schiff base function replaced by a guanylhydrazone group (LIV b) are the subject of antimalarial patent claims (BAYER 1979), with activity against *P. berghei* at a dose of 50 mg/kg. The activity of these compounds is claimed to be enhanced by addition of either antifolates or the glucose transport inhibitor 2,6-dihydroxy-2-(β-D-glucosido)β-(4-hydroxyphenyl)propiophenone dihydrate.

XVIII. Thiosemicarbazones and Sulphides

Following the discovery of antimalarial activity for the 2-acetylpyridine thiosemicarbazone derivative (LV a) a large number of thiosemicarbazone derivatives of aromatic ketones and aldehydes were prepared and their antimalarial properties evaluated. However, of the aldehydes and ketones used, only 2-acetyl- and 2-propionyl-pyridine gave derivatives with antimalarial activity. Since the semicarbazone corresponding to LV a was inactive, the sulphur atom would appear to be necessary for activity.

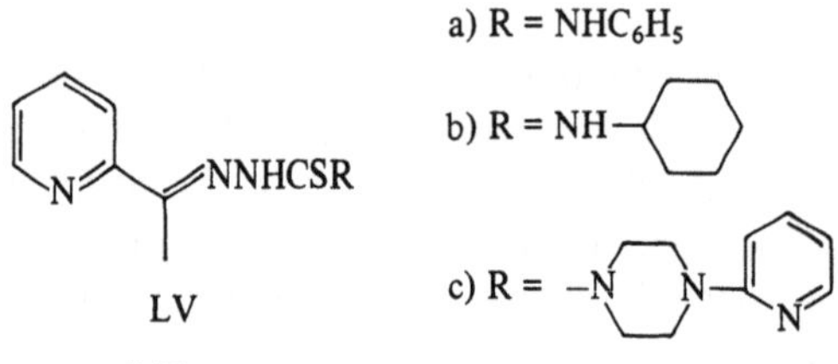

LV

Fig. 28. Chemical structure LV

Substitution of the phenyl substituent on the 4′-position of the thiosemicarbazone did not result in enhancement of the activity and neither did its replacement by linear aliphatic groups or heterocycles. However, some cycloaliphatic groups such as adamantyl and, especially, cyclohexyl (LV b) were more active, the cyclohexyl analogue showing curative activity against *P. berghei* in mice at a single subcutaneous dose of 160 mg/kg (KLAYMAN et al. 1979 a). It was subsequently found that compounds which are disubstituted at the 4′-position of the thiosemicarbazone were more active than the monosubstituted ones. While dialkyl derivatives were toxic, mixed alkyl and cycloalkyl substituted compounds gave cures in the 80- to 320-mg/kg range with toxicity at the higher dosage levels. For compounds where the 4′-nitrogen atom formed part of a ring, the six-membered heterocycle gave optimum activity, with simple alkyl substitution about the ring having a profound effect on the activity. Like the piperidino compounds, the activity of the 4-substituted piperazino derivatives was strongly dependent on the nature of the substituents, the most active compounds being those substituted with 4-fluorophenyl, ethoxycarbonyl and 2-pyridyl (LV c). The latter compound was curative at 20 mg/kg while toxicity appeared only at dose levels of 320 mg/kg (KLAYMAN et al. 1979 b).

The ability of disulphides of amino alkylthiols to bind reversibly to DNA, RNA and other nucleoproteins could result in a decrease in the rate of DNA replication in the presence of these compounds. The implications of this hypothesis for antimalarial therapy were examined for a series of *N*-heterocyclic alkyl disulphides and thiosulphates which were tested against *P. berghei* and *P. gallinaceum*. Activity in the series was limited by toxicity but two compounds (LVI a, LVI b) showed activity against *P. berghei* in mice at dose levels of 160 mg/kg and 320 mg/kg respectively (FOYE et al. 1975).

The blocking action of disulphides on mercapto groups was also explored in a series of substituted bis-quinoline disulphides (LVII) where the compounds prepared were derivatives of the 4-aldehyde group such as styryl, phenylhydrazone or acrylic acid while the substituent R_1 is limited to H, CH_3, or OCH_3 and R_2 is limited to H or Cl (ZAYED et al. 1978).

The metalloprotein oxygenase inhibitor tetraethylthiuram disulphide (Antabuse) (LVIII) and its reduction product diethyldithiocarbamate could favour se-

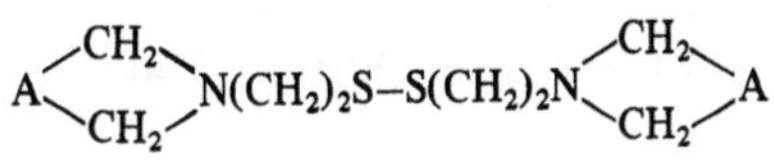

LVI

a) A = $-(CH_2)_2-$

b) A = $-(CH_2)_2CH(CH_3)-$

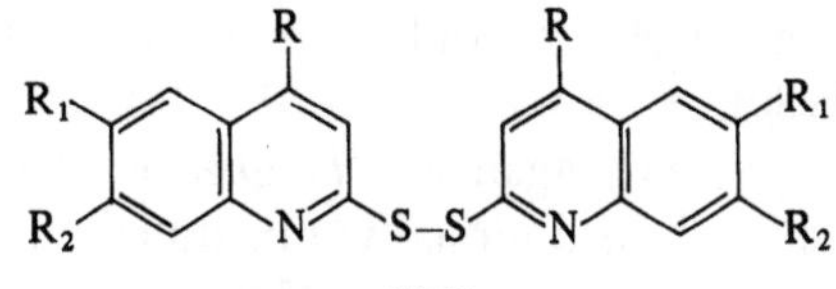

LVII

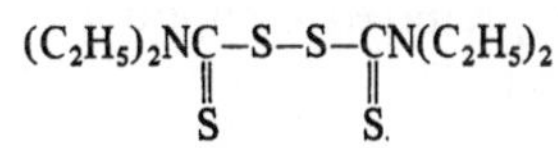

LVIII

Fig. 29. Chemical structures LVI–LVIII

lective toxicity to the malaria parasite. It is therefore of interest that they inhibited the growth of *P. falciparum* in vitro at all levels tested, the lowest being 0.1 μg/ml (SCHEIBEL et al. 1979).

Other chelating agents with activity against metalloproteins and with similar lipophilic characteristics to Antabuse were tested against *P. falciparum* in vitro. Both 8-hydroxyquinoline (LIX) and 2-mercaptopyridine-*N*-oxide (LX) rapidly inhibited the growth of the parasite at concentrations of ca. $10^{-4} M$, with lower levels being inhibitory over a longer time period. 2-Methyl-8-hydroxyquinoline, which is a less effective chelator of cations than 8-hydroxyquinoline itself, was also less active in inhibiting the growth of *P. falciparum* in vitro. Other compounds which are good

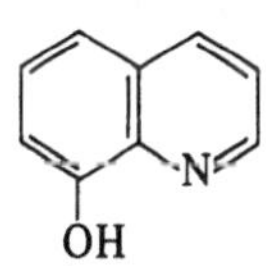

LIX

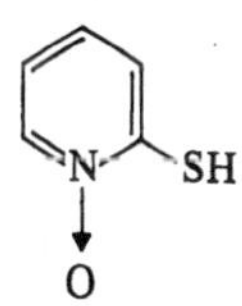

LX

Fig. 30. Chemical structures LIX and LX

$R_1NHCSS(CH_2)_nCO_2R_2$

LXI

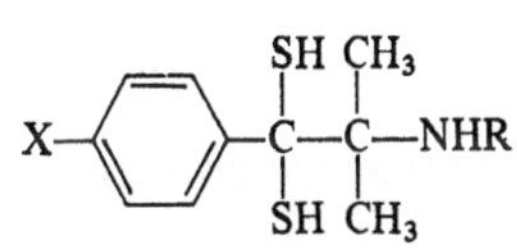

LXII

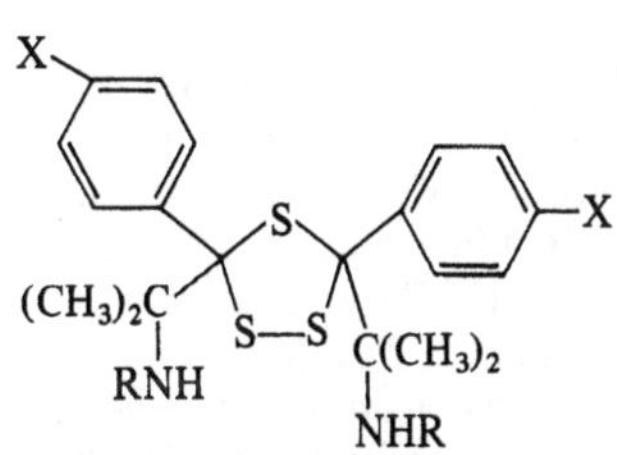

LXIII

Fig. 31. Chemical structures LXI–LXIII

metal chelators could also be selectively toxic to plasmodia (SCHEIBEL and ADLER 1980).

Activity against *P. berghei* has been claimed for aryldithiocarbamates (LXI) where R_1 is optionally substituted phenoxyphenyl or phenylaminophenyl and R_2 is H or lower alkyl (CIBA GEIGY 1975).

Antimalarial patent claims have been made for aryldimercaptoethylamine derivatives (LXII) and their trithiolane cyclisation products (LXIII).

The preferred compounds have X=H or Cl and $R=C_2H_5$ or C_4H_9 (ASH STEVENS 1972).

References

Abbott (1974) United States Patent 3821379

Alving CR, Schneider I, Swartz GM, Steck EA (1979) Sporozoite induced malaria: therapeutic effects of glycolipids in liposomes. Science 205:1142–1144

American Cyanamid (1971) South African Patent 7008675

American Cyanamid (1973a) British Patent 1304164

American Cyanamid (1973b) United States Patent 3749780

American Cyanamid (1975) United States Patent 3901944

Archer S, Osei-Gyimah P, Silbering S (1980) 4-[(Aminoalkyl)amino]-1,2-dimethoxynaphthalenes as antimalarial agents. J Med Chem 23:516–519

Aron Samuel (1973) German Patent 2240887

Ash Stevens (1972) United States Patent 3694498

Bayer AG (1979) German Patent 2736064

Bekhli AF, Kozyreva NP, Moshkovskii Sh D, Rabinovich SA, Maksakovskaya EV, Gladkikh VF (1977) Synthesis of benzo(g) quinoline derivatives XIV. New benzo(g)quinoline derivatives possessing antimalarial activity. Medskaya Parazit 46:71–72. (Trop Dis Bull 1977, 74, Abs. 2009)

Chaykovsky M, Lin M, Rosowsky A, Modest EJ (1973) 2,4-Diamino-thieno [2,3-d]-pyrimidines as antifolates and antimalarials. 2. Synthesis of 2,4-diaminopyrido-[4′,3′,4,5]thieno[2,3-d]pyrimidines and 2,4-diamino-8*H*-thiopyrano[4′,3′,4,5]thieno[2,3,-d[pyrimidines. J Med Chem 16:188–191

Christiaens A (1978) Belgian Patent 865704

Ciba AG (1970) German Patent 1934172

Ciba Geigy (1974) Swiss Patent 547820

Ciba Geigy (1975) Netherlands Patent 7607204

Ciba Geigy (1978) European Patent 3833

Clyde DF, McCarthy VC, Miller RM (1974) Inactivity of RC-12 as a causal prophylactic and relapse inhibitor of *Plasmodium vivax* in man. Trans R Soc Trop Med Hyg 68:167–168

CM Industries (1977) French Patent 2327783

Cranfield R, Goodford PJ, Norrington FE, Richards WHG, Sheppey GC, Williams SG (1974) The selection of arylamidinourea antimalarials by their predicted physicochemical properties. Br J Pharmacol 52:87–92

Das BP, Boykin DW (1977) Synthesis and antiprotozoal activity of 2,5 bis(4-guanylphenyl)-furans. J Med Chem 20:531–536

Ekanem OJ (1978) Has *Azadirachta indica* (Dongoyaro) any antimalarial activity? Niger Med J 8:8–10 (Trop Dis Bull 1979, 76: abs. 681)

Elslager EF, Johnson J, Werbel LM (1973) Synthesis of 5,5′-[(3(Dimethylamino)-propyl)imino]bis[3(trichloromethyl)-1,2,4-thiadiazole] and related thiadiazoles as antimalarial agents. J Heterocycl Chem 10:611–622

Farbwerke Hoechst (1975) German Patent 2337474
Foye WO, Lanzillo JJ, Lowe YH, Kauffman JM (1975) Synthesis and antimalarial activity of heterocyclic alkyl disulphides, thiosulphates and dithio acid derivatives. J Pharm Sci 64:211–216
Garg HG, Singhai A, Mathur JML (1973) Synthesis and biological activity of 1,5-diphenyl-4-arylazopyrazoles and 5,5-dimethylcyclohexane-1,2,3-trione bishydrazones. J Pharm Sci 62:494–496
Geigy SA (1972) Netherlands Patent 7205668
Gershon H, Krull IS (1979) Dipeptides of *O*-methyl-L-threonine as potential antimalarials. J Med Chem 22:877–879
Gilbert D, Goodford PJ, Norrington FE, Weatherley BC, Williams SG (1975) Forecasting the antimalarial activities of arylamidinoureas from their measured physicochemical properties. Br J Pharmacol 55:117–124
Goodford PJ, Norrington FE, Richards WHG, Walls LP (1973) Predictions of the antimalarial activity of arylamidinoureas. Br J Pharmacol 48:650–654
Hamer M, Batzer OF, Moats MJ, Wu CC, Lira EP (1975) Synthesis of 2-pyridyl-α-toluenesulphonates as antimalarials. J Pharm Sci 64:1961–1964
Herrin TR, Pauvlik JM, Schuber EV, Geiszler AO (1975) Antimalarials. Synthesis and antimalarial activity of 1-(4-methoxy-cinnamoyl)-4-(5-phenyl-4-oxo-2-oxazol-in-2-yl)-piperazine. J Med Chem 18:1216–1222
Hoechst AG (1979) German Patent 2748333
Hynes JB (1970) Hydroxylamine derivatives as potential antimalarial agents. 1. Hydroxamic acids. J Med Chem 13:1235–1237
Hynes JB, Gratz RF (1972) Hydroxylamine derivatives as potential antimalarial agents. 3. 1,2,4-oxadiazoles. J Med Chem 15:1198–1200
Johnson JL, Whitney B, Werbel LM (1980) Synthesis of 6-(arylthio)- and 6-(arylmethylthio)-1,2,4,5-tetrazine-3-amines and *N*-phenyl- and *N*-(phenylmethyl)-1,2,4,5-tetrazine-3,6-diamines as potential antimalarial agents. J Heterocycl Chem 17:501–506
Kai YC, Li Y, Yu PL, Cheng YP, Wang TS, Chen IS, Li LC (1978) Studies on the active principles of Shian-Ho-Tsao. IV. Synthesis of the analogues of agrimol. Hua Hsueh Hsueh Pao 36:143–148 (Chem Abs 89:197115)
Klayman DL, Bartosevich JF, Griffin TS, Mason CJ (1979a) 2-Acetylpyridine thiosemicarbazones 1. A new class of potential antimalarial agents. J Med Chem 22:855–862
Klayman DL, Scovill JP, Bartosevich JF, Mason CJ (1979b) 2-Acetylpyridine thiosemicarbazones 2. N^4N^4-Disubstituted derivatives as potential antimalarial agents. J Med Chem 22:1367–1373
Langer BW, Canfield CJ (1971) Methionine analogue metabolism in malaria. Trans R Soc Trop Med Hyg 65:100–101
Levy MR, Chou SC (1975) Inhibition of macromolecular synthesis in the malarial parasites by inhibitors of proteolytic enzymes. Experientia 31:52–54
Li Y, Yu PL, Chen YX, Li LQ, Gai YZ, Wang DS, Zheng YP (1979) Synthesis of some derivatives of artemisinine.Kexue Tongbao 24:667–669 (Chem Abs 91:211376: Trop Dis Bull 77: Abs 1724)
Markley LD, Van Heertum JC, Doorenbos HE (1972) Antimalarial activity of Clopidol, 3,5-dichloro-2,6-dimethyl-4-pyridinol and its esters, carbonates and suphonates. J Med Chem 15:1188–1189
McCaustland DJ, Chien PL, Cheng CC (1973) Deaza analogues of some 4-, 6-, and 8-aminoquinolines. J Med Chem 16:1311–1314
McCaustland DJ, Chien PL, Burton WH, Cheng CC (1974) A structural modification study of the antimalarial 2-(*p*-chlorophenyl)-2-(4-piperidyl)tetrahydrofuran. J Med Chem 17:993–1000
McCormick GJ, Canfield CJ, Willet GP (1974) *In vitro* antimalarial activity of nucleic acid precursor analogues in the simian malaria *Plasmodium knowlesi*. Antimicrob Agents Chemother 16:16–21
Merck (1976) United States Patent 4173631
Merck (1977) United States Patent 4053602

Merck (1978) United States Patent 4091094
Nickel P, Fink E (1972) Antimalarial 6-aminoquinolines III. 1,2,3,4-Tetrahydro-6-aminoquinolines. Arch Pharm Ber Dtsch Pharm Ges 305:442–448
Nickel P, Fink E (1976) Antimalarial 6-aminoquinolines V. 2-, 3-, and 4-mono-, di- and trimethyl derivatives of 6-(4-diethylamino-1-methyl butylamino)-5,8-dimethoxyquinoline. Justus Liebigs Ann Chem p. 367–382
Omar MS, Collins WE (1974a) The antimalarial activity of RC-12 against gametocytes and sporogony of *Plasmodium cynomolgi*. Trans R Soc Trop Med Hyg 67:423–424
Omar MS, Collins WE (1974b) Studies on the antimalarial effects of RC-12 and WR 14997 on the development of *Plasmodium cynomolgi* in mosquitoes and rhesus monkeys. Am J Trop Med Hyg 23:339–349
Peters W (1980) Antimalarial studies on Qinghaosu. Trop Dis Bull 77:555–558 (Abstract of paper in Chinese Medical Journal 92:811–816)
Peters W, Pietrowska H, Serafin B, Urbanski T (1975) Antimalarial compounds XIII. New derivatives of phenylchloromethyl-sulphone. Pol J Pharmacol Pharm 27:283–287
Raether W, Fink E (1979) Antimalarial activity of Floxacrine (Hoe 991). Studies on blood schizonticidal action of floxacrine against *P. berghei, P. vinckei* and *P. cynomolgi*. Ann Trop Med Parasitol 73:505–526
Razdan RK, Bruni RJ, Mehta AC, Weinhardt KK, Papanastassiou ZB (1978) A new class of antimalarial drugs: Derivatives of benzothiopyrans. J Med Chem 21:643–649
Richards WHG, Williams SG (1975) Malaria studies *in vitro* III. The protein synthesising activity of *P. falciparum in vitro* after drug treatment *in vivo*. Ann Trop Med Parasitol 69:135–140
Scheibel LW, Adler A (1980) Antimalarial activity of selected aromatic chelators. Mol Pharmacol 18:320–325
Scheibel LW, Adler A, Trager W (1979) Tetraethylthiuram disulphide (Antabuse) inhibits the human malaria parasite *Plasmodium falciparum*. Proc Nat Acad Sci USA 76:5303–5307
Schmidt LH (1979) Antimalarial properties of Floxacrine, a dihydroacridinedione derivative. Antimicrob Agents Chemother 16:475–485
Shoeb HA, Korkor MI, Tammam GH (1978) Synthesis and molluscicidal activity evaluation of some nitroquinolines. Pharmazie 33:581–583
Stogryn EL (1971) Antimalarials related to aminopyrocatechol dialkyl ethers. Conformational effects. J Med Chem 14:171–173
Tang SR, Wu YF, Fang CS (1980) Isolation and identification of the antimalarial constituents of *Gynura segetum* (Lour). Merr. Chung Ts'ao Yao 11:193–195 (Chem Abs 94:36187)
Temple C Jr, Rose JD, Montgomery JA (1974a) Amodiaquine analogues. Synthesis of 6-[[3-(*N,N* diethylamino)-methyl-4-hydroxy]anilino] 5,8-dimethoxy-2,4-dimethylquinoline and related compounds. J Med Chem 17:972–977
Temple C Jr, Rose JD, Montgomery JA (1974b) Synthesis of potential antimalarial agents. Preparation of some 6-amino-5,8-dimethoxyquinolines and the corresponding 6-amino-5,8-quinolinediones. J Med Chem 17:615–619
Thu NV, Kim NV, Nhu TV, Hoan DB, Mai TM, Thanh DT (1979) Effectiveness of *Brucea sumatrana* plant against malaria. Duoc Hoc 4:15–17 (from Chem Abs 92:191396)
Trager W, Robert-Gero M, Lederer E (1978) Antimalarial activity of *S*-isobutyl adenosine against *Plasmodium falciparum* in culture. FEBS Lett 85:264–266
Trager W, Tershakovec M, Chiang PK, Cantoni GL (1980) *Plasmodium falciparum:* Antimalarial activity in culture of Sinefungin and other methylation inhibitors. Exp Parasitol 50:83–89
US Secretary of the Army (1973) United States Patent 3733319
Wellcome Foundation (1974a) British Patent 1366855
Wellcome Foundation (1974b) German Patent 2537122
Wellcome Foundation (1977) British Patent 1476422
Wellcome Foundation (1980) European Patent 7529

Werbel LM, McNamara DJ, Colbrey N, Johnson JL, Degnan MJ, Whitney B (1979) Antimalarial drugs 42. Synthesis and antimalarial effects of *N,N*-dialkyl-6-(substituted-phenyl)-1,2,4,5-tetrazine-3-amines. J Heterocycl Chem 16:881–894

Yan SJ, Burton WH, Chien PL, Cheng CC (1978) Potential causal prophylactic antimalarial agents. Synthesis of quinoxaline, benzimidazole and alkoxybenzene derivatives containing a novoldiamine moiety. J Heterocycl Chem 15:297–300

Zayed A, Zoorob HH, El-Wassimi MT (1978) Novel substituted quinolines with possible antimalarial activity. Pharmazie 33:572–575

Zheng XY, Xia Y, Gao FH, Guo HZ, Chen C (1979) Synthesis of 7351, a new antimalarial drug. Yao Hsueh Hsueh Pao 14:736–736 (Chem Abs 93:132397)

Prevention of Drug Resistance

CHAPTER 16

Use of Drug Combinations

W. PETERS

A. Introduction

A general account of the different types of drug combination was given in this part, Chap. 6, and other references have appeared in other chapters, notably Part I, Chap. 14 and this part, Chaps. 4, 5, 7 and 13.

One of the major problems facing us today in malaria is how to protect the few available compounds that are in current use, if indeed it is not already too late and, even more essential, how to minimise the risk that the malaria parasites of man will become resistant to any new antimalarial drugs that may become available in the future. Drug combinations are therefore discussed here in the context of the prevention of resistance. First however the following general point must be made. It would be quite illusory to believe that *any* antimalarial drug or drug combination will ever provide the complete answer to the control of malaria in the individual or the community. Malaria control must be based on an informed programme, "tailor-made" to the local situation, containing both antivector and antiparasite measures, as well as the vital element of health education at *all* levels from Ministers of Health down to the simplest members of the community. It is very unlikely that reliance simply upon chemoprophylaxis or chemotherapy, no matter how effective the drug or drugs, will make a lasting impact upon the vicious cycle of malaria transmission, even if supplemented with whatever malaria vaccine may emerge from current research efforts in that direction over the next decade or two.

The history of the use of drug combinations in malaria control programmes for the prevention of drug resistance, and its dismal failure, were recounted by PETERS (1970) and will not be repeated here in detail. It is unfortunate that the extensive use of various combinations of 4-aminoquinolines with pyrimethamine that were advocated by WHO (e.g. WHO 1966), and vigorously promoted by several pharmaceutical companies, was based not on sound experimental evidence of their value, but on pure hypothesis. In the following pages are reviewed some of the experimental data that perhaps indicate how some, but not all, combinations may be of value in diminishing the risk of the emergence of drug resistance in *Plasmodium*.

B. Drugs with Additive Effects

I. Combinations with Mepacrine

At the time that resistance of *P. falciparum* to chloroquine was being recognised in a rapidly widening geographical area the important role of resistance transfer

(R) factors was being intensively studied in bacteria (MITSUHASHI 1977). The spread of chloroquine resistance in malaria through the mediation of some similar factor was postulated by the writer. In view of reports such as that of SEVAG (1964) and WARREN et al. (1967) that mepacrine prevented the development of resistance to antibiotics and other antibacterial agents, experiments were set up to see whether mepacrine would influence the rate at which *P. berghei* would become resistant to a sulphonamide, or vice versa. PETERS (1965a) had already described the ready development of a strain of this parasite with a high level of resistance to mepacrine when that drug was used alone. This strain proved unstable in the absence of drug selection pressure (PETERS 1966), much as did the highly chloroquine-resistant RC strain, and lacked malaria pigment. Unlike the RC strain, resistance to mepacrine, which was produced by slowly increasing the drug level over successive

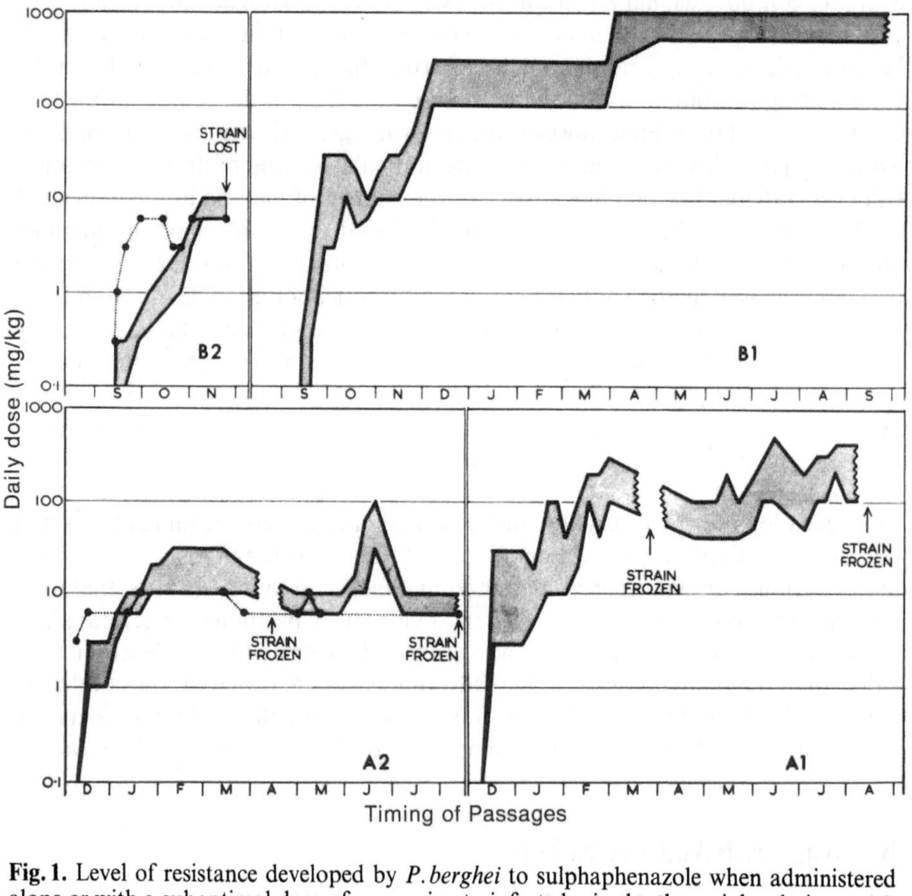

Fig. 1. Level of resistance developed by *P. berghei* to sulphaphenazole when administered alone or with a suboptimal dose of mepacrine to infected mice by the serial technique. *A 1, A 2,* sulphaphenazole alone; *B 1, B 2,* sulphaphenazole with mepacrine. *Points* indicate dose levels of mepacrine, *shaded areas* range of dose levels of sulphaphenazole. Resistance developed more rapidly to the sulphonamide and to a higher level when it was used alone. (PETERS 1969)

passages, remained an unstable character, perhaps because of the antimutagenic properties of this compound.

When *P. berghei* N-strain parasites in mice were exposed to sulphaphenazole alone, resistance developed rapidly so that the parasites survived in animals receiving a dose level of at least 1000 mg/kg daily for 5 days of each weekly passage. When the sulphonamide was administered together with mepacrine the dose of neither drug could be increased beyond about the 10 mg/kg level over the course of about 8 months (Fig. 1).

Quite a different picture may have emerged had this experiment commenced with a strain of *Plasmodium* that was inherently resistant to chloroquine at a low level. PETERS and GREGORY (1973) showed that *P. yoelii nigeriensis* N 67 rapidly developed a high level of resistance to mepacrine by the relapse technique (see Part I, Chap. 18), and that this resistance was completely stable in the absence of drug selection pressure. It was almost certainly due to pre-existing mutants. The experiment to see whether this strain (which bears a resemblance to chloroquine-resistant *P. falciparum* in man) would develop more slowly in the presence of a sulphonamide has not yet been carried out. Nor have any other mepacrine combinations, e.g. with pyrimethamine, been studied.

II. Combinations with Sulphonamides or Dihydrofolate Reductase Inhibitors

1. Chloroquine

Among the rodent malaria parasites *P. berghei* and *P. yoelii* ssp. have been most frequently used in drug resistance studies, the latter possessing an innate low level resistance to chloroquine and other 4-aminoquinolines. Lines of *P. berghei* resistant to proguanil (ROLLO 1951) and pyrimethamine (ROLLO 1952) developed readily when a relapse-type technique was employed, but even with this procedure *P. gallinaceum* proved somewhat less rapid. Resistance to sulphonamides had proved to be easy to accomplish, the earliest report being that of BISHOP and BIRKETT (1947) in *P. gallinaceum*, the species from which they had already derived a proguanil-resistant line the previous year. Following the first report by RAMAKRISHNAN et al. (1957), numerous workers published data on chloroquine-resistant lines of *P. berghei*. All shared the common experience that resistance to this parasite emerged quite rapidly, and indeed the paper of SAUTET et al. (1959) would suggest that resistant parasites were present in virtually the first passage. Subsequent studies indicated that chloroquine resistance in fact develops relatively slowly in true *P. berghei*, but that it is an innate character of *P. yoelii* (WARHURST and KILLICK-KENDRICK 1967). [There is now strong evidence that the original Keyberg 173 and other isolates of *P. berghei* such as NK 65 contain very small numbers of a second parasite, a member of the *P. yoelii* complex, which is readily selected out under heavy chloroquine selection pressure (PETERS et al. 1978).]

Chloroquine resistance does not develop readily in *P. vinckei* or *P. chabaudi*. Both POWERS et al. (1969) with the former parasite and ROSARIO (1976) with the latter only succeeded if they started with lines that were already resistant to pyrimethamine. Starting with a line of *P. berghei* that was already highly resistant to chloroquine PETERS (1965 b) superimposed a high level of resistance to cycloguanil which was maximal within about 15 passages.

When it became apparent that the simultaneous administration of chloroquine and pyrimethamine to man had failed to prevent the emergence of pyrimethamine resistance in Africa, and multiple resistance (to both drugs) in Southeast Asia and the New World, experiments were commenced with these two drugs and, for comparison, with a combination of chloroquine and a sulphonamide. Using the technique of slowly increasing drug selection pressure (see Part I, Chap. 18) PETERS et al. (1973) found that, as in the combination of mepacrine and sulphaphenazole referred to above, resistance to a combination of chloroquine and sulphaphenazole developed equally reluctantly (Fig. 2). In sharp contrast to this, combining chloroquine with pyrimethamine made virtually no difference to the rate at which the parasites acquired resistance to the pyrimethamine component.

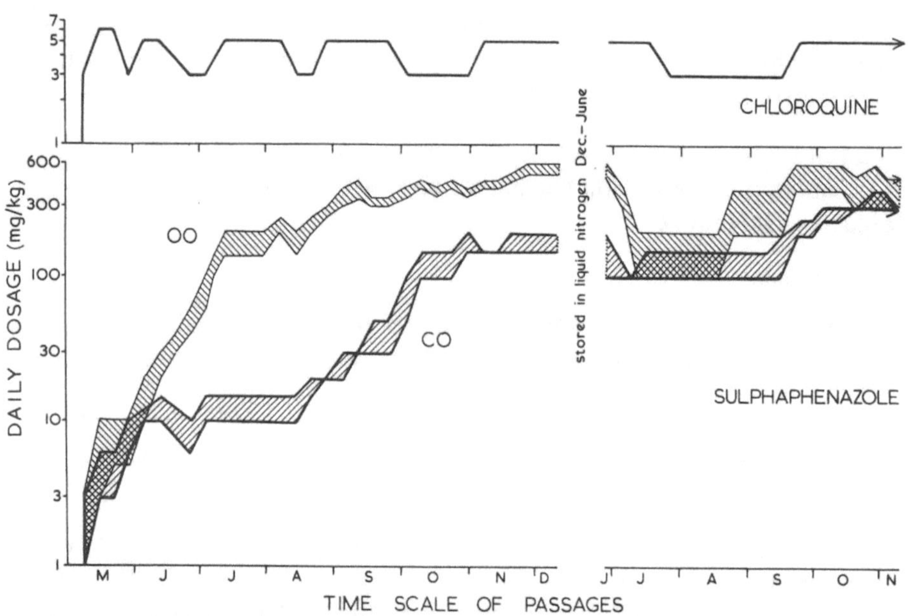

Fig. 2. The inhibiting effect of a sulphaphenazole and chloroquine mixture on the development of resistance to the individual components by *P. berghei* NK 65 in mice, using the serial technique (cf. Fig. 1, Chap. 6). (PETERS et al. 1973)

These observations would appear to substantiate other data [e.g. RABINOVICH (1965) also failed to slow down resistance to chloroquine in *P. berghei* when using a chloroquine-pyrimethamine mixture] and warnings by various authorities that a chloroquine-pyrimethamine combination should not be widely disseminated without experimental backing. Certainly it is usual now to find that strains of *P. falciparum* that are resistant to chloroquine are also resistant to pyrimethamine and to proguanil, but sensitive to sulphonamides. The explanation may lie in the shared ability of parasites resistant either to chloroquine or to pyrimethamine to utilise substrates provided by the host cells of which they are deprived in the presence of either drug (which would by itself of course kill drug-sensitive parasites).

2. Mefloquine

In a study of the mode of action of mefloquine PETERS et al. (1977 a) demonstrated that this compound has probably only an additive effect against *P. berghei* in mice when administered together with pyrimethamine, sulphaphenazole or primaquine. Resistance to mefloquine was readily produced in this parasite by the relapse (or serial passage) technique (Fig. 3), and even more readily in the slightly chloroquine-resistant NS line (which we now believe to be a subspecies of *P. yoelii*). The rate at which resistancc developed (using the serial passage technique) in *P. berghei* was greatly slowed when mefloquine was administered with pyrimethamine, sulphaphenazole or primaquine (PETERS et al. 1977 b). Moreover in any of these combinations resistance both to mefloquine and the accompanying compound were affected. This situation contrasts sharply with that seen when chloroquine and pyrimethamine were combined (compare Figs. 3 and 4).

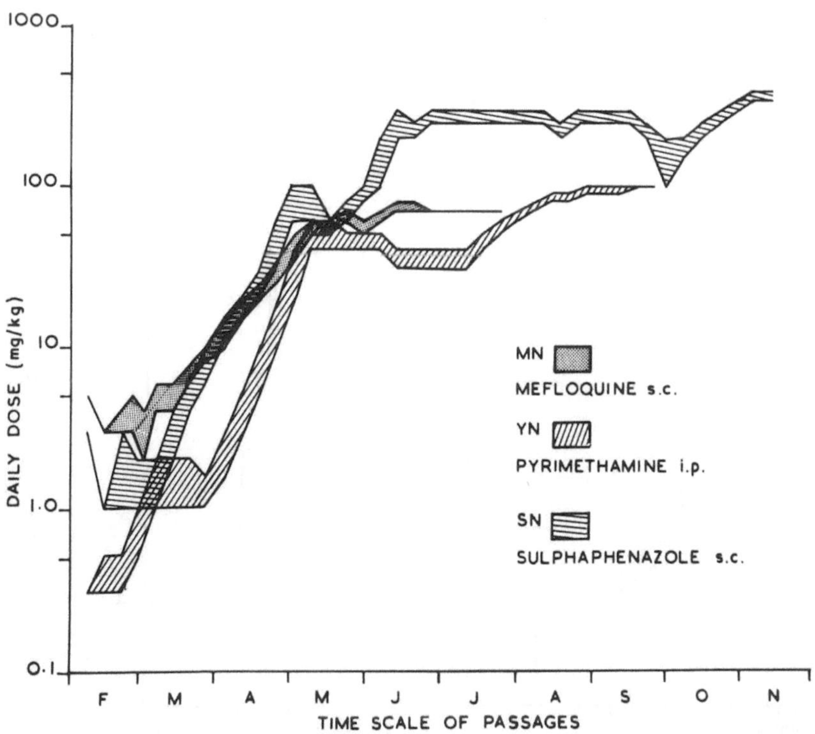

Fig. 3. Production of resistance to mefloquine, pyrimethamine and sulphaphenazole used alone, by *P. berghei* NK 65 in mice, serial technique. Compare the rapid rate of increase in daily dosages with Fig. 4. (PETERS et al. 1977 b)

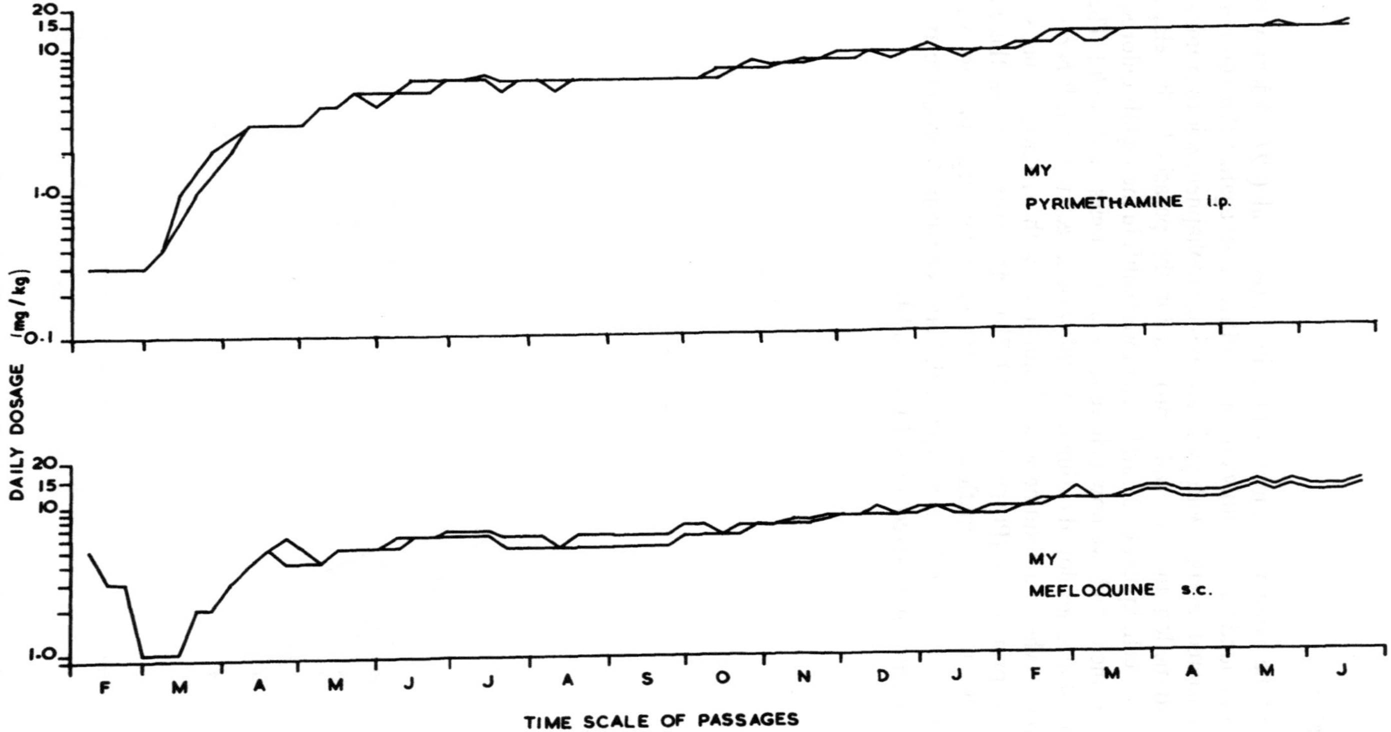

Fig. 4. Ibhibition of development by *P. berghei* NK 65 in mice of resistance to mefloquine and to pyrimethamine when the two compounds are given as a mixture. (PETERS et al. 1977b)

C. Potentiating Combinations

The general topic of potentiating combinations and various examples of these were dealt with in Chap. 6. THOMPSON et al. (1965) reported that resistance of *P. berghei* to a combination of cycloguanil and dapsone developed significantly more slowly than did resistance to either drug used alone. These observations were confirmed and the theme extended by RICHARDS (personal communication), who studied the rate at which *P. berghei* developed resistance to pyrimethamine, trimethoprim, sulphadoxine, sulphalene and dapsone, alone and in various combinations. Resistance developed, for example, to a sulphadoxine-pyrimethamine combination far more slowly than to any other combination examined. Similar data were obtained by PETERS (1974).

D. The Use of Triple Combinations

I. For the Control of Mixed *P. falciparum-P. vivax* Populations

A particular practical problem exists in areas such as Thailand where most strains of *P. falciparum* are resistant to chloroquine and pyrimethamine, and where *P. vivax* is probably resistant to pyrimethamine. The prophylactic use of a sulphonamide-antifol combination, or its application for the treatment of an acute malarial attack, will usually be effective against *P. falciparum* (although the therapeutic response may be slow), but may not be effective against *P. vivax*. It will be recalled that the latter species is innately less sensitive to sulphonamides than is *P. falciparum*. Although mefloquine has been shown to be an effective suppressive or curative agent against both parasites (see ROZMAN and CANFIELD 1979), it is, at the time of writing, not generally available. Thus the ideal combination for prophylaxis of malaria at the present time would appear to be a triple combination of chloroquine (against *P. vivax*) and a sulphonamide-pyrimethamine combination (e.g. Fansidar) (against *P. falciparum*). The choice of drug for treatment should be based on a diagnosis of the infecting species. A single dose of primaquine (45 mg base) as a gametocytocide should be given to patients with falciparum infection following treatment with, e.g., Fansidar (or quinine and Fansidar in clinically severe cases) *in order to minimise the transmission of drug-resistant gametocytes* through local anophelines. (Primaquine will also be needed of course as a radical curative agent in vivax infections treated with chloroquine.) The use of primaquine in travellers should also be considered as a preventive measure in view of the frequency of malaria infection in people flying from one endemic area to another, and the very real risk that drug-resistant parasites they carry with them may be transmitted locally in malaria receptive areas to set up new foci of resistance. This may be what is happening at the present time in parts of East Africa.

II. For the Protection of Existing and New Antimalarials

The demonstration that the use of a potentiating combination such as pyrimethamine with a sulphonamide would slow down the rate at which resistance developed to the individual component drugs (see above), and that a combination of chloroquine with a sulphonamide also had this desirable action, led us to experi-

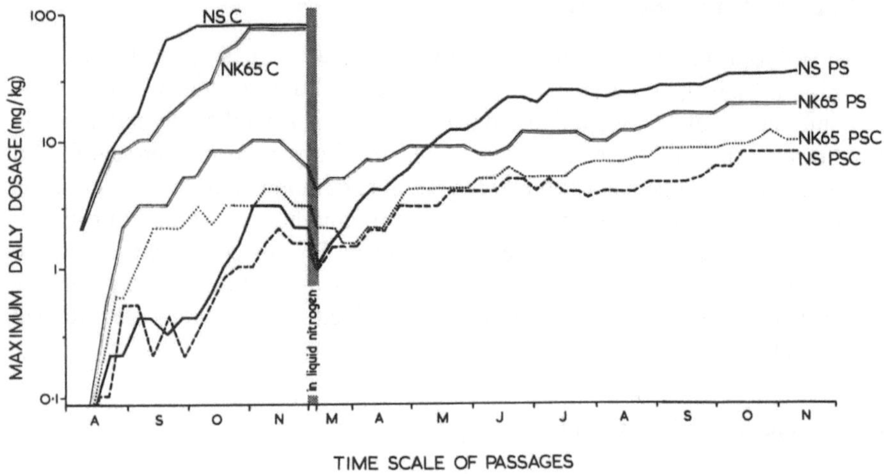

Fig. 5. Development of resistance to chloroquine, pyrimethamine and sulphadoxine used alone or in various combinations against the chloroquine-sensitive *P. berghei* NK 65 line and mildly chloroquine-resistant *P. berghei* NS line. NS C and NK 65 C exposed in serial technique to chloroquine alone (note rapid acquisition of resistance); PS lines exposed to a mixture of pyrimethamine and sulphadoxine; PSC lines exposed to a triple mixture of pyrimethamine, sulphadoxine and chloroquine. (PETERS 1974)

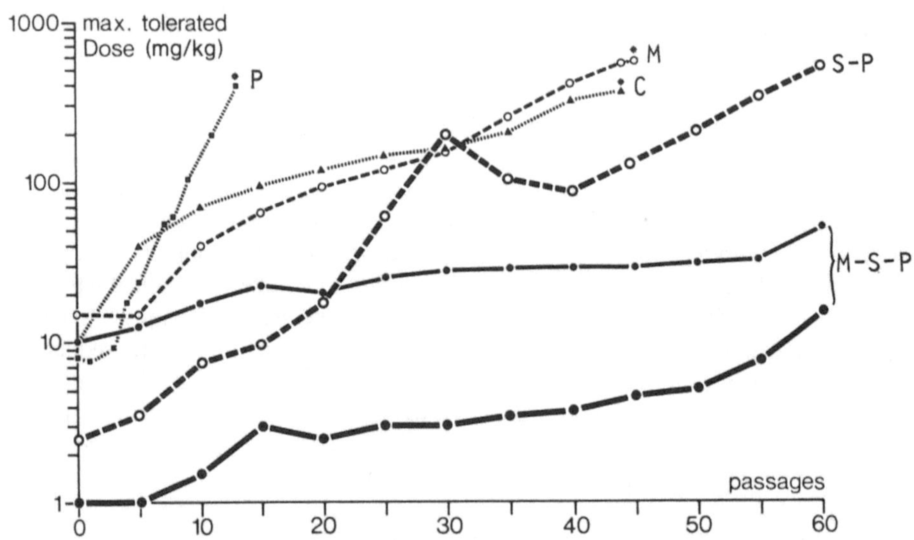

Fig. 6. Development of resistance to mefloquine, pyrimethamine and sulphadoxine by *P. berghei* K 173 in mice by the serial technique. Lines were exposed to the drugs as follows: *P*, pyrimethamine; *C*, chloroquine; *M*, mefloquine; *S-P*, a 2:1 sulphadoxine-pyrimethamine mixture; *M-S-P*, mefloquine (*top line*) with a 2:1 S-P mixture (*bottom line*); * toxic limit for host. MERKLI and RICHLE 1980)

ment with a *triple* combination of chloroquine-sulphadoxine-pyrimethamine (PETERS 1974). It was found that, starting either with the drug-sensitive NK 65 strain of *P. berghei* or the slightly chloroquine-resistant NS line of *P. yoelii* ssp., resistance developed only slowly to pyrimethamine and sulphadoxine and to only a low level when the parasites were submitted to all three drugs together (Fig. 5). *No resistance developed to chloroquine in these lines.*

In view of the success obtained by combining mefloquine with either pyrimethamine or a sulphonamide, MERKLI et al (1980) made a similar study of the triple combination mefloquine-pyrimethamine-sulphadoxine, with equally good results and a great reduction in the rate of development and level of drug resistance developed by *P. berghei* (Fig. 6).

These authors showed that, while of course pyrimethamine and sulphadoxine formed a potentiating pair, the addition of mefloquine had simply an additive effect.

E. Conclusion

The experiments recorded above indicate clearly the value of *appropriate* combinations of antimalarial drugs in slowing down, if not preventing, the development of resistance to them by *Plasmodium*. So far the only combinations that have been used in man with this aim in mind have been mixtures of sulphonamides or sulphones with pyrimethamine or other dihydrofolate reductase inhibitors. Experience with the injectable repository mixture of cycloguanil embonate and diacetyldapsone unfortunately failed, for a variety of reasons, to prevent the emergence of strains of *P. falciparum* resistant to dapsone or proguanil in New Guinea (RIECKMANN 1967) (where, incidentally, multiple drug-resistance is now common), and there are also data indicating that *P. falciparum* infections are no longer responding in parts of Southeast Asia, East Africa and Brazil to pyrimethamine- sulphadoxine, as was forecast by TIGERTT and CLYDE (1976).

It is most unfortunate also that several antifol-sulphonamide pairs are being promoted at the present time for the prophylaxis or treatment of malaria (chloroquine-resistant or otherwise), that are *not* ideally suited for this purpose. Among these are sulphamethoxazole-trimethoprim (co-trimoxazole), which is an excellent antibacterial agent and should be retained for the therapy of antibiotic-resistant bacterial infections, and sulphalene-pyrimethamine, in which the effective half-lives of the two components differ greatly (BRUCE-CHWATT 1981). The indiscriminate use of these and similar double combinations (including sulphadoxine-pyrimethamine) should be discouraged. The latter combination, on the basis of its proven efficacy and well-matched pharmacokinetic characteristics, is probably the best available at the present time. Its use should be restricted to areas where the presence of multiple-resistant *P. falciparum* renders alternative, single compounds ineffective (CHIN et al. 1966; SCHMIDT et al. 1977; BRUCE-CHWATT et al. 1981).

There is a great reluctance on the part of drug-regulatory agencies today to permit the use in man of fixed drug combinations, and even such a valuable combination as co-trimoxazole had a hard path to plough before becoming widely accepted. The use of a triple combination of antimalarial drugs will undoubtedly meet even greater barriers before it becomes an officially acceptable practice; yet the most logical, and experimentally demonstrable, way of "protecting" a new compound, be it mefloquine or some other compound yet to be discovered, is by using it as a component of a triple mixture. Today it would be unthinkable to treat a disease such as tuberculosis with even two drugs, much less a single one, and multiple drug combinations are becoming the rule rather than the exception in many bacterial infections and in cancer chemotherapy. In spite of all the measures that have been applied to control it, malaria remains and will remain for many years to come, a major challenge to the inhabitants of large parts of the tropics and subtropics, and to all who visit such places. New drugs will come and, if we do not take active steps to prevent it, will rapidly go again. Vaccines, new insecticides, all will be developed and will contribute, for a time, to control of the level of malaria in these communities. In spite of this, there is every likelihood that *Plasmodium,* with its highly complex genetic repertoire, will survive, and that we will still depend heavily on specific antimalarial drugs many years from now to protect us against the ravages of these wily protozoa.

References

Bishop A, Birkett B (1947) Acquired resistance to paludrine in *Plasmodium gallinaceum.* Acquired resistance and persistence after passage through the mosquito. Nature 159:884–885

Bruce-Chwatt LJ (ed), Black RH, Canfield CJ, Clyde DF, Peters W, Wernsdorfer W (1981) Chemotherapy of malaria, 2nd edn. WHO, Geneva

Chin W, Contacos PG, Coatney GR, King HK (1966) The evaluation of sulfonamides, alone or in combination with pyrimethamine, in the treament of multi-resistant falciparum malaria. Am J Trop Med Hyg 15:823–829

Merkli B, Richle RW (1980) Studies on the resistance to single and combined antimalarials in the *Plasmodium berghei* mouse model. Acta Trop (Basel) 37:228–231

Merkli B, Richle R, Peters W (1980) The inhibitory effect of a drug combination on the development of mefloquine resistance in *Plasmodium berghei.* Ann Trop Med Parasitol 74:1–9

Mitsuhashi S (ed) (1977) R factor drug-resistant plasmid. University of Tokyo Press, Tokyo

Peters W (1965 a) Mepacrine- and primaquine-resistant strains of *Plasmodium berghei,* Vincke and Lips, 1948. Nature 208:693–694

Peters W (1965 b) Drug resistance in *Plasmodium berghei,* Vincke and Lips, 1948. III. Multiple drug resistance. Exp Parasitol 17:97–102

Peters W (1966) Drug responses of mepacrine- and primaquine-resistant strains of *Plasmodium berghei,* Vincke and Lips, 1948. Ann Trop Med Parasitol 60:25–30

Peters W (1969) Partial inhibition by mepacrine of the development of sulphonamide resistance in *Plasmodium berghei.* Nature 223:858–859

Peters W (1970) Chemotherapy and drug resistance in malaria. Academic, London

Peters W (1974) Prevention of drug resistance in rodent malaria by the use of drug mixtures. Bull WHO 51:379–383

Peters W, Gregory KG (1973) The chemotherapy of rodent malaria. XVI: primary resistance to mepacrine in the N 67 strain of *Plasmodium berghei*-type parasite. Ann Trop Med Parasitol 67:133–141

Peters W, Portus JH, Robinson BL (1973) The chemotherapy of rodent malaria. XVII: dynamics of drug resistance, part 3. Influence of drug combinations on the development of resistance to chloroquine in *P. berghei.* Ann Trop Med Parasitol 67:143–154

Peters W, Howells RE, Portus JH, Robinson BL, Thomas S, Warhurst DC (1977 a) The chemotherapy of rodent malaria. XXVII: studies on mefloquine (WR 142, 490). Ann Trop Med Parasitol 71:407–418

Peters W, Portus J, Robinson BL (1977b) The chemotherapy of rodent malaria. XXVIII: the development of resistance to mefloquine (WR 142, 490). Ann Trop Med Parasitol 71:419–427

Peters W, Chance ML, Lissner R, Momen H, Warhurst DC (1978) The chemotherapy of rodent malaria. XXX: the enigmas of the "NS lines" of *P. berghei*. Ann Trop Med Parasitol 72:23–36

Powers KG, Jacobs RL, Good WC, Koontz LC (1969) *Plasmodium vinckei:* production of chloroquine-resistant strain. Exp Parasitol 26:193–202

Rabinovich SA (1965) Experimental investigations of antimalarial drug Haloquine. III Investigation of the possibility to restrain the development of chemoresistance to chloridine (Daraprim) by combined administration of chloridine with Haloquine. Medskaya Parazit 34:434–439 [in Russian]

Ramakrishnan SP, Satya Prakash Choudhury DA (1957) Selection of a strain of *Plasmodium berghei* highly resistant to chloroquine ("Resochin"). Nature 179:975

Rieckmann KH (1967) A new repository antimalarial agent, CI-564 used in a field trial in New Guinea. Trans R Soc Trop Med Hyg 61:189–198

Rollo IM (1951) A 2:4-diamino pyrimidine in the treatment of proguanil-resistant laboratory malarial strains. Nature 168:332–333

Rollo IM (1952) "Daraprim" resistance in experimental malarial infections. Nature 170:415

Rosario VE (1976) Genetics of chloroquine resistance in malaria parasites. Nature 261:585–586

Rozman RS, Canfield CJ (1979) New experimental antimalarial drugs. Adv Pharmacol Chemother 16:1–43

Sautet J, Aldighieri J, Aldighieri R, Arnaud G, Ausseil M; Rampal C, Castelli C (1959) Etudes sur la production expérimentale de la résistance a divers produits antimalariques d'une souche de *Plasmodium berghei*. Bull Soc Path Exot Filiales 52:331–345

Schmidt LH, Harrison J, Rossan RN, Vaughan D, Crosby R (1977) Quantitative aspects of pyrimethamine-sulfonamide synergism. Am J Trop Med Hyg 26:837–849

Sevag MG (1964) Prevention of the emergence of antibiotic-resistant strains of bacteria by atabrine. Arch Biochem Biophys 108:85–88

Thompson PE, Bayles A, Olszewski B, Waitz JA (1965) Studies on a dihydrotriazine and a sulfone, alone and in combination, against *Plasmodium berghei* in mice. Am J Trop Med Hyg 14:198–206

Tigertt WD, Clyde DF (1976) Drug resistance in the human malarias. Antibiot Chemother 20:246–272

Warhurst DC, Killick-Kendrick R (1967) Spontaneous resistance to chloroquine in a strain of rodent malaria (*Plasmodium berghei yoelii*). Nature 213:1048–1049

Warren GH, Gregory FJ, Healey EMH, Flint SF (1967) Effect of mixtures of atabrine and antibacterial agents on the emergence of resistant strains of *Mycobacterium tuberculosis*. Nature 215:526–527

Who (1966) WHO Expert Committee on Malaria. 12th Report. WHO Tech Rep Ser :324 (1966)

[illegible]

Subject Index

Handbook of Experimental Pharmacology

Continuation of "Handbuch der experimentellen Pharmakologie"

Springer-Verlag
Berlin
Heidelberg
New York
Tokyo

Volume 22: Part 1
Die Gestagene I

Part 2
Die Gestagene II

Volume 23
Neurohypophysial Hormones and Similar Polypeptides

Volume 24
Diuretica

Volume 25
Bradykinin, Kallidin and Kallikrein

Volume 26
Vergleichende Pharmakologie von Überträgersubstanzen in tiersystematischer Darstellung

Volume 27
Anticoagulantien

Volume 28: Part 1
Concepts in Biochemical Pharmacology I

Part 3
Concepts in Biochemical Pharmacology III

Volume 29
Oral wirksame Antidiabetika

Volume 30
Modern Inhalation Anesthetics

Volume 32: Part 2
Insulin II

Volume 34
Secretin, Cholecystokinin Pancreozymin and Gastrin

Volume 35: Part 1
Androgene I

Part 2
Androgens II and Antiandrogens/Androgene II und Antiandrogene

Volume 36
Uranium - Plutonium - Transplutonic Elements

Volume 37
Angiotensin

Volume 38: Part 1
Antineoplastic and Immunosuppressive Agents I

Part 2
Antineoplastic and Immunosuppressive Agents II

Volume 39
Antihypertensive Agents

Volume 40
Organic Nitrates

Volume 41
Hypolipidemic Agents

Volume 42
Neuromuscular Junction

Volume 43
Anabolic-Androgenic Steroids

Volume 44
Heme and Hemoproteins

Volume 45: Part 1
Drug Addiction I

Part 2
Drug Addiction II

Volume 46
Fibrinolytics and Antifibronolytics

Handbook of Experimental Pharmacology

Continuation of
"Handbuch der experimentellen
Pharmakologie"

Springer-Verlag
Berlin
Heidelberg
New York
Tokyo

Volume 47
Kinetics of Drug Action

Volume 48
Arthropod Venoms

Volume 50: Part 1
Inflammation

Part 2
Anti-Inflammatory Drugs

Volume 51
Uric Acids

Volume 52
Snake Venoms

Volume 53
Pharmacology of Ganglionic Transmission

Volume 54: Part 1
Adrenergic Activators and Inhibitors I

Part 2
Adrenergic Activators and Inhibitors II

Volume 55
Psychotropic Agents

Part 1
Antipsychotics and Antidepressants I

Part 2
Anxiolytics, Gerontopsychopharmacological Agents and Psychomotor Stimulants

Part 3
Alcohol and Psychotomimetics, Psychotropic Effects of Central Acting Drugs

Volume 56
Cardiac Glycosides

Part 1
Experimental Pharmacology

Part 2
Pharmacokinetics and Clinical Pharmacology

Volume 57
Tissue Growth Factors

Volume 58
Cyclic Nucleotides

Part 1: **Biochemistry**

Part 2: **Physiology and Pharmacology**

Volume 59:
Mediators and Drugs in Gastrointestinal Motility

Part 1: **Morphological Basis and Neurophysiological Control**

Part 2: **Endogenous and Exogenous Agents**

Volume 60
Pyretics and Antipyretics

Volume 61
Chemotherapy of Viral Infections

Volume 62
Aminoglycoside Antibiotics

Volume 64
Inhibition of Folate Metabolism in Chemotherapy

Volume 65
Teratogenesis and Reproductive Toxicology

Volume 66
Part 1: **Glucagon I**
Part 2: **Glucagon II**

Volume 67
Part 1
Antibiotics Containing the Beta-Lactam Structure I

Part 2
Antibiotics Containing the Beta-Lactam Structure II

MIX
Papier aus verantwortungsvollen Quellen
Paper from responsible sources
FSC® C105338

If you have any concerns about our products,
you can contact us on
ProductSafety@springernature.com

In case Publisher is established outside the EU,
the EU authorized representative is:
Springer Nature Customer Service Center GmbH
Europaplatz 3, 69115 Heidelberg, Germany

Printed by Libri Plureos GmbH
in Hamburg, Germany